AF897367

NOVEL ASPECTS ON EPILEPSY

Edited by **Humberto Foyaca-Sibat**

Novel Aspects on Epilepsy
Edited by Humberto Foyaca-Sibat

Published by InTech

Janeza Trdine 9, 51000 Rijeka, Croatia

Copyright © 2011 InTech

All chapters are distributed under the Creative Commons Attribution 3.0 license, which allows users to download, copy and build upon published articles even for commercial purposes, as long as the author and publisher are properly credited, which ensures maximum dissemination and a wider impact of our publications. After this work has been published by InTech, authors have the right to republish it, in whole or part, in any publication of which they are the author, and to make other personal use of the work. Any republication, referencing or personal use of the work must explicitly identify the original source.

As for readers, this license allows users to download, copy and build upon published chapters even for commercial purposes, as long as the author and publisher are properly credited, which ensures maximum dissemination and a wider impact of our publications.

Notice

Statements and opinions expressed in the chapters are these of the individual contributors and not necessarily those of the editors or publisher. No responsibility is accepted for the accuracy of information contained in the published chapters. The publisher assumes no responsibility for any damage or injury to persons or property arising out of the use of any materials, instructions, methods or ideas contained in the book.

Publishing Process Manager Dragana Manestar

Technical Editor Teodora Smiljanic

Cover Designer InTech Design Team

Additional hard copies can be obtained from orders@intechopen.com

Novel Aspects on Epilepsy, Edited by Humberto Foyaca-Sibat
p. cm.
ISBN 978-953-307-678-2

We are IntechOpen, the world's leading publisher of Open Access books

Built by scientists, for scientists

4,100+
Open access books available

116,000+
International authors and editors

120M+
Downloads

151
Countries delivered to

Our authors are among the
Top 1%
most cited scientists

12.2%
Contributors from top 500 universities

WEB OF SCIENCE™

Selection of our books indexed in the Book Citation Index
in Web of Science™ Core Collection (BKCI)

Interested in publishing with us?
Contact book.department@intechopen.com

Numbers displayed above are based on latest data collected.
For more information visit www.intechopen.com

For EU product safety concerns:
IN TECH d.o.o., Prolaz Marije Krucifikse Kozulić 3, 51000 Rijeka, Croatia,
info@intechopen.com or visit our website at intechopen.com.

Meet the editor

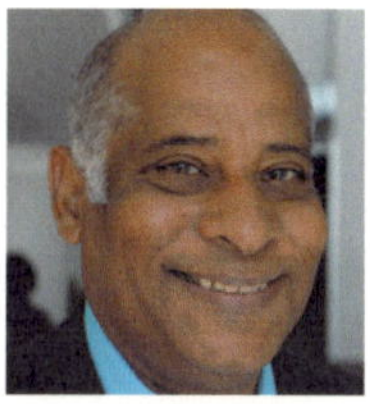

Professor Humberto Foyaca Sibat was born on May 03, 1948 in Havana City, Republic of Cuba. He graduated as a Medical Doctor in Havana University in 1971 soon after he assessed his first epileptic patient. He became specialist in neurology in 1975 and higher level specialist in 1984. He is married and has three daughters and one son. His one daughter tragically passed away in 1979. Currently Dr. Foyaca has been an Associate Professor of Walter Sisulu University for more than 14 years, and he is also Master in Sciences and Associate Investigator of Cuban Academy of Sciences. Dr. Foyaca is a member of 15 Medical Societies from all over the world; he presented more than 350 papers in different scientific events and he published more than 70 manuscripts in peer-review journals. He is the Chief-Editor of The Internet Journal of Neurology, currently the largest electronic journal of neurology worldwide. He received and delivered many short training courses and organized many National and International conferences.

Contents

Preface

Epilepsy continues to be a major health problem throughout the planet affecting millions of people, mainly in developing countries where parasitic zoonoses are more common and cysticercosis as a leading cause, is endemic.

We decided to edit this book because we found another way to approach this problem, covering novel aspects of epilepsy without ignoring its foundation and therefore, apart from the classic issues that cannot be missing in any book about epilepsy, we introduced novel aspects related with epilepsy and neurocysticercosis as a leading cause of epilepsy in developing countries. Of course, the publication of this book could not have been possible but for the ungrudging efforts put in by a large number of individuals working in the field of epilepsy and many people from many countries, ethnic, religious and socioeconomic groups that coincidentally confluence in Epilepsy.

As can be seen in other books on epilepsy, we also cover those topics related to history, classification of seizure and epileptic syndromes, associated sleep disorders and novel aspects on epileptic channelopathies. Social aspects related to epilepsy in three different chapters are included as well.

We are looking forward with confidence and pride in the vital role that this book has to play for a new vision and mission. Therefore, we introduce novel aspects of epilepsy related to its impact on reproductive functions, oral health and epilepsy secondary to tuberous sclerosis, mithocondrial disorders and lisosomal storage disorders.

It was a great sense of delight to include in this book two chapters about combined neuro-cardiogenic epilepsy syndromes and sudden unexpected death in epilepsy, and other three chapters about epilepsy and neglected parasitic zoonotic diseases, including a description of epileptic seizures not reported in the medical literature before and the role of the pig industry. It will push this book to a higher level of acceptance because the most common cause of epilepsy in developing countries is linked to the parasitic infections of the brain and in this regard, new knowledge is delivered in this book.

Some chapters and the edition job were entirely made in a rural setting and this edition is aimed at health care professionals including general practitioners, family doctors, internists, neurologists, epileptologists, neurosurgeons, psychiatrists, medical students, nursing students, and students of the professions allied to medicine among others.

More than 150 abstracts were submitted for review from all over the world, about 50 % were selected during the first phase of this editorial process. All materials for this edition has been thoroughly revised, and updated. Many specialists have provided expert advice on changes in their field and their help has been invaluable to us in our efforts to keep the relevance of the book for our readership community. All chapters were reviewed by each author twice after submission, the final version was peer-reviewed by two experts and recommendations were made. Nevertheless, some advices of contributors may differ from the approach of the editors or even the neurologic community. However, we kept and supported it as part of our policy of respect to all scientific criteria, mainly those that still remain controversial. The future will decide who was wrong. On the other hand, we also encourage other authors who are experts in the field, to report their personal experience, expertise, and obtained results.

Knowing that authors from many countries may have different experience and scientific results, in order to achieve a high degree of scientific content with a standard level of acceptance, we took a detailed overview of all important novel information. We all tried to keep the high prestige of our Editorial Company as a main priority and we declare our happiness in writing this book in the electronic era with a full-text website allowing us to display our scientific messages to an even larger global readership apart from all benefits of print format.

Our aim has been to produce a reference book in which this information is presented in an integrated and rapidly accessible format.

We all attempted to bring in valuable updated information about novel aspects of epilepsy, some of which has not been previously reported in the medical literature, as well as other new knowledge in epilepsy to our readership.

Akcnowledgements

Many people helped support the writing of this book. First, I'd like to thank all of technical reviewers. These folks check to make sure the examples work, look for technical errors, and make many suggestions on writing quality. It's not possible to write a quality medical book without quality scientific reviewers.

We are extremely grateful for the skill and support of our Publishing Process Managers Natalia Reinic and Dragana Manestar who have meticulously co-ordinated the whole project with unfailing good mood and patience and to the INTECH Open Access Publisher for giving us the opportunity to address this book to our medical community, mainly to those working for millions of epileptic patients in rural and sub-urban areas.

Furthrmore, I'd like to extend my gratitude to Dr. Roberto Gonzalez Martin Vice-Minister of the Cuban Ministry of Health (CMH), Dra Luisa Maria Diaz National Director of Postgraduate (CMH) and Dr. Jorge Delgado Bustillo Deputy Head of National Unit of International Collaboration (CMH), Prof. PhD Nereyda Cantelar del Castillo, Dr. PhD Reinaldo Menendez and Lic Maribel Chao from the National Institute of Tropical Medicine "Pedro Kouri", Prof. MM Balintulo Vice-Chancellor and Principal of Walter Sisulu University (WSU) in Mthatha, South Africa, Prof CL Obi Deputy Vice Chancellor, Academic Affairs and Research, Prof. G Buijs Deputy Chancellor, Planning, quality Assurance and Development, Prof. KJ Mammen Director, Directorate of Post Graduate Studies, Prof. GE Ekosse Director: Research Development (WSU); Prof K Mfenyana Executive Dean of Faculty of Health Sciences (WSU), Prof JE Iputo Director of the School of Medicine (WSU), Prof. A Awotedu Chairman of the Department of Medicine (WSU) , Dr. Xamlashe CEO and Dr. TM Madiba Head: Clinical Governance of Mthatha Hospital Complex and all my friends, colleagues and collaborators my deepest sense appreciation.

Finally, I'd like to thank to my first daughter Zayra Susana (died in 1979), who is my inspiration in life, to my wife Lourdes de Fátima, for her unconditional support and active participation in this book, to my second daughter, Lic. Lorna María (Who is also an excellent lawyer), my little daughter Fatima Susana Adolfina (2 years old) and my little son Thabo Humberto Jorge (3 years old) because writing chapters and editing a book takes a lot of time, and they were very understanding when I needed to work. They also understood when I was writing a chapter during our holidays at home and I had to move from one hotel to another looking for Internet access trying to download more than 150 abstracts. To my lovely father and my sister Lilia Teresa, Mayra Alejandra and Lorna Irene who always supported me, and the rest of my family: thanks very much indeed.

Many thanks also to family, relatives, and friends of all collaborators for their patience and acceptance of the lost evenings, nights, weekends, and holidays.

Prof. Humberto Foyaca- Sibat
Walter Sisulu University, Mthatha
South Africa

1

Psychosocial and Cultural Aspects of Epilepsy

Hamdy Fouad Moselhy
Faculty of Medicine and Health Sciences, UAE University, United Arab Emirates

1. Introduction

Epileptic activity within the brain has an effect on the behavior, mood, and cognitive functions of the epileptic patient. Additionally, his/her behavior and mood may be affected by the attitude of others to his/her disability. Furthermore, the patient's social and psychological adaptations may modify his/her epileptic experiences. As a consequence of the interaction between these aspects patients with epilepsy face many cultural and psychosocial problems (Betts et al., 1976). The definition of the term psycho-social in dictionaries is "pertaining to or concerning the mental factors or activities which determine the social relations of an individual" (Webster, 2011). Meanwhile, the definition of culture is all the knowledge and values shared by a society (Webster, 2011). As many as possible previously published studies on the psychosocial and cultural aspects of epilepsy were identified from various parts of the world by using multiple search strategies. Published literatures cover varieties of areas, including: psychiatric problems (e.g. mood disorders, anxiety, psychotic disorders); feeling of shame, fear, and worry; low self-esteem; problems related to education, employment, dating, marriage, child-bearing, poor quality of life, and stigma (Lai, 2007). Publications on the link between culture and epilepsy show the believed etiology of epilepsy, public awareness, understanding and attitude toward epilepsy (Fong & Hung, 2002). Although some of these aspects have been considered in earlier chapters, at the risk of some repetition, we aim in this chapter to introduce an overview of different psychosocial areas related to epilepsy and examining the public awareness, understanding and attitudes of different cultures to epilepsy.

2. Psychological effects of being epileptic

To be epileptic is to be stressed and stress can influence the incidence of fits. Under stress many people develop anxiety symptoms which may be seen as a fight or flight reaction, some become depressed, and others show obsessive ritualistic behavior. There are those who develop temporary psychotic states or acute conversion (hysterical) reactions which effectively isolate them from the stressful situation (Betts et al., 1976). Beside the significance of the stress to the epileptic, the reaction of individual depends on several factors. Firstly, the support which a person has from family and friends affects his ability to cope. Secondly, the genetic constitution of the individual and the responsiveness of his autonomic nervous system to stress may play an important part (Slater & Shields, 1969, as cited in Betts et al., 1976). Thirdly, stress responses are influenced by educational and cultural background. Finally, reactions are acquired and learnt as a part of growing up. Children are influenced greatly by the social mores of their family and the example of their parents (Betts et al., 1976).

Diagnosis of epilepsy can result in many psychological difficulties. Grief at the realization of being disabled goes through stages of shock, anxiety, bargaining and denial, mourning and depression, internalized anger, externalized anger, acknowledgement and finally acceptance and adjustment (Buchanan, 2002). Such grieves can occur either at onset or on realization of difference. Guilt can result in affective disorder. Anxiety combined with guilt can grow to become depression (Mendez, 1996). Depression appears to be the most common psychiatric comorbidity (Gilliam et al., 2003). The literature published has identified general mood disturbance, depression, and pathological distress, which are independent of seizure control, as significant predictors of quality of life impairment among people with epilepsy (Gilliam et al., 2003). Anxiety related emotions, which are very common in the epilepsy population, are amongst the most pathogenic secondary consequences (Mitan, 1983). However, anxiety disorders have not been extensively investigated. Many patients are afraid of dying during an epileptic attack, or seriously hurting themselves. These are feelings that are difficult to cope with both for the patient and the relatives. Also the experience of losing control is difficult to handle, rendering feelings of helplessness and being "reigned over" by the epilepsy (Siegler, 1981).

With regard to the more severe psychopathologies, the schizophrenia-like psychoses appear to be recorded and represented in India, Africa, and Japan. Interestingly, the rather characteristic features that Slater and Beard in 1963 described, namely that preponderance of positive over negative symptoms, and the high prevalence of first-rank symptoms, seem to be reported in the series that have examined these cases (Trimble & Krishnamoorthy, 2003). In Africa, Gureje, 1991, examined an unselected sample of 204 patients with epilepsy and noted that 37% were classified as having a psychiatric illness, and in almost a third, this was psychosis. Matsuura & Trimble, 2000, reviewed the Japanese studies that related to psychoses. Prevalence rates of psychosis varied with different institutions, from 0.9 to 9.1%. Finally there is a need for well-designed epidemiological studies of the psychological consequences and the comorbid psychiatric disorders in epilepsy. Coordinated protocols that attempt to explore these issues across cultures are desirable to understand the interface between behavior and the brain.

3. The social effects of being epileptic

To be epileptic means being exposed to the fear of having attacks, being at a disadvantage in terms of work and personal relationships, being open to prejudice, this exists both in the lay public and in the medical and nursing professionals. Unpredictability in connection with epilepsy is a source of fear and insecurity, giving the patient a constant feeling of being under threat. Fear of social exposure of fits and feelings of disgrace often lead to social isolation. Mitan, 1983, reports that between 50 to 75 per cent of the patients participating in an epilepsy research project in Los Angeles spent almost all their time at home. Many epileptic patients develop an extreme dependence upon their relatives, and this dependence interferes with the development of social skills. Public ignorance and fear of the unknown is another important source for the epileptic patients' problems. It is frightening to see a person having an epileptic attack, losing control of himself, and the simplest way to prevent such fear is to avoid the person with epilepsy. The consequence is even more social isolation and difficulty with employment for the patient as well. In Norway the employment rate was

21 per cent below the general population (Sletmo, 1982). Unemployment is higher among people with epilepsy, by up to 50% in developed countries if seizures are not fully controlled and up to 100% in developing countries. This can be caused by employer prejudice resulting from stigma and a lack of information, a belief that machinery should be avoided by the people with epilepsy, inability to drive, or poorer academic achievement. Disclosure to an employer is therefore a difficult decision. Unemployment commonly results in a lower self-esteem, lessened well-being and a lower quality of life (Bishop & Hermann, 2000; Gumnit, 1997). In addition to feelings of loneliness, as a consequence of Social isolation, about 20 % of the patients reported that they lacked close friends (Hills, 2007). Dansky & Andermann, found that the marriage rate for women with epilepsy was 86% of that in the normal population, and for men with epilepsy it was 59%. Emotional problems are the most common hindrances to marriage (Dansky & Andermann, 1980).
Across the world and throughout history, epilepsy has been a culturally devalued condition. Such devaluing often leads to people with epilepsy being stigmatized and bearing psychosocial burden (de Boer et al., 2008). Stigmatization leads to discrimination, and people with epilepsy have been the target of prejudicial behavior in many sphere of life, over many centuries and in many cultures (Pahl & de Boer, 2005). The experience of stigma occurs when individuals possess a socially relevant and significant difference that others in the general population use as a reason to set them apart, resulting in the individuals' experience of status loss and discrimination (Link &Phelan, 2006). The original Colony for epilepsy was founded at Chalfont in 1893 in a quite part of what was then rural England, in order to provide employment for people with epilepsy. People with epilepsy were all too often an outcast and epilepsy carried the stigma of insanity. As time went on, conditions in the open community improved for those with epilepsy. Anticonvulsants were affecting much better control of fits. Epilepsy was no longer considered as a form of insanity (Laidlaw & Laidlaw, 1976). Finally, epilepsy is not just a clinical disorder but a social label; and a wealth of research supports the view that the social prognosis of epilepsy may be less optimistic than the clinical one, particularly for the four-fifths of affected people who live in the world's resource poor countries (WHO, 2011), and for those with intractable seizures (Jacoby & Baker, 2000). Although progress continues to be made in relation to medical management of epilepsy, including the development of new antiepileptic drugs, attention to the social adjustment of individuals with the condition is still limited. Traditionally, the outcome of health conditions has been measured in terms of mortality. More recently, new indexes have been developed. These attempts to define better the need for health services and related interventions, to define health outcomes in terms of body, person, and social functioning, and to provide a common framework for research, clinical work, and social policy (de Boer et al., 2008).

4. Culture aspects of epilepsy

One of the leading brain disorders in developing countries is represented by epilepsy. It is estimated that 80% of people suffering from epilepsy around the world, reside in developing world such as Africa (WHO, 2004). In developed countries, the lifetime prevalence rate for epilepsy ranges from 3.5 to 10.7 per 1,000 person-years (Forsgren et al., 2005; Teodore et al., 2006). In the other hand, the lifetime prevalence rates for active epilepsy varied from 1.5 to 14 per 1,000 person-years in Asia (Mac et al., 2007), from 5.1 to 57.0 per 1,000 person-years in Latin America (Burneo et al., 2005), and from 5.2 to 74.4 per 1,000 person-years in sub-Saharan Africa (Preux & Druet-Cabanac, 2005). It is uncertain whether these broad variations between environmental regions are attributable to varying definitions of epilepsy or whether they are related to geographically relevant risk factors such as poverty, illiteracy, poor sanitation, inaccessibility of medical care, birth-related trauma or cerebral cysticercosis (de Bittencourt et al., 1996). Cultural interpretation contributes to exclude epileptic patients from the educational and productive fields, aggravating the burden they face and favoring a treatment gap estimated to 80% (WHO, 2004). Treatment gap is the difference between the number of people with active epilepsy and the number whose seizures are being appropriately treated in a given population at a given point in time, expressed as a percentage (Meinardi et al., 2001).

4.1 Epilepsy in Africa

The reaction to epilepsy in Africa is shaped by traditional indigenous beliefs which are surprisingly similar, in some way or other, throughout most of the African continent and result in severe psychological hardship. The African epilepsy sufferers have a hard time to achieve positive feelings about themselves and frequently suffer deprivations without protest (Jilek et al., 1997). In 1970 Osuntokun & Odeku, reviewed 522 Nigerian epilepsy sufferers and observed that the patients suffered psychosocial handicaps including suicidal tendency because they themselves considered epilepsy a social disgrace. Modern treatment for epilepsy is often unavailable in Africa. The reason might be lack of treatment facilities, but also the general belief that epilepsy is of supernatural causation and therefore not treatable by Western medicine (Osuntokun & Odeku, 1970). Behavior often of sudden impulsive onset and discharge of bursting seizures make the victim become visible as if in the hold of an eccentric power. This provokes powerful panic in those present and has most likely done much to be responsible for the belief that epilepsy is caused by evil spirits or other supernatural forces.

Although Africa is a diverse continent, and represents people of different cultural background, a widely held notion is that epilepsy may be caused by evil spirits (Carod-Artal & Vazquez-Cabrera, 2007). Other beliefs include witchcraft and contagious fears from bodily secretions (saliva, stool, or urine) that could potentially transmit seizures to bystanders (Carod-Artal & Vazquez-Cabrera, 2007). An added cause cited by Mauritania Moorish populations is the diet; the term "iguindi" refers to all clinical manifestations including seizures attributed to excessive eating (Traore et al., 1998). In Nigeria, Africa's most populous country, epilepsy is thought to be contagious, and that belief is even popular among medical school students (Awaritefe, 1989). A belief of the Bini of Nigeria is that epilepsy is a disease where the heart gets blocked by foam, restricting circulation and resulting in a seizure. In Uganda epilepsy is thought to be a result of a lizard spinning around in circles in the head disturbing the brain causing dizziness, usually followed by a seizure. In Malawi epilepsy is thought to be due to an insect moving inside the stomach. In Swaziland epilepsy is thought to be caused by sorcery, which sends evil animals or spirits into the body, causing convulsion (Andermann, 2011). A connection between the phases of the moon and convulsive attacks has been made since ancient times. It was, and still, is believed that either the new or the full moon is directly influencing and provoking seizure activity (Jilek, 1979).

Sub-Saharan Africa- and the continent of Arica as a whole- attach a huge social stigma to epilepsy (Jilek et al., 1997). Prejudice against the disease is common, persons with epilepsy are usually stigmatized and even pronunciation of the word 'epilepsy' is a taboo (Carod-

Artal & Vazquez-Cabrera, 2007). To suffer from epilepsy in Africa often means to also suffer from a very specific psychological and social trauma (Jilek-Aall & Jilk, 1989). It will drastically change the way a person perceives life and his or her position within the family unit. Additionally, because of the belief that epilepsy may be contagious or caused by supernatural forces, epilepsy sufferers are shunned and feared by their fellow men, and they themselves are ashamed and frightened (Jilek et al., 1997).

The traditional indigenous beliefs and traditional treatment of epilepsy in Africa contribute to the under-utilization of the medical health services, to discrimination and social isolation (Diop et al., 2003). In Africa preventable causes of epilepsy are more frequent than elsewhere, including infectious disease, head trauma, insufficient perinatal care and consanguinity (WHO, 2004). In 1997 the Global Campaign against epilepsy was launched to bring epilepsy 'out of shadows' to reduce treatment gap and social and physical burden, educate health personnel, dispel stigma, and support prevention (Diop et al., 2003). The Global Campaign against epilepsy consists of providing a platform for general awareness and assist departments of health in developing national epilepsy programs (Diop et al., 2003). The aim of reducing the treatment gap needs to take into consideration the cultural environment. Information and education of the public in general is important in order to enable and empower people to make informed choices. Cultural aspects should be studied with regard to patients' perceptions, attitudes and practices in relation to epilepsy, as well as their socio-familial relations. They provide the background for appropriate information, education and treatment programmes to be adapted in a holistic way to cultural specificities with a great chance of success. Furthermore research should be done to find out how apparent conflicts between cultural and scientific concepts can be resolved (WHO, 2004).

4.2 Epilepsy in Asia

Although substantial economic development and improvement of health services have occurred, Asia is a heterogeneous and resource-constrained continent. Over half of the 50 million people with epilepsy worldwide are estimated to live in Asia (Mac et al., 2007). There are some biological differences in epilepsy between Asia and the West, mainly related to the young average age and smaller physique among Asians. This probably partly explains the smaller doses of antiepileptic drugs found effective in some trials involving Asians (Yang et al., 2007). The climate differences partly account for the higher prevalence of Japanese encephalitis and malaria, which remains important causes of acute symptomatic seizures in parts of Asia (Tan, 2007). Numerous studies on knowledge and attitudes towards epilepsy have been done in Asia, particularly in Chinese communities within and outside china. Many communities remain negative towards people with epilepsy, with a third to half thought that a person with epilepsy cannot work like other people (Mac et al., 2007).

Some studies in Asia have looked into some specific research topics. The gender issue has been studied in Pakistan, showing that there are many more difficulties for female patients with epilepsy in coping with pressure from society and family, and female epileptic patients tend to internalize the prejudice and discrimination (Aziz et al., 1997). In Sri Lanka, marriage is most often arranged between the parties. Most men are unwilling to accept proposal from a girl who has epilepsy. A history of epilepsy often results in breaking proposals. Thus, women with epilepsy often remain single. When epilepsy is concealed and subsequently exposed after marriage, the wife is either ill-treated or sent back to her parent's home. Women with epilepsy are often beaten and divorced by their husbands.

Epilepsy is legally a valid reason for divorce in Sri Lanka (Gamage, 2004). In addition, there is misbelieving that women with epilepsy cannot bear children. Finally many women with epilepsy come from lower socioeconomic background and had very little formal education. They are often unskilled and have great difficulty in finding suitable employment (Gamage, 2004). In Korea actual discriminatory practices in the employment of patients with epilepsy are prevalent, and there are 24.5% who have been treated unfairly at work. More than half of those who disclosed their disease to employers report that they have been refused a job because of epilepsy (Lee, 2005).

In conclusion, what discriminate epilepsy in Asia from other regions is probably not so much genetic or biological differences of Asians or environmental factors that control the causes of acute symptomatic seizures and epilepsy, but the psychosocial, cultural, economic, political and organizational factors that influence epilepsy causation, management and outcome.

4.3 Epilepsy in native tribes from central and South America

American beliefs about epilepsy differ from those observed in African or Asian cultures. Epilepsy was a well-recognized disease in pre-Columbian cultures, as Spanish chroniclers of the sixteenth century reported (Carod-Artal & Vazquez-Cabrera, 2007). Several native societies persist in Central and South America with a traditional medical system, empiricism, rites and initiations, whose knowledge is orally transmitted (Carod & Domenech, 1995). Epilepsy is caused by an attack suffered by an animal spirit who accompanies the person, after a fight between the spirits who serve the forces of good and evil (Carod-Artal & Vazquez-Cabrera, 2007). People with chronic epilepsy are considered witches. Epilepsy is called "teawarup" by Kamayura, and is caused by the revenge of the spirit (mama'e) of the armadillo killed by a huntsman. It is treated with two roots. Epilepsy is called "tukuri" by Chipaya people, and is originated by a witchcraft that enters into the nose and the head, as a wind. Tukuri is treated with a ritual animal sacrifice called willancha, and by taking several dried insect infusions and bird's blood (Carod-Artal & Vazquez-Cabrera, 2007). For the hunter-fisher-gatherer tribe of Amerindians, epilepsy may be caused by an accident, the rupture of an animal-hunting taboo, familial violence, or due to witchcraft. Epilepsy cannot be dissociated from religious beliefs. Malefic powers can be originated either from the direct action of a harmful shaman or by interactions with the Devil. "Nahualism", the disruption of the accompanying animal spirit of the person, is an explanation for epilepsy in many Meso-American cultures (Carod-Artal & Vazquez-Cabrera, 2007).

4.4 Spirituality and religion in epilepsy

Convulsions had an historical association with spirits and religion, primarily through the concept of spirit possession (Reis, 1994). Epileptic seizures initially attributed to voodoo spirit possession (Carrazana et al., 1999). The religious aspects of epilepsy have been observed in traditional African cultures (Baskind & Birbeck, 2005) as occurred in South American cultures (Carod-Artal & Vazquez-Cabrera, 2007). Even in deeply different and distant cultures such as the Greco-Roman, Judeo-Christian, Islamic, Hindu, and Voodoo traditions, epilepsy has consistently been seen as an infliction or possession by a supernatural power, be it a god or a demon (Magiorkinis et al., 2010). The Greeks referred to epilepsy as the Sacred Disease, and over the millennia, the disorder has been associated with prophets, mystics, diviners, and the like (Temkin, 1971). Hippocrates began his discourse on the "sacred disease" by refuting the connection between epilepsy and the divine; he argued against the widespread beliefs of prophetic and mystical powers attributed persons with epilepsy and the disorder's divine causation. However, Hippocrates attempt to dissociate epilepsy and religion was unsuccessful. Subsequent religious figures were asked to heal people with epilepsy. The New Testament gospels of Matthew (17: 14-20), Mark (9: 14-29), and Luke (9:37-43), who was a physician; recount how Jesus cast out the evil spirit from a boy with epilepsy who just had a seizure, thereby curing him (DeToledo & Lowe, 2003). Throughout the Middle-Ages and the Renaissance, religious and magical treatments of epilepsy predominated (Temkin, 1971), and in the nineteenth century the religiosity of persons with epilepsy was stressed by physicians such as Esquirol, Morel, and Maudsley (Devinsky & Lai, 2008). Hyperreligiosity has been described in people with epilepsy by many early writers, including Echeverria, Clouston, Howden, and Kraeplin (Trimble & Freeman, 2006). One of the more influential investigators of recent times was Slater, who noted that mystical delusions were common in his series of patients with epilepsy and psychosis (Slater & Beard, 1963). Additionally, Dewhurst and Beard, 1970, reported on a series of patients with epilepsy who underwent religious conversions. All six had temporal lobe epilepsy, and none had been particularly religious before their conversion. More recently an investigation of religiosity in patients with temporal lobe epilepsy was done by Trimble and Freeman, 2006. They examined the religious experiences of 28 patients with epilepsy and religiosity, 22 patients with epilepsy and no expressed interest in religion, and 30 volunteer regular churchgoers. Members of the epileptic religious group were significantly more likely to have had past episodes of postictal psychosis and to have bilateral cerebral dysfunction. Finally, literature surveys have revealed that between 0.4% and 3.1% of partial epilepsy patients had ictal religious experiences; higher frequencies are found in systematic questionnaires versus spontaneous patients reports. Among patients with ictal religious experiences, there is a predominance of patients with right temporal lobe epilepsy. Postictal and interictal religious experiences occur most often in temporal lobe epilepsy patients with bilateral seizure foci (Davinsky & Lai, 2008). Although psychological and social factors such as stigma may contribute to religious experiences with epilepsy, a neurological mechanism most likely plays a large role. The limbic system is also often suggested as the critical site of religious experience due to the association with temporal lobe epilepsy and the emotional nature of the experiences. Neocortical areas also may be involved, suggested by the presence of visual and auditory hallucinations, complex ideation during many religious experiences, and the large expanse of temporal neocortex. In contrast to the role of the temporal lobe in evoking religious experiences, alteration in frontal functions may contribute to increased religious interests as personality trait (Davinsky & Lai, 2008).

5. Conclusion

Epileptic activity within the brain has an effect on the behavior, mood, and cognitive function of the patients. Problems related to areas such as overprotection, education, employment, marriage, child bearing, and psychiatric disturbances will vary according to the stage of epilepsy and the level of understanding in the society. There is widespread prejudice against epilepsy in almost all cultures. Among some cultures in Africa and Asia people with epilepsy are regarded with hostility and denied access to what medical and

social care may be available. Epileptic patient may become an exile from his society, exposed to social and religious taboo, isolated, sometimes denied the right to have children except with other epileptics. This reaction to epilepsy is essentially one of rejection.
People with epilepsy, sometimes along with their family members, are often stigmatized. This stigmatization generates a hidden burden, which discourages patients from seeking the diagnosis and care they need and deserve. Additional fallout of stigmatization is the discrimination, as people who experience seizures but are able to work are unemployed; and many who are able to find employment are underemployed. It is often said that social attitude towards the disorder often causes more distress to the person with epilepsy and the near ones than the disease itself.

6. References

Awaritefe, A. (1989). Epilepsy: the myth of a contagious disease. *Culture, Medicine and Psychiatry, Vol.* 13, pp. 449-456

Andermann, L.F. (March 2011). Epilepsy in different cultures: epilepsy in developing countries, In: *Epilepsy awareness,* 2.03.2011, available from http://www.epilepsytoronto.org/people/eaupdate/vi10-1.html

Aziz, H.; Akhtar, S.W.; & Hasan, K.Z. (1987). Epilepsy in Pakistan: stgma and psychosocial problems. A population-based epidemiologic study. *Epilepsia* Vol. 38, pp. 1069-1073

Baskind, R. & Birbeck, G. (2005). Epilepsy care in Zambia: a study of traditional healers. *Epilepsia, Vol.* 46, pp. 1121- 1126

Betts, T.A.; Merskey, H. & Pond, D.A. (1976). Psychiatry. In: *textbook of epilepsy,* Laidlaw J & Richens A. Churchill Livingstone, pp 145-184, ISBN 0443014264, Edinburgh, UK

Bishop, M. & Hermann, B. (2000). Impact of epilepsy on quality of life: a review. In: *quality of life in epilepsy: beyond seizure counts in assessment and treatment,* Baker GA, Jacoby A, Harwood Academic, pp. 103-120,Amsterdam

Buchanan, N. (2002). *Understanding epilepsy: what it is and how it can affect your life.* New ed. Simon Schuster, pp. 102-119, Sydney

Burneo, J.G.; Tellez-Zenteno, J. & Wiebe, S. (2005). Understanding the burden of epilepsy in Latin America: a systematic review of its prevalence and incidence. *Epilepsy Research, Vol.* 66, pp. 63-74

Carod-Artal, F.J. & Vazquez-Cabrera, C.B. (2007). An anthropological study about epilepsy in native tribes from Central and South America. *Epilepsia, Vol.* 48, No. 5, pp. 886-893

Carod, F.J. & Domenech, E. (1995). Treatment of epilepsy among the Guarine (Palenque) tribes. *Neurologia, Vol.* 9, pp. 394-395

Carrazana, E.; DeToledo, J.; Tatum, W.; Rivas-Vasquez, R.; Rey, G. & Wheeler, S. (1999) Epilepsy and religious experiences:voodoo possession. *Epilepsia, Vol.* 40, pp. 1041-1046

Dansky, L.V. & Andermann, F. (1980) Marriage and fertility in epileptic patients. *Epilepsia, Vol.* 27, pp. 261-271

de Boer, H.M.; Mula, M. & Sander, J.W. (2008). The global burden and stigma of epilepsy. *Epilepsy & behavior, Vol.* 12, pp. 540-546

de Bittencourt, P.; Adamolkun, B.; Bhurucha, N.; Carpio, A.; Cossio, O.; Danesi, M.; Dumas, M.; Femandes, J.; Genton, P.; Manreza, M.; Meinardi, H.; Ordinario, A.; Senanayake, N.; Shakir, R.; Singhal, B.& Sotelo, J.(1996). Epilepsy in the tropics: 1. Epidemiology, socioeconomic risk factors and etiology. *Epilepsia, Vol.* 37, pp. 1121-1127

DeToledo, J.C. & Lowe, M.R. (2003) Epilepsy, demonic possessions, and fasting: another look at translations of Mark 9:16. *Epilepsy Behavior, Vol.* 4, pp. 338-339

Devinsky, O. & Lai, G. (2008). Spirituality and religion in epilepsy. *Epilepsy & Behavior, Vol.* 12, pp. 636-643

Dewhurst, K. & Beard, A.w. (1970). Sudden religious conversions in temporal lobe epilepsy. *British J Psychiatry, Vol.* 117, pp. 497-507

Diop, A.G.; de Boer, M.; Mandlhate, C.; Prilipko, L. & Meinardi, H. (2003) The global campaign against epilepsy in Africa. *Acta Tropica, Vol.* 87, pp. 149-159

Fong, C.G. & Hung, A. (2002). Public awareness, attitude, and understanding of epilepsy in Hong Kong Special Administrative Region, China. *Epilepsia, Vol.* 43, pp. 311-316

Forsgren, I.; Beghi, E.; Oun, A. & Sillanpaa, M. (2005) The epidemiology of epilepsy in Europe: a systematic review. *European Neurology* Vol. 12, pp. 245-253

Gamage, R. (2004). Women and epilepsy, psychosocial aspects in Sri Lanka. *Neurology Asia, Vol.* 9, supp 1, pp. 39-40.

Gilliam, F.; Hecimovic, H. & Sheline, Y. (2003). Psychiatric comorbidity, health, and function in epilepsy. *Epilepsy & Behavior, Vol.* 4, pp. S26-S30

Gumnit, R.J. (1997). *Living well with epilepsy,* Demos Vermande, pp.173-181, New York

Gureje, O. (1991). Interictal psychopathology in epilepsy: Prevalence and pattern in a Nigerian clinic. *British Journal of Psychiatry,* Vol. 113, 1375-1379

Hills, M.D. (2007). The psychological and social impact of epilepsy. *Neurology Asia, Vol.* 12, supp 1, pp.10-12

Jacoby, A. & Baker, GA. (2000). Quality of life issues in intractable focal epilepsy. In: *intractable focal epilepsy,* Oxbury J, Polkey C, Duchowny M. WB Saunders, pp. 419-436 London

Jilek-Aall, L.M. & jilek, W.G. (1989). Epilepsy and its psychosocial implications in Africa. In *clinical psychology in Africa,* K. Peltzer and PO Ebigbo, pp. 353-364. University of Nigeria, Enugu, Nigeria

Jilek-AAI, L.; Jilek, M.; Kaaya, J.; Mkombachepa, L. & Hilary, K. (1997). Psychosocial study of epilepsy in Africa. *Social Science Medicine,* Vol. 45, No. 5, pp. 783-795

Jilek, W.G. (1979). The epileptic's outcast role and its background: a contribution to the social psychiatry of seizure disorders. *Journal of Operational Psychiatry,* Vol. 10, pp. 127-133

Lai, C.W. (2007). Epilepsy research priorities in Asia: psycho-social and cultural issues. *Neurology Asia,* Vol.12, Supp. 1, pp. 18-20

Laidlaw, J. & Laidlaw, M. (1976). People with epilepsy-living with epilepsy: in *textbook of epilepsy,* Laidlaw J & Richens A. Churchill Livingstone, pp 355-385, ISBN 0443014264, Edinburgh, UK

Lee, S.A. (2005). What we confront with employment of people with epilepsy in Korea. *Epilepsia,* Vol. 46, suppl. 1, pp. 57-8

Link, B.G. & Phelan, J.C. (2006). Stigma and its public health implications. Lancet, Vol. 367, pp. 528-529

Mac, T.L.; Tran, D.; Odematt, P.; Preux, P.; & Tan, C.T. (2007). Epidemiology, aetiology, and clinical management of epilepsy in Asia: a systematic review. *The Lancet Neurology,* Vol. 6, No.6, pp. 533-543

Magiorkinis, E.; Sidiropoulou, K. & Diamantis, A. (2010). Hallmarks in the history of epilepsy: epilepsy in antiquity. *Epilepsy Behavior,* Vol. 17, pp. 103-108

Matsuura, M. & Trimble, M. (2000). Psychoses in epilepsy: a review of Japanese studies. *Epilepsy & Behavior,* Vol. 1,pp. 315-326

Meinardi, H.; Scott, R.; Reis, R. & Sander, S. (2001). The treatment Gap in epilepsy: the current situation and ways forward. *Epilepsia,* Vol. 42, No.1, pp. 136-149

Mendez, M. (1996). Disorders of mood and affect in epilepsy, In: *Psychological disturbances in epilepsy*, Sackellares JC, Berent S, pp. 125-141, Butterworth-Heinemann, Boston.

Mitan, R.J. (1983). Patient's fears about seizures: a greater psychosocial stressor? Paper presented at *International epilepsy symposium*, Washington DC, USA

Osuntokun, B.O. & Odeku, E.L. (1970). Epilepsy in Ibadan, Nigeria. *African Journal of Medical Sciences,* Vol. 1, pp. 185- 200

Pahl, K. & de Boer, H.M.. (2005). Epilepsy and rights. In: *Atlas: epilepsy care in the world.* pp.72-73, WHO Press, Geneva

Preux, P.M. & Druet-Cabanac, M. (2005). Epidemiology and etiology of epilepsy in sub-Saharan Africa. *Lancet Neurology*, Vol. 4, 21-31

Reis, R. (1994). Evil in the body, disorder of the brain. Interpretations of epilepsy and treatment gap in Swaziland.*Tropical and Geographical Medicine,* Vol. 46, S40-S43

Siegler, R.G. (1981). Impairments of control and competence in epileptic children and their families. *Epilepsia,* Vol. 22, pp. 339-346

Slater, E.; Sheilds, J. (1969). Genetical aspects of anxiety, In: *studies of anxiety.* Edited by MH Ladder, Headly Brothers, Ashford, Kent, UK

Slater, E. & Beard, A.W. (1963). The schizophrenia-like psychoses of epilepsy. *British J Psychiatry,* Vol. 109, pp. 95-150

Sletmo, A. (1982). Rehabilitation in epilepsy, *Advances in epileptology.* XIIIth epilepsy international symposium, Raven Press, New York, USA

Tan, C.T. (2007). Differences in epilepsy and seizures between Asia and the West. *Neurology Asia,* Vol. 12, pp. 59-60

Temkin, O. (1971). *The falling sickness: a history of epilepsy from the Greeks to the beginnings of modern neurology,* John Hopkins University Press, London, UK

Theodore, W.H.; Spencer, S.; Wiebe, S.; Langf, H.; Ali, A.; Shafer, P.; Berg, A. & Vickrey, B. (2006). Epilepsy in North America: a report prepared under the auspices of the Global Campaign against epilepsy, the International Bureau for Epilepsy, the International League Against Epilepsy, and the World Health Organization. *Epilepsia,* Vol. 47, pp. 1700-1722

Traore, H.; Diagana, M.; Debrock, C.; Ba, A.; Algad, B. & Preux, P.M. (1998). Sociocultural approach to epilepsy in Mauritania. *Medecine tropcale: revue du Corps de santé colonial,* Vol. 58, pp. 365-368

Trimble, M. & Krishnamoorthy, E. (2003). Neuropsychiatric disorders in epilepsy: some transcultural issues. *Epilepsia,* Vol. 44, suppl. 1, pp. 21-24

Trimble, M. & Freeman, A. (2006). An investigation of religiosity and the Gastaut-Geschwind syndrome in patients with temporal lobe epilepsy. *Epilepsy & behavior,* Vol. 9, pp. 407-414

WHO. (2011). Epidemiology, etiology and prognosis, in: *fact sheet number 165,* accessed Feb 2011, available from: htt://www. WHO.unt.

WHO. (2004). Epilepsy in the WHO Africa Region, Bridging the gap: the global campaign against epilepsy, *out of the shadows,* WHO Press, Geneva

Webster's Online Dictionary. (2011). Definition, in: *Webster's Online Dictionary,* accessed 14 March, 2011, available from:
http://www.websters-online-dictionary.org/definitions

Yang, L.,; Xuefeng, W.; Qihua, L.; Jingmei, L. & Yong, Y. (2007). Tolerability and safety of topiramate in Chinese patients with epilepsy: an open-label, long-term, prospective study. *Clinical drug investigation,* Vol. 27, 683-690

2

Tuberous Sclerosis Complex

Teguh Haryo Sasongko[1], Nik Mohd Ariff Nik Abdul Malik[1],
Nur Farrah Dila Ismail[1] and Salmi Abd. Razak[2]
[1]Human Genome Center and
[2]Department of Pediatrics, School of Medical Sciences,
Universiti Sains Malaysia
Malaysia

1. Introduction

TSC (OMIM#191100) is an autosomal dominant disorder characterized by a broad phenotypic spectrum including epilepsy, mental retardation, skin lesions and tumors in various organs. The broad phenotypic spectrum reflected the development of hamartomas in multiple organs throughout the body (Schwartz et al., 2008). The incidence of TSC has been reported to be 1 in approximately 6000 (Osborne et al., 1991). However, its true incidence is not known because of a number of undiagnosed cases consisting mostly of mildly affected or asymptomatic individuals (Osborne et al., 1991).

Two-thirds of TSC patients have sporadic mutations and only about one-thirds is familial. The genes in which abnormalities are found are called *TSC1* and *TSC2*. Both genes have been studied by multigenerational linkage analysis (Fryer et al., 1987 and Kandt et al., 1992). *TSC1* is located at position 9q34, and encodes a protein called hamartin, with an mRNA transcript of 8.6 kb containing 23 exons and encompassing 55 kb of DNA (van Slegtenhorst et al., 1997). *TSC2* is located at position 16p13.3, and encodes a protein called tuberin, with an mRNA transcript of 5.5 kb, containing 41 exons and encompassing 40 kb of DNA (Eur TS Consortium, 1993).

2. Clinical diagnosis of tuberous sclerosis complex

There are major and minor clinical features (Table 1) that enable clinicians to clinically diagnose TSC. The clinical diagnosis is made when two major features, or one major and two minor ones, can be shown (Table 2). Sometimes, an antenatal diagnosis can be made based on fetal ultrasound and MRI, which show cardiac and brain lesions (Roach et al., 1998).

Most patients are diagnosed in infancy or early childhood. A **definitive** diagnosis of TSC can be made when two major features or one major feature plus two minor features are demonstrated (Hyman, 2000 and Roach, 1998). Additional diagnostic categories include **probable** TSC when one major feature and one minor feature are present, and **possible** TSC when either one major feature or two or more minor features are present (Hyman, 2000 and Roach, 1998). However, as hamartomas are individually rare in the population without TSC, the presence of hamartomas in two different organ systems is considered by some clinicians to be sufficient for the diagnosis (O'Callaghan, 2000).

MAJOR FEATURES					MINOR FEATURES			
Features	Description	Diagnosis, location	Age of onset	Prevalence	Features	Description	Diagnosis, location	Preva-lence
Facial angiofibromas or forehead plaque (Schwartz et al., 2007)	Red to pink papules with a smooth surface, symmetrically distributed over the centrofacial areas, sparing the upper lips	Histologic (head)	Second to fifth year of life; more promi-nent with age	74.5%	Multiple, randomly distributed pits in dental enamel (Mennel et al., 2007)	Dental pits are pits in the enamel of the permanent teeth. They occur more frequently in individuals with TSC than in people who do not have TSC.	Direct inspection of the labial surfaces of the incisor and canine teeth	48 - 100%.
Non-traumatic ungula or periungual fibroma (Schwartz et al., 2007)	Skin-colored or reddish nodules seen on the lateral nail groove, nail plate, or along the proximal nail folds; more commonly found on the toes than on the fingers	Histologic (fingers and toes)	Puberty or soon after; more common with age	15.1%	Hamarto-matous rectal polyps (Young & Povey, 1998)	These polyps are common and do not cause symptoms. Their distinctive appearance and distribution readily distinguish them from other types of rectal polyp and emphasize their importance as a potentially useful clinical marker of TSC	Histologic (rectum)	78%
Hypomelanotic macules (three or more) (Schwartz et al., 2007)	Leaf-shaped or polygonal white spots, enhanced by Wood's lamp examination; more common on the trunk and buttocks	Histologic (skin)	At birth or infancy Earliest cuta-neous lesion appeared	97.2%	Cerebral white matter radial (Xu et al., 1996)	Most lesions are best seen on proton density-weighted images as bright spots.	MRI (brain)	15%
Shagreen patch (connective tissue nevus) (Schwartz et al., 2007)	Slightly elevated patch or plaque, usually found on the dorsal body surfaces, especially the lumbosacral area; its rough surface resembles an orange peel. Represents a connective tissue nevus, sometimes called collagenoma	Histologic (skin)	Rare during infancy, tend to increase in size and number with age	48.1%	Gingival fibromas (Mennel et al., 2007)	These small fibrous nodules of the oral cavity are most commonly evident on the gingiva, especially in the anterior segment of the upper jaw but also on the buccal mucosa and dorsal surface of the tongue.	Oral (gums)	32%
Multiple retinal nodular hamartomas (Xu et al., 1995)	Retinal hamartoma is a common finding in tuberous sclerosis, but the symptomatic changes of this lesion have rarely been described.	Ocular (eyes)	Infancy	9.7%	Non-renal hamarto-ma (Mennel et al., 2007)	Homartomatous formation in other organs than the kidney.	Histologic (Liver, spleen)	
Cortical tuber (Mennel et al., 2007)	Cortical tubers are the most characteristic lesions of tuberous sclerosis at pathologic examination. Varying in size from millimeters to several centimeters, tubers are rounded or wart-like protrusions of single or adjacent gyri, very firm to touch and pale in color	MRI (brain)	During fetus develop-ment	95%	Retinal achromic patch (Mennel et al., 2007)	Greyish or yellowish-white lesion in the back of the globe on the ophthalmic examination. A differential diagnosis for a calcified globe mass on a CT scan.	CT Scan (eyes)	12%

MAJOR FEATURES					MINOR FEATURES			
Features	Description	Diagnosis, location	Age of onset	Prevalence	Features	Description	Diagnosis, location	Preva-lence
Subependymal nodule (Mennel et al., 2007)	Occur in the third and fourth ventricular walls, but most are found in the lateral ventricular walls, near the sulcus terminalis, with their deeper parts embedded in the caudate or thalamus.	MRI (brain)	Increases with the age of the patient	95%	Confetti-like skin lesions (Mennel et al., 2007)	Multiple, 1-2 mm white spots symmetrically distributed over extremities	Histologic (skin)	2.8%
SEGA (Mennel et al., 2007) (SEGAs)	This type of tumor develops in approximately 15% of individuals with tuberous sclerosis. Typically, SEGAs do not occur in very young children, and the chance for their growth decreases after age 20.	Radio-graphy (brain)	Child to adole-scent	15%	Multiple renal cysts (Inoue, 1998)	Like AMLs, they are frequently multiple and bilateral. However, renal cysts are more likely to become symptomatic than AMLs. Polycystic kidney disease may also occur. It is a more severe, distinct entity with innumerable cysts that enlarge, replace renal parenchyma, and cause renal insufficiency and hypertension typically at an early age	Histologic (kidney)	17% (children) 47% (adults)
Cardiac rhabdomyoma, single or multiple	Rhabdomyomas are benign tumors of striated muscle	Echocardio-graphy	Grow during the second half of preg-nancy and regress after birth	90% (newborn) 20% (adult)				
Lymphangio myomatosis (Schwartz et al., 2007)	Rare lung disease that results in a proliferation of disorderly smooth muscle growth (leiomyoma) throughout the bronchioles, alveolar septa, perivascular spaces, and lymphatics	Histologic (lung)	Adole-scent to adult	49%				
Renal angiomyolipom a (Schwartz et al., 2007)	Renal angiomyolipoma is a benign neoplasm that may grow massive in TSC patients.	Histologic (kidneys)	Adole-scent to adult	80%				

Table 1. Major and Minor Features of Tuberous Sclerosis Complex.

Clinical Diagnosis	Characteristic
Definite TSC	Either two major features or one major plus two minor features
Probable TSC	One major plus one minor features
Possible TSC	Either one major features or two or more minor features

Table 2. Clinical Diagnosis of TSC. There are several differential diagnosis of TSC :

a. Multiple Endocrine Neoplasia type I (MEN-I) in which multiple angiofibromas, confetti-like hypopigmented macules, and multiple gingival papules are also seen.
b. Hypopigmented macules in TSC resemble nevus anemicus and nevus depigmentosus.
c. Renal Carcinoma may also be caused by mutations within VHL (cause VHL disease) or MET (cause HPRC) genes, although with different pathologic findings. The renal cell carcinomas in TSC are morphologically heterogenous, including clear cell, papillary, and chromophobic tumors. VHL patients almost exclusively develop clear cell carcinoma, while HPRC patients develop almost exclusively papillary tumors.

3. Epilepsy in tuberous sclerosis complex

Epilepsy was once included in tuberous sclerosis triad along with mental retardation and adenoma sebaceum (Provenzale, 1991). Although removed from the diagnostic criteria, epilepsy remains a dominant feature in tuberous sclerosis, covering up to 60% - 90% of TSC cases. Genetic factors play important contributions in the manifestation of epilepsy in TSC. It has recently been described that inactivation of *TSC2* causes more severe epilepsy phenotype than inactivation of *TSC1* in a mouse model of tuberous sclerosis and suggested that the difference in phenotype may be related to the degree to which *TSC1* and *TSC2* inactivation causes abnormal mTOR activation (Zheng, 2010).

Based on clinical features alone, TSC patients may experience a wide variety of ictal symptoms. Two syndromes are usually noted: infantile spasms (Christophea et al., 2000), which then evolve into partial or mixed epilepsies (Dabora et al., 2001) and partial seizures, typically starting later in childhood. The high incidence of infantile spasms in TSC has long been emphasized. Infantile spasms have been reported to be the presenting symptoms in up to 69% of patients with TSC. Infantile spasms in TSC usually have their onset between 4 to 6 months of age (Curatolo et al., 2001 and Fukushima et al 2001). TSC has been found in 7%–25% of infants with symptomatic West syndrome. West syndrome classically consists of the clinical-electroencephalographic triad of spasms (the seizure type), hypsarrhythmia and mental deficiencies. The main types of spasms (flexor, extensor, mixed) may occur in infant with TSC, but focal features such as head turning, nystagmus, tonic eye deviation or unilateral limb movement differentiate them from classical infantile spasms. Partial seizures predominate with the increasing age (Curatolo, 2001 and Jambeque et al., 1991).

Location of tubers on MRI often correlates with EEG discharges. Tubers consist of dysplastic neurons and glial cells that distort the normal cortical architecture, causing them to be highly epileptogenic (Christopher et al., 2000). Jambaque and collegues found that an initial presentation with infantile spasms, refractory seizures and mental retardation or behaviour disorder were all more likely in children with greater numbers of cortical tubers. The classic interictal EEG pattern of patients with epileptic spasm is hypsarrhythmia. Hypsarrhythmia was originally defined by Gibbs and Gibbs in 1950 as completely chaotic and disorganized background pattern consisting of high amplitude slow waves and spikes that are asynchronous, non-rhythmic and variable in duration and topography. The spikes usually alternate randomly between focal, multifocal and generalized discharges at different moments within a brief record. It is most pronounced in slow-wave sleep. Ictal recordings of spasms can demonstrate a focal increase in spikes and polyspikes at the onset, with an abrupt generalized slow followed by electro decrement or generalized lower amplitude fast activity coincident with the spasm itself. Curatolo has theorized the following sequence of events. Electrographic onset of spasms is more common from the posterior temporal and occipital regions than from other locations. Subsequent partial seizures tend to arise from the frontal or anterior temporal regions.

Drug selection should be tailored to both clinical and EEG attributes observed. Antiepileptic drug monotherapy is used whenever possible. Vigabatrin may be especially effective for infantile spasms in patients with TSC, with some series reporting complete control occurring in about 95% of patients (Aicardi, 1996 and Hancock, 1999). Vigabatrin produces its antiepileptic effect by irreversibly inhibiting the enzyme GABA-aminotransferase. This results in increased brain and spinal fluid concentration of the inhibitory neurotransmitter GABA. Unfortunately, recent reports of visual-field constriction associated with vigabatrin therapy may limit its use and may prevent from becoming an approved treatment in United States and other countries (Krauss et al., 1998). Other evidence from randomized controlled studies includes using ACTH and corticosteroids for infantile spasms. Chronic use of benzodiazepines and barbiturates should be avoided if possible owing to their cognitive and behavioural adverse effects. Other medications useful to treat seizures in TSC include lamotrigine, felbamate, topiramate, carbamazepine and levetiracetam. When anticonvulsant options have been exhausted, alternative treatment such as ketogenic diet may be tried. If severely disabling seizures are present with consistent electroclinical and imaging data suggesting a confined area of seizure onset, surgical treatment should be considered. The most common surgical procedures offered to TSC patient include topectomies, gyrectomies or wider lobar resection as well as multiple subpial transection. Vagal nerve stimulation is a surgical option restricted to TSC patients with intractable epilepsy who fail to meet the criteria for resective surgery.

4. Molecular diagnosis of tuberous sclerosis complex

Despite the comprehensive criteria for clinical diagnosis of TSC, molecular analyses of both causing genes remain of importance. Mutation analysis in TSC patients is useful 1) to confirm a clinical diagnosis of TSC, especially in young patients in whom many clinical features have yet to develop, 2) in families with sporadic cases of TSC, mutation analysis may provide reassurance that the rest of the family members do not carry the mutation. However, such testing does not provide complete reassurance in regard to the possibility of having the second child with TSC, even when the parents do not appear to carry the mutation, and 3) to perform prenatal diagnosis, in families with either a child or a parent with a known mutation.

5. *TSC1* and *TSC2* genes variation spectrum

Table 3 and 4 summarized updates on the variation spectrum within *TSC1* and *TSC2* and review their characteristics. The information was accessed from the LOVD for Tuberous Sclerosis (http://chromium.liacs.nl/LOVD2/TSC/ home.php) on 3 April 2011 (Fokkema et al, 2005). There are 468 unique *TSC1* sequence variations and 1222 unique *TSC2* sequence variations reported. Tables 1 and 2 listed up all unique sequence variations of *TSC1* and *TSC2* respectively, along with their variation types and information of pathogenicity.

Types / Pathogenicity (R/C)*	Substitution	Insertion	Deletion	Duplication	Insertion / Deletion	**Total**
-/-	12	Nil	Nil	1	Nil	**13**
-/-?	Nil	1	2	1	Nil	**4**
-/?	1	Nil	Nil	Nil	Nil	**1**
-/+?	1	Nil	Nil	Nil	Nil	**1**
-?/-	1	Nil	Nil	Nil	Nil	**1**
-?/-?	9	Nil	Nil	Nil	Nil	**9**
-?/?	6	Nil	Nil	Nil	Nil	**6**
-?/+?	1	Nil	Nil	Nil	Nil	**1**
?/-	5	Nil	Nil	Nil	Nil	**5**
?/-?	5	Nil	Nil	Nil	Nil	**5**
?/?	23	Nil	Nil	Nil	Nil	**23**
?/+?	2	Nil	1	Nil	Nil	**3**
?/+	Nil	Nil	Nil	1	Nil	**1**
+?/?	5	Nil	2	Nil	Nil	**7**
+?/+?	4	Nil	Nil	Nil	Nil	**4**
+?/+	2	Nil	Nil	1	Nil	**3**
+/-	4	Nil	Nil	Nil	Nil	**4**
+/?	3	1	3	Nil	1	**8**
+/+?	16	Nil	7	2	Nil	**25**
+/+	133	12	146	51	2	**344**
Total	**233**	**14**	**161**	**57**	**3**	**468**

*R/C = Reported/Concluded. "Reported Pathogenicity" refers to the pathogenicity as published by the authors in the original paper or as submitted to the LOVD-TSC database if the data has not been published. "Concluded Pathogenicity" refers to the pathogenicity that the curators of the database have assigned to the variant. (Personal Communication with the LOVD-TSC Database Curator; Dr. Rosemary Ekong). "-" = no known pathogenicity; "-?" = probably no pathogenicity; "+" = pathogenic; "+?" = probably pathogenic; "?" = unknown pathogenicity.

Table 3. *TSC1* sequence variations and their pathogenicity.

Types / Pathogenicity (R/C)*	Substitution	Insertion	Deletion	Duplication	Insertion / Deletion	**Total**
-/-	154	2	8	6	1	**171**
-/-?	42	1	2	2	Nil	**47**
-/?	96	Nil	Nil	Nil	Nil	**96**
-/+?	1	Nil	Nil	Nil	Nil	**1**
-?/-	7	Nil	Nil	Nil	Nil	**7**
-?/-?	14	Nil	Nil	Nil	Nil	**14**
-?/?	1	Nil	Nil	Nil	Nil	**1**
?/-	5	Nil	1	Nil	Nil	**6**
?/-?	17	Nil	1	Nil	Nil	**18**
?/?	46	1	5	3	1	**56**
?/+?	13	Nil	1	Nil	Nil	**14**
?/+	13	Nil	4	2	Nil	**19**
+?/?	15	1	1	1	1	**19**
+?/+?	19	1	6	Nil	Nil	**26**
+?/+	1	1	5	1	1	**9**
+/-	6	Nil	2	Nil	Nil	**8**
+/?	22	Nil	5	3	Nil	**30**
+/+?	60	2	16	3	7	**88**
+/+	303	33	148	103	Nil	**587**
-/+	1	Nil	1	Nil	Nil	**2**
+?/-	1	Nil	Nil	Nil	Nil	**1**
+?/-?	1	Nil	Nil	Nil	Nil	**1**
+/-?	1	Nil	Nil	Nil	Nil	**1**
Total	**839**	**42**	**206**	**124**	**11**	**1222**

*R/C = Reported/Concluded. "Reported Pathogenicity" refers to the pathogenicity as published by the authors in the original paper or as submitted to the LOVD-TSC database if the data has not been published. "Concluded Pathogenicity" refers to the pathogenicity that the curators of the database have assigned to the variant. (Personal Communication with the LOVD-TSC Database Curator; Dr. Rosemary Ekong). "-" = no known pathogenicity; "-?" = probably no pathogenicity; "+" = pathogenic; "+?" = probably pathogenic; "?" = unknown pathogenicity.

Table 4. *TSC2* sequence variations and their pathogenicity.

In *TSC1*, the most prevalent types of variations found are substitution (49.8%) followed by deletion (34.4%). Of 468 unique variations reported in *TSC1*, 73.5% (344) had their pathogenicity determined. In *TSC2*, the most prevalent types of variations found are also substitution (68.7%) followed by deletion (16.9%). Of 1222 unique variations reported in *TSC2*, only less than half (48%) had their pathogenicity determined. Different gene sizes of *TSC1* and *TSC2* may explain the fact that more variations occurred in *TSC2* than in *TSC1*.

Perhaps because of more chances of the variations to occur along considerable length of intronic portions within *TSC2*, less pathogenicity variations can be conclusively determined. The tables showed that of 1690 *TSC1* and *TSC2* variations reported, only 27.7% (468) were found in *TSC1*. There are some explanations for the fact that up to date more *TSC2* variations were found compared to *TSC1*:

a. According to Knudson's hypothesis, loss of heterozygosity (LOH) of a tumor suppressor gene is necessary for tumor progression. Recent investigations of somatic mutations in a variety of TSC hamartomas support classification of the TSC genes as tumor suppressor genes. Loss of Heterozygosity (LOH) in *TSC1* hamartomas are rare compared to that in *TSC2* hamartomas (Cheadle et al., 2000). This may reflect the low frequency of *TSC1* diseases.
b. Several large studies reported that *TSC1* mutations are presented with less severe phenotype than *TSC2* mutations. In 1991, Osborne and colleagues outlined that although TSC incidence is reported as 1 in approximately 6000, the true incidence of TSC is not known because of a number of undiagnosed cases consisting mostly of mildly affected or asymptomatic individuals. It is probable that this portion of patients harbored *TSC1* mutations, accounting for the small number of *TSC1* mutations found until today.
c. *TSC2* coding region is about 1.5 times longer than *TSC1* and has approximately twice the number of splice sites, affording a proportionally increased opportunity for all manner of small mutations.

6. Molecular pathogenesis of TSC

Up to 85% of TSC cases are due to mutations in either *TSC1* or *TSC2* genes which lead to a truncated protein with a loss of function mechanism. Investigation of somatic mutations in a variety of TSC hamartomas supports classification of the *TSC1* and *TSC2* as tumor suppressor genes (Cheadle et al., 2000). Mutations in *TSC1* and *TSC2* affect neuronal proliferation, differentiation, and migration (Crino et al., 1999). The identification of the *TSC1* and *TSC2* genes and their encoded proteins, hamartin and tuberin respectively, has aided in understanding the molecular pathogenesis of TSC where hamartomatous formation is the outcome.

Both hamartin and tuberin are widely expressed in normal tissues including brain, liver, and kidney. Hamartin is highly expressed in G0-arrested cells and throughout the ongoing cell cycle (Crino, 2004). Alterations in tuberin expression have been reported in patients with TSC. Immunoreactivity of tuberin is reduced in the brain with TSC. Loss of hamartin and tuberin formation due to *TSC1* and *TSC2* mutations can enhance proliferation of neural and astrocytic precursor cells and increased in cell size characteristic of dysplastic neurons and giant cells. When either of the *TSC1* or *TSC2* genes is inactivated, G1 is shortened and tissues become hypertropic (Potter et al., 2001). Over-expression of either hamartin or tuberin can lengthen G1 and inhibits cell proliferation (Tapon et al., 2001).

Many studies indicated that hamartin and tuberin, encoded by *TSC1* and *TSC2* genes respectively, function as a complex. The complex has a stable interaction with stoichiometry of 1:1. The tight binding interaction between the two proteins formed a tumour suppressor heterodimer (Kwiatkowaki, 2008). Hamartin and tuberin have been found to physically associate with one another in vivo. Disruption in either one of the two genes may result in a truncated protein with the loss in controlling the cell growth and proliferation. The 130 kDa hamartin contains a putative transmembrane domain. Hamartin's membrane bound protein

and two coiled-coil domains are necessary for its association with tuberin (van Slegtenhorst et al., 1997 and van Slegtenhorst et al., 1998).
Although *TSC1*- or *TSC2*-specific functions are possible, it seems that the predominant biochemical activity of these proteins is exerted by an equimolar complex, which regulates the state of GTP-loading of the rheb GTPase, and thereby regulates mTOR activation in the cell. As most hamartomas in TSC develop through a two-hit inactivation mechanisms (Knudson's hypothesis for tumor suppressor genes, including *TSC1* and *TSC2*), it appears likely that somatic mutations in *TSC1* are less common than those in *TSC2*, just as the rate of germline mutation in *TSC1* is much lower than that in *TSC2*. Thus, fewer and/or less severe clinical manifestations would be seen in *TSC1* patients.
LOH is very common within TSC hamartomas, except for cardiac or brain. In both organs, study says that wildtype hamartin and tuberin are present. LOH is an event by which within the affected cells, the genomic DNA loss its heterozygosity, becoming homozygous for the mutation. In other cells (unaffected cells) the genomic DNA shows heterozygous for the mutation. To analyze the occurrence of LOH it is necessary to perform mutation analysis on the genomic DNA extracted from the affected cells as well as from the unaffected cells.
After the discovery of *TSC1* and *TSC2* and their encoded proteins, several downstream protein cascades that might be affected by the pathogenesis of the disease, such as the pathway of mTOR (mammalian target of rapamycin), were identified.

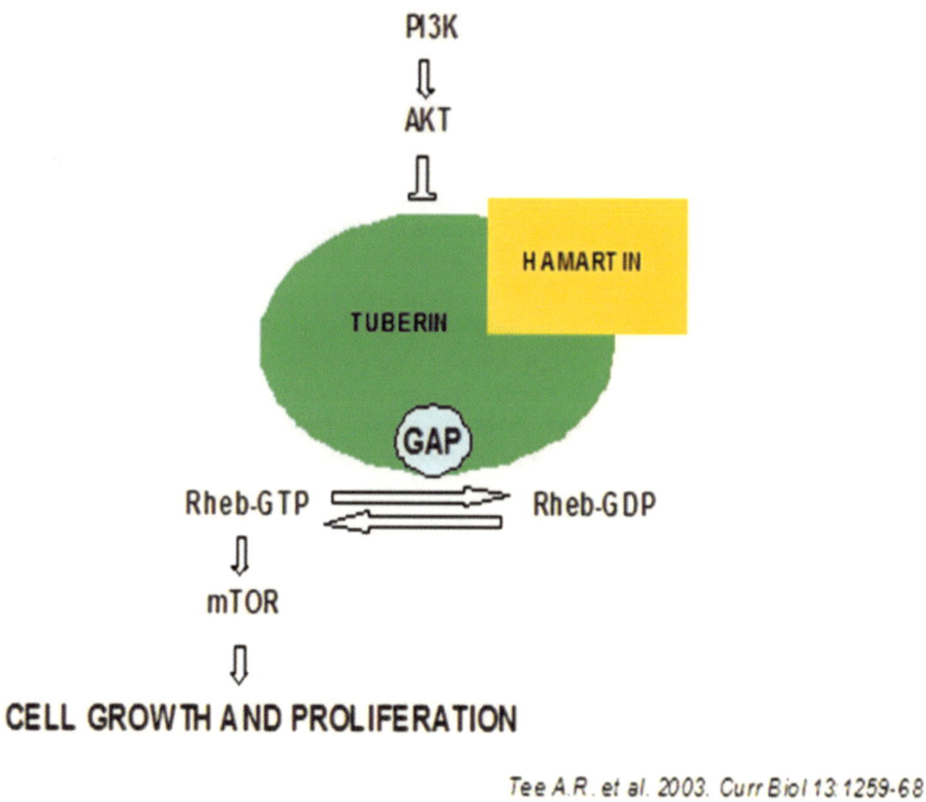

Fig. 1. Hamartin and tuberin as tumor suppressor gene.

Figure 1 illustrated the roles of hamartin and tuberin in cell metabolism describing that disruption in either of both genes may result in loss of the control of cell growth and proliferation. Hamartin-tuberin complex inhibits the mTOR which is a key regulator in the signalling pathway of cell proliferation and organ size (Kwiatkowski, 2008). It has been reported that the complex regulates mTOR via hydrolysis of Rheb-GTP into its inactive GDP bound state, Rheb-GDP (Rosner et al., 2004 and Tee et al., 2003).

Tuberin and hamartin form an intracellular complex which activates GTPase, reducing stimulation of mTOR. mTOR detects signals of nutrient availability, hypoxia, or growth factor stimulation, and is part of many cell processes, such as cell-cycle progression, transcription and translation control, and nutrient uptake. It phosphorylates, among other proteins, S6K1 and eukaryotic translation initiation factor 4E-BP1. S6K1 is a kinase that activates ribosomal subunit protein S6, leading to ribosome recruitment and protein translation. 4E-BP1 inhibits activity of eukaryotic translation initiation factor 4E (eIF4E) and, when phosphorylated by mTOR, releases eIF4E from its control.

The complex inhibits mTOR by acting as a GAP toward Rheb, which promotes hydrolysis of Rheb-GTP, converting it to an inactive GDP bound state. Without its active GTP bound state, Rheb cannot stimulate mTOR-mediated signalling to downstream components S6K1 and 4E-BP1. The mechanism is reversed with the presence of amino acids which activates Rheb-GEF. RhebGEF converts Rheb-GDP to its active Rheb-GTP and promotes mTOR signalling. Akt inactivates TSC tumor suppressor complex by phosphorylation of *TSC2* (Tee et al., 2003).

Common *TSC2* mutations result in the loss of the GAP domain of tuberin through C-terminal truncations, whereas some point mutations are clustered within the GAP domain. It is also reported that, an intact GAP domain of tuberin is crucial for association with hamartin in the formation of tuberin-hamartin heterodimers. The heterodimers will inhibit Rheb-induced mTOR signalling and can also function as a GAP toward Rheb. Higher proportion of the active GTP bound form of Rheb can likely be found within TSC patients. It is the result of non-functional tuberin-hamartin heterodimers where the genes failed to encodes for a functional protein (van Slegtenhorst et al., 1998).

The 200kDa (1806 amino acids) tuberin is homologous to the GTPase activating proteins (GAP) rap1GAP and mSpa1 where it contains relatively hydrophobic N-terminal domain and conserved 163 amino acids region close to the C-terminus. Rap1GAP is the member of Ras-related protein and functions in regulation of DNA synthesis and cell-cycle transition. The GAP activity of functional tuberin can regulate the effects of Rap1 on G to S phase transition during cell division. Thus, it implies that *TSC2* mutations may result in constitutive activation of Rap1 (Wienecke et al., 1996 and Wienecke et al., 1997).

Tuberin also has been demonstrated to interact with rab5. Rab5 is a cytosolic protein, is an effector for the endosomal small GTPase and therefore involved in endocytic fusion events (Stenmark et all., 1995). Consistently with the finding, tuberin has also been shown to act as a GTPase activating protein for rab5 and reduce the fluid-phase endocytosis (Xiao et al., 1997).

As for 130 kDa (1164 amino acids) hamartin, it has hydrophilic protein with no significant homology to tuberin or other known vertebrate protein. Van Slegtenhorst and colleagues have investigated the association between endogenous hamartin and tuberin and they found out that both proteins play a closely related role (van Slegtenhorst et al., 1998). The methods used in the study suggest that inactivation of hamartin and tuberin may prevent the formation of a functional protein complex.

Hamartin was recently identified as an interactor with the cytoskeletal proteins, ERM family (Lamb et al., 2000). The function loss can alternatively compromise neural migration via interaction with ERM or actin binding proteins. It was also shown to activate the GTPase Rho and regulates focal adhesion and stress fiber formation. Hamartin activates the GTPase Rho via the overlapping region of Rhos's amino acid and hamartin's tuberin-interaction domain (Lamb et al., 2000). The dysregulation of signalling by the Rho family of GTPase is said to have a critical role in cancer cell migration, invasion, and metastasis (Clark et al., 2000; Evers et al., 2000; Royal et al., 2000 and Schmitz et al., 2000).

It has also been recently shown that the functional complex interact with G2/M cyclin-dependant kinase 1 and its regulatory cyclins. Thus, mutation in either both genes may alter the kinetics of cell divisions (Catania et al., 2001). The functional heteromeric complex of hamartin and tuberin also plays important role in modulating the pathways of insulin receptor-or insulin-like growth factor-mediated signalling. The pathway functions downstream of the cell signalling molecule Akt, also play roles in regulating cell growth and potentially cell size.

7. Studies on therapeutics options for TSC

At present, the management of TSC is symptomatic. Some of TSC manifestations have been subjected to drug therapies but they are still in the developmental stage (Yates et al., 2006). Table 5 summarized several drugs under investigation for their efficacy towards Tuberous Sclerosis Complex.

The discovery of mTOR (mammalian target of rapamycin) pathway upregulation in tuberous-sclerosis-associated tumours presents new possibilities for treatment strategies. A TSC mouse treated with rapamycin, also known as sirolimus, was found to have its learning and memory deficits improved (Ehninger et al., 2008).

Sirolimus is a macrolide antibiotic that acts as an mTOR kinase inhibitor. It is isolated from *Streptomyces hygroscopicus*. Sirolimus and its analogs have been shown to make the dysregulated mTOR pathway return to normal in cells that lack *TSC1* or *TSC2*. Several results from in-vitro or in-vivo animal studies suggest that sirolimus or its analogues might be effective in the treatment of various manifestations of tuberous sclerosis such as skin lesions (Rauktys et al., 2008), lymphangioleiomyomatosis (Goncharova et al., 2006 and Bissler et al., 2008), renal angiomyolipomas (Lee et al., 2006; Herry et al., 2007 and Wienecke et al., 2006), renal-cell carcinoma (Robb et al., 2007), subependymal giant-cell astrocytomas (Franz et al., 2006) or even polycystic kidney disease (Weimbs et al., 2006).

However, angiomyolipomas increased in volume after the therapy was discontinued, and some patients taking sirolimus experienced serious adverse events (Bissler et al., 2008; Herry et al., 2007 and Wienecke et al., 2006).

Recently, other classes of drugs have also been found to be possible therapeutic options for TSC. Interferon gamma and interferon alpha interact with mTOR, leading to deactivation of the translational repressor 4E-BP1, which could be beneficial for the treatment of tuberous sclerosis (Kaur et al., 2007). Other classes of drugs ranging from those which can alter amino acids metabolism, inhibit VEGF signalling and inhibit microtubules were also studied. Presence or absence of amino acids is an important regulator of mTOR pathway signalling (Avruch et al., 2006).

For example, L-asparaginase, a hydrolase enzyme and one of the most important agents used in multidrug chemotherapy for the treatment of cancer. It is mainly used to treat human leukemic cells in acute lymphoblastic leukemic. L-asparaginase has been found to

Drug	Mechanism of action	Treatment	Adverse effects	Studies
Sirolimus/ Everolimus	Bind to cytosolic protein FK-binding protein 12 (FKBP12) and inhibits mTOR pathway by directly binding to mTOR complex 1	-Specifically subependymal giant cell astrocytomas in a dults and angiomyolipomas in children	Increase risk of nephrotoxicity and opportunistic infections	Rauktys et al., 2007; Lee et al., 2006; Lee et al., 2007; Kenerson et al., 2005; Smowleski et al., 2005; Woodrum et al., 2010; Messina et al., 2007
Interferon gamma/ Interferon alpha	Deactivate translational repressor 4E-BP1 and inhibits mTOR pathway	-Mostly patient with angiomyolypomas	Immunosupression, particularly through netropenia and certain ifections	Lee et al., 2006; Lee et al., 2007; Kenerson et al., 2005
L-Asparaginase/ Asparaginase	and 4E-BP1	-Mainly lymphoma (Hodgkin lymphoma and acute lymphoblastic leukemia) -Possible treatment for TSC	Can cause allergic and hypersensitivity, possible anaphylaxis	Iiboshi et al., 1999; Woodrum et al., 2010
Sorafenib in combination with rapamycin	Block VEGF-R	Advance renal cell and hepatocellular carcinoma	Possible skin-rash, hand-foot skin reactions, diarrhea and hypertension	Brugarolas et al., 2003; Lee et al., 2009
Sunitinib	Targets VEGF-R and platelet derived growth factor receptor (PDGF-R)	-Metastatic renal cell carcinoma (Motzer et al., 2007) gastrointestinal stromal tumors -Possible treatment for TSC	Generally well-tolerated, manageable and low incidence. Possible fatigue, diarrhea, nausea, hypertension and stomatitis	Motzer et al., 2007; Demetri et al., 2006 ; Woodrum et al., 2010
Bevacizumab	Can binds to all VEGF isoforms and produce inhibitory effects	-Colon, breast, normal lung cancer and glioblastoma -Possible treatment for TSC	Possible coronary artery disease, peripheral artery disease and hypertension	Yang et al., 2003; Wang et al., 2004; Woodrum et al., 2010

Table 5. Potential drugs under investigations for the therapy of TSC.

reduce the levels of mTOR pathway's target p70 S6 kinase and 4EBP-1 (Iiboshi et al., 1999). The reduction indicates that L-Asparaginase can be a possible therapeutic option for TSC.
VEGF is thought to play important role in the pathogenesis of TSC since tumors associated with TSC are vascular. *TSC2* has also been found to have association with increased levels of VEGF in cultured cells (Brogarolas et al., 2002). Since VEGF signalling is important in the TSC pathogenensis, combination of VEGF inhibitors with mTOR inhibitor analogs may provide a promising treatment.
Sorafenib is one of VEGF inhibitors. It is an oral targeted kinase inhibitor that blocks VEGF-R. In TSC tumor preclinical study by Lee and colleagues, combination of Sorafenib and Sirolimus was found more effective than single agent (Lee et al., 2009). Other VEGF inhibitor is Sunitinib which also inhibit platelet derived VEGF-R. It is a receptor tyrosine kinase inhibitor. Bevacizumab, a recombinant humanised monoclonal antibody, is also a VEGF-R inhibitor. Both Sunitinib and Bevacizumab produce inhibitory effects to VEGF-R signalling pathway and may be useful for TSC treatment.

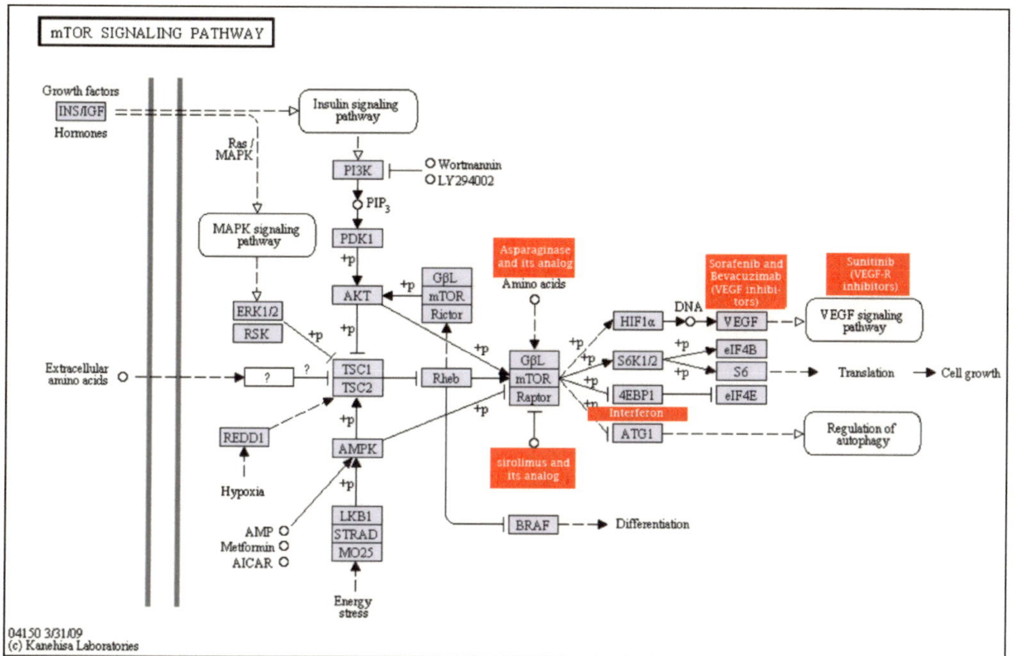

Fig. 2. Interaction of possible therapeutic options with various pathways in TSC pathogenesis (http://www.genome.jp/dbget-bin/www_bget?map04150).

8. Abbreviations

4E-BP1	: 4E Binding Protein 1
ACTH	: adrenocorticotrophic hormone
AML	: angiomyolipoma
DNA	: deoxyribonucleidc acid
EEG	: Electroencephalography
ERM	: Exin-radixin-moesin

GABA	: gamma-aminobutyric acid
kb	: kilobase pair
LOH	: Loss of Heterozygosity
LOVD	: Leiden Open Variation Database
MRI	: Magnetic Resonance Imaging
mRNA	: messenger ribonucleic acid
mTOR	: mammalian target of rapamycin
Rheb	: Ras homologue enriched in brain
TSC	: Tuberous Sclerosis Complex
TSC1	: Tuberous Sclerosis Complex gene 1
TSC2	: Tuberous Sclerosis Complex 2
VEGF	: vascular endothelial growth factor
VEGF-R	: vascular endothelial growth factor receptor

9. References

Aicardi, J., Mumford, J.P., Dumas, C. and Wood, S. (1996). Vigabatrin as initial therapy for infantile spasms: a European Retrospective Survey, *Epilepsia*, 37(7):638-42.

Avruch, J., Hara, k., Lin, Y., Liu, M., Long, X., Ortiz-Vega, S. & Yonezawa, K. (2006). Insulin and amino-acid regulation of mTOR signalling and kinase activity through the Rheb GTPase, *Oncogene*. 25:6361-72.

Bissler, J.J., McCormack, F.X., Young, L.R., Elwing, JM., Chuck, G., Leonard, J.M., Schmithorst, V.J., Laor, T., Brody, A.S., Bean, J., Salisbury, S. & Franz, D.N. (2008). Sirolimus for angiomyolipoma in tuberous sclerosis complex or lymphangiomeiomyomatosis, *N Engl J Med*. 358(2):140-51.

Brugarolas, J.B., Vazquez, F., Reddy, A., Sellers, W.R. & Kaelin, W.G.Jr. (2003). *TSC2* regulates VEGF through mTOR-dependent and –independent pathways, *Cancer Cell*. 4(2):147-58.

Catania MG, Mischel PS and Vinters HV. (2001). Hamartina and tuberin interaction with the G2/M cyclin-independent kinase CDK1 and its regulatory cyclins A and B, *J Neuropathol Exp Neurol*. 60(7):711-23.

Catania, M.G., Johnson, M.W., Liau, L.M., Kremen, T.J., deVillis, J.S. & Vinters, H.V. (2001). Hamartin expression and interaction woth tuberin in tumour cell lines and primary cultures, *J Neurosci Res*. 63:276-83.

Cheadle, J.P., Reeve, M.P., Sampson, J.R. & Kwiatkowski, D.J. (2000). Molecular genetics advances in tuberous sclerosis, *Hum Gen*. 107(2):97-114.

Christophea, C., SeAkhrab, T., Rypensc, F., Ziereisena, F., Chrisriaensb, F., & Dan, B. (2000). MRI spectrum of cortical malformations in tuberous sclerosis complex, *Brain & Development* 22. 487±493, 18.

Christophea, C., Sekhara, T. & Rypens, F. (2000). MRI spectrum of cortical malformations in tuberous sclerosis complex, *Brain Dev*. 22:487 -493.

Clark, G.J., Kinch, M.S., Rogers-Graham, K., Sebti, S.M., Hamilton, A.D. & Der, C.J. (1997). The RAs-related protein Rheb is farnesylated and antagonizes Ras signalling and transformation, *J Biol Chem*. 272:10608-10715.

Crino, P.B. & Henske, E.P. (1999). New developments in the neurobiology of the tuberous sclerosis complex, *Neurology*. 53(7):1384-90.

Crino, P.B. (2004). Molecular pathogenesis of tuber formation in tuberous sclerosis complex, *J Child Journal*. 4:105(3):357-68.

Curatolo, P. (1996). Neurological manifestation of tuberous sclerosis complex, *Childs Nerv Syst.* 12: 515 - 521

Curatolo, P. (2001). Infantile spasms in tuberous sclerosis complex, *Brain Dev.* 173:502-507

Curatolo, P. (2001). Vigabatrin for tuberous sclerosis complex, *Brain dev.* 23:649-653

Dabora, S.L., Jozwiak, S. &Franz, D.N. (2001). Mutational analysis in a cohort of 224 tuberous sclerosis patients indicates increased severity of *TSC2*, compared with TSC1, disease in multiple organs, *Am J Hum Genet.* 68: 64–80.

Demetri, G.D., van Oosterom, A.T., Garrett, C.R., Blackstein, M.E., Shah, M.H., Verweij, J., McArthur, G., Judson, I.R., Heinrich, M.C., Morgan, J.A., Desai, J., Fletcher, C.D., George, S., Bello, C.L., Huang, X., Baum, C.M. & Casali, P.G. (2006). Efficacy and safety of sunitinib in oatients with advanced gastrointestinal stromal toumour after failure of imatinib: a randomised controlled trial, *Lancet.* 368(9544):1329-38.

Ehninger, D., Han, S., Shilyansky, C., Zhou, Y., Li, W., Kwiatkowski, D.J., Ramesh, V. & Silva, A.J. (2008). Reversal of learing deficits in a *TSC2+/-* mouse model of tuberous sclerosis, *Nat Med.* 14(8):843-8.

European Chromosome 16 Tuberous Sclerosis Consortium. (1993). Identification and characterization of the tuberous sclerosis gene on chromosome 16, *Cell* 75: 1305–15.

Evers, E.E., Zondag, G.C., Malliri, A., Price, L.S., ten Klooster, J.P., van der Kemmen, R.A. & Collard, J.G. (2000). Rho family proteins in cell adhesion and cell migration, *Eur J Cancer.* 36(10):1269-74.

Fokkema, I.F.A.C., Den Dunnen, J.T. & Taschner, P.E.M. (2005). LOVD: easy creation of a locus-specific sequence variation database using an "LSDB-in-a-Box" approach, *Hum Mutat.* 2005 Aug;26(2):63-8.

Franz, D.N. (1998). Diagnosis and management of tuberous sclerosis complex, *Sem Pediatr Neurol.* 5:253-268

Franz, D.N., Leonard, J., Tudor, C., Chuck, G., Care, M., Sethuraman, G., Dinopoulos, A., Thomas, G. & Crone, K.R. (2006). Rapamycin causes regression of astrocytomas in tuberous sclerosis complex, *Ann Neurol.* 59:490-498.

Fryer, A.E., Chalmers, A. & Connor, J.M. (1987). Evidence that the gene for tuberous sclerosis is on chromosome 9, *Lancet 1*: 659–61.

Fukushima, K., Inoue, Y. & Fujiwara, T. (2001). Long term follow up study on Wst syndrome associated with tuberous sclerosis, *Brain Dev* 23:698-704.

Goncharova, E.A., Goncharova, D.A., Spaits, M., Noonan, D.J., Talovskava, E., Esterhas, A. & Krymskava, V.P. (2006). Abnormal growth of smooth muscle-like cells in lymphangioleiomyomatosis: Role for tumor suppressor TSC, *Am J Respir Cell Mol Biol,* 34(5):561-72.

Hancock, E., Tomkins, S., Sampson, J. & Osborne, J. (1999). Lymphangioleiomyotosis and tuberous sclerosis (original research articles), *Respiratory medicine,* volume 96, issue 1, January 1999, 7-13.

Herry, I., Neukirch, C., Debray, M.P., Mignon, F. & Crestani, B. (2007). Dramatic effect of sirolimus on renal angiomyolipomas in a patient with tuberous sclerosis complex, *Eur J Intern Med,* 18:76-77.

Hymann, M. & Whittemore, V. (1996). Tuberous Sclerosis Complex: A Review: Diagnosis, *Clinical Genetics* ;150:36-40.

Iiboshi, Y., Papst, P.J., Hunger, S.P. & Terada, N. (1999). L-asparaginase inhibits the rapamycin-targeted signalling pathway, *Biochem Biophys Res Commun,* 260(2):534-9.

Inoue, Y., Nemoto, Y., Murata, R., Tashiro, T., Shakudo, M., Kohne, K. & et al. (1998). CT and MR imaging of Cerebral Tuberous Sclerosis, *Brain & Development,* 209–221 (3).

Jambaque, I., Cusmai, R. & Curatolo, P. (1991). Neuropsychological aspects of tuberous sclerosis in relation to epilepsy and MRI findings, *Dev Med Child Neurol* 33:398 -705.

Jiang, X. & Yeung, R.S. (2006). Regulation of microtubule-dependant protein transport by the *TSC2*/mammalian target of rapamycin pathway, *Cancer Res,* 66(10):5258-69.

Kandt, R.S., Haines, J.L. & Smith, M. (1992). Linkage of an important gene locus for tuberous sclerosis to a chromosome 16 marker for polycystic kidney disease, *Nat Genet* 2: 37–41.

Kanehisa Laboratory, pathway map04150, mTOR signalling pathway[Online]. [Accessed on 8th March 2011]. Available from GenomeNet: http://www.genome.jp/dbget-bin/www_bget?map04150

Kaur, S., Lal, L., Sassano, A., Majchrzak-Kita, B., Srikanth, M., Baker, D.P., Petroulakis, E., Hay, N., Sonenberg, .N, Fish, E.N. & Platanias, L.C. (2007). Regulatory effects of mammalian target of rapamycin-activated pathways in type I and type II interferon signalling, *J Biol Chem,* 282(3):1757-68.

Kenerson, H., Dundon, T.A. & Yeung, R.S. (2005). Effects of rapamycin in the Eker rat model of tuberous sclerosis complex, *Pediatr Res,* 57:67-75.

Kenerson, H.L., Aicher, L.D. & True L. (2002). Activated mammalian target of rapamycin pathway in the pathogenesis of tuberous sclerosis complex renal tumours, *Cancer Res,* 62:5645-5650.

Kwiatkowski, D.J. (2003). Tuberous sclerosis: from tubers to mTOR, *Ann Hum Genet* ;67:87–96

Kwiatkowski, D.J. (2005). *TSC1, TSC2,* TSC3? Or mosaicism, *Eur J Hum Genet,* 13(6):695-6.

Lamb, R.F., Roy, C. & Diefenbach, T.J. (2000). The *TSC1* tumour suppressor hamartin regulates cell adhesion through ERM proteins and the GTPase Rho, *Nat Cell Biol,* 2:281-287.

Lee, L., Sudentas, P. & Dabora, S.L. (2006). Combination of a rapamycin analog (CCI-779) and interferon-gamma is more effective than single agents in treating a mouse model of tuberous sclerosis complex, *Gene Chromosome Cancer,* 45:933-944.

Lee, L., Sudentas, P., Donohue, B., Asrican, K., Worku, A., Walker, V., Sun, Y., Schmidt, K., Albert, M.S., El-Hashemite, N., Lader, A.S., Onda, H., Zhang, H., Kwiatkowski, D.J. & Dabora, S.L. (2005). Efficacy of rapamycin analog (CCI-779) and IFN-gamma in tuberous sclerosis mouse models, *Genes Chromosomes Cancer,* 42:213-227.

Lee, N., Woodrum, C., Nobil, A., Rauktys, A., Messina, M.P. & Dabora, S.L. (2009). Rapamycin weekly maintenance dosing and the potential efficacy of combination sorafenib plus rapamycin but not atorvastatin or deoxyxycline in tuberous sclerosis preclinical models, *BMC Pharmacol,* 9:8.

McManus, E.J. & Alessi, D.R. (2002). A complex tale of PKB mediated S6K regulation, *Nat Cell Biol,* 4:E214-E216.

Mennel, S., Meyer, C.H., Peter, S., Schmidt, J.C. & Kroll, P. (2007). Current treatment modalities for exudative retinal hamartomas secondary to tuberous sclerosis: Review of the literature, *Acta Opthalmol Scand;* 85(2):127-32

Messina, M.P., Rauktys, A., Lee, L. & Dabora, S.L. (2007). Tuberous sclerosis preclinical studies: timing of treatment, combination of a rapamycin analog (CCI-779) and interferon-gamma, and comparison of rapamycin to CC1-779, *BMC Pharmacol,* 7:14.

Motzer, R.J., Hutson, T.E., Tomczak, P., Michaelson, M.D., Bukowski, R.M., Rixe, O., Oudard, S., Negrier, S., Szczylik, C., Kim, ST., Chen, I., Bycott, P.W., Baum, C.M. & Figlin, R.A. (2007). Sunitinib versus interferon alfa in metastatic renal cell carcinoma, *N Engl J Med,* 356(2):154-24.

O'Callaghan, F. (2000). Tuberous sclerosis complex, *Paedeatrics and Child Health,* 18:1.

Osborne, J.P., Fryer, A. & Webb, D. (1991). Epidemiology of tuberous sclerosis, *Ann N Y.Acad Science* ;615:125-7

Potter, C.J., Huang, H. & Xu, T. (2001). Drosophila *TSC1* functions with TSC2 to antagonize insulin signalling in regulating cell growth, cell proliferation and organ size, *Cell,* 4:105(3):357-68.

Provenzale, J. & DeLuca S.A. (1991). Tuberous Sclerosis, *Am Fam Physician* 43:470-2.

Rauktys, A., Lee, N., Lee, L. & Dabora, S.L. (2008). Topical rapamycin inhibits sclerosis tumor growth in a nude mouse model, *BMC Dermatology,* 8:1 doi:10.1186/1471-5945-8-1.

Roach, E.S., Gomez, M.R. & Northrup, H. (1998). Tuberous sclerosis complex consensus conference: revised clinical diagnostic criteria, *J Child Neurol* 13: 624–28.

Rosner, M., Freilinger, A. & Hengstschlager, M. (2004). Proteins interacting with tuberous sclerosis gene products, *Amino Acids,* 27(2):119-28.

Royal, I., Lamarche-Vane, N., Lamorte, L., Kaibuchi, K. & Park, M. (2000). Activation of cdc42, rac, PAK, and rho-kinase in response to hepatocyte growth factor differentially regulates epithelial cell colony spreading and dissociation, *Mol Biol Cell,* 11(5):1709-25.

Schmitz, A.A., Govek, E.E., Bottner, B. & Aelst, L. (2000). Rho GTPases: signalling , migration and invasion, *Exp Cell Res,* 261(1):1-12.

Schwartz, R.A., Fernandez, G., Kotulska, K. & Jozwiak, S. (2007). Tuberous Sclerosis Complex. Advances in diagnosis, genetics and managements (Review articles), *Journal of the American Academy of Dermatology,* volume 57, Issue 2, 189-202.

Smolewski, P. (2006). Recent developments in targeting the mammalian target of rapamycin (mTOR) kinase pathway, *Anticancer Drugs,* 17:487-494.

Stenmark, H,. Vitale, G,. Ullrich, P. & Zerial, M. (1995). Rabaptin-5 is a direct effector of the small GTPase Rab5 in endocytic membrane fusion, *Cell,* 83(3):423-32.

Tapon, N., Ito, N., Dickson, J.B., Treisman, J.E. & Hariharan, I.K. (2001). The drosophila tuberous sclerosis complex gene homologs restrict cell growth and cell proliferation, *Cell,* 105(3):345-55.

Tee, A.R., Anjum, R. & Blenis, J. (2003). Inactivation of the tuberous sclerosis complex-1 and -2 gene products occurs by phosphoinositide s-kinase/Akt-dependent and -independent phosphorylation of tuberin, *J Biol Chem,* 278(39):37288-96.

Tee, A.R., Fingar, D.C., Manning, B.D., Kwiatkowski, D.J., Cantley, L.C. & Blenis, J. (2002). Tuberous sclerosis complex-1 and -2 gene products function together toi inhibit mammalian target of rapamycin (mTOR)-mediated downstream signalling, *Proc Natl Acad Sci USA 99,* 13572-13576.

Tee, A.R., Manning, B.D., Roux, P.P., Cantley, L.C. & Blenis, J. (2003). Tuberous sclerosis gene products, *Amino Acids* 27:119-128.

Tee, A.R., Manning, B.D., Roux, P.P., Cently, L.C. & Blenis, J. (2003). Tuberous sclerosis compelx gene products, Tuberin and Hamartin, control mTOR signalling by acting as GTPase activating protein complex toward Rheb, *Curr Biol,* 13(15):1259-68.

van Slegtenhorst, M., de Hoogt, R. & Herman, C. (1997). Identification of the tuberous sclerosis gene *TSC1* on chromosome 9q34, *Science,* 277:805-808.

van Slegtenhorst, M., de Hoogt, R., Hermans, C., Nellist, M., Janssen, B., Verhoef, S., Lindhout, D., van den Ouweland, A., Halley, D., Young, J., Burley, M., Jeremiah, S., Woodward, K., Nahmias, J., Fox, M., Ekong, R., Osborne, J., Wolfe, J., Povey, S., Snell, R.G., Cheadle, J.P., Jones, A.C., Tachataki, M., Ravine, D., Sampson, J.R., Reeve, M.P., Richardson, P., Wilmer, F., Munro, C., Hawkins, T.L., Sepp, T., Ali,

J.B., Ward, S., Green, A.J., Yates, J.R., Kwiatkowska, J., Henske, E.P., Short, M.P., Haines, J.H., Jozwiak, S. & Kwiatkowski, D.J. (1997). Identification of the tuberous sclerosis gene, *TSC1* on chromosome 9q34, *Science,* 277(5327):805-8.

van Slegtenhorst, M., Nellist, M., Nagelkerken, B., Cheadle, J., Snell, R., van den Ouwland, A., Reuser, A., Sampson, J., Halley, D. & van der Sluijs. (1998). Interaction between hamartin and tuberin, the *TSC1* and *TSC2* gene products, *Hum Mol Genet,* 7(6):1053-7.

Wang, Y., Fei, D., Vanderlaan, M. & Song, A. (2004). Biological activity of bevazimucab, a humanized anti-VEGF antibpdy in vitro, *Angiogenesis,* 7(4):335-45.

Weimbs, T. (2006). Regulation of mTOR by polycystin-1: is polycystic kidney disease a case of futile repair?, *Cell cycle,* 5(21):2425-9.

Wienecke, R., Fackler, I., Linsenmaier, U., Mayer, K., Licht, T. & Kretzler, M. (2006). Antitumoral activity of rapamycin in renal angiolyolipoma associated with tuberous sclerosis complex, *Am J Kidney Dis,* 48:e27-9.

Wienecke, R., Maize, J.C.Jr., Reed, J.A., de Gunzburg, J., Yeung, R.S. & DeClue, J.E. (1997). Expression of the *TSC2* product tuberin and its target Rap1 in normal human tissues, *Am J Pathol,* 150(1):43-50.

Wienecke, R., Maize, J.C.Jr., Shoarinejad, F., Vass, W.C., Reed, J., Bonafacino, J.S., Resau, J.H., de Gunzburg, J., Yeung, R.S. & DeClue, J.E. (1996). Co-localization of the *TSC2* product tuberin with its target Rap1 in the golgi apparatus, *Oncogene,* 13(5):913-23.

Woodrum, C., Nobil, A. & Dabora SL. (2010). Comparison of three rapamycin dosing schedules in A/J *Tsc2+/-* mice and improved survival with angiogenesis inhibitor or asparaginase treatment in mice with subcutaneous tuberous sclerosis related tumors, *Journal of Translational Medicine,* 8:14.

Xiao, G.H., Shoarinejad, F., Jin, F., Golemis, E.A. & Yeung, R.S. (1997). The tuberous sclerosis 2 gene product, tuberin, function as a Rab5 GTPase activating protein (GAP) in modulating endocytosis, *J Biol Chem,* 272(10):6097-100.

Xu, L., Sterner, C., Maheshwar, M.M., Wilson, P.J., Nellist, M., Short, P.M., Haines, J.L., Sampson, J.R. & Ramesh, V. (1995). Alternative splicing of the tuberous sclerosis 2 (*TSC2*) gene in human and mouse tissues, *Genomics* 27:475–480

Xu, L., Sterner, C., Maheshwar, M.M., Wilson, P.J., Nellist, M., Short, P.M., Haines, J.L., Sampson, J.R. & Ramesh, V. (1995) New insights into the role of the tuberous sclerosis genes in leukemia. Leukemia Research 33 (2009) 883–885. Alternative splicing of the tuberous sclerosis 2 (*TSC2*) gene in human and mouse tissues, *Genomics* 27:475–480

Yang, J.C., Haworth, L., Sherry, R.M., Hwu, P., Schwartzentruber, D.J., Topalian, S.L., Steinberg, S.M., Chen, H.X. & Rosenberg, S.A. (2003). A randomized trial of bevacizumab, an anti-vascular endothelial growth factor antibody, for metastatic renal cancer, *N Engl J Med,* 349(5):427-34.

Yates, J.R. (2006). Tuberous sclerosis, *Eur J Hum Genet,* 14(10):1065-73.

Young, J. & Povey, S. (1998). The genetic basis of tuberous sclerosis, *Mol. Med.* 313–319.

Young, L.R., Inoe, Y. & McCormack, F.X. (2008). Diagnostic potential of serum VEGF-D for lymphangioleiomyomatosis, *N Engl J Med,* 358(2):199-200.

Zheng, L.H., Rensing, N.R., Zhang, B., Gutmann, D.H., Gambello, M.J. & Wong, M. (2010). *TSC2* gene inactivation in a mouse model of Tuberous Sclerosis Complex, *Hum Mol Genet; Nov 9 [Epub ahead of print]*,20(3):445-54.

3

Daytime Sleepiness and Changes of Sleep in Patients with Epilepsy

Katarína Klobučníková and Branislav Kollár
I st Department of Neurology University Hospital of Medical Faculty, Comenius University,Bratislava, Slovak Republic

1. Introduction

It is well known, that patients with epilepsy suffer from excessive daytime sleepiness, fatigue and insufficient sleep. These problems are often overlooked or referred to epileptic seizures or antiepileptic drugs. It should be noticed, that patients with epilepsy suffer from sleep disorders more often than general population (Bazil 2003). Health outcome of patients with comorbidity of epilepsy and sleep disorders is worse as sleep disorders may aggravate epilepsy. Changes in amount and severity of epileptic seizures may lead to pharmacoresistency of epilepsy in patients with untreated sleep disorders. That is the reason why attention to quality of sleep and daytime vigility in patients with epilepsy should be payed. The cooperation of neurologist, pneumologist, somnologist and psychologist is very important in correct management of patients with epilepsy and sleep disorders.

Daytime sleepiness is defined as the inability to stay awake during waking episodes of the day. It results in unintended lapses into drowsiness or sleep. Sleepiness occurs mainly in boring situations. Sometimes it is associated with increase of total amnount of sleep without feeling of restoration. In most cases excessive daytime sleepiness (EDS) is a chronic symptom and it must occur for at least three months prior to diagnosis (ICSD-2, 2005).

Excessive daytime sleepiness is often result of self-imposed sleep deprivation espetially in young people. More often it is effect of disturbed nocturnal sleep or misaligned circadian rhytms. It may be side effect of many often-used drugs, for example hypnotics or alcohol. Nocturnal sleep disturbances, which lead to EDS, should be carefully assessed and treated. In several conditions EDS is not an outcome of night-sleep loss and should be considered as primary hypersomnia of central origin. These hypersomnias according to ICSD-2 include narcolepsy with or without cataplexy, recurrent hypersomnia, idiopathic hypersomnia with or without long sleep time and hypersomnias due to different medical and neurological conditions. Narcolepsy with cataplexy is characretized with daytime sleepiness and unwanted episodes of sleep, which occur several times a day. The duration of episodes may vary from a few minutes to more than an hour, patients wake up refreshed. Cataplexy is paroxyzmal, abrupt and reversible loss of muscule tone often elicited with emotional experience. Manifestations of disociated REM sleep (sleep paralysis and hypnagogic halucinations) are also exposed (Chokverty, 1994). Narcolepsy without cataplexy is associated with snoozing in daytime, sleep paralysis and hypnagogic hallucinations may occur. Secondary narcolepsy may be caused by tumors of brain or multiple sclerosis, if

hypothalamus is harmed. Recurrent hypersomnia, Kleine-Levin syndrome, is characterized by atacs of hypersomnia, which lasts for several days and occur several times per year. Episodes are accompanied by disturbances of behaviour (agression), bulimia and hypersexiality. Idiopathic hypersomnia with long sleep time is characterized by constant and sever EDS with unrefreshing naps of up to four hours and prolonged major sleep episode up to 10 - 14 hours. There are great difficulties with morning waking up and sleep drunkeness. Idiopathic hypersomnia without long sleep time, or essential hypersomnia is characterized with constant and sever EDS, which results in unintended naps of nonrefreshing nature. Cataplexa is absent. The major sleep episode is either normal, or slightly prolonged (to 10 hours). Post-wakening confusion of often reported.
Behaviorally induced insufficient sleep syndrome is another reason of EDS. A therapeutic trial of a longer sleep episode can reverse the symptoms. Hypersomnia has been described also in association with a large range of medical conditions, including head trauma, stroke, encephalitis, inflammatory conditions, tumors and neurodegenerative diseases as M.Parkinson (ICSD-2), (Overeem & Readings , 2010).

1.1 Diagnostic evaluation of sleepiness in patient with epilepsy

Obtaining an accurate 24-hour-sleep-wake history is extremly important. History should be focused also on relevant factors as medical history, compensation of epilepsy, type and frequency of epileptic seizures, their incidence according to circadian cycle and actual antiepileptic medication, or other drug and medication use. Also social, enviromental or psychological conditions, which may interfere with sleep quality, should be evaluated.
Neurological examination in connection with neuroimaging methods (MRI) can detect cerebral leasions as the reason of sleep problems. Standard EEG evaluation is recommended to detect abnormalities in EEG activity and interictal epileptic discharges. Epworth Scale of Sleepiness (ESS) is widely used questionnaire to quantify severity of daytine sleepiness. Score above 9 indicates elevated daytime sleepiness (Johns, 1991).
Multiple Sleep Latency Test (MSLT) can objectively evaluate daytime sleepiness. When used as diagnostic prosedure of central hypersomnia it should be done during the day after polysomnographically documented adequate night sleep, which lasts at least six hours and after two weeks of regular sleep. (Carscadon & Dement, 1982, American sleep disorders association, 1992) (ICSD-2, 2005). Evaluation of MSLT starts 1,5-3 hours after morning awakening and consists of 5, or at least 4 records of polysomnography, each lasting 20minutes (Littner et al., 2005). Latency of sleep and occurence and latency of REM sleep is in each record noted. A mean sleep latency below five minutes is generally considered as indicative of sleepiness, latency over ten minutes is generally considered indicative of normal alertness (American Sleep Disorders Association, 1992).

1.2 Correlation of sleep and epilepsy

Relationship of sleep and epilepsy is complex and reciprocal. Epilepsy may distrub sleep with night and also daytime epileptic seizures. On the other hand sleep modulates probabality of epileptic discharges and seizures in different sleep stages.
Specific types of epilepsy are bounded to specific part of sleep-wake cycle, as night sleep, awakening, or appear randomly during circadian rhytm. Typical night epilepsy is for example nocturnal frontal lobe epilepsy (Zucconi, 2007), juvenile myoclonical epilepsy is typically connected to awakening. Sleep deprivation elevates probabality of epileptic seizure (Bazil,

Malow & Sammaritano, 2002), what is widely used in EEG evaluation. Influence of antiepileptic medication on daytime vigility and quality of sleep is also important. Unrecognised primary sleep disorders, which cause fragmentation of sleep, may aggravate epilepsy and increase amount of epileptic seizures. Distinction of sleep-related epileptic seizures and non-epileptic paroxymal events in sleep is frequently problematic and requires careful diagnostic approach with video-polysomnography (Moráň, 2005).

Unrecognised sleep-related generalised epileptic seizures disturb sleep achritecture as they cause arousals. Generalized epileptic seizures reduce total sleep time and elongate latency to REM sleep. Amount of NREM1 and NREM2 stages may be extended (Foldvary-Schaefer, 2002). Partial epileptic seizures during sleep do not disrupt night sleep markedly, only in case of their secondary generalization (Dasheiff, 2003). Epileptic seizures during daytime influence night sleep too. They reduce REM sleep, what may be cause of fatigue in postparoxysmal period (Bazil, Castro & Walczak, 2000).

Antiepileptic therapy is considered to have influence on daytime vigility and quality of sleep. Barbiturates and benzodiazepines have sedative effect and cause daytime sleepiness (Bazil, 2003, Rang & Dale, 1991). Carbamazepine also induces daytime sleepiness, elongates slow-wave sleep and reduces REM sleep, mainly in the beginning of medication. Approximately after one month of medication these effects are not more noticeable (Placidi et al., 2000). Valproate according to literature elongates NREM1 and abbreviates NREM2 (Foldvary-Schaefer, 2009). It elevates number of arousals and elongates slow-wave sleep (Moráň, 2005). Put on weight may be unfavorable for patients with sleep apnoe syndrome (Moráň, 2003).

Primidone abbreviates latency of sleep and may improve quality of sleep. Phenytoin extends NREM1 and NREM2, shorten REM period and multiplies arousals. Gabapentin improves sleep stability and elongates slow-wave sleep as well as REM sleep (Foldvary-Schaefer, 2009). Lamotrigine reduces NREM3 and NREM4 and elongates REM sleep (Foldvary, 2002). As alerting drug should be dosed early in the day. Sleep latency may be shortened by topiramate (Foldvary-Schaefer, 2009). Levetiracetam consolidates sleep and does not modify vigilance (Cicolin, 2006). According to othe study (Cho, Kim & Motamendi, 2011) levetiracetam increase sleep efficiency without major effects on sleep structure. Antiepileptic drugs may be helpful in treatment of some sleep disorders. For example gabapentin, carbamazepine or lamotrigine have good effect on restles leg syndrome (Garcia-Borreguero et al, 2002).

1.3 Sleep disorders and epilepsy

Exact evidence about incidence of sleep disorders in patients with epilepsy is not available, but it is supposed, that the amount is higher in patients with epilepsy than in general population. For example patients with partial epilepsy have twice higher appearence of sleep disorders as in healthy group (39% vs 18%) (Bazil, 2003). According to this study higher presence of sleep disorders did not correlate with antiepileptic therapy.

According to Foldvary-Schaefer (2002) patients with epilepsy have problems with initialization of sleep and have worse quality of sleep. Meatiness of these problems, as well as wores control of epileptic seizures, was higher in group of patients with partial epilepsy.

Some literature indicates, that patients with epilepsy have also higher appearance of sleep related breathing disorders than general population. Sleep apnoe syndromes are present in 0,8 - 2,2% of general adult population (Marin et at., 1997), however 28-55% patients with epilepsy suffer for sleep related disorders (Foldvary, 2002).

Even 33% pacients with medically refractory epilepsy have sleep apnoe syndrome (Malow et al., 2000). Reason of higher appearance of sleep related breathing disorders in patients with epilepsy is not clear. It may be connected with higher weight of patients as effect of anticonvulsant therapy (Manni & Terzaghi, 2010), or changes of endocrine system (valproate). Sleep apnoe syndrome leads to fragmented macroarchitecture of sleep with repeated hypoxemia of brain in consequence of repeated apnoic episodes. This may cause higher frequency of epileptic seizures. It is important, that correct therapy of sleep apnoe syndrome (reduction of weight, indication of CPAP or BiPAP) may bring improvement of epilepsy (Foldvary, 2002).

Sleep disorders should be considered especially when patient with epilepsy indicates hypersomnia, but has low frequency of epileptic seizures, is treated with monotherapy of antiepileptic drug and has low blood levels of medication.

1.4 Management of patient with epilepsy and sleep disorders

Patient with epilepsy and EDS reguires accurate evaluation to detect reason of hypersomnia. Compensation of epilepsy should be examined. EEG during daytime and overnight-EEG should detect interictal or ictal discharges. This may cause microarousals and fragmentation of sleep with secondary hypersomnia. Adjusting of antiepileptic medication should reduce amount of epileptic seizures and improve sleep. It is recommended to avoid antiepileptic therapy with sedative effects (barbiturates, benzodiazepines) and useless combination of too many antiepileptic drugs.

Correct sleep hygiene and life-style with regular and sufficient night-sleep and optimal surroundings is also important (Bazil, 2003, Happe, 2003).

Hypersomnia in patients with epilepsy may be caused by sleep apnoe syndrome. This should be considered particulary in obese patients with morning headache and hypertension. Diagnosis is estimated by polysomnography. According to literature 1/3 patients with refractory epilepsy have obstructive sleep apnoe syndrome (Malow et al., 2000). Correct therapy of sleep related breathing disorders may improve quality of sleep. Antiepileptic therapy, which increase weight (valproate) should be avoided, as it may worsten sleep apnoe syndrome (Bazil et al., 2002).

Insomnia is another possible reason of daytime hypersomnia and fatigue of patients with epilepsy. It should be treated by behavioral and relaxation methods, improvement of sleep habits or by sedative drugs. If antiepileptic therapy is considered as reason of insomnia, then it should be taken only in morning.

2. Objectives

Targets of this study were:

- to determine daytime sleepiness in patients with epilepsy by Epworth scale of sleepiness and Multiple Sleep Latency Test and compare it with healthy controls
- to investigate sleep architecture of patients with epilepsy and compare changes with healthy controls
- to find out, if detected changes of sleep architecture correlate with some characteristics of epilepsy

3. Methodology

All patients underwent standard EEG evaluation with 21 canal EEG machine and distribution of electrodes according to system 10-20, duration of record was 20 minutes.

Noticed abnormalities were rated as regional or generalised, with continual of intermitent occurence. Appearance of epileptiform ictal or interictal discharges was noted.

3.1 Methods used to examine daytime sleepiness

In both groups (patients with epilepsy and healthy controls) we used a questionnaire Epworth Scale of Sleepiness (ESS) (Johns, 1991). By answering eight questions about probability of falling asleep in standard situations we came to the result, i.e. score of daytime sleepiness ranging from 0 to 24. Rate 0-9 is considered as normal value, above 9 as elevated daytime sleepiness and value above 16 is considered as remarkably elevated daytime sleepiness (Watanabe et al., 2003).

All patients with epilepsy were evaluated by Multiple Sleep Latency Test (MSLT) (Carscadon & Dement, 1982) in order to objectivise the daytime sleepiness. The latency of sleep was measured in five 20 minute polysomnographic registrations in this test. Between the registrations the patient should be awake (Usui et al., 2008). Mean latency of sleep and appearance of REM sleep was noticed. Mean latency of sleep shorter than 6 minutes was considered as indicative of elevated sleepiness (American sleep disorders association, 1992).

3.2 Methods used to register sleep architecture

Nocturnal polysomnografy was used in both groups to evaluate quality of sleep. We used program Brain Quick System 98 for polysomnography. Scoring of sleep stages was done with Sleep View Rembrandt Sleep Analysis Program.

Registration and scoring of sleep stages was done according to criteria of Manual of Standardized Terminology, Techniques and Scoring System for Sleep Stages of Human Subjects (Rechtschaffen & Kales, 1968). We used four electrodes (C3, C4, O1, O2, A1, A2) in EEG registration. When topographical localization of epileptiform discharges was needed, we used 19 EEG electrodes located according to international system 10-20. Standard localization of electrodes for electrooculogram and electromyogram m.mentalis was used.

The result of sleep analysis was hypnogram, amount of sleep stages (NREM S1, NREM S2, NREM S3+-S4, REM) in %, total sleep time in minutes and efficiency of sleep in %was marked.

For purpose of registration of different abnormal movement manifestations (epilepsy, REM behavior diseases etc.), a video was recorded simultaneously with polysomnography.

3.3 Characteristics of the group of patients with epilepsy

We examined 100 patients with epilepsy who were admitted to the I. Neurology Clinic of Comenius University Hospital in Bratislava for diagnostic or therapeutic reasons in the period from January 2004 to January 2009. The group consisted of 49 men and 51 women, with the average age of 34.68 ± 13.55 years. Patients of the age 9 - 61 were included. Average duration of illness was 9.31 ± 9.93 years, ranging from 0.5 to 47 years. Medical history of duration and type of epilepsy was taken. International classification of epileptic seizures (1981, 1989) and International classification of epilepsy (1989) was used.

According to this classification 50 patients had focal symptomatic epilepsy, 26 patients had focal cryptogenic epilepsy. Generalised symptomatic epilepsy was diagnosed by 15 pacients and 9 patients had generalised cryptogenic or idiopathic epilepsy (see Fig.1).

Etiology of epilepsy was evaluated. Idiopathic or cryptogenic epilepsy have 35% patients and symptomatic epilepsy have 65% of patients. Detailed analysis of reasons of epilepsy in group of symptomatic patients showed these factors:

- vascular (stoke) had 13 patients (20%)
- perinatal lesion of brain had 13 patients (20%)
- prenatal damage of brain had 10 patients (15,4%)
- injury and posttraumatic lesion had 6 patients (9,2%)
- tumors of brain had 8 patients (12,3%)
- multiple sclerosis and other demyelinization diseases of brain - 5 patients (7,7%)
- residual damage of brain after inflammatory disease - 5 patients (7,7%)
- arteriovenous malformation - 3 patients (4,6%)
- exotoxic encefalopathy - 2 patients (3%)

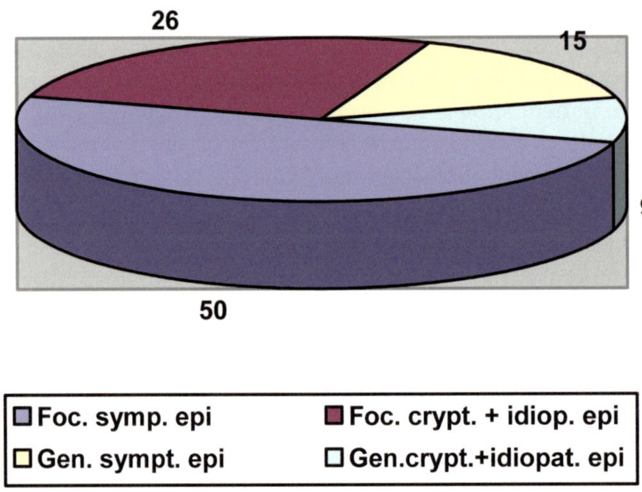

Fig. 1. Amount of patients according to type of epilepsy

Compensation of epilepsy was evaluated according to Diagnostic and therapeutic standard of epilepsy (Donáth, 1996). As insufficiently compensated epilepsy were rated patients with several epileptic seizures during last month. Partially compensated epilepsy had patients with minimally half of year seizure free period and fully compensated epilepsy had patients, who had not for last 3 years an epileptic seizure. According to these criteria 80 patients had insufficiently compensated epilepsy and 20 patients were rated as having partially or fully compensated epilepsy.

All patients were treated by antiepileptic medication. Monotherapy used 59 patients (59%), 29 pacients (29%) were treated by two antiepileptic drugs (AEDs) and 12 pacients (12%) have three and more AEDs (see Fig.2).

Most frequently used monotherapy was carbamazepine, which used 31 patients (it was 52,5% of patients treated by monotherapy). Valproate as monotherapy used 14 pacients (23,7% of patients on monotherapy), 10 patient (16,9%) used lamotrigin, one pacient (1,7%) used primidon, one patient (1,7%) was treated by clonazepam, one patient (1,7%) gabapentin and one patient phenytoin (1,7%) (see Fig.3).

Two AEDs were used by 29 patients. Most frequent combination of EADs was carbamazepine /valproate, which used 9 patients (31 % of all patients on combination of two AEDs). Next most commonly used combination of two AEDs was valproate/ lamotrigine used by 6 patients (20,7% of all patients on combination of two AEDs). Three patients used combination of lamotrigine/topiramate. Two patients used combination of carbamazepine/lamotrigine, carbamazepine/topiramate and combination valproate/topiramate. One patient used combination carbamazepine/levetiracetam, carbamazepine/gabapentin, carbamazepine/pregabalin, valproate/levetiracetam and topiramate/zonisamid (see Table 1).

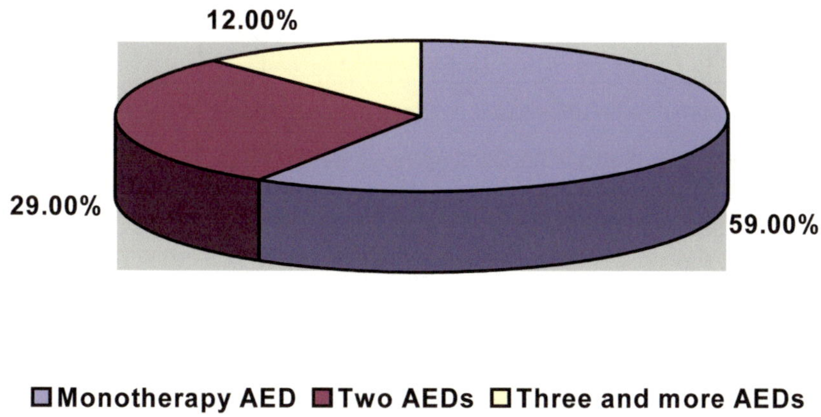

Fig. 2. Antiepileptic therapy in group of epileptic patients.

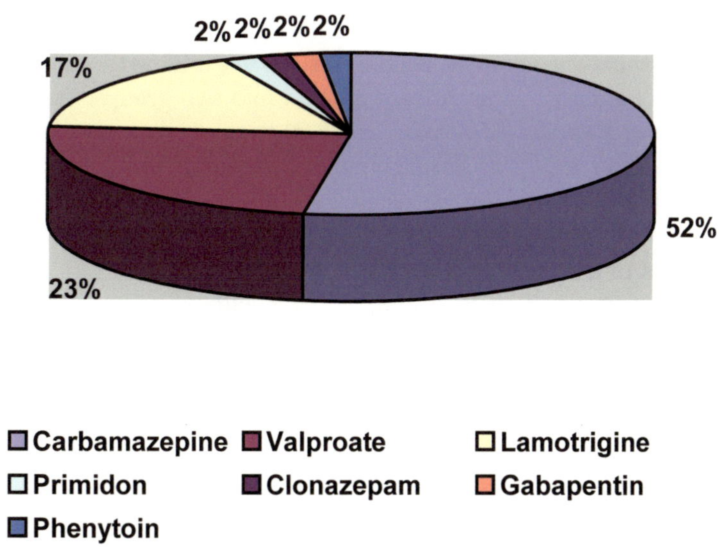

Fig. 3. Antiepileptic monotherapy in group of epileptic seuzures.

Carb.	+	+	+	+	+	+	+	+	+	+	+	+	+	+	+	+													
Valpr.	+	+	+	+	+	+	+	+	+								+	+	+	+	+	+	+	+	+				
Lamic.										+	+						+	+	+	+	+	+				+	+	+	
Topir.												+	+										+	+		+	+	+	+
Levet.														+											+				
Zonis.																													+
Gabap															+														
Pregab																+													

Table 1. Combinations of two AEDs used in the group of patients with epilepsy.

Combination of three and more AEDs was used by 11 patients. Most commonly used combination of AEDs was carbamazepine/ valproate/lamotrigine, which used 7 pacientov, next combinations see in table 2.

Carbam.	+	+	+	+	+	+	+	+	+	+	+	+
Valproate	+	+	+	+	+	+	+	+	+	+	+	
Lamotrig.	+	+	+	+	+	+	+					+
Topiramate										+		+
Levetirac.											+	
Clonazepam								+	+			
Benzodiaz.												+

Table 2. Combinations of three and more AEDs used in the group of patients with epilepsy.

The relation of seizures and sleep or waking state was examined in all patients suffering from epilepsy. On this basis, patients were divided into two groups. The first group of 17 patients had seizures between 10.00 p.m. and 7.00 a.m. which means during sleep or on awakening. The second group of 83 patients had predominantly or exclusively seizures related to waking hours.

3.4 Characteristics of the control group

Control group was composed by 80 healthy persons without anamnesis of epilepsy. They were admitted to the I. Neurology Clinic of Comenius University Hospital in Bratislava for low back pain and in time of evaluation were without pain, which could interfere with sleep. The group consisted of 45 women and 35 men with everage age 38,75 ±14,32 year, including 17 - 78 years.

4. Stastistical methods

The standard box-and-whisker plots were used for graphical representation of the parameter distribution in the particular groups of patients (Rousseeuw et al., 1999). Normality of data was verified by the Lilliefors test (Conover, 1999). To compare the observed parameters, the parametric method unpaired Student's group t-test was used

(Kirkwood, 2003; Dušek, 2009). As the non-parametric statistical methods we used the Kruskal - Wallis H test and the Kolmogorov-Smirnov test. (Gibbons and Subhabrata, 2003)

5. Results

5.1 Changes in daytime sleepiness

Mean value of ESS in the group of patients with epilepsy was 7,11 ± 4,54, in control group 5,53 ± 2,15. Both mean values were in physiological range (under 9). Through that mean value of ESS was higher in group with epilepsy and the difference against control group was significant on p< 0,05 confirmed by all three used stastistical methods (see figure 4, table 3, 4). This result is assesed as significant tendency to daytime sleepiness in patients with epilepsy.

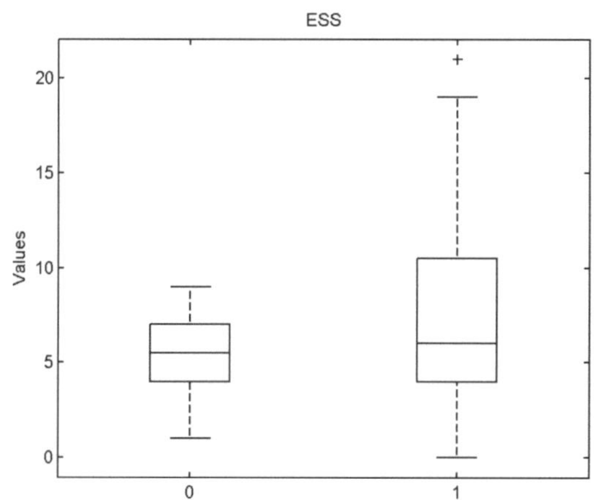

Fig. 4. Values of score Epworth Scale of Sleepiness (ESS) in the control group (0) and in the group of patients with epilepsy (1). The difference is statistically significant (p<0,05).

	nubmer	Mean value	SD	Min value	Max value	Median	Lilliefors test (p)
ESS control group	80	5,53	2,15	1	9	5,5	0,003488
ESS Epilep.	100	7,11	4,54	0	21	6,0	0,001938

Table 3. Values of score ESS and statistical parameters in cotrol group and group of patients with epilepsy.

	t-test	Kruskal-Wallis	Kolmogorov-Smirnov
p	0,00261226*	0,047123469*	0,000152915*

Table 4. Statistical comparison of values ESS by Students t-test, Kruskal-Wallis test a Kolmogorov-Smirnovov test. All result are statistically significant.

5.2 Changes in sleep architecture

In control group and group of patients with epilepsy statistical parameters as effectivity of sleep, amount of NREM S1, S2, S3+4, REM, latency to NREM S1 and latency to REM sleep were evaluated. Normality of distribution of data was tested by Lilliefors test and tests like Student's t-test, Kruskal-Wallis test and Kolmogor-Smirnov test were used (see tables 5a, 5b, 5c)

	nubmer	average	SD	Min value	Max value	Median	Lilliefors (p)
Eff. of sleep /%/	80	87,38	9,89	50	99	90,5	0,001
S1 /%/	80	26,39	12,62	1,4	60,7	25,2	0,5
S2 /%/	80	29,40	10,10	12,3	49,9	28,7	0,14
S3,S4 /%/	80	21,02	9,34	0,1	48,9	19,35	0,002
REM /%/	80	23,06	9,96	0	47,8	24,95	0,02
Lat. to S1 /min/	80	27,58	28,18	2	123,5	15,5	0,001
Lat. to REM /min/	79	132,64	67,04	21,5	372	118	0,001

(SD - standard deviation)

Table 5a. Descriptive characteristics in the control group

	nubmer	average	SD	Min value	Max value	Median	Lilliefors (p)
Eff. of sleep /%/	100	77,10	15,06	30	98	80	0,001
S1 /%/	99	22,75	11,29	1,3	48,5	21	0,34
S2 /%/	100	38,77	12,83	12,8	68,9	36,55	0,17
S3,S4/%/	100	19,13	9,28	0,23	43	17,95	0,003
REM /%/	100	18,82	9,06	1,9	54,3	18,05	0,30
Lat. to S1 /min/	100	41,55	60,23	1,5	386,5	20,5	0,001
Lat. to REM /min/	98	163,26	94,75	33	454,5	137	0,001

(SD - standard deviation)

Table 5b. Descriptive characteristics in the group of patients with epilepsy

	t-Test (p)	Kruskal-Wallis (p)	Kolmogorov-Smirnov (p)
Eff. of sleep /%/	**1,3509E-07***	**6,23404E-07***	**3,84773E-05***
S1 /%/	0,046	0,066	0,230
S2 /%/	**1,42639E-07***	**1,29334E-06***	**1,04321E-05***
S3,S4/%/	0,179	0,163	0,304
REM /%/	**0,004***	**0,001***	**0,0008***
Lat. to S1 /min/	0,042	0,346	0,346
Lat. to REM /min/	**0,013***	**0,047***	**0,004***

Table 5c. Comparison of observed characteristics in the control group and in the group of patients with epilepsy

Patients with epilepsy have significantly lower effectivity of sleep than healthy controls on statistical significance p< 0,001* (see figure 5a). Furthermore patients with epilepsy have significantly more NREM S2 sleep, fewer REM sleep and have significantly longer latency to first REM sleep in comparison to healthy controls (see figures 5b, 5C, 5d). Other differences were not significant.

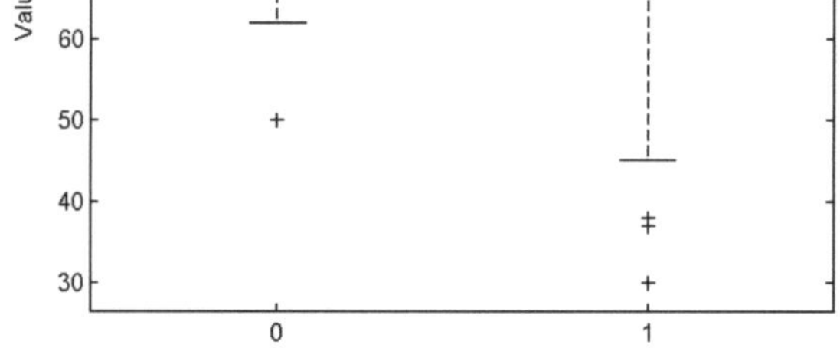

Fig. 5a. Effecitvity of sleep in the control group (0) and in the group of patients with epilepsy (1). The difference is statistically significant (p< 0,001).

Significant changes in sleep architecture of patients with epilepsy were observed. Lower effectivity of sleep together with higher amount of NREM S2 sleep and fewer REM sleep may have considerable consequences on quality of life of patients with epilepsy.

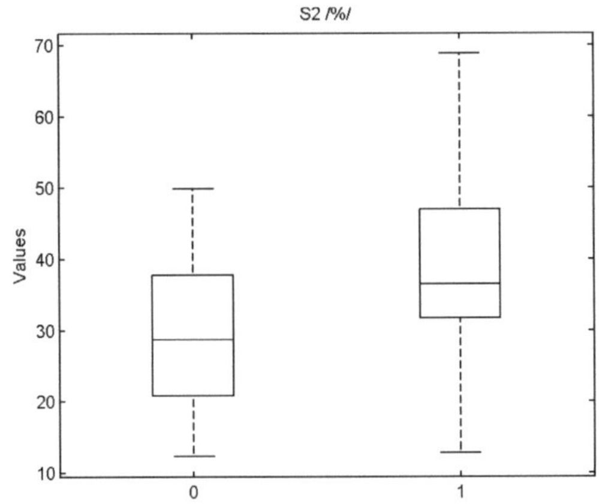

Fig. 5b. Value of NREM S2 (%) in the control group (0) and in the group of patients with epilepsy (1). The difference is statistically significant (p< 0,001).

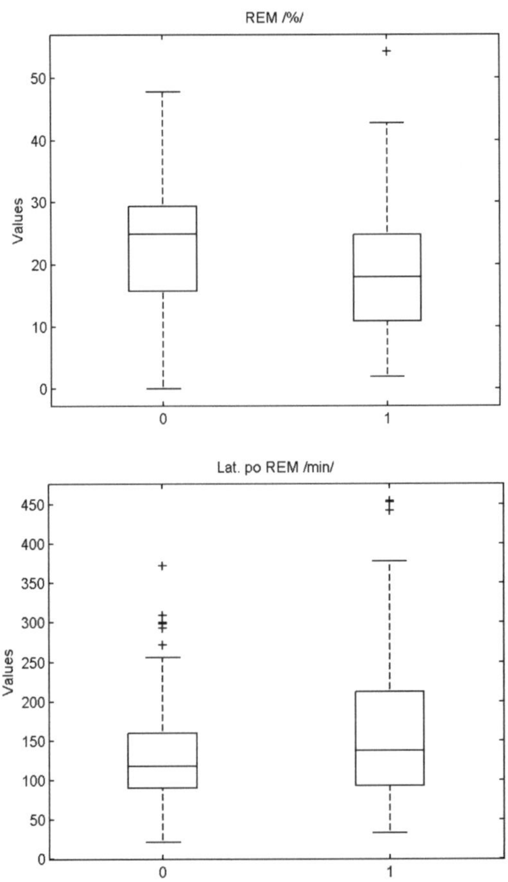

Fig. 5c., 5d. Value of REM (%) and latency to REM sleep (minutes) in the control group (0) and in the group of patients with epilepsy (1). The differences are statistically significant.

5.3 Evaluation of factors with possible influence on sleep architecture of patients with epilepsy

Some characteristics of epilepsy, like type of epilepsy, it's etiology, antiepileptic medication, actual compensation of seizures or evidence of ictal discharges may have influence on quality of sleep. We have chosen some of these factors with purpose to try to find reasons of different characteristics of sleep in patients with epilepsy. Parameters of ESS, MSLT and sleep macroarchitecture were evaluated and statistically compared.

5.3.1 Influence of antiepileptic medication on daytine sleepiness and architecture of sleep

All patients with epilepsy in monitored group were treated by AEDs. As the first step 55 patients with monotherapy AEDs were evaluated. In this group 14 patients were treated by valproate, 31 patients by carbamazepine and 10 patients by lamotrigine. Parameters of ESS, MSLT, effectivity of sleep, % portions of sleep stages NREM S1, S2, S3+4, REM sleep and latency to NREM S1 sleep and latency to REM sleep were examined and statistically compared. No significant differences were ascertained, only patients treated by carbamazepine had higher score of ESS, more % portion of S1 NREM stage, less % portion of deep S3+S4 NREM sleep and had longer latency to first REM stage in comparison with patients treated only by valproate or lamotrigine (see figures 6a, 6b, 6c and 6d). These results may indicate some negative effect of carbamazepine on quality of daytime vigility and sleep.

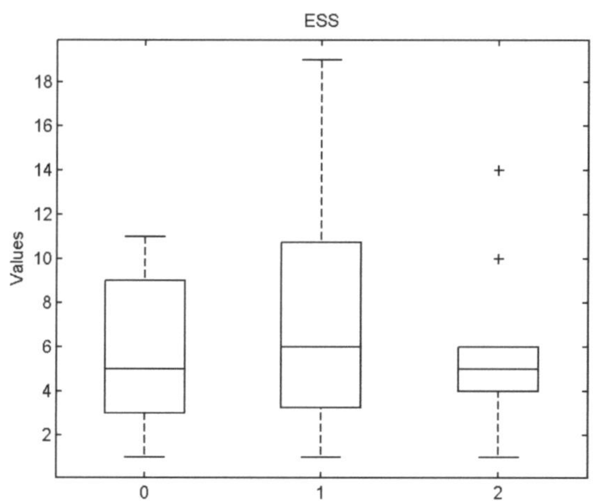

Fig. 6a. Values of ESS in the group of patients with valproate (0), carbamazepine (1) and lamotrigine (2). Differences are not statistically significant.

As the next step, characteristics of daytime sleepiness and quality of sleep in the group of patients with monotherapy and the group of patients on two and more AEDs were evaluated and compared. We supposed, that combination of two and more AEDs could disturb night sleep and worsten daytime vigility. Group of patients using monotherapy consisted of 55 parients, in next group with more AEDs were 45 patients. Observed parameters are presented in tables 6a, 6b.

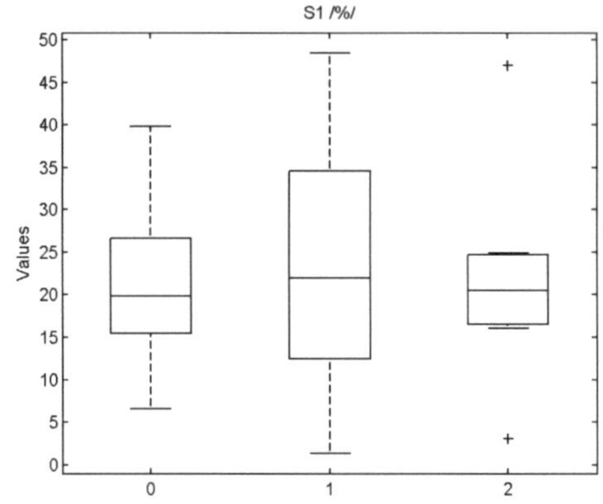

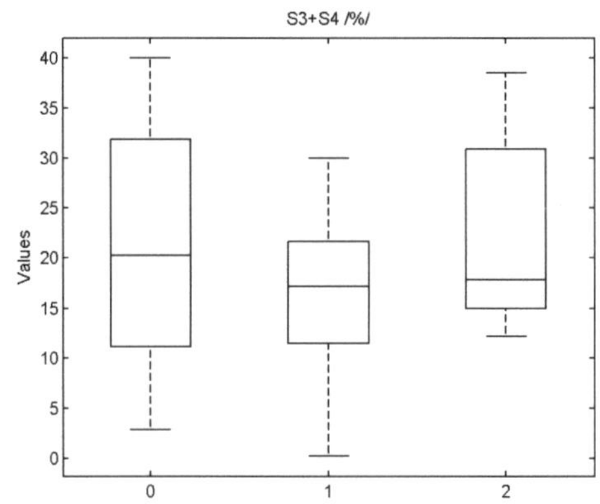

Fig. 6b., 6c. Portion of S1 NREM sleep and S3+S4 NREM sleep in the group of patients with valproate (0), carbamazepine (1) and lamotrigine (2). Differences are not statistically significant.

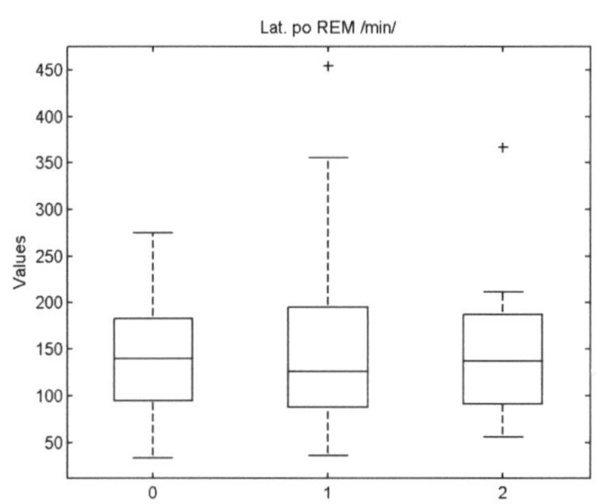

Fig. 6d. Latency to first REM sleep in the group of patients with valproate (0), carbamazepine (1) and lamotrigine (2). Differences are not statistically significant.

	number	mean	SD	Min value	Max value	Median	Lilliefors test (p)
ESS	55	6,58	4,36	1	19	6	0,001
MSLT /min/	38	12,87	5,18	3,2	20	14,1	0,09
Eff. of sleep /%/	55	76,45	15,08	30	98	79	0,012
S1 /%/	55	22,99	11,45	1,3	48,5	20,8	0,039
S2 /%/	55	38,39	13,29	15,3	67,9	36,7	0,5
S3+S4 /%/	55	18,50	9,63	0,23	40	17,3	0,23
REM /%/	55	19,75	9,79	1,9	54,3	20	0,40
Lat. to S1 /min/	55	40,12	58,08	1,5	386,5	18,5	0,001
Lat. to REM /min/	55	161,38	90,79	33	454,5	139,5	0,002

(SD –standard deviation)

Table 6a. Descriptive characteristics of patients with monotherapy of antiepileptic drugs.

	number	mean	SD	Min value	Max value	Median	Lilliefors test (p)
ESS	45	7,88	4,73	0	21	8	0,46
MSLT	33	12,9	5,15	3,1	20	13,6	0,30
Ef.sp. /%/	45	78,02	15,17	38	98	81	0,05
S1 /%/	45	22,39	11,20	1,6	46,6	23,3	0,23
S2 /%/	45	39,33	12,28	12,8	68,9	36,4	0,14
S3+S4 /%/	45	20,04	8,79	7,9	43	18,7	0,002
REM /%/	45	17,49	7,80	7,4	32,7	15,7	0,22
Lat.po S1 /min/	45	43,61	63,88	2	386,5	23,5	0,001
Lat.po REM /min/	45	165,88	101,08	49	453	125	0,001

(SD –standard deviation)

Table 6b. Descriptive characteristics of patients with therapy of two and more AEDs.

Table 6c shows statistical comparison of evaluated parameters in both groups. Differences are not significant.

	t-Test (p)	Kruskal-Wallis (p)	Kolmogor-Smirnov (p)
ESS	0,17	0,12	0,06
MSLT	0,98	0,96	0,10
Eff. of sleep /%/	0,61	0,49	0,90
NREM S1 /%/	0,79	0,88	0,72
NREM S2 /%/	0,72	0,96	0,57
NREM S3+S4 /%/	0,41	0,50	0,66
REM /%/	0,20	0,29	0,28
Lat. to S1 /min/	0,78	0,63	0,63
Lat. to REM /min/	0,82	0,10	0,89

Table 6c. Comparison of observed parameters in the group of patients on monotherapy and the group with two and more AEDs.

Though patients in the group with combination of AEDs have lightly elevated score ESS (ESS 7,88 ± 4,74) in comparison of patients on monotherapy (ESS 6,58 ± 4,36), the difference was not significant (see figure 7). Neither of other evaluated differences was significantly different.

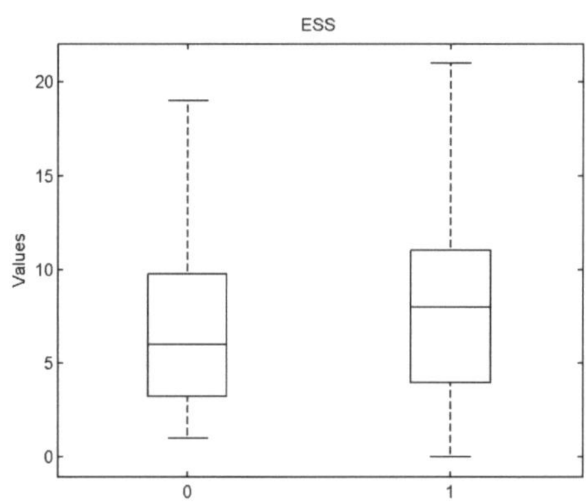

Fig. 7. Values of ESS in the group with monotperapy (0) and the group with two and more AEDs (1). The difference is not significant.

5.3.2 Influence of type of epilepsy (focal/generalized) on daytime sleepiness and quality of sleep

Epileptogenesis of focal and generalized epilepsy is diverse. In focal epilepsy epileptic discharge is localizated and placement of epileptic focus is important as well as possible secondary generalization. Primary generalized epilepsies have different mechanism of epileptigenesis with involvement of bigger areas of the brain. It was expected, that focal and generalized epilepsies have also different influence on sleep architecture. Group of 100 patients with epilepsy was divided in two groups. Group of patients with focal epilepsy inclosed 76 patients, in group of generalized epilepsy were 24 patients. Tables 7a, 7b and 7c describe results of ESS, MSLT, effectivity of sleep and other characteristics of sleep.

	number	mean	SD	Min value	Max value	Median	Lilliefors test (p)
ESS	76	7,22	4,50	0	21	6	0,008
MSLT	56	12,64	5,02	3,1	20	13,15	0,30
Eff. of sleep /%/	76	78,60	13,78	38	98	81	0,007
S1 /%/	75	23,88	11,54	1,3	48,5	22,9	0,5
S2 /%/	76	39,34	12,88	12,8	68,9	36,95	0,14
S3+S4 /%/	76	17,80	8,61	0,23	43	17,1	0,006
REM /%/	76	18,79	9,55	1,9	54,3	17,45	0,37
Lat. to S1 /min/	76	36,67	52,87	1,5	386,5	18,5	0,001
Lat. to REM /min/	75	165,61	101,05	36	454,5	125	0,001

Table 7a. Descriptive characteristics of group with focal epilepsy.

	numbert	mean	SD	Min value	Max value	Median	Lilliefors test (p)
ESS	24	6,75	4,73	0	15	5,5	0,05
MSLT	15	13,79	5,59	3,2	20	15	0,05
Eff.of sleep /%/	24	72,32	18,07	30	98	76,5	0,45
S1 /%/	24	19,22	9,89	3,1	39,8	19,9	0,50
S2 /%/	24	36,97	12,77	15,3	57,4	35,65	0,50
S3+S4 /%/	24	23,35	10,23	2,5	40	21,9	0,33
REM	24	18,92	7,47	6,9	34,8	19,1	0,50
Lat. to S1 /min/	24	57	78,58	3	386,5	36,75	0,001
Lat. to REM /min/	23	155,61	71,81	33	333	139,5	0,05

Table 7b. Descriptive characteristics of group with primary generalized epilepsy.

	t-test (p)	Kruskal-Wallis (p)	Kolmogor-Smirnov (p)
ESS	0,67	0,61	0,89
MSLT	0,48	0,37	0,45
Eff. of sleep /%/	**0,02***	**0,01***	**0,005***
NREM S1 /%/	0,06	0,10	0,43
NREM S2 /%/	0,43	0,50	0,36
NREM S3+S4 /%/	**0,02***	**0,01***	**0,008***
REM /%/	0,94	0,69	0,82
Lat. to S1 /min/	0,24	0,09	0,16
Lat. to REM /min/	0,61	0,74	0,42

Table 7c. Comparison of observed parameters in the group with focal epilepsy and the group with generalized epilepsy.

It was detected, that patients with generalized epilepsy have lower effectivity of sleep and patients with focal epilepsy have fewer deep sleep stages of NREM sleep. These differences are statistically significant. Figures 8a, 8b show these results.
This may be result of different mechanism of epileptogenesis in both types of epilepsy, though further study should be done to exlpain these differences.

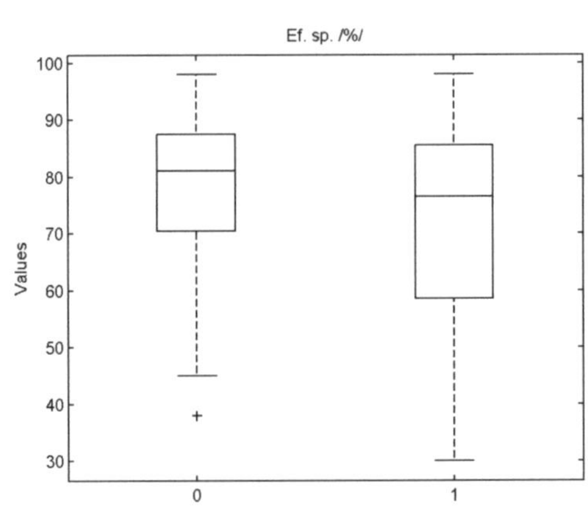

Fig. 8a. Effectivity of sleep in the group of focal epilepsy (0) and the group of generalized epilepsy (1). The difference is statistically significant.

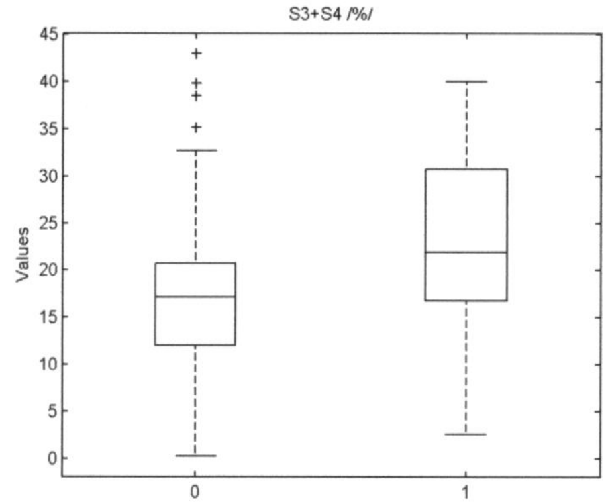

Fig. 8b. Portion of S3+S4 NERM sleep in the group of focal epilepsy (0) and the group of generalized epilepsy (1). The difference is statistically significant.

5.3.3 Influence of localization of epileptic focus on daytime sleepiness and architecture of sleep

Localization of epileptic focus in the group of patients with focal epilepsy was determined by EEG evaluation. Correct localization of epileptic focus was possible by 72 patients. The rest of patients had multiple foci or normal EEG.

Group of 72 patients was divided into two parts. In the first group 61 patients had focus in temporal or temporoparietal region. Next group of 11 patients had focus in frontal or frontotemporal region. Characteristics of daytime vigility and night sleep were compared in both groups. Results are presented in tables 8a, 8b and 8c.

	Number	Mean	SD	Min value	Max value	Median	Lilliefors test (p)
ESS	61	7,28	4,39	0	19	6	0,02
MSLT	44	12,20	4,84	4,5	20	11,9	0,42
Eff. of sleep /%/	61	78,36	13,49	38	98	81	0,002
S1 /%/	60	23,34	11,83	1,3	48,5	21,9	0,50
S2 /%/	61	39,21	13,03	12,8	68,9	36,7	0,14
S3+S4 /%/	61	17,84	8,90	0,23	43	16,9	0,002
REM /%/	61	19,40	9,86	1,9	54,3	18,8	0,50
Lat. to S1 /min/	61	38,09	56,28	1,5	386,5	19,5	0,001
Lat. to REM /min/	60	163,59	97,35	36	454,5	135	0,007

(SD –standard deviation)

Table 8a. Descriptive characteristisc of group with temporal, or temporoparietal focus.

	Number	Mean	SD	Min value	Max value	Median	Lilliefors test (p)
ESS	11	7,54	5,25	1	21	7	0,48
MSLT	9	14,27	5,57	3,1	20	15,25	0,03
Eff. of sleep /%/	11	79,08	15,47	50	98	79	0,22
S1 /%/	11	26,32	9,63	11,6	40	24,9	0,50
S2 /%/	11	41,02	12,90	15,9	67,9	37,8	0,39
S3+S4 /%/	11	17,13	8,05	1,1	30,6	17,1	0,50
REM /%/	11	15,47	7,87	5,1	32,7	15	0,50
Lat. to S1 /min/	11	25,50	25,74	1,5	97	17	0,07
Lat. to REM /min/	11	164,39	114,51	36	378	112,5	0,03

Table 8b. Descriptive characteristisc of group with frontal of frontotemporal focus.

	t-test (p)	Kruskal-Wallis (p)	Kolmogor-Smirnov (p)
ESS	0,87	0,98	0,99
MSLT	0,26	0,19	**0,04***
Ef.sp. /%/	0,88	0,93	0,77
S1 /%/	0,34	0,28	0,66
S2 /%/	0,65	0,53	0,51
S3+S4 /%/	0,78	0,96	0,96
REM /%/	0,13	0,19	0,52
Lat. to S1 /min/	0,22	0,68	0,76
Lat. to REM /min/	0,98	0,80	0,94

Table 8c. Comparison of observed parameters in the group with temporal or temporoparietal focus and the group with frontal or frontotemporal focus.

Kolmogov-Smirnov test showed significant difference in mean latency of sleep by MSLT as patients with temporal or temporoparietal focus have significantly shorter time in MSLT in comparison with group of patients with frontal or frontotemporal focus (see figure 9). Though medians of both MSLT tests are in normal range (> 10 minutes), distribution of datas in the group with temporal and temporoparietal localization of focus is more disperzed as well as values of short mean latency are presented. This may indicate some tendency to elevated daytime sleepiness in the group of patients with temporal or temporoparietal localization of epileptic focus.

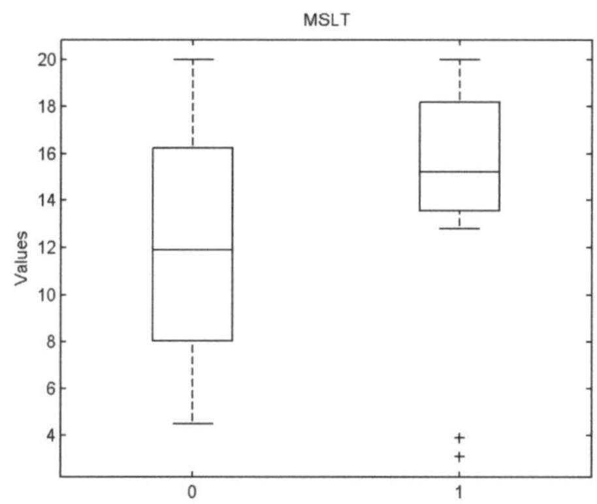

Fig. 9. Mean values of latencies in MSLT in the group with temporal or temporoparietal focus (0) and in the group with frontal and frontotemporal focus (1). The difference is significant.

6. Discussion

Patients in our study as well as control group didn't have elevated daytime sleepiness according to results of Epworth scale of sleepiness (ESS). This result is in accordance with literature, where ESS of epileptic patients and healthy controls did not differ significantly (Malow et al., 1997; Manni et al., 2000; Watanabe et al., 2003). Patients with epilepsy in our group had significantly higher score of ESS than control group. This result was assessed as tendency to daytime sleepiness in patients with epilepsy.

Reason of tendency to problems with vigility in epileptic patients is probably multifactorial. We suppose that detemining cause is fragmentation of sleep architecture with failure of its restorative functions. We found out significant changes in sleep architecture of epileptic patients, which correlate with literature data (Bazil, 2003; Niedermeyer, 1982; Sammaritano et al., 1994; Touchon et al., 1991), as significantly lower effectivity of sleep, significantly more NREM S2 stage sleep, fewer REM sleep and longer latency to REM sleep. According to literature these changes are caused by epileptic seizures, antiepileptic therapy and severity of epilepsy (Bazil, Malow & Sammaritano, 2002). We did not prove influence of antiepileptic therapy on quality of sleep and daytime vigility. This might be influenced by that patients were using medication for longer time before evaluation. Further evaluation should be done in this area to determine influence of specific antiepileptic drugs on sleep architecture.

According to different mechanizms of epileptogenesis in focal and generalized epilepsies various centers of brain involved in regulation of sleep may be influenced (Faber, 1995). This probably correlates with our results of significant reduction of S3 and S4 NREM sleep in the group of patients with focal epilepsy and significant decrement of effectivity of sleep in patients with generalized epilepsy. Changes of sleep in focal epilepsy are probably influenced by localization and ethiology of laesion, in generalized epilepsy thalamocortical circuits involved in epileptogenesis probably influence wider areas of brain.

That is why localization of epileptic focus was also evaluated in correlation with daytime sleepiness and quality of sleep. Significantly shorter mean latency in MSLT was detected in patients with temporal focus in comparison with patients with extratemporal epileptic focus.

Similar results were published by De Almeida et al. (2003), who referred that patients with temporal lobar epilepsy have fragmentation of sleep and reduction of REM sleep.

7. Conclusion

Significant changes in sleep architecture of patients with epilepsy were observed, as lower effectivity of sleep together with higher amount of NREM S2 sleep and fewer REM sleep. These may negatively influence daytime vigility, mental abilities and also compensation of epilepsy.

It was also detected, that patients with generalized epilepsy have lower effectivity of sleep and patients with focal epilepsy have fewer deep sleep stages of NREM sleep.

Some tendency to elevated daytime sleepiness in the group of patients with temporal or temporoparietal localization of epileptic focus was proved.

We recommend awareness among clinicians of the comorbidity of epilepsy and sleep disorders as correct diagnostic and therapeutic approach may improve quality of life of patients.

8. Acknowledgement

This article was published with support of UCB s.r.o, Slovakia.

9. References

American Sleep Disorders Association: The clinical use of the Multiple sleep latency test. *Sleep,*Vol.15, No.3, (Mar., 1992), pp. 268-276, ISSN 0161-8105

Bazil CW. Epilepsy and sleep disturbance. *Epilepsy & Behavior*, Vol.4, Supplement 2, (Oct., 2003), pp. 39-45, ISSN 1525-5050.

Bazil CW, Castro LHM, Walczak TS. (2000). Reduction of Rapid Eye Movement Sleep by Diurnal and Nocturnal Seizures in Temporal Lobe Epilepsy. *Arch neurol,* Vol. 57, No. 3, (Mar. 2000), pp. 363-368, ISSN ISSN:0003-9942.

Bazil CW, Malow BA, Sammaritano MR (2002). *Sleep and Epilepsy:the Clinical Spectrum.* Elsevier Science B.V., ISBN: 0-444-50479-6, Amstedram.

Carscadon MA, Dement WC. (1982). The multiple sleep latency test: what does measure? *Sleep: Journal of Sleep research & Sleep Medicine,* vol.5, (Suppl 2, 1982), pp. 67-72. ISSN 0161-8105.

Cicolin A, Magliola U, Giordano A, Terreni A., Bucca C, Mutani R. (2006). Effects of levetiracetam on nocturnal sleep and daytime vigilance in healthy volunteers. *Epilepsia,* Vol. 47., No. 1, (Jan., 2006), pp.82-5, ISSN 0013-9580.

Commission report: Proposal for revised classification of epilepsies and epileptic syndromes: Commission on Classification and Terminology of the International League Against Epilepsy (1989). *Epilepsia,* Vol. 30., No. 4, pp. 389-399, ISSN 0013-9580.

Conover W. (1999). *Practical Nonparametric Statistics* (3rd edition), John Wiley&Sons, Inc., ISBN 0471160687, New York, p.45.

Dasheiff RM, Kofke WA. (2003). Primarily generalised seizures are more effective than partial seizures in arousing patients from sleep. *Neurol Res.* Vol. 25, No.1, (Jan., 2003), pp. 63-67. ISSN 0161-6412.

De Almeida CA, Lins OG, Lins SG, Laurentino S, Valenca MM. (2003). Sleep disorders in temporal lobe epilepsy. *Arq Neuropsiquiatr.* Vol. 61, No.4, (Dec., 2003), pp. 979-987. ISSN 0004-282X

Donáth V, Karovičová M, Kuchar M, Bratský L, Piťhová B, Sýkora P. (1996). *Diagostický a terapeutický štandard epilepsie.* EPI-Stop, Mediforum, Bratislava, p.17.

Dušek L, Pavlík T, Koptíková J. (2009). Analýza dat v neurologii. *Česká a Slovenská neurologie a neurochirurgie,* Vol. 4, No. 1, (Jan., 2009), pp. 389-393, ISSN 1210-7859.

Faber J. (1995). *Epilepsie a epileptózy.* Maxdorf-Jesenius, ISBN 80-85912-02-3, Praha, p.9.

Foldvary-Schaefer N.(2002). Sleep complaints and epilepsy: the role of seizures, antiepileptic drugs and sleep disorders. *Journal of Clinical Neurophysiology,* Vol. 19, No. 6, (Dec., 2002), pp. 514-521, ISSN 1388-2457.

Foldvary-Schaefer N, Grigg-Damberer M. (2009). Sleep and Epilepsy. *Seminars in Neurology,* Vol. 29, No. 4, (Jan., 2009), pp. 419-428. ISSN 0271-8235.

Garcia-Borreguero D, Larrosa O, de la Llave Y, Verger K, Masramon X, Hernandez G. (2002). Treatment of restless legs syndrome with gabapentin: a double-blind, crossover study. *Neurology,* Vol. 59, No. 10, (Nov.,2002), pp. 1573-1579, ISSN 10158618.

Gibbons JD, Chakraborti S. (2003). *Nonparametric Statistical Inference,* (4th edition), CRC Press, ISBN: 0824740521, New York.

Happe S.(2003). Excessive daytime sleepiness and sleep disturbances in patients with neurological diseases: epidemiology and management. *Drugs.* Vol. 63, No. 24, (Dec., 2003), pp. 2725-2737. ISSN 0012-6667.

Cho YW, Kim DH, Motamendi GK. (2011). The effect of levetiracetam monotherapy on subjective sleep quality and objective sleep parameters in patients with epilepsy: Compared with the effect of carbamazepine-CR monotherapy. *Seizure.* Vol. 20, (Feb., 2011), pp.-in press, ISSN 1059-1311.

Chokroverty S. (1994). *Sleep Disorders Medicine: Basic Science, Technical Considerations, and Clincal Aspects.* Butterworth-Heinemann, p. 27. ISBN:0-7506-9002-X. Stoneham.

Johns MW. (1991). A new method for measuring daytime sleepiness: the Epworth sleepiness scale. *Sleep.* Vol. 14, No. 6, (Dec.,1991), pp. 540-545, ISSN 0161-8105.

Kirkwood B.R., Sterne J.A.C. (2003). *Essential Medical Statistics.* Blackwell Science Ltd. 1988, Blackwell Publishing company, ISBN 0-86542-871-9, pp. 64-70, Malden, Massachusetts, USA.

Littner M, Kushida C, Wise M, et al. (2005). Practice parameters for clinical use of the Multiple Sleep Latency Test. *Sleep,* Vol. 28, No. 1, (Jan., 2005), pp.113-121, ISSN 0161-8105.

Malow BA, Bowes RJ, Lin X. (1997). Predictors of sleepiness in epilepsy patients. *Sleep.* Vol. 20, No. 12 (Dec., 1997), pp. 1105-1110, ISSN 0161-8105.

Manni R, Politini L, Sartori I et al. (2000). Daytime sleepiness in epilepsy patients: evaluation by means of the Epworth sleepiness scale. *J Neurol.,* Vol. 247, No. 9, (Apr., 2000), pp. 716-17. ISSN 0340-5354.

Manni R, Terzahgi M. (2010). Comorbidity between epilepsy and sleep disorders. *Epilepsy Research,* Vol.90, No.3, (May,,2010), pp.171-177, ISSN 0920-1211.

Malow BA, Levy K, Maturen K, Bowes R. (2000). Obstructive sleep apnea is common in medically refractory epilepsy patients. *Neurology,* Vol. 55, No. 7, (Oct.,2000), pp. 1002-1007, ISSN 0028-3878

Marin JM, Gascon JM, Carrizos M, Gispen J. (1997). Prevalence of Sleep Apnoe Syndrome in Spanish Adult Population. *International Journal of Epidemiology,* Vol. 26, No. 2, (Feb.,1997), ISSN 0300-5771, pp.381-386.

Moráň M. (2003). *Praktická epileptologie.* Triton, p. 54, ISBN 80-7254-352-0, Brno.

Moráň M. (2005). Spánek a epilepsie. *Neurol. prax,* Vol.6, No.1, (Jan., 2005), pp. 45-51, ISSN 1335-9592.

Niedermeyer E. Epileptic seizure disorders. In: Bazil CW, Malow BA, Sammaritano MR. (2002). *Sleep and Epilepsy:the Clinical Spectrum.* Elsevier Science B.V., ISBN: 0-444-50479-6, Amsterdam, p.149.

Overeem S, Readings P. (2010). *Sleep Disorders in Neurology. A clinical approach.* Willey-Blackwell, ISBN 978-1-4051-8843-2, Singapore, p.5.

Placidi F, Diomedi M, Scalise A, Marciani MG, Romigi A, Gigli GL. (2000). Effect of anticonvulsants on nocturnal sleep in epilepsy. *Neurology,* Vol. 54, No.5,Suppl 1, (Jan,2000), pp. 25-32, ISSN 0340-5354.

Rang HP, Dale MM. (1991). *Pharmacology.* Churchill Livongstone, ISBN 0-443-04110-5, New York, p.689.

Rechtschaffen A, Kales A. (1968). *Manual of standardized terminology, techniques and scoring system for sleep stages of human subjects.* NIH Publication No.204, Washington, D.C., p.2-11.

Sammaritano M, Levtova V, Samson-Dolfus D. (1994). Modifications of sleep architecture in patients with temporal lobe epilepsy. *Epilepsia.* Vol. 35, No. 8, (Dec., 1994), p.124, ISSN 0013-9580.

American Academy of Sleep Medicine . (2005). *The International Classification of Sleep Disorders, Diagnostic and Coding Manual.* Second Edition. One Westbrook Corporate Center, ISBN:0-9657220-2-3, Suite 920, Westchester, IL, 60154, USA.

Touchon J, Baldy-Moulinier M, Biliard M, Besset A, Cadhillac J. (1991). Sleep organization and epilepsy. *Epilepsy Res.* Suppl. 2, (1991), pp. 73-81, ISSN 0920-1211.

Rousseeuw PJ, Ida Ruts and John W. Tukey. (1994). The bagplot: A Bivariate Boxplot. *The American Statistician.* Vol. 53, No. 4, (Nov., 1999), pp. 382–387, ISSN 0003-1305.

Usui A, Kitahara Y, Matsushita Y, Kitajima M, Sakamoto R, Watanabe T, Motohashi N. (2008). Do you perform the multiple sleep latency test according to the guidelines? A case with multiple sleep onset REM periods. *Sleep and Biological Rhytms.* Vol. 6, No. 1, (Jan., 2008), pp.53-55, ISSN 1446-9235.

Watanabe M, Matsuura M, Sano T, Matsuda R, Matsuda T, Kojima T. (2003). Daytime sleepiness in hypersomniac patients, epileptic patients, and in healthy subjects. *Sleep and Biological Rhytms.* Vol. 1, No. 2, (June, 2003), pp. 137-138. ISSN 1446-9235.

Zucconi M. (2007). Nocturnal Frontal Lobe Epilepsy – An Update on Differential Diagnosis with Non-rapid Eye Movement Parasomnia. *European neurological Disease.* Issue 2, (2007), pp.62-64, ISSN: 1753-3953

4

The Impact of Epilepsy on Reproductive Functions

Cemal Tamer Erel and Onur Guralp
Istanbul University, Cerrahpasa School of Medicine,
Department of Obstetrics and Gynecology,
Division of Reproductive Endocrinology
Turkey

1. Introduction

1.1 Regulation of female reproductive system

Regulation of female reproductive system consists of very complex interactions between the hypothalamus, neurohypophysis and ovaries. Beginning from the embryologic stage, female reproductive system is regulated by the brain. Ovarian hormone production is supressed by the hypothalamo-hypophyseal control mechanism till the end of the childhood period when the puberty begins. During puberty, menstrual cyclicity and timely ovulation, which are the result of the precise integration within different components of the reproductive system, are achieved. After puberty, comes the reproductive period which generally lasts about 30-35 years. During reproductive period, from daily social behavior to sexual life and reproduction, many important issues depend on normal ovarian folliculogenesis and hormonogenesis. Menopause refers to the final menstrual period accompanying the permanent cessation of ovarian function and menstruation.

Gonadotropin releasing hormone receptor (GnRHR) is secreted from hypothalamus and delivered to the anterior pituitary via the hypophyseal portal circulation where it binds to the GnRHR on the surface of gonadotropes triggering the synthesis and secretion of the gonadotropins, follicle stimulating hormone (FSH) and luteinizing hormone (LH). In the female, LH stimulates the production of androgens by the thecal cells that surround the growing ovarian follicle. During the terminal stages of follicular growth, LH also drives the production of progesterone from the granulosa cells of the preovulatory follicle. FSH binds to receptors on the surface of ovarian granulosa cells stimulating the expression of aromatase enzymes that convert thecal androgens to estradiol. The Hypothalamus-hypophysis-gonadal (HPG) axis is subject to both positive feed-forward and negative feedback regulation at several levels. At the level of the hypothalamus, early recognition of the pulsatile nature of gonadotropin releasing hormone secretion led to the notion of a central "pulse generator", the inherent oscillatory activity of which controls the secretory rhythm of GnRH neurons (Knobil, 1980). Hypothalamic pulse generator is extensively modulated by a multitude of higher level inputs including photoperiod, environmental stress, metabolic state and nutritional status, as well as various endocrine mediators. (Bliss, 2010)

1.2 Impact of epilepsy on female reproductive system

Epilepsy is a neurological disorder clinically characterized by recurrent seizures ranging from a very mild form of disruption in attention for a few seconds, to a severe form of muscle spasms and loss of consciousness. Epilepsy is a major public health problem worldwide. The prevalence of epilepsy increases with age (Brodie et al, 2009; Wallace et al, 1998) from 90 per 100,000 people of age 65–70 years, to 150 per 100,000 in those older than 80 years. The treatment goals are suppression and prevention of the seizures. For these purposes, antiepileptic drugs (AED) are used.

Epilepsy has a gender-related pathophysiology and consequences. Therefore, being a woman with epilepsy is not the same as being a man with epilepsy (Taubøll et al, 2008); in fact, the frequency and severity of seizures can increase on certain days of the menstrual cycle (Herzog et al, 1997). Seizures generally exacerbate during the 3 different periods of the menstrual cycle: in perimenstrual and periovulatory periods in normal cycles, and in inadequate luteal phase in abnormal cycles (Figure 1). This type of epilepsy is defined as catamenial epilepsy and is under the influence of estrogen and progesterone. Estrogen has been shown to increase seizure activity, while progesterone decreases it by raising the seizure threshold level (Frye, 2008). Progesterone is converted to allopregnanolone in the brain. Allopregnanolone has been suggested as a primary compound responsible for decreased seizure susceptibility (Scharfman and MacLusky, 2006).

Estrogen acts as a proconvulsant in several animal models of epilepsy, including amygdalal kindling and pentylenetetrazol administration in ovariectomized rats (Hom and Buterbaugh, 1986). Estrogen induces the formation of new excitatory synapses in the CA1 region of the hippocampus; and further, this estrogenic induction involves activation of N-methyl-Daspartate (NMDA) receptors (McEwen, 2002). Increasing the complexity of hippocampal synaptic density is likely a mechanism for the proconvulsant activity of estrogen. Standard hormone replacement in postmenopausal women with epilepsy, which includes estrogen and a progestin, can be postulated to have an effect on seizures that is more evident than that of oral contraceptives in cycling women with epilepsy. This is because reproductive hormone levels during menopause are low and unchanging. Therefore, the brain hormonal milieu in which exogenous hormones are introduced is markedly different in menopause from that in menstruating women.

In the ovariectomized animals, however, the hormonal changes in the animals are abrupt in contrast to the gradual hormonal changes found in the menopausal transition. It might be the concerted lack of estradiol and progesterone that facilitate the seizure susceptibility. Both estradiol and progesterone affect γ-amino butyric acid (GABA) ergic function (Scharfman et al, 2005; Nakumura et al, 2005; Kokate et al, 1994). The simultaneous decrease of estrogen and progesterone may thereby lead to a decrease in GABAergic inhibition, facilitating seizures. Recently published results by Lavaque et al (2006) suggest age-related focal production of sex hormones especially prominent in the hippocampus and cerebral cortex. The expression of the steroidogenic acute regulatory protein was found to increase particularly in these areas. The hippocampus and cerebral cortex are areas associated with seizure initiation and propagation. It is therefore discussed how pathological disturbances in the local estrogen production after menopause may contribute to an increase in seizures in some women (Veliskova, 2007).

Estrone is the primary estrogen after menopause, and its main source is subcutaneous fat. This might be of importance for overweight women with epilepsy. Little is known on the influence of estrone on epilepsy. An altered ratio of estradiol/estriol/estrone might be of importance; however, this has not been investigated. Most likely, however, the hormonal changes in menopause may not affect the different types of epilepsy in the same way.

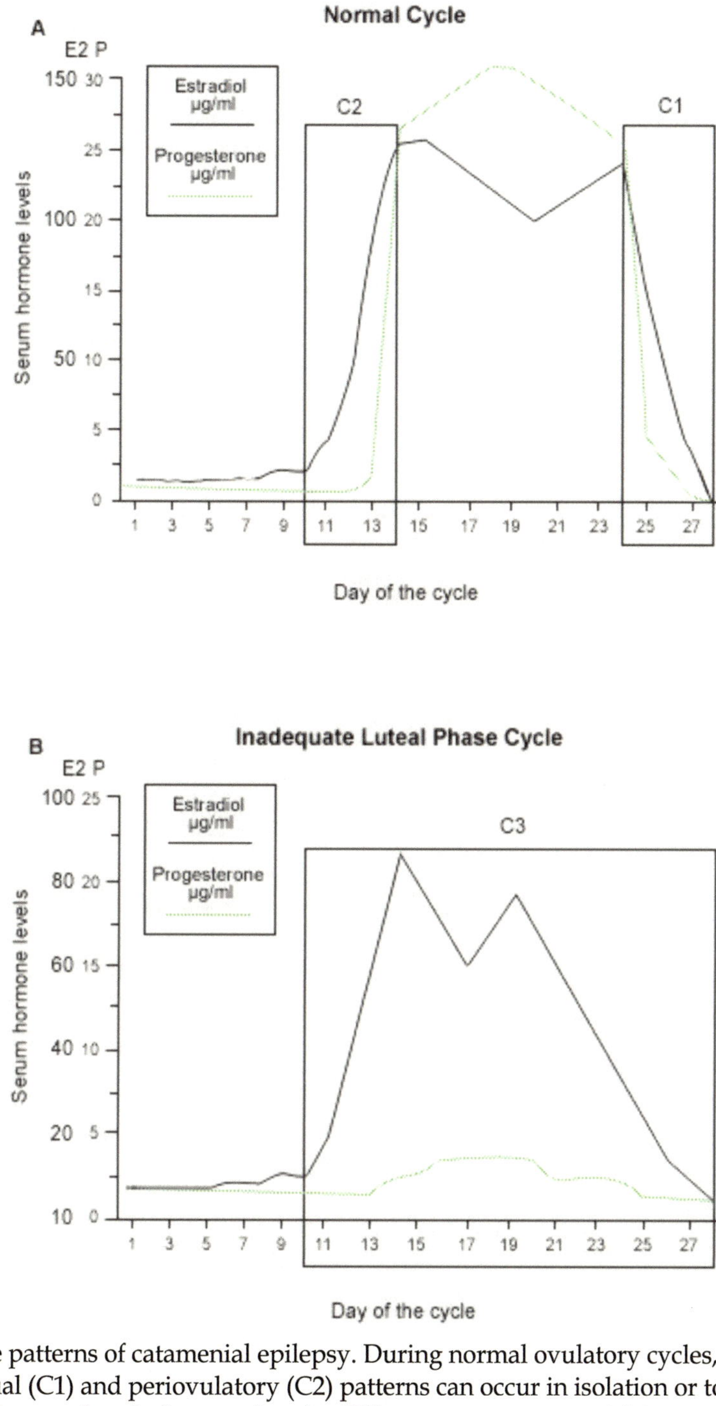

Fig. 1. Three patterns of catamenial epilepsy. During normal ovulatory cycles, both perimenstrual (C1) and periovulatory (C2) patterns can occur in isolation or together. During inadequate luteal phase cycles, the (C3) pattern can occur with increased seizures during the entire second half of the cycle. (Herzog AG. Catamenial epilepsy: definition, prevalence pathophysiology and treatment. Seizure 2008;17:151)

Reproductive dysfunction is common among women with epilepsy primarily due to the dysfunction in the temporolimbic system. This system has integral roles in reproductive endocrine regulation and feedback as well as in sexual and reproductive function (Herzog, 1989). Consequently, the development of epileptiform discharges in medial temporal lobe structures may disrupt hypothalamic regulation of pituitary secretion and, hence, alter gonadal function.

In addition, most of the AEDs (carbamazepine, oxcarbazepine, phenobarbital, phenytoin, and topiramate) may also alter endocrine function by inducing the cytochrome P450 isoenzyme 3A4 in women with epilepsy (Luef, 2009). Therefore, certain AEDs may accelerate hepatic elimination of hormonal preparations and decrease the serum concentrations of bioactive sex steroids.

Epileptic women have increased risk of polycystic ovary syndrome (PCOS), premature ovarian failure (POF), and hormonal contraceptive failure; as well as osteoporosis (Figure 2).

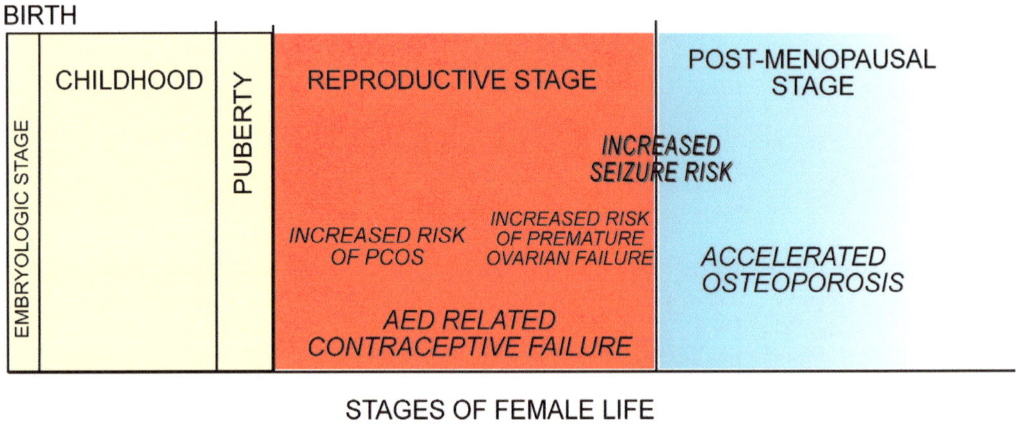

Fig. 2. Possible changes in epileptic women according to different stages of female life
AED, anti-epileptic drug; PCOS, polycystic ovary syndrome.

2. Epilepsy and polycystic ovary syndrome

PCOS is characterized by enlarged ovaries with multiple small cysts and a hypervascularized, androgen-secreting stroma leading to the associated signs of androgen excess (hirsutism, alopecia, acne), obesity, and menstrual-cycle disturbance (oligo or amenorrhea) (Balen, 1999). The most common reproductive endocrine disorder in women with epilepsy, as well as in women in the general population, is PCOS. PCOS occurs in 10-20% of women with epilepsy compared to 5-6% of women in the general population (Bauer et al, 2008; Knochenhauer et al, 1998; Herzog, 2002; Herzog et al, 2003). The prevalence of PCOS in women with epilepsy is greater, even if they are not taking AEDs; and it is more frequent in women who take valproic acid (VPA), primarily if initiated before the age of 20.

PCOS is probably not a single nosological entity, but rather the common endpoint for a number of pathophysiological mechanisms, some of which may be attributable to epilepsy itself (Herzog et al, 1986, 2003) or to the use of AEDs, most notably valproate. PCOS represents the failure of the ovarian follicle to complete normal maturation during the menstrual cycle or a series of cycles -- a failure that is perhaps related to the presence of inadequate levels of pituitary follicle-stimulating hormone (FSH); whereas levels of luteinizing hormone (LH) are normal or elevated (Isojärvi, 2008; Herzog, 2008).

The brain controls reproductive function primarily through hypothalamic regulation of pituitary secretion. The left and right vagus nerves exert different modulatory influences on ovarian structure and function (Gerendai & Halasz, 1997). The reproductive neuroendocrine system, like many other brain systems, shows a lateralized asymmetry that might, by virtue of ipsilaterally predominating effects, contribute to the development of distinct reproductive endocrine disorders in association with unilateral left- and right-sided epileptic foci (Herzog, 2007). Unilateral temporolimbic discharges are associated with laterally differing, consistent, predictable, stochastic directional changes in hormonal secretion at all levels of the reproductive neuroendocrine axis, that is, hypothalamus, pituitary, and ovary (Herzog et al, 2003). These directional changes are consistent with the finding that different reproductive disorders may develop in relation to left- and right-sided temporolimbic epilepsy. Specifically, left temporal lobe epilepsy (LTLE) is associated with significantly higher pulse frequencies of GnRH secretion (Herzog et al, 2003; Herzog, 2008). Higher GnRH pulse frequency, in turn, is associated with higher LH/FSH ratios and higher serum testosterone levels. This combination of neuroendocrine changes characterizes PCOS and is consistent with the previously suggested association between left unilateral TLE and PCOS.

Antiepileptic drugs, on the other hand, also have substantial and differential effects on reproductive hormone levels. The first report suggesting a high incidence of menstrual disorders linked to obesity, hyperandrogenism, and polycystic ovaries in women taking VPA for epilepsy was published in 1993 (Isojarvi). Changes in serum androgen levels have been detected before and during pubertal development in young girls taking VPA for epilepsy (Vainionpää, 1999).

Studies by Murialdo et al (1997) have also reported a high prevalence of menstrual disorders and hyperandrogenic anovulation in VPA treated women with epilepsy. However, the study by Bauer et al (2008) did not show any differences between carbamazepine- and VPA-treated women with epilepsy with respect to reproductive endocrine parameters. Although the interpretation of the results of this study is difficult, because the age of the patients, the duration of medication, and seizure frequency in the different treatment groups were not given (Isojärvi, 2005). Other studies have also addressed the issue of reproductive endocrine function in women with epilepsy. Luef et al (2002) reported similar frequencies of menstrual disorders and PCOS in women taking carbamazepine and VPA for epilepsy. It has been suggested that obesity and associated hyperinsulinemia could be implicated in the development of PCOS and hyperandrogenism in women taking VPA. It seems that obesity and related hyperinsulinemia may exacerbate the VPA-related reproductive endocrine disorders in women with epilepsy. It seems likely that VPA has a direct effect on ovarian androgen production, or as an enzyme inhibitor, it may inhibit the metabolism of sex steroids and thereby lead to increased serum androgen levels (Isojärvi et al, 2005).

Several studies have suggested that the reproductive endocrine effects of AEDs may be reversible if the medication is discontinued. In a prospective study, the replacement of VPA with lamotrigine resulted in normalization of endocrine function during a 1-year follow-up in 12 women with a previously identified endocrine disorder (PCOS or hyperandrogenism, or both) likely to be related to VPA. Serum insulin and testosterone levels returned to normal 2 months after VPA was discontinued, and the levels remained normal thereafter (Isojärvi et al, 2005).

3. Epilepsy and premature ovarian failure

POF is characterized by amenorrhea, cessation of ovarian function, and elevated gonadotropin levels before 35 years of age and younger. Ovarian failure due to POF may not be absolute; hence, this condition needs to be differentiated from premature menopause because the latter reflects a "permanency" of the ovarian failure.

Indeed, women with POF often continue to have some residual ovarian function for many years after diagnosis (Kodaman, 2010, Kalantaridou&Nelson 2000). Both sporadic ovulation and occasional pregnancy are possible with POF; (Nelson et al, 1994, Alper et al, 1986) in fact; up to half of women affected by POF have intermittent follicular development, 25% may occasionally ovulate, and 5 to 10% will conceive and deliver (Nelson et al, 1994, Rebar&Connolly, 1990, Rebar, 2009). The term menopause thus should be avoided in the context of counseling these patients, and more recently, the term POF has also fallen into disfavor because it implies finality and gives a further negative connotation to an already devastating diagnosis for a young woman to come to terms with. POF, the term first coined by the endocrinologist Fuller Albright almost 70 years ago, is now the preferred nomenclature for this entity. (Albright et al, 1942, Welt, 2008, Nelson, 2009) The incidence of POF increases with age, affecting 0.01%, 0.1%, and 1% of women <20, 30, and 40 years of age, respectively (Coulam, 1986). Given the association of chemoradiation therapy with subsequent ovarian insufficiency and the increasing successes with childhood and early adulthood malignancy treatments, it has been predicted that the number of cases of POF will increase significantly in the future (Sklar, 2006, Panay&Fenton, 2008). Etiologies for POF are heterogeneous and, for the most part, poorly understood. The etiology for up to 90% of cases of POF remains elusive (Kodaman, 2010).

POF occurs more commonly in women with epilepsy. Klein et al (2001) evaluated the incidence of POF in 50 women with epilepsy, aged 38 to 64, compared with control women. Premature menopause was defined as amenorrhea for greater than 1 year with elevated day 3 FSH levels in women younger than 42 years. Premature perimenopause was defined by the presence of perimenopausal symptoms. Of the women with epilepsy, 14% had premature perimenopause or menopause, compared with only 3.7% of the control women ($P = 0.042$). They did not find an association with epilepsy duration, seizure severity, or AEDs; although women with premature menopause were more likely to have had catamenial exacerbation of their seizures than women without POF ($P = 0.02$). Harden et al (2003) also found in their multicentric cohort study that premature menopause was associated with epilepsy. In another study, the median age at menopause in the group of women with epilepsy was 47 years, compared with the median age of 51.4 years in the general US population (Gold, et al, 2001). When the investigators divided the patients into low, intermediate, and high seizure frequency groups, there was an increasingly lower age at menopause with a negative correlation between the age at menopause and seizure group based on estimated lifetime seizures ($P = 0.014$). They also found no influence of enzyme-inducing AEDs. The authors concluded that the association of lifetime number of seizures with the timing of cessation of reproductive cycling may occur as a result of direct disruption of hypothalamic and pituitary function by the seizures.

Women with epilepsy have an increased risk of experiencing an early onset of perimenopausal symptoms. Some studies draw attention to the increased frequency of POF in women with epilepsy. However, no association has been detected so far between the POF and epilepsy duration, seizure severity, or use of enzyme-inducing AEDs. POF may occur as a result of direct disruption of hypothalamic and pituitary function by the seizures. It has been suggested that women with POF were more likely to have catamenial exacerbation of their seizures than women without POF.

4. Contraception and epilepsy

Contraceptive methods can be divided into two subgroups as hormonal and non-hormonal. Hormonal contraceptives include combined-oral contraceptives, progestin only pills, hormonal implants, progestin releasing intrauterine systems, depomedroxyprogesterone acetate injections, and vaginal rings. Non-hormonal contraceptive methods include male and female condoms, copper intrauterine device, tubal ligation and vasectomy of the companion.

Combined oral contraceptives are a widely used and well accepted form of contraception. Combined-oral contraceptives are highly effective when used consistently and correctly, and are well tolerated by most women. Combined-oral contraceptives contain a combination of an estrogen and a progestin. Since their introduction, several progestins have been developed for use in combined-oral contraceptives. Conversely, the estrogen component has remained largely unchanged, with the vast majority of combined-oral contraceptives containing ethinylestradiol (EE) or, more commonly in the past, mestranol, the 3-methyl ether of EE. The estrogen component of combined-oral contraceptives is responsible for suppressing FSH, providing endometrial stability, and potentiating the activity of the progestin component, e.g., by increasing progestin receptor concentrations. However synthetic progestins may directly influence ovarian function by a direct inhibition of the ovarian steroid biosynthesis. Modern combined-oral contraceptives have two components: EE and a progestin. Both are on their own able to inhibit ovulation. In modern combined-oral contraceptives ovulation inhibition is mainly achieved by the progestin and not by ethinylestradiol. The typical daily progestin dose in today's combined-oral contraceptives is about 1.5–2 times the ovulation-inhibiting dose (Schwenkhagen&Stodieck, 2008).

The choice of a contraceptive drug can be challenging for women with epilepsy due to possible interactions between AEDs and hormonal contraception. Enzyme-inducing AEDs can cause hormonal contraception to fail and can increase the risk of teratogenicity. Higher doses of oral contraceptives can overcome pharmacologic failure but may create additional risks (Burakgazi et al, 2009).

In women with epilepsy failure rates of oral contraceptives may increase to 6% depending on the antiepileptic drug they are taking (Morell, 1996). Drugs such as phenobarbital (PB), primidone (PRM), phenytoin (PHT), carbamazepine (CBZ), oxcarbazepine (OXC) at doses above 600 mg daily and topiramate (TPM) at doses above 200 mg (Doose et al, 2003) may cause induction of hepatic cytochrome P450, reducing the effects of contraceptives to block ovulation. VPA and felbamate (FBM) inhibit the hepatic microsomal system and do not reduce, and can even increase, the levels of the steroid hormones of oral contraceptives. Other drugs such as gabapentin (GBP), lamotrigine (LTG), tiagabine (TGB), pregabalin (PGB), vigabatrin (VGB), and levetiracetam (LEV) do not affect the serum concentrations of contraceptives (Tatum et al, 2004) (Table 1). To avoid lack of efficacy of contraception used in a patient that is on therapy with enzyme-inducing AEDs when the "morning-after pill" is used at the same time, the first dose of levonogestrel should be 1.5 mg (twice the usual dose of 750 μg), and after 12 hours the recommended 750 μg are reinstated (Mayor, 2004; Perruca, 2004). Moreover, oral contraceptives can reduce levels of LTG by 25% to 70%. If the woman is taking AEDs, which reduce steroid hormone levels, oral contraceptives must contain a minimum of 50 µg of EE. If there is a hemorrhage, the dose should be raised to 75 or 100 µg. During the first months of oral contraceptive use, and once ovulation has been eliminated, complementary contraceptive methods are recommended. To improve contraceptive efficacy, the use of a combined-oral contraceptives that contains a progestin well above the dose needed to inhibit ovulation may be recommended. Ovulation-inhibiting doses of progestins are given in table 1.

Progestin	**mg/day**
Chlormadinone acetate	1.7
Cyproterone acetate	1.0
Desogestrel/3-keto-desogestrel	0.06
Dienogest	1.0
Drospirenone	2.0
Gestodene	0.04
Levonorgestrel	0.06
Norethisterone	0.4
Norethisterone acetate	0.5
Nomegestrol acetate	5.0

Table 1. Ovulation-inhibiting doses of progestins (without additional estrogen) (Kuhl, 2005)

Commonly used AEDs which do and do not interact with oral contraceptives are given in Table 2.

Drugs which do not reduce the effects of oral contraceptives	**Drugs which reduce the effects of oral contraceptives**
Clonazepam	Barbiturates
Ethosuximide	Carbamazepine
Felbamate	Oxcarbazepine
Gabapentin	Phenytoin
Levetiracetam	Primidone
Lamotrigine	Topiramate (>200 mg/day)
Tiagabine	
Valproate	

Table 2. Commonly used AEDs which do and do not interact with oral contraceptives

Most drug–drug interaction studies have focused on the effect of AEDs on oral contraceptive safety. Much less is known about the result of a co-prescription of hormonal contraceptives on AEDs, which is surprising, since it is known for a long time that oral contraceptives have a strong influence on drug metabolizing enzymes. (Schwenkhagen&Stodieck, 2008).

In combined oral contraceptives, during the period "on the pill" lamotrigine levels decrease by approximately 50%, followed by an increase of lamotrigine levels in the contraceptive-free week up to 80– 100% of the baseline lamotrigine level. This is often clinically relevant and may result in an increased risk of seizure recurrence especially in week 2 and 3 on the pill or in concentration-dependent adverse effects at the end of the pill-free interval (Sabers et al, 2001, 2003; Stodieck &Schwenkhagen, 2004; Christensen, 2007). These fluctuations are most likely due to an induction of UGT1A4, the enzyme responsible for the glucoronidation of lamotrigine, by EE. VPA levels also seem to be reduced by the concomitant use of hormonal contraceptives (Herzog et al, 2005; Galimberti, 2006). Just as with lamotrigine the magnitude of observed fluctuations of the VPA levels appear to vary interindividually. Hormonal contraceptives which are adversely affected by hepatic cytochrome P450 enzyme-inducing AEDs are given in Table 3.

Oral
Various combined estrogen/progesterone preparations
Progestin only pill
Morning after pill
Transdermal patch (norelgestromin and ethinyl estradiol)
Vaginal ring (etonorgestrel/ethinyl estradiol ring)
Implants (etonorgestrel)

Table 3. Hormonal contraceptives which are adversely affected by hepatic cytochrome P450 enzyme-inducing AEDs

In addition to induction of cytochrome P450 enzyme system, several AEDs induce the production of sex hormone binding globulin (SHBG) to which the progestins are tightly bound, resulting in lower concentrations of free progestin that may also lead to combined-oral contraceptive failure (Dutton C, Foldvary-Schaefer, 2008).

While higher dose combined-oral contraceptives are one contraceptive option for women on enzyme-inducing AEDs, a variety of other options are available. Injectable contraception (depot medroxyprogesterone acetate) appears effective with AED use, but the potential for bone mineral density loss is a concern. (Dutton C, Foldvary-Schaefer, 2008)

Non-hormonal contraceptive methods are not contraindicated in women with epilepsy. If contraception is addressed as a permanent measure, the safest method is tubal ligation or vasectomy of the companion. Intrauterine devices are an alternative to pharmacologic approaches because they lack drug-drug interactions and side effects (Burakgazi et al, 2009). There is no evidence that combined-oral contraceptives increase seizures in women with epilepsy (Dutton C, Foldvary-Schaefer, 2008).

5. Epilepsy and menopause

Ovarian reserve shrinks throughout life and reaches a critical threshold level at the inception of the menopause. At this point, a woman notes her first skipped menstrual period. The menopausal transition begins with the onset of first menstrual irregularity, or skipped menses, and ends with the final menstrual period. Progressive loss of ovarian follicles results in decreased production of inhibin and a loss of restraint on FSH secretion. The monotropic increase in FSH leads to variable hormonal patterns, depending on the available ovarian follicles and their degree of responsiveness. Once follicles reach a critically low level, ovulation becomes progressively less likely and prolonged amenorrhea ensues. In addition to ovarian factors that contribute to reproductive senescence in women, there is accumulating evidence that as in rodents, hypothalamic-pituitary dysfunction accompanies reproductive aging and contributes to the process. As knowledge about the menopausal transition increases, it may turn out that the ovary is not the only area that should be studied—the brain may undergo changes as well (Santoro, 2005).

During the perimenopausal period, the frequency of catamenial epileptic seizures may increase (probably due to hyperestrogenism) and then decrease after menopause. According to current data, hormone replacement therapy (HRT) may increase the frequency of epileptic seizures. Changes in serum concentrations of sex steroid hormones are frequently observed when enzyme-modulating AEDs (VPA, CBZ, phenytoin, or phenobarbital) are used. It is generally accepted that long-term treatment with VPA and CBZ may lead to reproductive endocrine disorders in patients with epilepsy. VPA can increase biologically active sex hormone levels (e.g., hyperandrogenism) independent of associated weight gain, more commonly seen in women before the age of 20. In contrast, CBZ may decrease free serum testosterone concentrations through the induction of SHBG. If the woman is taking AEDs, which reduce steroid hormone levels, OCs must contain a minimum of 50 µg of EE. If there is a hemorrhage, the dose should be raised to 75 or 100 µg.

Indications for HRT are dealing with menopausal symptoms and conservation of bone mass and fracture prevention. As epilepsy is affected by sex steroids, careful consideration must be given to the regimen used. However, the data are extremely limited (Harden et al, 2006; Shen & Stearns 2009). The details of the only randomized trial double-blind, placebo-controlled trial are now described (Harden et al, 2006). This was undertaken in postmenopausal women with epilepsy who are taking stable doses of AEDs and are within 10 years of their last menses. After a 3-month prospective baseline, subjects were randomized to placebo, Prempro (0.625 mg of conjugated equine estrogens plus 2.5 mg of medroxyprogesterone acetate or CEE/MPA) daily, or double-dose CEE/MPA daily for a 3-month treatment period. Twenty-one subjects were randomized after completing baseline. The subjects' ages ranged from 45 to 62 years (mean, 53 years), and the number of AEDs used ranged from none to three (median, one). Five (71%) of seven subjects taking double-dose CEE/MPA had a worsening seizure frequency of at least one seizure type, compared with four (50%) of eight taking single-dose CEE/MPA, and one (17%) of six taking placebo ($p = 0.05$). An increase in seizure frequency of the subject's most severe seizure type was associated with increasing CEE/MPA dose ($p = 0.008$). An increase in complex partial seizure frequency also was associated with increasing CEE/MPA dose ($p = 0.05$). Two subjects taking lamotrigine had a decrease in lamotrigine levels of 25–30% while taking CEE/MPA. The authors concluded that CEE/MPA is associated with a dose-related increase in seizure frequency in postmenopausal women with epilepsy. CEE/MPA may decrease lamotrigine levels. There are no data with other regimens with different estrogens and progestogens or transdermal or vaginal administration. It is not known whether women with epilepsy need higher doses of estrogen or whether transdermal rather than oral therapy is preferred depending on their AED use. Based on the randomized trial, it would be prudent to closely monitor women who start HT as their AED needs may change (Erel et al, 2010).

Non-estrogen based treatments are used to treat hot flushes and symptoms of urogenital atrophy (Erel et al, 2010). Drug interactions need to be carefully assessed before using pharmacotherapy. Interventions to consider include clonidine, selective serotonin reuptake inhibitors (SSRIs) and serotonin and noradrenaline reuptake inhibitors (SNRIs), gabapentin, and vaginal lubricants and mosturizers (Shen et al, 2009). While bisphosphonates will conserve bone mass, there are little data in women with epilepsy and there are concerns about the safety of long term use (Drezner, 2004).

As vitamin D and calcium metabolism can be affected by AEDS, supplements should be considered. Herbal preparations should be avoided as their efficacy is uncertain and they may interact with AEDs (Erel et al, 2010).

6. Epilepsy and osteoporosis

The cessation of ovarian function at the menopause is associated with a phase of rapid bone loss which probably lasts from 5 to 10 years (Genant et al, 1982; Recker et al, 2000). This rapid bone loss results from an increase in bone turnover in association with a negative remodelling imbalance (Compston, 2001); whilst reduced bone formation undoubtedly contributes to the latter, there is evidence that increased osteoclastic activity also plays a role, particularly in the earlier stages of menopausal bone loss (Compston et al, 1995). The combination of increased bone turnover and increased resorption depth results in disruption of bone microarchitecture, with loss of connectivity of cancellous bone and thinning of the cortices, which also show increased porosity.

Osteoporosis and fractures may increase due to hypoestrogenism in menopause and cytochrome P450 inducing AEDs. Recent studies suggest lower bone mineral density (BMD) in adults and children with epilepsy, irrespective of AED treatment.

Both idiopathic epilepsy and symptomatic epilepsy are associated with reduced BMD, with the greatest reduction in symptomatic generalized epilepsy (Sheth & Hermann, 2008). However, the pathophysiological underlying mechanisms are far from understood and likely multifactorial. Potential risk or predisposing factors include physical impairment, genetic factors, AED treatment with enzyme-inducing drugs, AED polytherapy, impact of seizures on the hypothalamus-hypophysis-adrenal (HPA) axis, and vitamin D deficiency/insufficiency. As growth and sexual maturation in adolescence are regulated by a complex neuroendocrine system including the HPA axis, potential AED-related abnormalities may be reflected in growth and bone metabolism in childhood epilepsy. In adults and children treated with enzyme-inducing AEDs, vitamin D deficiency/insufficiency (up to 50% of patients) and low BMD have been reported in most, but not all, studies (Petty et al, 2007; Farhat et al, 2002; Pack et al, 2005; Verrotti et al, 2000).

However, and in particular in children, it is unclear whether non-enzyme-inducing AED monotherapy (lamotrigine, sulthiame) or minimal enzyme-inducing AED monotherapy (oxcarbazepine) seem to have any adverse effects on linear growth or to cause vitamin D deficiency in otherwise healthy children with epilepsy (Luef & Rauchenzauner, 2008). In contrast to adults, there is controversy over the association of chronic AED use with an increased incidence of fractures in children (Souverein et al, 2005; Petty, et al, 2007). Recent studies suggest lower BMD in adults and children with epilepsy, irrespective of AED treatment (Pack, 2008; Sheth et al, 2008a, 2008b; Pack & Walczak, 2008; Sheth & Hermann, 2008).

7. Conclusion

In conclusion, in gynecological practice, women with epilepsy deserve special care with a multidisciplinary approach. Women with epilepsy should be questioned routinely about menstrual cycles, infertility, excessive weight gain, hirsutism, galactorrhea, and changes in sexual life. If abnormalities are detected, hormone determinations, pelvic ultrasound, and neuroimaging of pituitary gland should be assessed. If the cause of the problem is AED-related, a therapeutic alternative should be addressed, taking into account seizure control possibilities versus side effects.

Seizures generally exacerbate during the 3 different periods of the menstrual cycle: in perimenstrual and periovulatory periods in normal cycles, and in inadequate luteal phase in abnormal cycles. This type of epilepsy is defined as catamenial epilepsy and is under the influence of estrogen and progesterone. Estrogen has been shown to increase seizure activity, while progesterone decreases it by raising the seizure threshold level.

The prevalence of PCOS in women with epilepsy is 10-20%, which is greater than the normal population, even if epileptic women are not taking AEDs. PCOS is more frequent in women who take VPA, primarily if initiated before the age of 20.

Women with epilepsy have an increased risk of experiencing an early onset of perimenopausal symptoms. Some studies draw attention to the increased frequency of POF in women with epilepsy, although this relationship needs to be further investigated.

In women with epilepsy, failure of oral contraceptives may increase to 6% depending on the antiepileptic drug they are taking. Barbiturates, Carbamazepine, Oxcarbazepine, Phenytoin, Primidone, and Topiramate (>200 mg/day) may reduce the efficacy of oral contraceptives. Clonazepam, Ethosuximide, Felbamate, Gabapentin, Levetiracetam, Lamotrigine, Tiagabine, and VPA do not seem to interact with oral contraceptives. During the first months of oral contraceptive use, and once ovulation has been eliminated, complementary contraceptive methods are recommended. Non-hormonal contraceptive methods are not contraindicated in women with epilepsy. There is no evidence that combined-oral contraceptives increase seizures in women with epilepsy.

During menopause, 27% of the epileptic women had improvement, 33% did not modify their seizure pattern, and 40% worsened. Monitoring for osteoporosis is recommended, particularly if treatment is with AEDs which reduce steroid hormone levels. According to the The European Menopause and Andropause Society (EMAS) position statement, epileptic women starting hormone therapy should be closely monitored as their AED needs may change; calcium and vitamin D supplements should be considered, and herbal preparations should be avoided as their efficacy is uncertain and they may interact with AEDs (Erel et al, 2010).

8. References

Albright F, Smith PH, Fraser R. A syndrome characterized by primary ovarian insufficiency. Am J Med Sci 1942;204:625–648

Alper MM, Jolly EE, Garner PR. Pregnancies after premature ovarian failure. Obstet Gynecol 1986;67(3, Suppl):59S–62S

Balen A. Pathogenesis of polycystic ovary syndrome—the enigma unravels? Lancet 1999;354:966–7.

Bauer J, Cooper-Mahkorn D. Reproductive dysfunction in women with epilepsy: menstrual cycle abnormalities, fertility, and polycystic ovary syndrome. Int Rev Neurobiol 2008;83:135–55. 23.

Bauer J, Stoffel-Wagner B, Flügel D, Kluge M, Elger CE. The impact of epilepsy surgery on sex hormones and the menstrual cycle in female patients. Seizure 2000;6:389–93.

Bilo L, Meo R, Nappi C, et al. Reproductive endocrine disorders in women with primary generalized epilepsy. Epilepsia 1988;29:612–9.

Bliss SP, Navratil AM, Xie J, Roberson MS. GnRH signaling, the gonadotrope and endocrine control of fertility. Front Neuroendocrinol. 2010 Jul;31(3):322-40. Epub 2010 May 6.

Brodie MJ, Elder AT,KwanP. Epilepsy in later life. Lancet Neurol 2009;8:1019–30.

Burakgazi E, Harden C, Kelly JJ. Contraception for women with epilepsy. Rev Neurol Dis. 2009 Spring;6(2):E62-7.

Christensen J, Petrenaite V, Atterman J, Sidenius P, Ohman I, Tomson T, et al. Oral contraceptives induce lamotrigine metabolism: evidence from a double-blind, placebo-controlled trial. Epilepsia March 2007;48(3):484 – 9.

Compston JE, Yamaguchi K, Croucher PI et al. The effects of gonadotrophin-releasing hormone agonists on iliac crest cancellous bone structure in women with endometriosis. Bone 1995; 16: 261–267.

Compston JE. Bisphosphonates and atypical femoral fractures: a time for reflection. Maturitas. 2010 Jan;65(1):3-4. Epub 2009 Nov 22.

Compston JE. Sex steroids and bone. Physiological Reviews 2001; 81: 419–447.

Coulam CB, Adamson SC, Annegers JF. Incidence of premature ovarian failure. Obstet Gynecol 1986;67(4):604–606

Doose DR, Wang SS, Padmanabhan M, et al. Effect of topiramate or carbamazepine on the pharmacokinetics of an oral contraceptive containing norethindrone and ethinyl estradiol in healthy obese and nonobese female subjects. *Epilepsia.* 2003;44:540 -549.

Drezner MK. Treatment of anticonvulsant drug-induced bone disease. Epilepsy Behav 2004;5(February (Suppl. 2)):S41–7.

Dutton C, Foldvary-Schaefer N. Contraception in women with epilepsy: pharmacokinetic interactions, contraceptive options, and management. Int Rev Neurobiol. 2008;83:113-34.

Erel CT, Brincat M, Gambacciani M, Lambrinoudaki I, Moen MH, Schenck-Gustafsson K, Tremollieres F, Vujovic S, Rozenberg S, Rees M. EMAS position statement: managing the menopause in women with epilepsy. Maturitas. 2010 Jul;66(3):327-8. Epub 2010 Apr 24.

Farhat G, Yamout B, Mikati MA, Demirjian S, Sawaya R, El-Hajj Fuleihan G. Effect of antiepileptic drugs on bone density in ambulatory patients. Neurology 2002;58:1348–53.

Frye CA. Hormonal influences on seizures: basic neurobiology. Int Rev Neurobiol 2008;83:27–77.

Galimberti CA, Mazzucchelli I, Arbasino C, Canevini MP, Fattore C, Perucca E. Increased apparent oral clearance of valproic acid during intake of combined contraceptive steroids in women with epilepsy. Epilepsia September 2006;47 (9):1569 – 72.

Genant HK, Cann CE, Ettinger B & Gilbert SG. Quantitative computed tomography of vertebral spongiosa: a sensitive method for detecting early bone loss after oophorectomy. Annals of Internal Medicine 1982; 97: 699–705.

Gerendai I, Halasz B. Neuroendocrine asymmetry. Front Neuroendocrinol 1997;18:354–81.

Gold EB, Bromberger J, Crawford S, et al. Factors associated with age at natural menopause in a multiethnic sample of midlife women. Am J Epidemiol 2001;153: 865–74.

Harden CL, Herzog AG, Nikolov BG, et al. Hormone replacement therapy in women with epilepsy: a randomized, double-blind, placebo-controlled study. Epilepsia 2006;47:1447–51.

Harden CL, Koppel BS, Herzog AG, et al. Seizure frequency is associated with age at menopause in women with epilepsy. Neurology 2003;61:451–5.

Herzog AG, Coleman AE, Jacobs AR, et al. Interictal EEG discharges, reproductive hormones and menstrual disorders in epilepsy. Ann Neurol 2003;54:625–37.

Herzog AG, Farina EL, Blum AS. Serum valproate levels with oral contraceptive use. Epilepsia June 2005;46(6):970 – 1.

Herzog AG, Klein P, Ransil BJ. Three patterns of catamenial epilepsy. Epilepsia 1997;38:1082–8.

Herzog AG, Schachter SC. On the association between valproate and polycystic ovary syndrome. Epilepsia 2001;42:311–5.

Herzog AG, Seibel MM, Schomer DL, et al. Reproductive endocrine disorders in women with partial seizures of temporal lobe origin. Arch Neurol 1986;43:341–6.

Herzog AG. A hypothesis to integrate partial seizures of temporal lobe origin and reproductive disorders. Epilepsy Res 1989;3:151–9.

Herzog AG. Disorders of reproduction in patients with epilepsy: primary neurological mechanisms. Seizure 2008;17:101–10.

Herzog AG. Is there a lateralized asymmetry in the sensitivity of the brain to hormones in epilepsy? Epilepsy Behav 2007;11:157–9.

Herzog AG. Reproductive endocrine regulation in men with epilepsy: effects on reproductive function and neuronal excitability. Ann Neurol 2002;51:539–42.

Hom AC, Buterbaugh GG. Estrogen alters the acquisition of seizures kindled by repeated amygdala stimulation or pentylenetetrazol administration in ovariectomized female rats. *Epilepsia* 1986;27:103–108

Isojärvi J. Disorders of reproduction in patients with epilepsy: antiepileptic drug related mechanisms. Seizure 2008;17:111–9.

Isojarvi JI, Laatkainen TJ, Pakarinen AJ, et al. Polycystic ovaries and hyperandrogenism in women taking valproate for epilepsy. N Engl J Med 1993;329:1383–8.

Isojärvi JIT, Tauboll E, Herzog A. Effect of entiepileptic drugs on reproductive endocrine function in individuals with antiepileptic. CNS Drugs 2005;19:207–23.

Kalantaridou SN, Nelson LM. Premature ovarian failure is not premature menopause. Ann N Y Acad Sci 2000;900:393–402

Klein P, Serje A, Pezzullo JC. Premature ovarian failure in women with epilepsy. Epilepsia 2001;42:1584–9.

Knobil E, The neuroendocrine control of the menstrual cycle, Recent Prog. Horm. Res. 1980,(36):53–88.

Knochenhauer ES, Key TJ, Kahsar-Miller M, et al. Prevalence of the polycystic ovary syndrome in unselected black and white women of the southeastern United States: a prospective study. J Clin Endocrinol Metab 1998;83:3078–82.

Kodaman PH. Early menopause: primary ovarian insufficiency and surgical menopause. Semin Reprod Med. 2010 Sep;28(5):360-9. Epub 2010 Sep 15.

Kokate TG, Svenssonn BE, Rogawski MA. Anticonvulsant activity of neurosteroids: correlation with gamma-aminobutyric acid-evoked chloride current potentiation. J Pharmacol Exp Ther 1994;270:1223 – 9.

Kuhl H. Pharmacology of estrogens and progestogens: influence of different routes of administration. Climacteric, August 2005;8(Suppl. 1):3 – 63.

Lavaque E, Sierra A, Azcoitia I, Garcia-Segura LM. Steroidogenic acute regulatory protein in the brain. Neuroscience 2006;138:741 – 7.

Luef G, Abraham I, Haslinger M, et al. Polycystic ovaries, obesity and insulin resistance in women with epilepsy: a comparative study of carbamazepine and valproic acid in 105 women. J Neurol 2002;249:835-41.

Luef G, Rauchenzauner M. Epilepsies in girls and women. In: Panayatopoulos CP, editor. The educational kit on epilepsies. Oxford: Medicinae Press; 2008. p. 73-82.

Luef G. Female issues in epilepsy: A critical review. Epilepsy Behav 2009;15:78-82.

Mayor S. NICE gives guidance on use of new antiepileptic drugs in children. *BMJ.* 2004;328:1093.

McEwen B. Estrogen actions throughout the brain. *Recent Prog Horm Res* 2002;57:357-384.

Morrell MJ. The new antiepileptic drugs and women: efficacy, reproductive health, pregnancy, and fetal outcome. *Epilepsia.* 1996;37(Suppl 6):S34 -S44.

Murialdo G, Galimberti CA, Magri F, et al. Menstrual cycle and ovary alterations in women with epilepsy on antiepileptic therapy. J Endocrinol Invest. 1997;9:519-26.

Nakumura NH, Rosell DR, Akama KT, McEwan BS. Estrogen and ovariectomy regulate mRNA and protein of glutamic acid decarboxylases and cation-chloride cotransporters in the adult rat hippocampus. Neuroendocrinology 2005;80:308 – 23. 19.

Nelson L, Anasti JN, Kimzey LM et al. Development of luteinized graafian follicles in patients with karyotypically normal spontaneous premature ovarian failure. J Clin Endocrinol Metab 1994;79:1470-1475

Nelson LM. Clinical practice. Primary ovarian insufficiency. N Engl J Med 2009;360(6):606-614

Pack A. Bone health in people with epilepsy: is it impaired and what are the risk factors? Seizure 2008;17:181-6.

Pack AM, Morrell MJ, Marcus R, et al. Bone mass and turnover in women with epilepsy on antiepileptic drug monotherapy. Ann Neurol 2005;57:252-7.

Pack AM, Walczak TS. Bone health in women with epilepsy: clinical features and potential mechanisms. Int Rev Neurobiol 2008;83:305-28.

Panay N, Fenton A. Premature ovarian failure: a growing concern. Climacteric 2008;11(1):1-3

Perucca E. NICE guidance on newer drugs for epilepsy in adults. *BMJ.* 2004;328:1273-1274.

Petty SJ, O'Brien TJ, Wark JD. Anti-epileptic medication and bone health. Osteoporos Int 2007;18:129-42.

Rebar RW, Connolly HV. Clinical features of young women with hypergonadotropic amenorrhea. Fertil Steril 1990;53(5): 804-810

Rebar RW. Premature ovarian failure. Obstet Gynecol 2009; 113(6):1355-1363

Recker R, Lappe J, Davies KM & Heaney R. Characterisation of perimenopausal bone loss: a prospective study. Journal of Bone Mineral Research 2000; 15: 1965-1973.

Sabers A, Buchholt JM, Uldall P, Hansen EL. Lamotrigine plasma levels reduced by oral contraceptives. Epilepsy Res November 2001;47(1 – 2):151 – 4.

Sabers A, Ohman I, Christensen J, Tomson T. Oral contraceptives reduce lamotrigine plasma levels. Neurology August 26, 2003;61(4):570 – 1.

Santoro N. The menopausal transition. Am J Med. 2005 Dec 19;118 Suppl 12B:8-13.

Scharfman HE, Goodman JH, Rigoulot M-A, Berger RE,Walling SG, Mercurio TC, et al. Seizure susceptibility in intact and ovariectomized female rats treated with the convulsant pilocarpine. Exp Neurol 2005;196:73 – 86. 18.

Scharfman HE, MacLusky NJ. The influence of gonadal hormones on neuronal excitability, seizures, and epilepsy in the female. Epilepsia 2006;47:1423–30.

Schwenkhagen AM, Stodieck SR. Which contraception for women with epilepsy? Seizure. 2008 Mar;17(2):145-50. Epub 2008 Jan 4.

Shen W, Stearns V. Treatment strategies for hot flushes. Expert Opin Pharmacother 2009;10:1133–44.

Sheth RD, Binkley N, Hermann BP. Gender differences in bone mineral density in epilepsy. Epilepsia 2008;49:125–31. (a)

Sheth RD, Binkley N, Hermann BP. Progressive bone deficit in epilepsy. Neurology 2008;70:170–6. (b)

Sheth RD, Hermann BP. Bone in idiopathic and symptomatic epilepsy. Epilepsy Res 2008;78:71–6.

Sklar CA, Mertens AC, Mitby P, et al. Premature menopause in survivors of childhood cancer: a report from the childhood cancer survivor study. J Natl Cancer Inst 2006; 98(13):890–896

Sklar CA, Mertens AC, Mitby P, et al. Premature menopause in survivors of childhood cancer: a report from the childhood cancer survivor study. J Natl Cancer Inst 2006; 98(13):890–896

Souverein PC, Webb DJ, Petri H, Weil J, Van Staa TP, Egberts T. Incidence of fractures among epilepsy patients: a population-based retrospective cohort study in the General Practice Research Database. Epilepsia 2005;46:304–10.

Stodieck SRG, Schwenkhagen A. Lamotrigine plasma levels and combined monophasic oral contraceptives (COC) or a contraceptive vaginla ring. A prospective study in 30 women. Epilepsia 2004;45:187.

Tatum WOt, Liporace J, Benbadis SR, et al. Updates on the treatment of epilepsy in women. *Arch Intern Med.* 2004;164:137–145.

Tauboll E, Luef G. Gender issues in epilepsy-the science of why it is special. Seizure 2008;17:99–100.

Vainionpää LK, Rättyä J, Knip M, et al. Valproate-induced hyperandrogenism during pubertal maturation in girls with epilepsy. Ann Neurol 1999;44:444–50.

Veliskova J. Estrogens and epilepsy: why are we so excited? Neuroscientist 2007;13:77—88.

Verrotti A, Greco R, Morgese G, Chiarelli F. Increased bone turnover in epileptic patients treated with carbamazepine. Ann Neurol 2000;47:385–8.

Wallace H, Shorvon S, Tallis R. Age-specific incidence and prevalence rates of treated epilepsy in an unselected population of 2,052,922 and age-specific fertility rates of women with epilepsy. Lancet 1998;352:1970–3.

Welt CK. Primary ovarian insufficiency: a more accurate term for premature ovarian failure. Clin Endocrinol (Oxf) 2008;68(4):499–509

5

The Classification of Seizures and Epilepsy Syndromes

Leslie A. Rudzinski[1] and Jerry J. Shih[2]
[1]*Emory University School of Medicine,*
[2]*Mayo Clinic Florida*
U.S.A.

1. Introduction

Understanding the classification of epileptic seizures is the first step towards the correct diagnosis, treatment and prognostication of the condition. The initial management of a patient with seizures begins with an understanding of the patient's seizure type and, if pertinent, epilepsy syndrome. Specific seizure types or syndromes often respond better to specific medications or surgical approaches. Some seizure types or syndromes carry a benign prognosis or high likelihood of seizure remission by a certain age. Other seizure syndromes may carry a far poorer prognosis, and early knowledge of this allows focused treatment and lifestyle modifications for patients and families.

The classification of epileptic seizures is still largely based on clinical observation and expert opinions. The International League Against Epilepsy (ILAE) first published a classification system in 1960. The last official update for seizures was published in 1981, and the last official update for the epilepsies was in 1989. By definition, epilepsy is diagnosed after a patient has two or more unprovoked seizures. The 1981 and 1989 updates form the officially accepted classification system, although there continues to be efforts to develop a clinically meaningful revision to the current system. A report in 2010 by the ILAE Commission on Classification and Terminology recommended that changes be made in the current conceptualization, terminology, and definitions of seizures and epilepsy. This chapter will focus primarily on the currently accepted standard based on the 1981 and 1989 reports, and discuss the recommendations of the 2010 ILAE report.

2. The classification of epileptic seizures

2.1 Partial seizures

Partial or focal seizures comprise one of the two main classes of epileptic seizures, with generalized seizures being the other. Partial seizures are subdivided between simple and complex partial seizures, which are distinguished by the presence or absence of impairment of consciousness. Simple partial seizures are defined as seizures without impairment of consciousness while complex partial seizures are defined as seizures with impairment of consciousness. Consciousness is defined as the "degree of awareness and/or responsiveness of the patient to externally applied stimuli". Responsiveness refers to the ability of the patient to respond to external stimuli, and awareness refers to the recall of events occurring during the ictal period. These two features of consciousness are usually tested during and after a seizure in an epilepsy monitoring unit. A patient may be able to follow commands during a seizure, but may not be able to recall portions of the event afterwards, which indicates intact responsiveness but impaired awareness.

Partial seizures manifest themselves in many different forms, depending on which area of the cortex is involved in the onset and spread of the ictal discharge. Partial seizures originate from a focal area of cerebral cortex and may spread to other cortical regions either unilaterally or bilaterally. A partial seizure may manifest with motor signs, autonomic symptoms, somatosensory or special sensory symptoms, or psychic symptoms. The term aura comes from the Latin word "breeze" and is synonymous with a simple partial sensory or psychic seizure. An aura often reflects the location of the seizure onset zone, although there are exceptions.

2.1.1 Simple partial seizures

Focal motor seizures can originate in the precentral gyrus or spread to the precentral gyrus from neighboring cortical regions. They can remain focal, causing right hand clonic activity for example, or can spread or "march" along the motor strip involving different areas of the motor homunculus. This type of seizure is known as a "Jacksonian seizure" and often clinically manifests as clonic activity originating in the hand and then marching up the ipsilateral arm, shoulder, face, and leg. After a focal motor seizure, post-ictal weakness (Todd's paralysis) can last for minutes to hours. The mechanism of Todd's paralysis is thought to be either from "neuronal exhaustion due to the increased metabolic activity of the discharging focus" or from "increased inhibition in the region of the focus." Epilepsia Partialis Continua (EPC) is defined as a continuous focal motor seizure which remains confined to a specific body part and usually consists of clonic movements which can persist for up to months with preserved consciousness (1981). EPC can be seen in Rasmussen Syndrome, focal lesions (cortical dysplasia, vascular lesions, or tumors), nonketotic hyperglycemia, and some inborn errors of metabolism (MERRF) (Engel, 2006).

In a series of 14 patients with focal motor seizures who underwent epilepsy surgery at Mayo Clinic, 11 patients were seizure-free post operatively (Sandok & Cascino, 1998). Other types of focal motor seizures originating from the language area include those with a motor speech arrest or vocalization. Versive seizures originating from the dorsolateral frontal cortex (frontal eye fields) involve contralateral head, eye, or trunk deviation. Tonic seizures originating from the SMA (supplementary motor area) involve abrupt bilateral or asymmetric posturing usually of the contralateral arm, where sometimes the contralateral arm is abducted, externally rotated, and elevated and the head is also deviated contralaterally. This has been termed the "fencing posture" or M2e sign. Consciousness is usually preserved.

Simple partial seizures can also have autonomic symptoms such as vomiting, sweating, piloerection, pupil dilation, pallor, flushing, borborygmi, and incontinence. Simple partial seizures with somatosensory symptoms originating from the post central gyrus may include feelings of focal paresthesias ("pins and needles"), numbness, warmth, or electrical shock-like sensations which can also spread like Jacksonian seizures (a sensory Jacksonian march). Simple partial seizures with somatosensory symptoms can also originate from the secondary sensory area which lies above the Sylvian fissure anterior to the precentral gyrus. Secondary sensory seizures are characterized by more widespread involvement of the sensation (contralateral, ipsilateral, and bilateral involvement) and may include symptoms of feeling cold, pain, or the desire to move (Penfield W et. al., 1950). Sensory seizures can also originate from the supplementary sensory area, which is just posterior to the supplementary motor area, and involve tingling, the desire for movement, feeling stiff, pulling, pulsing, and heaviness (Lim et al.,

1994). Finally, sensory seizures can also originate from the insular cortex. The symptoms often involve the naso-oropharyngeal-laryngeal regions and consist of throat paresthesias, warmth, tightening, or a sense of strangulation or suffocation (Nguyen et al., 2009).

Simple partial seizures with special sensory symptoms include visual, auditory, gustatory, olfactory, and vertiginous symptoms. Visual seizures can originate from primary visual cortex and consist of primary visual hallucinations such as flashing lights, spots, stars, or circles of colored light which can appear in the contralateral visual field or directly ahead. More complex visual hallucinations originate from visual association cortex and can include seeing persons or scenes. One patient described seeing Fred Flintstone and The Gingerbread Man at the onset of seizures. Post-ictal darkness or blindness can follow simple visual seizures. Auditory seizures which arise from the lateral temporal region, specifically the superior temporal gyrus and Heschl's gyrus, can include the clinical symptoms of buzzing, ringing, hearing a rushing sound, hyper- or hypoacusis, sound distortion, or hearing words or music. Olfactory seizures originating from the uncinate gyrus or mesial temporal region typically involve smelling unpleasant odors such as burning rubber, smoke, or sulfur. Gustatory sensations originating from the temporal lobe, insula, or parietal operculum can be pleasant or unpleasant and usually are described as a metallic taste but can also be bitter or sweet. On rare occasions, vertiginous symptoms may also be a type of simple partial seizure which originates from the lateral temporal region.

Simple partial seizures with psychic symptoms indicate a disturbance of higher cortical function. For example, dysphasic symptoms include expressive or receptive language disturbances and may involve repetition of a word or phrase (epileptic palilalia). Dysmnesic symptoms involve a distortion of memory and include déjà vu, jamais-vu, déjà-entendu, jamais- entendu, autoscopy, or panoramic vision (see Table 1). Other cognitive disturbances such as dreamy states, distorted time sense, derealization, or a sense of unreality may be present. Emotional symptoms include pleasure, fear, or anger which occurs in paroxysms lasting seconds to minutes. Illusions may be present which result in distorted perceptions of the person him or herself or objects around him or her. Structured hallucinations can take the form of music or scenes and may affect multiple sensory modalities (somatosensory, visual, olfactory, or gustatory). Primitive hallucinations originate from the corresponding primary sensory area whereas more complex and elaborate hallucinations originate from the corresponding association cortices. Psychic auras often originate from the temporal lobe.

Psychic Aura	Definition
Déjà vu	An illusion of a familiar memory
Jamais vu	When what should be a familiar visual experience becomes unfamiliar
Déjà entendu	An auditory illusion of something familiar
Jamais entendu	When what should be a familiar auditory experience becomes unfamiliar
Autoscopy	Seeing oneself in external space, as if the mind has left the body
Derealization	A feeling of unreality of the outside world; the world seems strange and unreal
Depersonalization	A feeling of unreality in one's sense of self; feeling as if in a dream or watching oneself act
Macro-/Micropsia	Objects appear larger or smaller than usual
Macr-/Micracusia	Sounds are louder or softer than usual

Table 1. Psychic Auras

2.1.2 Complex partial seizures

Complex partial seizures are partial seizures with impairment of consciousness. They may start as simple partial seizures (auras) and progress to complex partial seizures or may begin as complex partial seizures with impairment of consciousness at the onset of the seizure. They may or may not involve automatisms. The clinical features of the complex partial seizure depend on the region affected by abnormal electrical activity. Complex partial seizures usually originate in the frontal or temporal lobes but can occur in the parietal or occipital lobes.

3. Generalized seizures

Absence Seizures are characterized by a sudden onset behavioral arrest, a blank stare, unresponsiveness, and sometimes a brief upward rotation of the eyes. The duration is typically a few seconds to half a minute. There is little to no post-ictal confusion, and the patient typically resumes the activity he/she was doing prior to the seizures. This seizure type is also referred to as simple absence. The ILAE's 1981 classification also recognizes five subtypes of absence seizures: absence with impairment of consciousness only, with mild clonic components, with atonic components, with tonic components, and with automatisms. In absence with mild clonic components, there are subtle clonic movements of the eyelids, corner of the mouth, or upper extremities sometimes at a frequency of 3 Hz. In absence with atonic components, there is a loss of postural tone causing the head to drop, the trunk to slump forward, the arms to drop, or the grip to relax. Falls are rare. In absence with tonic components, tonic muscle contraction of the trunk and neck extensors may cause the head to extend and the trunk to arch, thus causing retropulsion. Tonic contraction of the neck muscles may cause the head or trunk to deviate to one side. In absence with automatisms, the patient engages in purposeful or semipurposeful repetitive movements while consciousness is impaired. Examples of automatisms may include lip licking, chewing, lip smacking, swallowing, grimacing, smiling, yawning, fumbling with the hands, picking, scratching, rubbing, or aimless walking. Absence with autonomic phenomena is another subtype with signs of tachycardia, pallor, flushing, piloerection, salivation, or urinary incontinence. A mixture of clonic, atonic, tonic, automatic, and autonomic features may occur which is also referred to as complex absence. The ictal EEG pattern in absence seizures is a 3 Hz generalized monomorphic spike and wave with abrupt onset and termination. Absence seizures in the EEG laboratory can be precipitated by hyperventilation and less commonly photic stimulation.

Atypical absence seizures are usually seen in patients with symptomatic generalized epilepsy. They are similar to absence seizures in that they have both simple and complex presentations. One distinguishing feature is that they are less abrupt in onset clinically. The seizures are usually less than 10 seconds but may be prolonged and result in absence status. They also are not usually induced by hyperventilation or photic stimulation. The ictal EEG pattern consists of a less monomorphic slow spike and wave discharge characterized by a blunt sharp wave and occurs at a frequency of < 2.5 Hz.

Tonic-clonic seizures, also known as grand mal seizures, are characterized by abrupt loss of consciousness followed by tonic contraction of the muscles. This leads to the ictal cry, where air is forcefully expired against a closed glottis. The mouth is forcefully closed which can result in a tongue bite. The pupils become dilated and the eyes deviate upwards. The upper extremities often symmetrically abduct and flex at the elbows while the lower extremities may briefly flex and then extend and adduct with the toes pointed. Clonic activity then ensues which is initially rapid and then slows. Gasping respirations occur as the respiratory muscles are involved in the clonic activity. The patient may become cyanotic. Urinary incontinence may occur. At the end of the seizure, the patient is unconscious for a brief period of time and then gradually recovers. Patients typically report generalized muscle soreness and sometimes a headache post-ictally.

Tonic-clonic seizures may occur independently, may arise from other generalized seizures, or may occur during secondary generalization of a partial onset seizure. The semiologic features of tonic-clonic seizures in primary generalized epilepsy may be bilaterally symmetric or may involve a forced head deviation to either side (Ochs et al., 1984). During secondarily generalized partial onset seizures, patients often assume a figure-4 posture where the contralateral arm extends, and the ipsilateral arm flexes at the elbow. This posture can occur with the legs as well. Tonic-clonic seizures may lead to injuries such as burns, head injuries, vertebral compression fractures, shoulder dislocations, and tongue and cheek lacerations.

Myoclonic seizures are generalized seizures characterized by brief, irregular, shock-like jerks of the head, trunk, or limbs. They can be symmetric or asymmetric and involve the whole body, regions of the body, or focal areas. They tend to occur close to sleep onset and upon awakening from sleep. Myoclonic seizures can be a feature of some idiopathic generalized epilepsies (Juvenile Myoclonic Epilepsy), symptomatic generalized epilepsies (Myoclonic-Astatic Epilepsy), the progressive myoclonic epilepsies (Lafora Disease), and infantile spasms. Myoclonus can be positive or negative. Negative myoclonus refers to the brief loss of postural tone when the body part is held against gravity. Consciousness is not impaired and there is no post-ictal confusion with single myoclonic jerks. Myoclonic seizures can occur in clusters and evolve into clonic-tonic-clonic seizures, with resultant loss of consciousness and postictal confusion. The ictal EEG pattern is characterized by brief generalized polyspike or polyspike and wave discharges which corresponds to the myoclonic jerk.

Tonic seizures are seizures which involve tonic contraction of the face, neck, axial, or appendicular musculature lasting from 10 seconds to one minute. They can involve extension or flexion of the muscles and often lead to falls and head injuries. They may be more subtle and involve only upward eye deviation. They often occur out of NREM sleep. They are usually seen in patients with symptomatic generalized epilepsy and are one of the common seizure types in patients with Lennox-Gastaut syndrome. They can also occur in epilepsy with myoclonic-astatic seizures. The ictal EEG usually shows a brief generalized attenuation of cerebral activity followed by generalized paroxysmal fast activity in the beta frequency range.

Clonic seizures are generalized seizures that are characterized by repetitive rhythmic clonic jerks (1-2 Hz) with impairment of consciousness and a short post-ictal phase. They can lead into a clonic-tonic-clonic seizure. It is thought that the repetitive discharges are due to rhythmic excitatory discharges from the cortex (1981; Engel, 2006). The ictal EEG demonstrates generalized polyspike and wave discharges or generalized fast activity.

Atonic seizures are characterized by a sudden loss of muscle tone which can lead to a head drop, a limb drop, or a drop of the whole body (a.k.a. – a drop attack). There is a brief loss of consciousness and injuries, particularly to the face, may occur (1981). Atonic seizures last less than 5 seconds, and there is minimal post-ictal confusion. Atonic seizures may be preceded by a brief myoclonic jerk or tonic component. Atypical absence seizures may have an atonic component. The criteria distinguishing between negative myoclonus, atonic seizures, and some atypical absences still needs to be developed (Engel 2006). Atonic seizures are usually seen in the symptomatic generalized epilepsies such as Lennox-Gastaut syndrome. The ictal EEG typically shows a high voltage spike and wave or slow wave followed by a generalized attenuation of cerebral activity or low voltage paroxysmal fast activity.

4. Unclassified epileptic seizures

This category listed in the ILAE's Classification of Epileptic Seizures (1981) includes all seizures that defy classification due to incomplete data. An example is seizure in infancy, which may involve chewing, swimming movements, eye movements, jittering, and apnea, and have not yet been subtyped.

5. The classification of epilepsies and epileptic syndromes

An epileptic disorder can be symptomatic, idiopathic, or cryptogenic. Symptomatic is a term that means the etiology is known—usually a structural lesion within the brain. Idiopathic is a term that refers to an epilepsy of presumed genetic etiology without a structural brain lesion or other neurological signs or symptoms. Cryptogenic is a term that refers to an epilepsy that is presumed to be symptomatic but the etiology is unknown (1989). The term cryptogenic has been replaced by "probably symptomatic"(Engel, 2001). The 1989 classification system is divided into four main categories: localization-related (focal, local, or partial), generalized, epilepsies and syndromes undetermined whether focal or generalized, and special syndromes (see Table 2).

1. Localization-related epilepsies and syndromes

1.1 Idiopathic
- Benign childhood epilepsy with centrotemporal spikes
- Childhood epilepsy with occipital paroxysms
- Primary reading epilepsy

1.2 Symptomatic
- Chronic progressive epilepsia partialis continua of childhood (Kojewnikow's syndrome)
- Syndromes characterized by seizures with specific modes of precipitation
- Temporal lobe epilepsies
- Frontal lobe epilepsies
- Parietal lobe epilepsies
- Occipital lobe epilepsies

1.3 Cryptogenic

2. Generalized epilepsies and syndromes

2.1 Idiopathic
- Benign neonatal familial convulsions
- Benign neonatal convulsions
- Benign myoclonic epilepsy in infancy
- Childhood absence epilepsy

- Juvenile absence epilepsy
- Juvenile myoclonic epilepsy
- Epilepsy with GTCS on awakening
- Other generalized idiopathic epilepsies not defined above
- Epilepsies with seizures precipitated by specific modes of activation

2.2 Cryptogenic or symptomatic

- West syndrome
- Lennox-Gastaut syndrome
- Epilepsy with myoclonic-astatic seizures
- Epilepsy with myoclonic absences

2.3 Symptomatic

2.3.1 Non-specific etiology

- Early myoclonic encephalopathy
- Early infantile epileptic encephalopathy with suppression burst
- Other symptomatic generalized epilepsies not defined above

2.3.2 Specific syndromes

- Diseases in which seizures are a presenting or predominant feature

3. Epilepsies and syndromes undetermined whether focal or generalized

3.1 With both generalized and focal seizures

- Neonatal seizures
- Severe myoclonic epilepsy in infancy
- Epilepsy with continuous spike-waves during slow wave sleep
- Acquired epileptic aphasia (Landau-Kleffner syndrome)
- Other undetermined epilepsies not defined above

3.2 Without unequivocal generalized or focal features (i.e. - Sleep related GTCS; when the EEG shows both focal and generalized ictal or interictal discharges, and when focal or generalized onset cannot be determined clinically)

4. Special syndromes

4.1 Situation-related seizures

- Febrile convulsions
- Isolated seizures or isolated status epilepticus
- Seizures occurring only when there is an acute metabolic or toxic event (alcohol, drugs, eclampsia, nonketotic hyperglycemia)

Table 2. ILAE's 1989 International Classification of Epilepsies and Epileptic Syndromes, from (1989). Proposal for revised classification of epilepsies and epileptic syndromes. Commission on Classification and Terminology of the International League Against Epilepsy. *Epilepsia,* Vol. 30, No. 4, (August 1989), pp. 389-99, ISSN 1528-1167

An epilepsy syndrome is defined as "a complex of signs and symptoms that define a unique epilepsy condition" (Engel, 2001). The groups of syndromes are: idiopathic focal epilepsies of infancy and childhood, familial (autosomal dominant) focal epilepsies, symptomatic (or probably symptomatic) focal epilepsies, idiopathic generalized epilepsies, reflex epilepsies, epileptic encephalopathies, progressive myoclonus epilepsies, and seizures not necessarily requiring a diagnosis of epilepsy (see Table 3). There are over 25 specific syndromes in the 1989 ILAE report. A discussion regarding a few of the more common syndromes affecting adolescents and adults follows.

Groups of syndromes	Specific syndromes
Idiopathic focal epilepsies of infancy and childhood	Benign infantile seizures • Benign childhood epilepsy with centrotemporal spikes • Early-onset benign childhood occipital epilepsy • Late-onset childhood occipital epilepsy
Familial (autosomal dominant) focal epilepsies	Benign familial neonatal seizures Benign familial infantile seizures Autosomal dominant nocturnal frontal lobe epilepsy Familial temporal lobe epilepsy Familial focal epilepsy with variable foci*
Symptomatic (or probably symptomatic) focal epilepsies	Limbic epilepsies • Mesial temporal lobe epilepsy with hippocampal sclerosis • Mesial temporal lobe epilepsy defined by specific etiologies • Other types defined by location and etiology Neocortical epilepsies • Rasmussen syndrome • Hemiconvulsion-hemiplegia syndrome • Other types defined by location and etiology • Migrating partial seizures of early infancy*
Idiopathic generalized epilepsies	Benign myoclonic epilepsy in infancy Epilepsy with myoclonic astatic seizures Childhood absence epilepsy Epilepsy with myoclonic absences Idiopathic generalized epilepsies with variable phenotypes • Juvenile absence epilepsy • Juvenile myoclonic epilepsy • Epilepsy with GTCS only Generalized epilepsies with febrile seizures plus*
Reflex epilepsies	Idiopathic photosensitive occipital lobe epilepsy Other visual sensitive epilepsies Primary reading epilepsy Startle epilepsy

Groups of syndromes	Specific syndromes
Epileptic encephalopathies	Early myoclonic encephalopathy Ohtahara syndrome West syndrome Dravet syndrome Lennox-Gastaut syndrome Landau-Kleffner syndrome Epilepsy with continuous spike-waves during slow-wave sleep
Progressive myoclonic epilepsies	Ceroid lipofuscinosis Sialidosis Lafora disease Unverricht-Lundborg disease Neuroaxonal dystrophy MERRF Dentatorubropallidoluysian atrophy
Seizures not necessarily requiring a diagnosis of epilepsy	Benign neonatal seizures Febrile seizures Reflex seizures Alcohol-withdrawal seizures Drug or other chemically induced seizures Immediate and early posttraumatic seizures Single seizures or isolated clusters of seizures Rarely repeated seizures (oligoepilepsy)

* Syndromes in development

Table 3. An Example of a Classification of Epilepsy Syndromes, from Engel, J., Jr. (2001). A proposed diagnostic scheme for People with epileptic seizures and with epilepsy: report of the ILAE Task Force on Classification and Terminology. *Epilepsia*, Vol.42, No. 6, (June 2001), pp. 796-803, ISSN 1528-1167

5.1 Temporal lobe epilepsies

Temporal lobe seizures are the most common type of partial epilepsy. Temporal lobe seizures often begin with an aura (Quesney, 1986). Auras may include viscerosensory symptoms (epigastric sensation, thoracic sensation, and warm ascending sensation) or sensory illusions or hallucinations. The ictal event is usually characterized by a blank stare, loss of contact with the environment, oroalimentary or vocal automatisms, hand automatisms, upper limb tonic or dystonic posturing, early head or eye deviation, and dysphasia. Oroalimentary automatisms are defined as stereotyped, repetitive movements of the mouth, tongue, lips, or jaw which have the appearance of chewing or lip-smacking. They may also involve gulping, swallowing, or spitting. Hand automatisms are repetitive, purposeless movements of the hands including grasping, fumbling, and searching movements. Both oroalimentary and hand automatisms often localize to the mesial temporal lobe. Table 4 lists other ictal signs with localizing and lateralizing value. In terms of lateralization (determining right vs. left hemispheric involvement), unilateral automatisms and post-ictal dysphasia were determined to have the highest predicative value. Unilateral automatisms are typically ipsilateral to region of seizure onset, and post-ictal dysphasia lateralized to the dominant hemisphere (Chee et al., 1993). Nondominant temporal lobe seizures can have preservation of language and responsiveness with minimal post-ictal confusion. Patients with right temporal lobe epilepsy due to MTS (mesial temporal

Clinical Event	**Localization/Lateralization**
Head turn	
• Early non-forced	Ipsilateral temporal
• Forced	
Early forced	Frontal
Late forced	Contralateral temporal (in process of generalizing)
Ocular version	Contralateral occipital
Focal clonic	Contralateral peri-rolandic or temporal
Dystonic limb	Contralateral temporal > frontal
Unilateral tonic limb	Contralateral hemisphere
M2e sign (fencing posture)	Contralateral frontal > temporal
Figure 4	Contralateral hemisphere (to extended arm)
Ictal paresis	Contralateral hemisphere
Todd's paresis	Contralateral hemisphere (extratemporal > temporal)
Unilateral blinking	Ipsilateral hemisphere
Unilateral limb automatism	Ipsilateral hemisphere
Postictal nose rubbing	Ipsilateral temporal > frontal (to hand used)
Postictal cough	Temporal
Bipedal automatisms	Frontal > temporal
Hypermotor	SMA (supplementary motor area)
Ictal spitting	Right temporal
Automatisms with preserved responsiveness	Right temporal
Gelastic	Hypothalamic, mesial temporal
Ictal vomiting/retching	Right temporal
Ictal urinary urge	Non-dominant temporal
Loud vocalization	Frontal > temporal
Ictal speech arrest	Temporal
Ictal speech preservation	Non-dominant hemisphere
Post-ictal aphasia	Language-dominant hemisphere

Table 4. Localization and Lateralization of Ictal Seizure Semiology

sclerosis) may be able to speak normally during the seizure. Patients with left temporal lobe seizures due to MTS often make prominent paraphasic errors during and after seizures. Specific semiological features are also helpful in distinguishing between mesial, mesial-lateral, and lateral temporal lobe epilepsy. Mesial temporal lobe seizures are often characterized by an initial epigastric sensation or viscerosensory sensation, fear, a dreamy state, longer seizure duration, delayed loss of contact, and delayed oroalimentary and upper limb automatisms while lateral temporal lobe seizures are characterized by an initial sensory illusion or hallucination (mainly auditory), an initial loss of contact, a shorter duration (< 1 minute), and frequent secondary generalizations. The mesial-lateral temporal lobe seizures were similar to the mesial temporal seizures but had an earlier loss of contact and earlier oroalimentary, verbal, and vocal automatisms (Maillard et al., 2004). It is important to distinguish between mesial (limbic) and lateral (neocortical) temporal lobe epilepsy if one is considering a surgical option such as a temporal lobectomy, as postsurgical seizure-freedom and complication rates differ.

5.2 Frontal lobe epilepsies

Frontal lobe seizures are the second most common type of focal epilepsy and occur in approximately 30% of patients with partial epilepsy (Bancaud & Talairach, 1992). Frontal lobe seizures are often confused with pseudoseizures due to the bizarre clinical semiology. Frontal lobe seizures are usually brief (less than 30 seconds), tend to occur in clusters, can occur multiple times per day, and often have minimal or no post-ictal confusion. The clinical semiology includes an abrupt onset of stereotyped hypermotor behavior and may include vocalizations, gestural or sexual automatisms, and bilateral leg automatisms consisting of pedaling or bicycling movements. The seizure semiology of frontal lobe seizures varies depending on what region of the frontal lobe is involved. The patient may have asymmetric tonic extension of the proximal extremities, as in SMA seizures, or clonic activity of the contralateral limb, as in seizures from the lateral convexity. Seizures originating from the mesial frontal region or SMA are characterized by vocalizations and abrupt tonic extension of the proximal extremities which may be bilateral and is often asymmetric. There is minimal impairment of consciousness or post-ictal confusion. Lateral dorsal frontal lobe seizures are characterized by speech arrest, forced thinking, contraversive head and eye deviation, and automatisms such as laughing, crying, sniffing, chewing, or kicking. Orbitofrontal seizures are characterized by prominent autonomic symptoms (flushing, mydriasis, tachycardia), automatisms, and loud vocalizations. They can also appear similar to mesial temporal lobe seizures due to rapid spread to this region. Cingulate gyrus seizures are similar to SMA seizures but also involve behavioral arrest, oroalimentary automatisms, gestural or sexual automatisms, mood changes, and sometimes urinary incontinence. Because of the extensive inter-regional connectivity within the frontal lobe and rapid seizure propagation, frontal lobe seizures are difficult to localize on the basis of clinical semiology.

5.3 Parietal lobe epilepsies

Parietal lobe seizures account for < 10% of focal seizures. Often they arise from clinically silent areas and only manifest symptoms when the seizure spreads to other functional cortical regions. They can spread to the occipital, temporal, or frontal regions. Clinically, patients may report somatosensory symptoms, most commonly in the face and hand, contralateral to the seizure focus. In nondominant parietal lobe seizures, patients can have spatial neglect of the contralateral body or environment. In dominant parietal lobe seizures, patients may have language dysfunction.

5.4 Occipital lobe epilepsies

Occipital lobe seizures also account for < 10% of focal seizures. They are characterized by elementary visual hallucinations of fixed or moving flashing white or colored lights which start in the contralateral visual field and can spread to the entire visual field. Patients may also report a "whiting out" or "blacking out" of their vision. The eyes may deviate contralaterally, and the eyelids may rapidly blink. The remainder of the seizure is characterized by where the seizure discharge spreads. If the seizure spreads to the posterior temporal region (area of visual association cortex), complex visual hallucinations may occur. Occipital seizures may also spread to the mesial temporal, parietal, and perirolandic regions and mimic seizures of those regions.

5.5 Autosomal dominant nocturnal frontal lobe epilepsy

Autosomal Dominant Nocturnal Frontal Lobe Epilepsy (ADNFLE) is a familial autosomal dominant focal epilepsy characterized by clusters of brief seizures (5-30 seconds) during NREM sleep (stages N2 and N3). They are often initially misdiagnosed as nightmares or parasomnias. The mean age of onset is around 12 years of age (range 1-30). The seizures themselves are characterized by brief motor attacks, usually with a dystonic or dyskinetic component. During a seizure patients may have complex and bizarre behaviors, shouting, bimanual and bipedal automatisms, mumbling, urinary incontinence, and rarely violent behavior. The ictal EEG may demonstrate a frontally predominant ictal discharge in approximately 30% of patients and focal background attenuation or focal rhythmic slowing over the anterior head regions in about 55% of patients (Oldani et al., 1998). The CHRNA4 gene on chromosome 20, which encodes the neuronal nicotinic acetylcholine receptor (nAChR) alpha 4 subunit, is mutated in patients with ADNFLE type 1. The CHRNB2 gene on chromosome 1 is mutated in patients with ADNFLE type 3. The molecular pathogenesis of how these mutations cause ADNFLE is unknown (Hirose et al., 2005).

5.6 Autosomal dominant partial epilepsy with auditory features

Autosomal Dominant Partial Epilepsy with Auditory Features (ADPEAF) or Autosomal Dominant Lateral Temporal Epilepsy (ADLTE) is also a familial autosomal dominant focal epilepsy characterized by lateral temporal lobe epilepsy and auditory aura. It is due to a mutation in the LGI1 gene (leucine-rich glioma-inactivated 1 gene) which is expressed in neurons in the neocortex and limbic regions (Hirose et al., 2005). Mutations in the LGI1 gene have been found in 50% of families with this type of epilepsy (Ottman et al., 2004). The age of onset is between 1 and 60 years with a mean of 18 years. The seizures are characterized by auditory auras (64%), complex visual (17%), psychic (16%), autonomic (12%), vertiginous (9%), other sensory (13%), and aphasia (17%). The majority of auditory auras are simple in nature (humming, buzzing, ringing). A minority of patients report complex hallucinations such as music or voices. The MRI of the brain is normal, and patients typically have a good response to treatment with antiepileptic drugs (Michelucci, 2003, 2009).

5.7 Mesial temporal lobe epilepsy with hippocampal sclerosis

Mesial temporal lobe epilepsy with hippocampal sclerosis (MTLE-HS) is a symptomatic focal epilepsy and subcategorized as a limbic epilepsy (vs. neocortical epilepsy). Mesial temporal lobe epilepsy is one of the most common types of epilepsy referred for epilepsy surgery and is often refractory to AEDs. The age of onset is between late childhood to mid adolescence. Patients often had febrile convulsions in infancy or early childhood. Most patients report an aura. Common auras include an epigastric sensation (a rising sensation, butterflies, nausea), fear, olfactory hallucinations, lightheadedness, and déjà vu (French et al., 1993). Complex partial seizure semiology may also consist of ipsilateral upper extremity automatisms and ipsilateral early non-forced head turn. Contralateral dystonic posturing, Todd's paralysis, and late forced head turn prior to secondary generalization can also be seen.

Hippocampal sclerosis is the most common pathological substrate found in patients with medial temporal lobe epilepsy who undergo surgical resection. Hippocampal sclerosis is strongly associated with prolonged febrile seizures in childhood, but the cause is still unknown. The majority of patients who undergo surgical resection for MTLE-HS become seizure free (Ozkara et al., 2008). Is an example of a patient with right mesial temporal sclerosis who was rendered seizure-free after a right temporal lobectomy.

5.8 Juvenile absence epilepsy

Juvenile absence epilepsy (JAE) is classified as an idiopathic generalized epilepsy. The age of onset is typically at or after puberty between the ages of 10-17. Unlike in childhood absence epilepsy (CAE) where absence seizures can occur hundreds of times per day, absence seizures in JAE may only occur sporadically. There is less impairment of consciousness with absence seizures in JAE compared to absences in CAE. Patients with JAE can have generalized tonic-clonic seizures (usually upon awakening), myoclonic seizures, and even absence status epilepticus. The ictal EEG pattern resembles that of CAE (3 Hz spike and wave) but the discharges tend to vary slightly in frequency (usually > 3 Hz), are more irregular, and include more polyspike discharges. There is a strong genetic component with linkage to chromosomes 5, 8, 18, and 21. The response to antiepileptic medication is usually excellent (Beghi et al., 2006).

5.9 Juvenile myoclonic epilepsy

Juvenile Myoclonic Epilepsy (JME) is also classified as an idiopathic generalized epilepsy. The age of onset is in the mid-teens between the ages of 12-18. Patients may present with myoclonic jerks upon awakening in the morning. Patients may first ignore the myoclonic jerks, often attributing them to clumsiness. Sometimes the diagnosis is not made until the patient has a generalized tonic-clonic seizure. The myoclonus usually involves the neck, shoulders, arms, or legs with the upper extremities being more frequently affected. Consciousness is usually not impaired during the myoclonic seizures. Generalized tonic-clonic and absence seizures are also seen. Generalized tonic-clonic seizures may also occur in the morning upon awakening and can be triggered by sleep deprivation, alcohol, and stress. Often, several myoclonic jerks may precede a generalized tonic-clonic seizure, which is known as a clonic-tonic-clonic seizure. Approximately 50% of patients can be photosensitive. The ictal EEG consists of generalized polyspike and wave discharges > 3 Hz. There is a strong genetic component with linkage to chromosomes 2, 3, 5, 6, and 15. The response to AED treatment is excellent but needs to be continued lifelong in most patients due to a high rate of relapse (Beghi et al., 2006).

5.10 Epilepsy with generalized tonic clonic seizures (GTCS) on awakening

This syndrome is also known as Epilepsy with generalized tonic-clonic seizures only and is classified as one of the idiopathic generalized epilepsies. The age of onset is the second decade of life. GTCS occur > 90% of the time, with absence and myoclonic seizures occurring less frequently. Seizures occur 1-2 hours after awakening from sleep or during periods of relaxation in the evening. Sleep deprivation, alcohol, and photic stimulation can be precipitating factors. The ictal EEG demonstrates frontally predominant fast rhythmic spiking. The prognosis is good if the patient is adequately treated with AED's and avoids provoking factors (1989; Beghi et al., 2006).

5.11 Lennox-Gastaut syndrome

Lennox-Gastaut Syndrome (LGS) is classified as an epileptic encephalopathy. The age of onset is usually before age 8 with a peak age of onset between 3-5 years of age. Rarely, the disorder can present in early adulthood. The syndrome is characterized by a triad of multiple seizure types (tonic and atypical absence are the most common), slow spike and wave on EEG (1-2.5 Hz), and some degree of mental retardation. The etiology can be symptomatic or cryptogenic. It may evolve from West syndrome. Tonic seizures are considered a prerequisite for the diagnosis. Atypical absence and atonic seizures are also common. Myoclonic, generalized tonic-clonic, unilateral clonic, and partial seizures can occur less frequently. Non-convulsive status epilepticus can occur in > 50% of patients and involves near continuous atypical absence seizures interrupted by brief tonic seizures. The interictal EEG is characterized by slow spike and wave complexes (< 2.5 Hz) and activation of generalized paroxysmal fast activity during sleep. The diagnosis may be difficult to make at first because not all features of the syndrome may be present. The seizures in LGS are typically refractory to medical treatment (Arzimanoglou et al., 2009).

5.12 Progressive myoclonic epilepsies (PME)

These diseases are characterized by myoclonic jerks, seizures (GTC, absence, clonic, partial) and dementia caused by cerebral and cerebellar atrophy. The myoclonus is termed "massive myoclonus" which can cause falls and lead into generalized tonic-clonic seizures. Patients may exhibit cerebellar dysfunction, action myoclonus, or extrapyramidal dysfunction. Childhood development is normal until the age of onset. The autosomal recessive forms include Lafora disease, Unverricht-Lundborg disease, the neuronal ceroid lipofuscinoses , sialidosis, Action Myoclonus-Renal Failure Syndrome (AMRF), and Gaucher disease. The autosomal dominant form is dentatorubropallidolluysan atrophy. PME is also seen in some mitochondrial cytopathies such as myoclonic epilepsy with ragged-red fibers (MERRF).

6. 2010 ILAE commission on classification and terminology report

The 1981 and 1989 ILAE classifications are based on concepts formulated prior to modern neuroimaging and genomic research. The 1989 classification was not a true scientific classification but rather an organized list built on concepts which no longer correspond to or accurately describe our increasing knowledge of seizures and the epilepsies. Numerous attempts have been made by the ILAE Committee (Engel, 2001, 2006) and individual investigators (Luders et al., 1998) to revise the current classification. These attempts have generated controversy, and the lack of consensus has blocked any formal revision until 2010 (Berg et al., 2010). The most recent ILAE Commission on Classification and Terminology report is an update and revision to the classification schemes which are now several decades old. It was devised to simplify the classification of seizures, as new concepts have emerged broadening our understanding of seizures and epilepsy syndromes. The 2010 ILAE report on revised terminology and concepts for organization of seizures and epilepsies is not a new classification of epilepsies but rather a reflection of new terminology and concepts that lead to a better understanding of the current neurobiology, clinical features, prognostic implications, and features relevant to clinical practice and research. The ILAE did not feel that there was adequate knowledge at this time to propose a new classification of seizures and the epilepsies. The following paragraphs are a summary of the ILAE's report on classification and terminology from 2010 (Berg et al., 2010).

6.1 Generalized and focal redefined

The new definition of generalized epileptic seizures is "originating at some point within, and rapidly engaging, bilaterally distributed networks" which include both cortical and subcortical structures, can appear localized but have inconsistent localization and lateralization, and can be asymmetric. Focal epileptic seizures originate "within networks limited to one hemisphere" and can originate in subcortical structures, can be localized or widely distributed, , and have a consistent site of ictal onset (Berg et al., 2010).

6.2 Changes to the ILAE's 1981 classification of seizures

There have been a few changes to the 1981 ILAE classification of seizures. First, neonatal seizures are no longer classified as a separate entity. Secondly, the subclassification of absence seizures was simplified to either typical, atypical, or absence with special features which now included myoclonic absence and eyelid myoclonia. Thirdly, epileptic spasms which were not previously acknowledged in the 1981 seizure classification are now included. It is still unknown whether epileptic spasms are focal in onset, generalized in onset, or both so they are classified as "unknown." Fourth, the distinction between simple partial and complex partial focal seizures was eliminated, however, the concept of impairment of consciousness/awareness is still recognized. Lastly, myoclonic astatic seizures are now termed "myoclonic atonic" seizures. (see Table 5).

6.3 Focal seizures should be described

Focal seizures should be described according to their specific elemental features and sequence of occurrence. The glossary of ictal semiology (Blume, et al., 2001) should be consulted for clearly defined and recommended descriptors. For example, the term "dyscognitive" corresponds to the old term complex partial seizure. (see Table 6).

6.4 Replacing idiopathic, symptomatic, and cryptogenic

The term idiopathic is replaced by the term "genetic." The epilepsy must be a direct result of a known or presumed genetic defect and the seizures a core symptom of the disorder. An example would be Dravet syndrome due to a mutation in the SCN1A mutation. Classifying an epilepsy as genetic does not exclude the possibility that environmental factors may contribute to expression of the disease.

The term symptomatic is replaced by the term "structural/metabolic." To be classified in this category, the epilepsy has to be associated with a structural lesion or metabolic disease that has been shown in previous studies to substantially increase the risk of developing

epilepsy. Examples of structural lesions include stroke, trauma, infection, tuberous sclerosis, and malformations of cortical development.
The term cryptogenic is replaced by the term "unknown cause." The epilepsies of unknown cause constitute over one-third of all epilepsies. These epilepsies are an area of active current research in the fields of genetics, immunology, and neuroimaging.

Classification of Seizures
Generalized seizures
Tonic-clonic
Absence
Typical
Atypical
Absence with special features
Myoclonic absence
Eyelid myoclonia
Myoclonic
Myoclonic
Myoclonic atonic
Myoclonic tonic
Clonic
Tonic
Atonic
Focal seizures
Unknown
Epileptic spasms

Table 5. The Classification of Seizures, from Berg, A.T., Berkovic, S.F, et. al. (2010). Revised terminology and concepts for organization of seizures and epilepsies: Report of the ILAE Commission on Classification and Terminology, 2005-2009. *Epilepsia*, Vol. 51, No. 4, (April 2010), pp. 676-685, ISSN 1528-1167

Descriptors of focal seizures according to degree of impairment during seizure	Replaces the term
Without impairment of consciousness or awareness	
With observable motor or autonomic components	Simple partial seizure
Involving subjective sensory or psychic phenomena only	Aura
With impairment of consciousness or awareness	Complex partial seizure
Evolving to a bilateral, convulsive seizure	Secondarily generalized seizure

Table 6. Replacement of the terms simple partial, complex partial, and secondarily generalized seizures, from Berg, A.T., Berkovic, S.F, et. al. (2010). Revised terminology and concepts for organization of seizures and epilepsies: Report of the ILAE Commission on Classification and Terminology, 2005-2009. *Epilepsia*, Vol. 51, No. 4, (April 2010), pp. 676-685, ISSN 1528-1167

6.5 Disease-syndrome groupings

Instead of using the terms "disease" or "syndrome" to classify the epilepsies, four distinct groupings were developed: electroclinical syndromes, constellations, structural/metabolic epilepsies, and epilepsies of unknown cause (previously termed cryptogenic). The electroclinical syndromes are defined as "a complex of clinical features, signs, and symptoms that together define a distinctive, recognizable clinical disorder." They are defined on the basis of age of onset, specific EEG findings, seizure types, and other features which combine to from a specific diagnosis. Constellations are groups of epilepsies defined by diagnostically meaningful specific lesions or other causes which often have treatment implications. Examples of constellations are: mesial temporal epilepsy with hippocampal sclerosis, gelastic seizures and hypothalamic hamartoma, epilepsy with hemiconvulsion and hemiplegia, and Rasmussen syndrome. Regarding epilepsies due to structural or metabolic causes, more emphasis should be given to the seizure etiology rather than localization because the structural or metabolic etiology lends to a better understanding of prognosis. Based on these new concepts, instead of defining an epilepsy as "symptomatic temporal lobe epilepsy" the new terminology would read "epilepsy with focal seizures secondary to a cavernous angioma in the temporal lobe." (See Table 7).

Electroclinical syndromes and other epilepsies
Electroclinical syndromes arranged by age at onset
Neonatal period
Benign familial neonatal epilepsy
Early myoclonic encephalopathy
Ohtahara syndrome
Infancy
Epilepsy of infancy with migrating focal seizures
West syndrome
Myoclonic epilepsy in infancy
Benign infantile epilepsy
Benign familial infantile epilepsy
Dravet syndrome
Myoclonic encephalopathy in nonprogressive disorders
Childhood
Febrile seizures plus
Panayiotopoulos syndrome
Epilepsy with myoclonic atonic (previously astatic) seizures
Benign epilepsy with centrotemporal spikes
Autosomal-dominant nocturnal frontal lobe epilepsy
Late onset childhood occipital epilepsy (Gastaut type)
Epilepsy with myoclonic absences
Lennox-Gastaut syndrome
Epileptic Encephalopathy with continuous spike-and-wave during sleep (CSWS)
Landau-Kleffner syndrome
Childhood absence epilepsy
Adolescence-Adult
Juvenile absence epilepsy

Juvenile myoclonic epilepsy
Epilepsy with generalized tonic-clonic seizures alone
Progressive myoclonus epilepsies
Autosomal dominant epilepsy with auditory features
Other familial temporal lobe epilepsies
Less specific age relationship
Familial focal epilepsy with variable foci
Reflex epilepsies
Distinctive constellations
Mesial temporal lobe epilepsy with hippocampal sclerosis
Rasmussen syndrome
Gelastic seizures with hypothalamic hamartoma
Hemiconvulsion-hemiplegia-epilepsy
Epilepsies attributed to and organized by structural-metabolic causes
Malformations of cortical development
Neurocutaneous syndromes (tuberous sclerosis complex, Sturge-Weber, etc.)
Tumor
Infection
Trauma
Angioma
Perinatal insults
Stroke
Etc.
Epilepsies of unknown cause
Conditions with epileptic seizures that are traditionally not diagnosed as a form of epilepsy per se
Benign neonatal seizures
Febrile seizures

Table 7. Electroclinical syndromes and other epilepsies, adapted from Berg, A.T., Berkovic, S.F, et. al. (2010). Revised terminology and concepts for organization of seizures and epilepsies: Report of the ILAE Commission on Classification and Terminology, 2005-2009. *Epilepsia*, Vol. 51, No. 4, (April 2010), pp. 676-685, ISSN 1528-1167

6.6 Pros and cons of the new ILAE classification (2010)

The new classification of seizures and epilepsy syndromes is both an update of the old and a radical restructuring of it. It is a work in progress and it remains to be seen whether this new classification will come to acceptance or require further revision. The older classifications were simplified and specific seizure types were added. The replacement of the term "idiopathic" by the term "genetic" may be problematic. First, genetic etiologies due to a single gene mutations are still rare. Secondly, many of the epilepsies may be defined by multiple gene mutations and not due to a specific genetic defect. Additionally, some of the epilepsies don't fit into a single category in the new classification system. An example would be the age-specific epilepsies, such as the primarily generalized epilepsies. Overall however, the changes to the classifications needed to be made. Although it may be difficult to come to a consensus and there will be disagreement in the future, revisiting the way we classify seizures and epilepsy is a step forward for the field. (Shinnar, 2010).

7. Conclusion

The current ILAE Classification System for seizures and the epilepsies has formed the basis for a worldwide standardized approach to diagnosing, treating, and studying seizure disorders. The seizure classification system is primarily based on clinical semiology and EEG correlation, with a major distinction made between focal and generalized seizures. Focal seizures are further subdivided into simple and complex partial seizures, with the presence or absence of impairment of consciousness distinguishing the two. Generalized seizures are divided into absence, tonic, tonic-clonic, myoclonic, or atonic seizures. The epilepsy classification system highlights specific syndromes defined from anatomic-pathological bases (mesial temporal lobe epilepsy with hippocampal sclerosis) to electroclinical bases (Lennox-Gastaut Syndrome). This system has been useful for both clinicians and researchers over the past 30 years, but new data from modern neuroimaging techniques, molecular biology studies, and genetics research has revealed the limitations of the 1981 and 1989 Classification systems. The 2010 ILAE report sets forth new concepts and terminology, with an emphasis on reducing the dichotomy between focal and generalized epilepsies. The 2010 ILAE report did not propose a new classification system, but noted its recommendations will likely be a precursor to a substantive revision of the current classification system in the near future.

8. References

Arzimanoglou, A., French, J., et al. (2009). Lennox-Gastaut syndrome: a consensus approach on diagnosis, assessment, management, and trial methodology. *Lancet Neurol* , Vol. 8, No.1, (January 2009), pp. 82-93, ISSN 1474-4422

Bancaud, J., & Talairach, J. (1992). Clinical semiology of frontal lobe seizures. *Adv Neurol,* Vol. 57, n.d., pp. 3-58, ISSN 0091-3952

Beghi, M., Beghi, E., et al. (2006). Idiopathic generalized epilepsies of adolescence. *Epilepsia, Vol.*47, Suppl.2, (November 2006), pp. 107-10, ISSN 1528-1167

Berg, A.T., Berkovic, S.F, et. al. (2010). Revised terminology and concepts for organization of seizures and epilepsies: Report of the ILAE Commission on Classification and Terminology, 2005-2009. *Epilepsia,* Vol. 51, No. 4, (April 2010), pp. 676-685, ISSN 1528-1167

Blume, W.T., Luders, H.O., et al. (2001). Glossary of ictal semiology. *Epilepsia,* Vol.42, No. 9, (September 2001), pp. 1212-1218, ISSN 1528-1167

Chee, M. W., Kotagal, P., et al. (1993). Lateralizing signs in intractable partial epilepsy: blinded multiple-observer analysis. *Neurology,* Vol. 43, No.12, (December 1993), pp. 2519-25, ISSN 0028-3078

Engel, J., Jr. (2001). A proposed diagnostic scheme for people with epileptic seizures and with epilepsy: report of the ILAE Task Force on Classification and Terminology. *Epilepsia, Vol.* 42, No.6, (June 2001), pp. 796-803, ISSN 1528-1167

Engel, J., Jr. (2006). Report of the ILAE classification core group. *Epilepsia,* Vol.47, No.9, (September 2006), pp. 1558-68, ISSN 1528-1167

French, J. A., Williamson, P.D., et al. (1993). Characteristics of medial temporal lobe epilepsy: I. Results of history and physical examination. *Ann Neurol,* Vol.34, No.6, (December 1993), pp. 774-80, ISSN 1531-8249

Hirose, S., Mitsudome, A., et al. (2005). Genetics of idiopathic epilepsies. *Epilepsia*, Vol. 46, Suppl. 1, (March 2005), pp. 38-43, ISSN 1528-1167

ILAE. (1981). Proposal for revised clinical and electroencephalographic classification of epileptic seizures. From the Commission on Classification and Terminology of the International League Against Epilepsy. *Epilepsia,* Vol.22, No. 4, (August 1981), pp. 489-501, ISSN 1528-1167

ILAE. (1989). Proposal for revised classification of epilepsies and epileptic syndromes. Commission on Classification and Terminology of the International League Against Epilepsy. *Epilepsia,* Vol.30, No.4, (August 1989), pp. 389-99, ISSN 1528-1167

ILAE. (2009). Revised terminology and concepts for organization of the epilepsies: Report of the Commission on Classification and Terminology, In: *ILAE website,* 28 July 2009, Available from: www.ilae-epilepsy.org/visitors/centre/ctf/ctfoverview.cfm

Lim, S. H., Dinner, D.S., et al. (1994). Functional anatomy of the human supplementary sensorimotor area: results of extraoperative electrical stimulation. *Electroencephalogr Clin Neurophysiol,* Vol.91, No.3, (September 1994), pp. 179-93, ISSN 1388-2457

Luders, H., Acharya, J., et al. (1998). Semiological seizure classification. *Epilepsia* , Vol.39, No.9, (September 1998), pp. 1006-13, ISSN 1528-1167

Maillard, L., Vignal, J.P., et al. (2004). Semiologic and electrophysiologic correlations in temporal lobe seizure subtypes. *Epilepsia,* Vol. 45, No.12, (December 2004), pp. 1590-9, ISSN 1528-1167

Michelucci, R., Pasini, E., et al. (2009). Lateral temporal lobe epilepsies: clinical and genetic features. *Epilepsia,* Vol. 50, Suppl. 5, (May 2009), pp. 52-4, ISSN 1528-1167

Michelucci, R., Poza, J.J., et al. (2003). Autosomal dominant lateral temporal epilepsy: clinical spectrum, new epitempin mutations, and genetic heterogeneity in seven European families. *Epilepsia,* Vol.44, No.10, (October 2003), pp. 1289-97, ISSN 1528-1167

Nguyen, D. K., Nguyen, D.B., et al. (2009). Revisiting the role of the insula in refractory partial epilepsy. *Epilepsia,* Vol.50, No.3, (March 2009), pp. 510-20, ISSN 1528-1167

Ochs, R., Gloor, P., et al. (1984). Does head-turning during a seizure have lateralizing or localizing significance? *Neurology,* Vol.34, No.7, (July 1984), pp. 884-90, ISSN 0028-3878

Oldani, A., Zucconi, M., et al. (1998). Autosomal dominant nocturnal frontal lobe epilepsy. A video-polysomnographic and genetic appraisal of 40 patients and delineation of the epileptic syndrome. *Brain,* Vol. 121, No.2, (February 1998), pp. 205-2, ISSN 1460-2156

Ottman, R., Winawer, M.R., et al. (2004). LGI1 mutations in autosomal dominant partial epilepsy with auditory features. *Neurology,* Vol. 62, No.7, (April 2004), pp. 1120-6, ISSN 0028-3878

Ozkara, C., Uzan, M., et al. (2008). Surgical outcome of patients with mesial temporal lobe epilepsy related to hippocampal sclerosis. *Epilepsia,* Vol. 49, No.4, (April 2008), pp. 696-9, ISSN 1528-1167

Quesney, L. F. (1986). Clinical and EEG features of complex partial seizures of temporal lobe origin. *Epilepsia,* Vol.27, Suppl. 2, (August 1986), pp. S27-45, ISSN 1528-1167

Sandok, E. K.., & Cascino, G.D. (1998). Surgical treatment for perirolandic lesional epilepsy. *Epilepsia* Vol.39, Suppl. 4, (April 1998), pp. S42-8, ISSN 1528-1167

Shinnar, S., (2010). The new ILAE classification. *Epilepsia,* Vol.51, No.4, (April 2010), pp. 715-717, ISSN 1528-1167

Vigevano, F., Fusco, L., et al. (2001). Neurophysiology of spasms. *Brain Dev,* Vol.23, No.7, (October 2001), pp. 467-72, ISSN 0387-7604

Wyllie , E., (Ed.). (2006). *The Treatment of Epilepsy: Principles & Practice.* Lippincott Williams & Wilkins, ISBN 0781749956, Philadelphia

6

Combined Neuro-Cardiogenic Epilepsy Syndromes and Novel Mechanistic Insights

S.E. Lehnart
[1]*Heart Research Center Göttingen,*
Dept. of Cardiology & Pulmonology,
University Medical Center Göttingen,
[2]*Center for Biomedical Engineering and Technology,*
University of Maryland Baltimore,
[1]*Germany*
[2]*U.S.A.*

1. Introduction

A large portion of patients with epilepsy without other obvious organ disease die unexpectedly. Epidemiological studies have estimated the rate of unexpected death in patients with epilepsy up to 24 times higher as compared to the general population (Ficker et al., 1998). However, in contrast to a significantly increased risk of sudden death in epilepsy patients, the underlying causes and pathophysiological mechanisms leading to sudden death are not well understood. This important problem is clinically identified as sudden unexplained death in epilepsy (SUDEP). Of note, SUDEP does not include death after prolonged seizures (e.g. status epilepticus) or due to other organ disease which excludes common cardio-pulmonary pathology. SUDEP occurs frequently in patients with idiopathic epilepsy with an estimated prevalence of 2% to 18% (Nashef et al., 2007; Tomson et al., 2008). It has been hypothesized that SUDEP and certain types of seizures may initiate a pathological signal to the heart, which subsequently triggers cardiac dysrhythmias and sudden death in epilepsy (Jehi & Najm, 2008; Surges et al., 2009). Alternatively, dysfunction of fast ion transport mechanisms, which directly control membrane excitability within the context of either the brain or the heart, may directly cause both neuronal or cardiac dysrhythmias. Importantly, if certain genetic defects in ion channel genes coexisted in the brain and heart, this may constitute a candidate mechanism of SUDEP and potentially precipitate life-threatening cardiac dysrhythmias (Nashef et al., 2007). Indeed, recent work has identified ion channelopathies in the context of generalized epilepsy that coexist in the brain and the heart. For the first time, defined molecular mechanisms of coexisting brain and heart dysrhythmias have been shown in genetically engineered rodent models with patient mutations which reproduce both neuronal and cardiac patient phenotypes. This article focuses on previous perspectives and recent insights about molecular epilepsy mechanisms, which underlie both dangerous dysrhythmias in the brain and heart. In addition, novel targeted treatment rationales based on molecular and cellular mechanisms of dysrhythmias are discussed.

2. Can existing genetic epilepsy mechanisms explain unexpected death?

Epilepsy is an episodic dysrhythmia of electrical brain activity in the cerebral cortex marked by abnormal neuronal network synchronization. Approximately 20 genes with major effects on susceptibility to epilepsy have been associated with different seizure syndromes. These epileptogenic genes define distinct as well as common modulatory pathways of neuronal network activity. One group of genetic variants appears to destabilize neuronal signaling through defects which affect the neurophysiology of electrical membrane excitability and synaptic transmission. Another group of genetic variants causes neurodevelopmental effects which perturb the balance between inhibitory and excitatory circuits. Unfortunately, none of the genetically defined epilepsy mechanisms can readily explain molecular pathways which lead to cardiac dysrhythmias as a hypothetical cause of unexpected death in epilepsy.

Due to a high rate of SUDEP in primary epilepsy patients with generalized seizures, it might be important to consider how epilepsy genes are identified and within which pathophysiological context a genetic defect has been further characterized. The following two principal strategies exist: 1) a candidate gene is identified in the context of inherited disorders in patients or animal models and 2) an incidental phenotype identifies a genetic epilepsy syndrome following targeted mutagenesis in animal models. Indeed, both strategies have contributed to a growing list of genes linked to inherited epilepsies. The diversity of distinct phenotypes and their causative gene mutations provides important clues both to a gene's physiological function as well as to a behavioral disease mechanism which might surprisingly reveal overlap with cardiac dysrhythmias. The list of epileptogenic genes spans from intrinsic membrane proteins underlying cell membrane excitability to nuclear transcription factors which control the fate of developing neuronal networks. Accordingly, mechanisms that underlie epilepsy may range from abnormal action potential firing to developmental abnormalities of specific neural circuits. Within the context of unexpected death in epilepsy, mechanisms which directly cause electrical membrane dysfunction and thereby alter fast action potential signaling seem promising to explain either or both brain and heart dysrhythmias. Indeed, recent insight from genetically engineered animal models has uncovered previously unknown epilepsy syndromes and genes in the context of cardiac dysrhythmia syndromes.

2.1.1 Consideration of previous perspectives to explain SUDEP

Risk factors for SUDEP include early onset of epilepsy from age 20 to 40 years, generalized seizures, resistance to anticonvulsant drug therapy, and poor patient compliance (Hitiris et al., 2007). Importantly, several clinical studies have documented abnormalities of the heart rhythm in SUDEP patients suggesting the possibility of co-existing or even synergistic neuro-cardiogenic mechanisms (Britton et al., 2006; Johnson et al., 2009; Nei et al., 2000; Opherk et al., 2002; Zijlmans et al., 2002). Indeed, sudden death caused by dysrhythmia of the heart (in cardiovascular sciences also referred to as *arrhythmia*) represents a frequent cause of electrical organ dysfunction in the general population. The phenotype of cardiac arrhythmia has been linked to a large spectrum of gene variants that include multiple ion channel genes (see 2.1.2). Therefore, a hypothetical mechanism of SUDEP could be that the identical ion channel gene expressed in the brain and the heart becomes dysfunctional due to a mutation, and causes a combined neuro-cardiogenic syndrome including unexpected death in epilepsy. Is there sufficient evidence for such a combined neuro-cardiogenic mechanism of SUDEP in patients?

In epilepsy patients and also in SUDEP victims a spectrum of cardiac dysrhythmias has been reported including arrhythmias of the atria as well as life-threatening ventricular arrhythmias. Thus, genetic ventricular arrhythmia syndromes may provide an opportunity to gain mechanistic insight about SUDEP if brain seizures coexisted. However, the originally proposed pathophysiological mechanism which starts from a primary neuronal defect which leads to secondary cardio-respiratory arrest and dangerous cardiac arrhythmias could not be established in patients. As alternative, if an epileptogenic gene defect were expressed both in the brain and heart, this would allow for investigation of the underlying dysrhythmia mechanisms separately in the brain and heart, and be tested for mechanistic links between cortical hyperexcitability and sudden unexpected death by unknown neuro-cardiogenic mechanisms. Before I outline such novel epilepsy mechanisms with potential mechanistic links between the brain and the heart, I will review existing evidence about gene defects associated either with brain or heart dysrhythmias, to assess if common denominators exist which may contribute to seizure susceptibility.

2.1.2 Genes of fast neuronal signaling associated with epilepsy

The identification of genes that determine the risk of epilepsy has very important implications for patients, clinical diagnosis, and basic research. Within this context it is important to consider that molecular testing for genetic defects in epilepsy at current is mainly used by hypothesis driven research for the following two reasons: 1) genetic defects such as mutations can significantly increase our understanding of the basic mechanisms underlying seizure susceptibility; and 2) genetic defects which cause seizures in patients often lead to important research insights about the fundamental role of a protein which has previously not been fully understood in a neurophysiological context. Readers with a special interest in clinical diagnostic testing may also refer to the up-to-date special report of the International League Against Epilepsy (ILAE) Genetics Commission (Ottman et al.,2010).

In epilepsy, the majority of gene defects affect voltage- and/or ligand-gated ion channels that have been linked to paroxysmal network synchronization in seizure syndromes. These epileptogenic genes include both the pore-forming and regulatory subunits of Na^+, K^+, and Ca^{2+} channels of the plasma membrane, as well as ligand-gated channels modulated by GABA, Ach, and other ligands. Additionally, certain transport proteins are affected by genetic defects include the Na^+/K^+-ATPase and an important glucose transporter of the brain. While analysis of some of these epileptogenic gene mutations in heterologous cell expression systems has provided important insights, it is important to note that considerable gaps remain in our understanding how a specific channelopathy may result in increased network excitability and abnormal network synchronization in the brain. Therefore, it is without doubt very challenging to mechanistically understand epilepsy syndromes associated with other paroxysmal neuronal disorders or even other organ dysfunction like cardiac arrhythmias as a hypothetical cause of SUDEP. Table 1 on the following page summarizes confirmed genetic epilepsy syndromes, which have been mostly linked to defects in ion transport. Although we do not understand the precise mechanisms of abnormal network synchronization behind most of the defects listed in table 1, a common denominator of these epilepsy genes are fast neurophysiological signaling mechanisms.

<table>
<tr><th colspan="5">Seizure syndromes that start within the first year of life</th></tr>
<tr><th>Syndrome</th><th>Gene</th><th>Protein</th><th>Defect</th><th>References</th></tr>
<tr><td rowspan="2">Benign familial neonatal seizures</td><td>KCNQ2</td><td>Kv7.2</td><td>I(K) ↓</td><td rowspan="2">(Biervert et al., 1998; Charlier et al., 1998; Singh et al., 1998)</td></tr>
<tr><td>KCNQ3</td><td>Kv7.2</td><td>I(K)</td></tr>
<tr><td>Benign familial neonatal-infantile seizures</td><td>SCN2A</td><td>Nav1.2</td><td>I(Na)</td><td>(Berkovic et al., 2004; Heron et al., 2002)</td></tr>
<tr><th colspan="5">Syndromes with prominent febrile seizures</th></tr>
<tr><th>Syndrome</th><th>Gene</th><th>Protein</th><th>Defect</th><th>References</th></tr>
<tr><td>Dravet syndrome (severe myoclonic epilepsy of infancy)</td><td>SCN1A</td><td>Nav1.1</td><td rowspan="3">I(Na)</td><td>(Claes et al., 2001; Nabbout et al., 2003)</td></tr>
<tr><td rowspan="3">Genetic (generalized) epilepsy with febrile seizures plus (GEFS+)</td><td>SCN1A</td><td>Nav1.1</td><td>(Escayg et al., 2000)</td></tr>
<tr><td>SCN1B</td><td>β1 SU</td><td>(Wallace et al., 1998)</td></tr>
<tr><td>GABRG2</td><td>γ2 SU</td><td rowspan="2">GABA$_A$ receptor</td><td>(Baulac et al., 2001)</td></tr>
<tr><td>Childhood absence epilepsy with febrile seizures</td><td>GABRG2</td><td>γ2 SU</td><td>(Kananura et al., 2002; Wallace et al., 2001)</td></tr>
<tr><th colspan="5">Idiopathic generalized epilepsies</th></tr>
<tr><th>Syndrome</th><th>Gene</th><th>Protein</th><th>Defect</th><th>References</th></tr>
<tr><td>Early-onset absence epilepsy</td><td>SLC2A1</td><td>GLUT1</td><td>Glucose uptake ↓</td><td>(Suls et al., 2009)</td></tr>
<tr><td>Juvenile myoclonic epilepsy</td><td>GABRA1</td><td>α1 SU</td><td>GABA$_A$ receptor ↓</td><td>(Cossette et al., 2002; Suzuki et al., 2004)</td></tr>
<tr><th colspan="5">Focal epilepsies</th></tr>
<tr><th>Syndrome</th><th>Gene</th><th>Protein</th><th>Defect</th><th>References</th></tr>
<tr><td rowspan="3">Autosomal dominant nocturnal frontal lobe epilepsy</td><td>CHRNA4</td><td>α4 SU</td><td rowspan="3">nACh receptor</td><td>(Steinlein et al., 1995)</td></tr>
<tr><td>CHRNB2</td><td>β2 SU</td><td>(De Fusco et al., 2000)</td></tr>
<tr><td>CHRNA2</td><td>α2 SU</td><td>(Aridon et al., 2006)</td></tr>
<tr><th colspan="5">Epilepsies associated with other paroxysmal disorders</th></tr>
<tr><th>Syndrome</th><th>Gene</th><th>Protein</th><th>Defect</th><th>References</th></tr>
<tr><td>Generalized epilepsy and paroxysmal dyskinesia</td><td>KCNMA1</td><td>K$_{Ca}$1.1</td><td>I(K)</td><td>(Du et al., 2005)</td></tr>
<tr><td>Epilepsy with paroxysmal exercise-induced dyskinesia</td><td>SLC2A1</td><td>GLUT1</td><td>Glucose uptake ↓</td><td>(Suls et al., 2008; Weber et al., 2008)</td></tr>
<tr><td>Absence epilepsy and episodic ataxia</td><td>CACNA1A</td><td>Cav2.1</td><td>I(Ca, P/Q) ↓</td><td>(Imbrici et al., 2004; Jouvenceau et al., 2001)</td></tr>
<tr><td>Focal epilepsy and episodic ataxia</td><td>KCNA1</td><td>Kv1.1</td><td>I(K)</td><td>(Eunson et al., 2000; Spauschus et al., 1999; Zuberi et al., 1999)</td></tr>
<tr><td>Familial hemiplegic migraine and epilepsy</td><td>ATP1A2</td><td>Na^+,K^+-ATPase</td><td>I(K) ↓</td><td>(Deprez et al., 2008; Vanmolkot et al., 2003)</td></tr>
</table>

Table 1. Genes identified in idiopathic epilepsy syndromes. Abbreviations: I, indicates ionic current (type); ↑ gain-of-function; ↓ loss-of-function.

To compare the above identified mechanisms of epilepsy syndromes with those of paroxysmal arrhythmia syndromes of the heart, we will next review confirmed monogenetic disorders of the heart, which have also been linked to ion transport dysfunction. Please note, that for clarity this chapter is focused on genes underlying different forms of membrane transport defects in epilepsy or cardiac arrhythmias.

2.2.1 Genetic defects underlying cardiac dysrhythmias

Europe and North America have a high annual incidence of sudden cardiac death (SCD) amounting to up to 100 per 100.000 in the general population (Byrne et al., 2008; Chugh et al., 2004). SCD is defined as a sudden and unexpected pulseless primary cardiac event (Chugh et al., 2008). Despite the presence of modern resuscitation chains for out-of-hospital SCD the overall survival rate is only 4.6% (Nichol et al., 2008). SCD is the outcome of electrical heart disease that manifests as fast ventricular arrhythmias or pulseless electrical activity. In a significant number of patients, cardiac dysrhythmia and SCD occur unexpected without prior warning and without a clinically identifiable triggering mechanism. Therefore, cardiac dysrhythmia and SCD risk prediction remain a major challenge. However, understanding of molecular mechanisms has significantly advanced for inherited cardiac channelopathies that predispose to SCD (Lehnart et al., 2007).

Cardiac ion channelopathies provide important rationales to understand mechanisms of cardiac dysrhythmias and the risk of SCD. The most common cardiac genetic channelopathies manifest as delayed ventricular repolarization seen as a prolonged QT interval by surface electrocardiogram (ECG), fast ventricular arrhythmias, recurrent syncope (loss of consciousness), and seizures. The Long QT syndrome (LQTS) is mostly caused by genetic ion channel defects resulting in abnormal prolongation of the cardiac action potential in approximately 1 in 2000 mutation carriers (Roden, 2008). Depending on the underlying gene defect and incompletely understood environmental factors, LQTS mutation carriers have a significantly increased risk for fatal ventricular arrhythmias and SCD. The majority of identified LQTS mutations cause ion channel dysfunction through mutations of pore-forming α or accessory β subunits as summarized in table 2. A recently discovered LQTS variant phenotype is Sudden Infant Death Syndrome (SIDS) caused by some of the same gene defects. Among known cardiac ion channelopathies K^+ and Na^+ channel mutations of the *KCNQ1*, *KCNH2*, and *SCN5A* genes stand out, because these cause the great majority of LQTS cases.

Although seizures occur in LQTS mutation carriers, these were previously considered to represent secondary events due to reduced blood perfusion of the brain during cardiac arrhythmias. However, it can be difficult to distinguish between a phenotype of syncope from cardiac dysrhythmias and primary neurogenic seizure auras with or without myoclonus (McKeon et al., 2006). In addition, simultaneous electroencephalogram (EEG) and ECG recordings revealed a surprisingly high prevalence of up to 44% of different types of cardiac arrhythmias in individuals with primary epileptic seizures (Britton et al., 2006; Johnson et al., 2009; McKeon et al., 2006; Nei et al., 2000; Opherk et al., 2002; Zijlmans et al., 2002). Recently, seizure phenotypes have been reported in approximately one third of confirmed LQTS mutation carriers (including 22% with the most prevalent form LQTS1) suggesting that LQTS genes may cause neuronal hyperexcitability independent from cardiac arrhythmias (Johnson et al., 2009). In addition, seizures have been reported in up to half of confirmed *RYR2* mutation carriers affected by stress-induced ventricular arrhythmias (Postma et al., 2005). Of note, in a given mutation carrier neuronal seizures and cardiac arrhythmias may occur simultaneously, or a brain dysrhythmia may secondarily trigger a cardiac arrhythmia through unknown mechanisms.

Sudden infant death syndrome (SIDS): starting within the first year of life				
Syndrome	**Gene**	**Protein**	**Defect**	**References**
SIDS1	*KCNH2*	Kv11.1	I(Kr) ↓	(Arnestad et al., 2007)
SIDS2	*KCNQ1*	Kv7.1	I(Ks) ↓	(Moss et al., 2007)
SIDS3	*KCNJ2*	Kir2.1	I(K1) ↓	(Arnestad et al., 2007)
SIDS4	*SCN5A*	Nav1.5	I(Na) ↑	(Plant et al., 2006; Van Norstrand et al., 2008)
Long QT syndrome (LQTS): prominent lengthening of the electrocardiogram QT interval				
Syndrome	**Gene**	**Protein**	**Defect**	**References**
LQTS1	*KCNQ1*	Kv7.1	I(Ks) ↓	(Moss et al., 2007; Wang et al., 1996)
LQTS2	*KCNH2*	Kv11.1	I(Kr) ↓	(Curran et al., 1995)
LQTS3	*SCN5A*	Nav1.5	I(Na) ↑	(Bennett et al., 1995; Wang et al., 1995)
LQTS5	*KCNE1*	β SU	I(Ks) ↓	(Sanguinetti et al., 1996; Splawski et al., 1997)
LQTS6	*KCNE2*	β SU	I(Kr) ↓	(Abbott et al., 1999)
LQTS7	*KCNJ2*	Kir2.1	I(K1) ↓	(Bendahhou et al., 2003; Plaster et al., 2001)
LQTS8	*CACNA1C*	Cav1.2 α1c	I(Ca,L) ↑	(Splawski et al., 2005; Splawski et al., 2004)
LQTS10	*SCN4B*	β4 SU	I(Na) ↑	(Medeiros-Domingo et al., 2007)
Short QT syndrome (SQTS): prominent shortening of the electrocardiogram QT interval				
Syndrome	**Gene**	**Protein**	**Defect**	**References**
SQTS1	*KCNH2*	Kv11.1	I(Kr) ↑	(Brugada et al., 2004; Hong et al., 2005a)
SQTS2	*KCNQ1*	Kv7.1	I(Ks) ↑	(Bellocq et al., 2004; Hong et al., 2005b)
SQTS3	*KCNJ2*	Kir2.1	I(K1) ↑	(Priori et al., 2005)
SQTS4	*CACNA1C*	Cav1.2 α1c	I(Ca,L) ↓	(Antzelevitch et al., 2007)
SQTS5	*CACNB2*	β2b SU	I(Ca,L) ↓	(Antzelevitch et al., 2007)
Timothy Syndrome (TS) and Autism Spectrum Disorder				
Syndrome	**Gene**	**Protein**	**Defect**	**References**
TS1	*CACNA1CA*	Cav1.2 α1c	I(Ca,L) ↑	(Splawski et al., 2004)
TS2	*CACNA1C*	Cav1.2 α1c	I(Ca,L) ↑	(Splawski et al., 2005)
Catecholaminergic Polymorphic Ventricular Tachycardia (CPVT)				
Syndrome	**Gene**	**Protein**	**Defect**	**References**
CPVT1	*RYR2*	RyR2	SR Ca leak ↑	(Laitinen et al., 2001; Priori et al., 2001)
CPVT2	*CASQ2*	Calsequestri n	SR Ca leak ↑	(Lahat et al., 2001; Postma et al., 2002)
CPVT3	*KCNJ2*	Kir2.1	I(K1) ↑	(Plaster et al., 2001; Tester et al., 2006)

Table 2. Genes identified in idiopathic ventricular arrhythmia syndromes. Abbreviations: I, indicates ionic current (type); SR, sarcoplasmic reticulum calcium store; ↑ gain-of-function; ↓ loss-of-function.

It is important to note that many genetic and phenotypic variations of cardiac channelopathy syndromes exist. In LQTS approximately 40% of family members who are confirmed carriers of a gene mutation are clinically silent with a normal or borderline QT interval (Bai et al., 2009; Hofman et al., 2007). In addition, some patients with borderline QT interval prolongation are negative for LQTS mutations, but positive for mutations linked to the syndrome CPVT (Tester et al., 2006; Tester et al., 2005). Furthermore, mutations in intronic regions have recently been identified as a cause of LQTS (Zhang et al., 2004). Of significance for molecular mechanisms, cardiac arrhythmias in LQTS1 and CPVT1 mutation carriers are both triggered by increased physical or emotional stress, indicating that the respective Kv7.1 and RyR2 defects may share the same regulatory pathways during arrhythmia triggers under control of the sympathetic nervous system (Lehnart et al., 2004). In contrast, LQTS3 mutation carriers experience cardiac arrhythmias during rest or sleep (Roden, 2008). Notably, for intermediate risk traits at the level of the general population genome-wide association studies have identified determinants of the QT interval including variants of the *KCNQ1*, *KCNH2*, and *SCN5A* genes (Albert et al.; Newton-Cheh et al., 2009). In analogy to the ILAE for epilepsy, the International Long QT Syndrome Registry facilitates insight and patient recommendations about genetic forms of cardiac arrhythmias (Moss & Schwartz, 2005).

2.2.2 Synopsis of existing genetic dysrhythmia mechanisms in the brain and heart

Excitability of the brain and heart is based on the same principles of ion transport. At the molecular level some of the same classes of ion channels, for example the *SCN* and *KCNQ* isoforms, exist in the brain and heart. However, comparison of tables 1 and 2 shows that previously established monogenic defects cannot readily provide a mechanistic association between neuronal and cardiac dysrhythmias. In addition, as outlined under 2.1.2 the prevailing research focus about a given organ disease like cardiac arrhythmias may introduce a phenotypic bias such that other organs like brain seizures may have not been comprehensibly studied. Indeed, prior to the age of genetic information epilepsy patients with frequent seizures were sometimes diagnosed with the syndrome of Catecholaminergic Polymorphic Ventricular Tachycardia (CPVT), however, the arrhythmias were thought to explain the seizure phenotype and epilepsy treatment was discontinued (Leenhardt et al., 1995). Within this context it is important to realize that the differential diagnosis of brain and heart seizure phenotypes is of historical significance and extends to famous scholars and patients including Napoleon Bonaparte (Osler, 1903). Thus, one must consider that accurate differentiation between neuronal and cardiac seizure phenotypes is challenging in patients and may need patience (McKeon et al., 2006).

Despite these difficulties, initial clues that LQTS gene mutations may also cause seizures originating from the brain came from studies of the cardiac sodium channel Nav1.5. As outlined in table 2, *SCN5A* mutations cause LQTS including ventricular arrhythmias and SCD (Chen et al., 1998; Wang et al., 1995). In addition, Nav1.5 is expressed in the entorhinal cortex and the amygdala, and other limbic brain regions which have been associated with a low threshold for abnormal network synchronization and brain seizures (Hartmann et al., 1999). Despite these early hypothetical associations, cardiac LQTS genes have subsequently not been mechanistically linked to the context of primary brain dysrhythmias. Therefore, despite a wealth of molecular and electrophysiological insights originating from genetic linkage studies, prediction and prevention of associated brain and heart dysrhythmias remain little understood. Clearly, additional and likely complex studies which integrate multiple investigative levels are needed, in particular to explore underlying mechanisms of potentially co-existing brain and heart dysrhythmias, and to elucidate mechanistic links between electrical brain and heart phenotypes. As will be discussed next, recent basic science research studies suggest an unprecedented level of complexity concerning ion transport dysfunction and molecular crosstalk within the context of excitable organ disease of the brain and heart.

2.3 Novel genetic mechanisms of associated brain and heart dysrhythmias

Completely new epilepsy mechanisms have recently been identified in mouse models with human cardiac arrhythmia symptoms of confirmed mutation carriers. Of note, through a bench-to-bedside approach these experimental studies strongly suggest that combined neuro-cardiogenic disease mechanisms exist. These neuro-cardiogenic syndromes may in principle also underlie SUDEP in patients. Notably, combined neuro-cardiogenic mechanisms have been implicated earlier in the genetic Timothy syndrome, a rare ion channelopathy causing multiple organ phenotypes including cardiac arrhythmias, autism, mental retardation and seizures. Patients with Timothy syndrome have de novo mutations of splice exon 8A of the main cardiac L-type Ca^{2+} channel pore-forming α-subunit Cav1.2 resulting in intracellular Ca^{2+} overload, which occurs in the heart and brain (Splawski et al., 2005). While the patient phenotype of Timothy syndrome is very complex due to multiple coexisting organ and metabolic disease processes, which makes elucidation of specific molecular SUDEP mechanisms difficult, it emphasizes the importance to consider both the brain and heart in seizure phenotypes.

Abnormal intracellular Ca^{2+} homeostasis has also been identified for a different epileptogenic mechanism due to mutations of the cardiac ryanodine receptor type 2 (RyR2). RyR2 forms the α-subunit of the tetrameric intracellular Ca^{2+} release channel, and is highly expressed in the heart and brain. In 2001 RyR2 missense mutations were identified in patients with syncope, seizures and SCD (Laitinen et al., 2001; Priori et al., 2001). Due to the characteristic dependence of the cardiac phenotype on physical and/or emotional stressors, the syndrome has been called Catecholaminergic Polymorphic Ventricular Tachycardia type 1 (CPVT1) (Priori et al., 2001). The phenotype of stress-induced cardiac arrhythmias is dependent on heart rate and reproducible for diagnostic purposes by exercise ECG testing in RyR2 mutation carriers (Lehnart et al., 2004). It has been assumed that in CPVT the syncope and seizures are not of primary neuronal origin, but due to decreased blood perfusion of the brain during ventricular arrhythmias (also known as Stokes-Adams attack)(Leenhardt et al., 1995). However, under experimentally controlled conditions behavioural and electrophysiological analysis of knockin mice with RyR2 missense mutations have shown that generalized seizures can occur independent from cardiac arrhythmias (Lehnart et al., 2008). As will be discussed below, RyR2 mutant mice provided the first evidence that the same molecular ion channel defect can cause generalized seizures and ventricular arrhythmias. RyR2 mutations cause abnormal intracellular Ca^{2+} signals in neurons and cardiac myocytes, which represents a novel genetic candidate mechanism of generalized seizures and of unexpected death in epilepsy.

Recently, a second mechanism of generalized seizures and cardiac arrhythmias has been identified in mice with *KCNQ1* mutations, which affects the pore-forming α-subunit of the cardiac delayed rectifier K^+ channel Kv7.1 (table 2). Kv7.1 forms the slow repolarizing membrane current I(Ks), which is active during the repolarizing phases 2 and 3 of the cardiac action potential. Kv7.1 loss-of-function mutations increase cardiac action potential duration (Wang et al., 1996; Wang et al., 1999; Westenskow et al., 2004). Kv7.1 mutations underlie the most common form of the cardiac Long QT syndrome (LQTS1) leading to syncope, stress-induced arrhythmias, seizures and SCD. Mouse models harbouring patient missense mutations of the *KCNQ1* gene have reproduced key aspects of the human cardiac LQTS1 phenotype (Casimiro et al., 2004). In addition, the LQTS1 mouse models reproduce sensory defects of the inner ear hair cells, which also express Kv7.1 channels (Casimiro et al., 2004; Kubisch et al., 1999). As will be discussed below, Noebels and colleagues have recently re-evaluated the same KCNQ1 knockin mice with patient missense mutations and identified a previously unknown generalized seizure phenotype (Goldman et al., 2009).

The same gene defects which have originally been identified in patients with cardiac arrhythmia phenotypes in the LQTS1 and CPVT1 syndromes, have recently been associated with generalized seizure phenotypes in the respective *KCNQ1* and *RYR2* knock in mouse models with patient mutations (Goldman et al., 2009; Lehnart et al., 2008). While LQTS1 mutations of Kv7.1 lead to prolongation of the cardiac action potential, CPVT1 mutation of RyR2 result in abnormal cardiac membrane depolarizations following the regular cardiac action potential, referred to as delayed afterdepolarizations (DADs). Notably, the clinical phenotypes of LQTS1 and CPVT1 patients both include syncope and seizures, which as mentioned earlier can be difficult to differentiate (McKeon et al., 2006). Indeed, in LQTS1 seizures have been reported in up to one-third of genotype-confirmed patients (Johnson et al., 2009) and in CPVT1 in up to half of confirmed RyR2 mutation carriers (Postma et al., 2005). Thus, genetic patient studies have shown that both LQTS1 and CPVT1 mutation carriers exhibit symptoms of neuronal hyperexcitability.

Despite significant conceptual advances through recent identification of ion channel gene variants, which cause combined seizure and arrhythmia syndromes, many questions remain unanswered and require further study. These questions concern the specific brain regions and neuron types, which show a decreased threshold for aberrant network synchronization, such that prolonged depolarization or delayed repolarization may initiate primary brain seizures. In addition, arrhythmias in LQTS1 and CPVT1 are characteristically modulated by the autonomous nervous system. If the autonomous nervous system is also affected by the same genes and modulates the phenotype defects needs further exploration. The following chapters will discuss recent advances in ion channel studies related to epilepsy and particular insight about combined neuro-cardiogenic phenotypes and mechanisms which may link the dysrhythmia phenotypes of the two separate organs. Already, these recent insights have motivated further research about diagnostic strategies to improve risk prediction and prevention in patients with seizure disorders of unknown origin. In addition, novel therapeutic strategies targeting the underlying molecular mechanisms are under development. Therefore, the following chapters will also discuss the translation of novel seizure mechanisms in neuro-cardiogenic syndromes into therapeutic rationales.

2.3.1 Ryanodine receptor mutations cause generalized seizures

Seizure models using pharmacological inducers have found intracellular Ca^{2+} abnormalities in inhibitory interneurons and astrocytes during seizure like activity (Tian et al., 2005). In addition, inositol 1,4,5-trisphosphate receptor type 1 (IP3R1) intracellular Ca^{2+} release channels, which localize to intracellular ER Ca^{2+} stores, have been associated with seizures in mice (Street et al., 1997). However, a mechanistic relationship between dysfunction of intracellular Ca^{2+} release channels and seizures has not been established. Ca^{2+} is an important neuronal signaling molecule and intracellular Ca^{2+} release channels are an important source including IP3R1-3 isoforms (Mignery et al., 1989; Street et al., 1997) and the related ryanodine receptor isoforms (RyR1-3)(Henzi & MacDermott, 1992; Kostyuk & Verkhratsky, 1994). Interestingly, mutation carriers with RyR2 mutations have been shown to exhibit syncope, seizures and cardiac arrhythmias (Postma et al., 2005).

RyR2 is the major Ca^{2+} release channel of the heart. Over 100 different *RYR2* mutations have been associated with Catecholaminergic Polymorphic Ventricular Tachycardia type 1 (CPVT) and ventricular arrhythmias (table 2). Importantly, early clinical descriptions of childhood CPVT documented initial presentations with seizures, loss of consciousness, convulsions, and involuntary incontinence in approximately 50% of patients (Leenhardt et al., 1995). A similar presentation has been confirmed in *RYR2* mutation carriers who have also presented with seizures in 50% of patients (Postma et al., 2005). Additionally, patients with CPVT2 caused by calsequestrin2 mutations also have seizures (Lahat et al., 2001). Indeed, RyR2 is highly expressed in the brain including the hippocampus dentate gyrus granule cell layer and the CA1-3 pyramidal cell layers (figure 1). These hippocampal areas have been associated with pharmacologically stimulated ryanodine receptor dysfunction and generalized tonic-clonic seizure activity (Mori et al., 2005).

We created knockin mice with RyR2 patient missense mutations (R2474S and N2386I) which have been linked to autosomal-dominant CPVT in families (Priori et al., 2001). The heterozygous *RYR2* mutant mice spontaneously developed recurring generalized tonic-clonic seizures during arousal as well as in the absence of obvious environmental changes. Generalized myoclonic seizures in *RYR2* mutant mice exhibited a rapid progression from freezing to partial behavioral abnormalities to generalized myoclonic and tonic-clonic behavior (Lehnart et al., 2008). Video-assisted analysis showed that generalized seizure activity lasted between 20 and 120 seconds. Simultaneous EEG-ECG recording showed bilateral voltage discharges including higher frequency sharp spikes and waves, however, no cardiac arrhythmias (figure 1; *lower, left*). These data unambiguously show that at least some of the seizures in *RYR2* mutation carriers are of primary neuronal origin. Importantly, recent studies have confirmed the a seizure phenotype in patients including *RYR2* mutation carriers (Johnson et al.,2009; Nagrani et al.,2011).

Pharmacological challenge with the seizure inducing drugs 4-aminopyridine and caffeine showed increased seizure susceptibility in *RYR2* mutant mice. Generalized tonic-clonic seizures occurred significantly earlier in *RYR2* mutant as compared to wild-type control mice. In addition, *RYR2* mutant mice showed a faster progression to more severe seizure stages. Moreover, the seizure phenotype was found in two independently generated *RYR2* mutant knockin mouse strains (R2474S and N2386I).

Extracellular local field potential (LFP) recording in acute hippocampal brain slices revealed significantly increased excitability following 4-aminopyridine treatment in *RYR2* mutant brain tissue as compared to wild-type control tissue sections (Lehnart et al., 2008). LFP recording showed discharges with higher burst frequency and duration in CA3 network regions of *RYR2* mutant brain tissue (figure 1; *lower, center*). Increased hippocampal CA3 seizure activity of *RYR2* mutant cells has been confirmed with confocal Ca^{2+} imaging of the somata in the principal cell layer in hippocampal brain slices (figure 1; *lower, right*). The Ca^{2+}

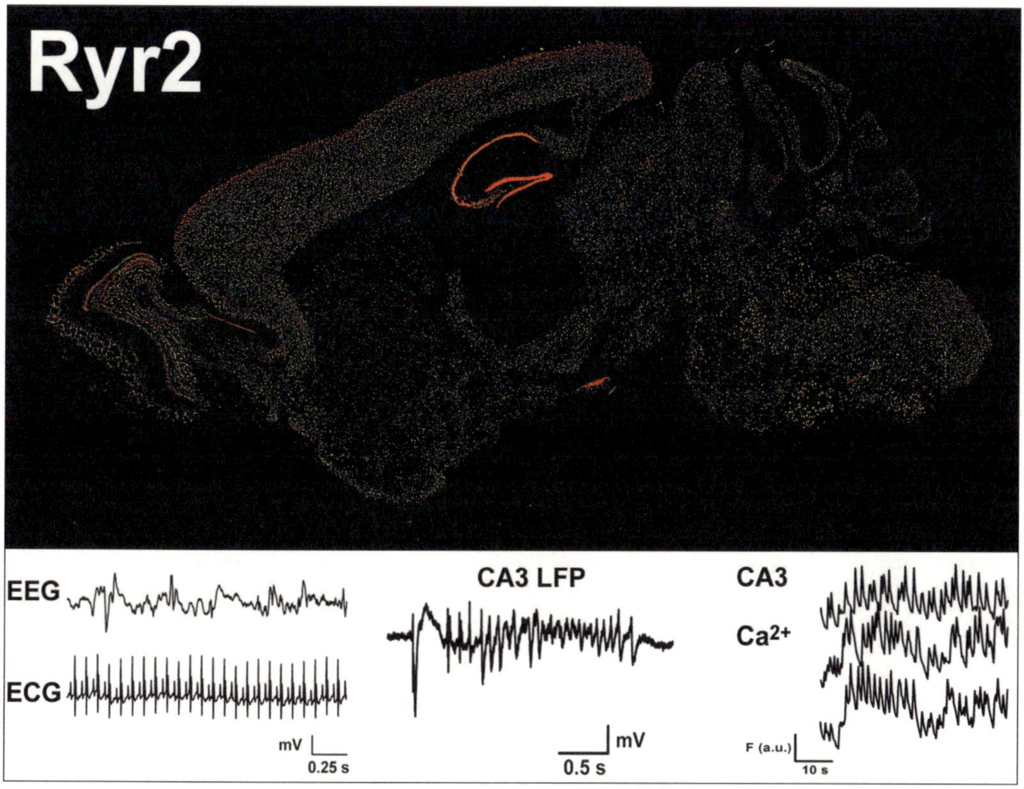

Fig. 1. Epileptogenic phenotype of *RYR2* knockin mice with orthologous patient mutations. *Top*: In situ RyR2 hybridization of a sagittal brain section from an adult male mouse brain. Red colour indicates maximal RyR2 mRNA expression as evidenced in the hippocampus and cerebral cortex. Image was prepared with the Allen Brain Atlas: http:www.brain-map.org; Seattle, WA: Allen Institute for Brain Science © 2006. *Bottom, left*: simultaneous EEG-ECG recording of awake heterozygous RyR2-R2474S mouse during start of generalized myoclonic seizure. *Bottom, center*: extracellular local field potential (LFP) recording of seizure-like events from CA3 region of hippocampal slices incubated in 10 μM 4-aminopyridine from heterozygous RyR2-R2474S mutant adult mouse showing abnormally complex and sustained bursting activity as compared to wild-type control (not shown). *Bottom, right*: continuous confocal fluo-4 Ca^{2+} fluorescence imaging of RyR2-R2474S mutant CA3 principal cell layer showing synchronized seizure bursting activity in low Mg^{2+} (0.5 mM)/high K^+ (8.5 mM) solution. Each trace represents the cytosolic Ca^{2+} signal from a local region of interest corresponding to the somata of three neighbouring CA3 pyramidal neurons. Reproduced from (Lehnart et al., 2008) with permission by "The American Society of Clinical Investigation" (www.jci.org) provided by Copyright Clearance Center, 2011.

imaging experiments revealed increased neuronal network synchronization in the CA3 region consistent with increased bursting activity of CA3 cells by LFP recording. In addition, single-channel bilayer recording, which were isolated from hippocampal tissue, showed a gain-of-function defect of RyR2-R2474S mutant channels consistent with abnormal intracellular Ca^{2+} leak, and consistent with abnormal confocal Ca^{2+} bursting activity in RyR2-R2474S brain slices (Lehnart et al., 2008). Because heterozygous RyR2-R2474S mice exhibited recurrent generalized tonic-clonic seizures and bilateral cortical EEG discharges in the absence of cardiac arrhythmias and in addition stress-induced ventricular arrhythmias in the absence of seizure activity, we proposed that RyR2 mutations cause a combined neuro-cardiogenic syndrome (Lehnart et al., 2008). As CPVT mutation carriers experience a very high mortality rate at young age which has been estimated between 33% and 50% at 35 years (Lehnart et al., 2004; Priori et al., 2002), *RYR2* is is a potential candidate gene for SUDEP.

2.3.2 Potassium channel mutations and generalized seizures

Unexpectedly, a LQTS patient study found that one third of confirmed mutation carriers have seizures including the relatively common *KCNQ1* mutation, indicating a potential link between cardiac arrhythmias and epilepsy (Johnson et al., 2009) However, *KCNQ1* expression in the brain is incompletely understood partially due to conflicting data. Importantly, *KCNQ1* mRNA and Kv7.1 protein expression, as well as expression of the accessory β-subunit minK have recently been confirmed in the human and mouse brain in the cortex and hippocampus (Goldman et al., 2009). Immunofluorescence staining as shown in figure 2 (*left*) further demonstrated that Kv7.1 is expressed within important hippocampal pathways including pyramidal neurons of the CA1 and CA3 regions, granule cells of the dentate gyrus, and hilar interneurons (Goldman et al., 2009). In addition, Kv7.1 positive neurons were found in the cortex, the thalamus, as well as brain stem nuclei which contribute parasympathetic outflow to the heart by the vagus nerve (Goldman et al., 2009). Thus, Kv7.1 protein expression has been confirmed in specific brain regions of the adult mouse, which are of potential significance for epileptogenesis.

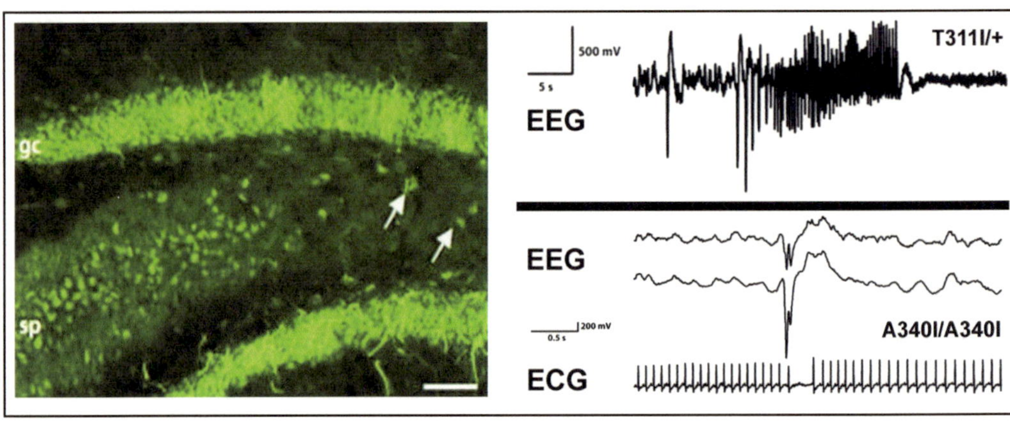

Fig. 2. Epileptogenic phenotype of *KCNQ1* knockin mice with orthologous patient mutations. *Left*: Kv7.1 immunofluorescence image of adult mouse brain section of the hippocampus dentate gyrus/hilar region showing positively stained granule cell layer (gc), CA3 pyramidal cell layer (sp), and hilar interneurons (arrows). Scale bar indicates 50 µm. *Right top*: EEG recording of a heterozygous Kv7.1-T311I mutant mouse during onset of a spontaneous convulsive seizure attack. *Right bottom*: Detail of combined EEG and ECG recording of a homozygous Kv7.1-A340I mutant mouse showing bilateral interictal discharges over the temporal cortex with coinciding AV conduction block in the ECG. Reproduced from (Goldman et al.,2009) with permission by "The American Association for the Advancement of Science" (www.sciencemag.org) provided by Copyright Clearance Center, 2011.

Two knockin mouse lines (T311I and A340E) with *KCNQ1* point mutations corresponding to human mutation carriers have previously been shown to reproduce the cardiac phenotype of LQTS1 (table 2) including ventricular arrhythmias (Casimiro et al., 2004). In addition, video-monitoring showed spontaneously occurring generalized seizures in one third of heterozygous mutant *KCNQ1* knockin mice, but never in wild-type control animals (Goldman et al., 2009). In addition, all heterozygous *KCNQ1* mutant animals showed partial seizures lasting less than 10 secs. The generalized seizures were characterized by sudden arrest of activity, followed by tonic extension and whole body convulsive movements, and simultaneous EEG showed bilateral rhythmic high voltage sharp wave discharges evolving into a higher frequency rhythmic discharges (figure 2, *right top*). In contrast, the partial seizures were characterized by behavioural arrest without prominent clonic movements, and the EEG showed coinciding low-voltage rhythmic slow activity interspersed with spike and wave discharges.

Registration of cortical activity by EEG in *KCNQ1* knockin mice with Kv7.1 mutations revealed epileptiform spike discharges and simultaneous ECG recording showed abnormal cardiac events consistent with slowing of the heart rhythm (Goldman et al., 2009). Awake, freely moving *KCNQ1* knockin mice exhibited frequent bilateral interictal epileptiform discharges including sharp waves and spikes, and prolonged runs of temporal focal slow waves. Interestingly, simultaneous ECG recording showed that approximately one fourth of cortical EEG discharges coincided with cardiac ECG abnormalities including prolonged beat-to-beat intervals, extrabeats, and even asystolie (complete block of ventricular rhythm) as shown figure 2 (*right bottom*). Of note, 62% of ECG abnormalities coincided with cortical EEG changes. Simultaneous EEG-ECG abnormalities are in agreement with autonomic dysregulation of impulse conduction as previously reported in SUDEP patients (Nei et al., 2004). In addition SCD was found in one homozygous T311I mouse, which died spontaneously from cardiac asystolie following prolonged seizures (Goldman et al., 2009).

2.4 Novel, targeted treatment strategies

Significant progress has been made to understand epilepsy through studies of monogenetic syndromes and the associated molecular mechanisms of seizures. Epilepsy genes have been identified in human mutations carriers and increasingly through animal models with distinct seizure phenotypes. Notably, the majority of identified epilepsy genes encode ion channels and associated subunits. These important insights have provided candidate treatment targets based on identified cellular and molecular mechanisms of epileptogenesis. In addition, epilepsy is increasingly recognized as heterogeneous syndrome of co-existing and even multi-organ syndromes, for example the neuro-cardiogenic syndromes discussed above. Advanced understanding of basic and complex seizure mechanisms has triggered development of new diagnostic and therapeutic approaches some of which are summarized here in the context of ion channelopathies.

Existing pharmacological and surgical therapies have been estimated to control seizure symptoms in approximately 60% of epilepsy patients. Therefore, development of novel therapies remains a major challenge. If one considers combined neuro-cardiogenic syndromes in the context of pharmacotherapies several important perspectives can be drawn from the mechanistic insights discussed in earlier chapters. Individuals at risk with SUDEP represent a major clinical challenge, and the gray area of undetected cardiac arrhythmia risk is potentially high due to lack of adequate screening strategies and awareness. Recent ECG studies showed that every fifth epilepsy patients experiences abnormally slow heart rhythms during seizures, culminating in 16% with asystolie which is potentially lethal (Rugg-Gunn et al., 2004). For confirmed *KCNQ1* mutation carriers implantable pacemaker therapy should be considered in the context of abnormally slow heart rhythms, and considering the possible changes of brainstem parasympathetic outflow to the heart recently identified in knockin mice with Kv7.1 mutations (Goldman et al., 2009). As β-blockers are therapeutically recommended in LQTS1 in confirmed *KCNQ1* mutation carriers with the potential side effect of slow heart rates, it is important to carefully monitor the heart rate behaviour in affected patients (Roden, 2008).

In addition, we have developed novel RyR2-specific compounds which permeate the blood-brain barrier and inhibit both neuronal seizures and cardiac arrhythmias (Lehnart et al., 2008). Different from conventional ion channel blockers, RyR2 stabilizing compounds like S107 have no effect on physiological channel function and do not alter intracellular Ca^{2+} signaling (Lehnart, 2007). In addition, S107 has not shown any significant side effects against other ion channels or enzymes in large screening panels (Lehnart et al., 2008). Similar to LQTS1, β-blocker therapy is recommended in patients with CPVT1 and confirmed *RYR2* mutation carrier status due to the characteristic dependence of cardiac arrhythmias on sympathetic outflow to the heart. In summary, the neuro-cardiological implications of idiopathic epilepsies are potentially important in mutation carriers, and comprehensive phenotype and genotype risk profiling may lead to improved therapy and prevention of fatal arrhythmias in affected epilepsy patients.

2.5 Summary of combined syndromes of neuronal and cardiac ion channelopathies

Recent studies have for the first time identified previously unrecognized brain ion channelopathies as the neurobiological basis of generalized seizures. While the epilepsy phenotypes represent primary brain discharges, the same molecular defects precipitate life-threatening cardiac arrhythmias. The following mechanisms have been proposed to underlie epilepsy in combined neuro-cardiogenic syndromes:

Kv7.1 dysfunction in *KCNQ1* mutation carriers with LQTS1 may alter the propensity of neurons and cardiac myocytes to repolarize following depolarization by an action potential. This results in a decreased repolarization capacity in the brain and heart. In the brain, a decreased repolarization capacity during action potential firing may result in seizures and brainstem autonomic dysfunction of parasympathetic outflow leading to heart rhythm block and asystolie for example at the level of the cardiac AV node. Dysfunction of brain stem parasympathetic outflow to the cardiac sinus and atrioventricular nodes as a cause of asystolie in epilepsy expands previously described arrhythmia mechanisms, since fast ventricular arrhythmias are characteristically triggered by increased sympathetic outflow in *KCNQ1* mutation carriers. Because Kv7.1 mutations can cause dangerous cardiac arrhythmias, *KCNQ1* is a molecular candidate mechanism and risk factor of SUDEP. These findings establish *KCNQ1* in neuronal hyperexcitability and epileptogenesis. Hundreds of *KCNQ1* mutations have been identified mostly leading to loss-of-function phenotypes. However, the correlation between Kv7.1 channel defects and the clinical phenotype in different organs is variable, and not all mutations may cause epilepsy or only when a permissive background or environmental condition exists.

RYR2 mutations appear to cause increased neuronal burst activity of the hippocampal CA3 region and seizure activity as evidenced by synchronous bursting Ca^{2+} signals of principal cells in hippocampal brain slices. Indeed, increased neuronal network synchronization in the CA3 region is consistent with a gain-of-function defect of RyR2-R2474S mutant channels which exhibit defective closure (Lehnart et al., 2008). A hippocampal seizure mechanism is also consistent with the progressive, generalized tonic-clonic seizures and bilateral cortical EEG discharges documented in *RYR2* mutant mice with patient mutations.

3. Conclusion

Recent advances in ion channelopathy studies related to epilepsy have achieved important new insights about combined neuro-cardiogenic phenotypes, and mechanisms which may link dysrhythmia phenotypes of the brain and heart through the autonomic nervous system. Already, these insights have motivated further research about diagnostic strategies to improve risk prediction and prevention in patients with seizure disorders of unknown origin. In addition, novel therapeutic strategies which target the underlying molecular mechanisms are under development. Despite significant new mechanistic insight about Kv7.1 and RyR2 ion channel mutations as the cause of combined neuro-cardiogenic seizure and arrhythmia syndromes, many questions remain unanswered and require further study. These questions concern the specific brain regions and neuron types, which show a decreased threshold for aberrant network synchronization, such that prolonged depolarization or delayed repolarization may initiate primary brain seizures. In addition, arrhythmias in LQTS1 and CPVT1 are characteristically modulated by the autonomous nervous system. If the autonomous nervous system is also affected by the same gene mutations and exacerbates the cardiac and/or neuronal phenotypes needs further exploration through multidisciplinary research teams. Clearly, the new insights about neuro-cardiogenic dysrhythmias should motivate both clinicians and researchers to critically inquire complex phenotypes beyond the borders of a given research discipline.

4. Acknowledgment

This work was supported by Deutsche Forschungsgemeinschaft through a clinical research unit KFO 155 subproject grant [LE 1313/2-1]. The research leading to these results has received funding from the European Community's Seventh Framework Program FP7/2007-2013 under grant agreement n° HEALTH-F2-2009-241526, EUTrigTreat.

5. References

Abbott, G.W., Sesti, F., Splawski, I., Buck, M.E., Lehmann, M.H., Timothy, K.W., Keating, M.T., & Goldstein, S.A. (1999). MiRP1 forms IKr potassium channels with HERG and is associated with cardiac arrhythmia. *Cell*, Vol. 97, pp. 175-187, ISSN 0092-8674

Albert, C.M., MacRae, C.A., Chasman, D.I., VanDenburgh, M., Buring, J.E., Manson, J.E., Cook, N.R., & Newton-Cheh, C. Common variants in cardiac ion channel genes are associated with sudden cardiac death. *Circ Arrhythm Electrophysiol*, Vol. 3, (2010/04/20), pp. 222-229, ISSN 1941-3084

Antzelevitch, C., Pollevick, G.D., Cordeiro, J.M., Casis, O., Sanguinetti, M.C., Aizawa, Y., Guerchicoff, A., Pfeiffer, R., Oliva, A., Wollnik, B., Gelber, P., Bonaros, E.P., Jr., Burashnikov, E., Wu, Y., Sargent, J.D., Schickel, S., Oberheiden, R., Bhatia, A., Hsu,

L.F., Haissaguerre, M., Schimpf, R., Borggrefe, M., & Wolpert, C. (2007). Loss-of-function mutations in the cardiac calcium channel underlie a new clinical entity characterized by ST-segment elevation, short QT intervals, and sudden cardiac death. *Circulation*, Vol. 115, (2007/01/17), pp. 442-449, ISSN 1524-4539

Aridon, P., Marini, C., Di Resta, C., Brilli, E., De Fusco, M., Politi, F., Parrini, E., Manfredi, I., Pisano, T., Pruna, D., Curia, G., Cianchetti, C., Pasqualetti, M., Becchetti, A., Guerrini, R., & Casari, G. (2006). Increased sensitivity of the neuronal nicotinic receptor alpha 2 subunit causes familial epilepsy with nocturnal wandering and ictal fear. *Am J Hum Genet*, Vol. 79, (2006/07/11), pp. 342-350, ISSN 0002-9297

Arnestad, M., Crotti, L., Rognum, T.O., Insolia, R., Pedrazzini, M., Ferrandi, C., Vege, A., Wang, D.W., Rhodes, T.E., George, A.L., Jr., & Schwartz, P.J. (2007). Prevalence of Long-QT Syndrome Gene Variants in Sudden Infant Death Syndrome. *Circulation*, ISSN 1524-4539

Bai, R., Napolitano, C., Bloise, R., Monteforte, N., & Priori, S.G. (2009). Yield of genetic screening in inherited cardiac channelopathies: how to prioritize access to genetic testing. *Circ Arrhythm Electrophysiol*, Vol. 2, (2009/10/08), pp. 6-15, ISSN

Baulac, S., Huberfeld, G., Gourfinkel-An, I., Mitropoulou, G., Beranger, A., Prud'homme, J.F., Baulac, M., Brice, A., Bruzzone, R., & LeGuern, E. (2001). First genetic evidence of GABA(A) receptor dysfunction in epilepsy: a mutation in the gamma2-subunit gene. *Nat Genet*, Vol. 28, (2001/04/28), pp. 46-48, ISSN 1061-4036

Bellocq, C., van Ginneken, A.C., Bezzina, C.R., Alders, M., Escande, D., Mannens, M.M., Baro, I., & Wilde, A.A. (2004). Mutation in the KCNQ1 gene leading to the short QT-interval syndrome. *Circulation*, Vol. 109, pp. 2394-2397, ISSN 1524-4539

Bendahhou, S., Donaldson, M.R., Plaster, N.M., Tristani-Firouzi, M., Fu, Y.H., & Ptacek, L.J. (2003). Defective potassium channel Kir2.1 trafficking underlies Andersen-Tawil syndrome. *J Biol Chem*, Vol. 278, pp. 51779-51785, ISSN 0021-9258

Bennett, P.B., Yazawa, K., Makita, N., & George, A.L., Jr. (1995). Molecular mechanism for an inherited cardiac arrhythmia. *Nature*, Vol. 376, pp. 683-685, ISSN 0028-0836

Berkovic, S.F., Heron, S.E., Giordano, L., Marini, C., Guerrini, R., Kaplan, R.E., Gambardella, A., Steinlein, O.K., Grinton, B.E., Dean, J.T., Bordo, L., Hodgson, B.L., Yamamoto, T., Mulley, J.C., Zara, F., & Scheffer, I.E. (2004). Benign familial neonatal-infantile seizures: characterization of a new sodium channelopathy. *Ann Neurol*, Vol. 55, (2004/03/30), pp. 550-557, ISSN 0364-5134

Biervert, C., Schroeder, B.C., Kubisch, C., Berkovic, S.F., Propping, P., Jentsch, T.J., & Steinlein, O.K. (1998). A potassium channel mutation in neonatal human epilepsy. *Science*, Vol. 279, (1998/02/07), pp. 403-406, ISSN 0036-8075

Britton, J.W., Ghearing, G.R., Benarroch, E.E., & Cascino, G.D. (2006). The ictal bradycardia syndrome: localization and lateralization. *Epilepsia*, Vol. 47, (2006/05/03), pp. 737-744, ISSN 0013-9580

Brugada, R., Hong, K., Dumaine, R., Cordeiro, J., Gaita, F., Borggrefe, M., Menendez, T.M., Brugada, J., Pollevick, G.D., Wolpert, C., Burashnikov, E., Matsuo, K., Wu, Y.S., Guerchicoff, A., Bianchi, F., Giustetto, C., Schimpf, R., Brugada, P., & Antzelevitch, C. (2004). Sudden death associated with short-QT syndrome linked to mutations in HERG. *Circulation*, Vol. 109, pp. 30-35, ISSN 1524-4539

Byrne, R., Constant, O., Smyth, Y., Callagy, G., Nash, P., Daly, K., & Crowley, J. (2008). Multiple source surveillance incidence and aetiology of out-of-hospital sudden cardiac death in a rural population in the West of Ireland. *Eur Heart J*, Vol. 29, (2008/04/22), pp. 1418-1423, ISSN 1522-9645

Casimiro, M.C., Knollmann, B.C., Yamoah, E.N., Nie, L., Vary, J.C., Jr., Sirenko, S.G., Greene, A.E., Grinberg, A., Huang, S.P., Ebert, S.N., & Pfeifer, K. (2004). Targeted point mutagenesis of mouse Kcnq1: phenotypic analysis of mice with point mutations that cause Romano-Ward syndrome in humans. *Genomics*, Vol. 84, pp. 555-564, ISSN 0888-7543

Charlier, C., Singh, N.A., Ryan, S.G., Lewis, T.B., Reus, B.E., Leach, R.J., & Leppert, M. (1998). A pore mutation in a novel KQT-like potassium channel gene in an idiopathic epilepsy family. *Nat Genet*, Vol. 18, (1998/01/13), pp. 53-55, ISSN 1061-4036

Chen, Q., Kirsch, G.E., Zhang, D., Brugada, R., Brugada, J., Brugada, P., Potenza, D., Moya, A., Borggrefe, M., Breithardt, G., Ortiz-Lopez, R., Wang, Z., Antzelevitch, C., O'Brien, R.E., Schulze-Bahr, E., Keating, M.T., Towbin, J.A., & Wang, Q. (1998). Genetic basis and molecular mechanism for idiopathic ventricular fibrillation. *Nature*, Vol. 392, pp. 293-296, ISSN 0028-0836

Chugh, S.S., Jui, J., Gunson, K., Stecker, E.C., John, B.T., Thompson, B., Ilias, N., Vickers, C., Dogra, V., Daya, M., Kron, J., Zheng, Z.J., Mensah, G., & McAnulty, J. (2004). Current burden of sudden cardiac death: multiple source surveillance versus retrospective death certificate-based review in a large U.S. community. *J Am Coll Cardiol*, Vol. 44, (2004/09/15), pp. 1268-1275, ISSN 0735-1097

Chugh, S.S., Reinier, K., Teodorescu, C., Evanado, A., Kehr, E., Al Samara, M., Mariani, R., Gunson, K., & Jui, J. (2008). Epidemiology of sudden cardiac death: clinical and research implications. *Progress in cardiovascular diseases*, Vol. 51, (2008/11/26), pp. 213-228, ISSN 1532-8643

Claes, L., Del-Favero, J., Ceulemans, B., Lagae, L., Van Broeckhoven, C., & De Jonghe, P. (2001). De novo mutations in the sodium-channel gene SCN1A cause severe myoclonic epilepsy of infancy. *Am J Hum Genet*, Vol. 68, (2001/05/19), pp. 1327-1332, ISSN 0002-9297

Cossette, P., Liu, L., Brisebois, K., Dong, H., Lortie, A., Vanasse, M., Saint-Hilaire, J.M., Carmant, L., Verner, A., Lu, W.Y., Wang, Y.T., & Rouleau, G.A. (2002). Mutation of GABRA1 in an autosomal dominant form of juvenile myoclonic epilepsy. *Nat Genet*, Vol. 31, (2002/05/07), pp. 184-189, ISSN 1061-4036

Curran, M.E., Splawski, I., Timothy, K.W., Vincent, G.M., Green, E.D., & Keating, M.T. (1995). A molecular basis for cardiac arrhythmia: HERG mutations cause long QT syndrome. *Cell*, Vol. 80, pp. 795-803, ISSN 0092-8674

De Fusco, M., Becchetti, A., Patrignani, A., Annesi, G., Gambardella, A., Quattrone, A., Ballabio, A., Wanke, E., & Casari, G. (2000). The nicotinic receptor beta 2 subunit is mutant in nocturnal frontal lobe epilepsy. *Nat Genet*, Vol. 26, (2000/11/04), pp. 275-276, ISSN 1061-4036

Deprez, L., Weckhuysen, S., Peeters, K., Deconinck, T., Claeys, K.G., Claes, L.R., Suls, A., Van Dyck, T., Palmini, A., Matthijs, G., Van Paesschen, W., & De Jonghe, P. (2008). Epilepsy as part of the phenotype associated with ATP1A2 mutations. *Epilepsia*, Vol. 49, (2007/11/22), pp. 500-508, ISSN 0013-9580

Du, W., Bautista, J.F., Yang, H., Diez-Sampedro, A., You, S.A., Wang, L., Kotagal, P., Luders, H.O., Shi, J., Cui, J., Richerson, G.B., & Wang, Q.K. (2005). Calcium-sensitive potassium channelopathy in human epilepsy and paroxysmal movement disorder. *Nat Genet*, Vol. 37, (2005/06/07), pp. 733-738, ISSN 1061-4036

Escayg, A., MacDonald, B.T., Meisler, M.H., Baulac, S., Huberfeld, G., An-Gourfinkel, I., Brice, A., LeGuern, E., Moulard, B., Chaigne, D., Buresi, C., & Malafosse, A. (2000). Mutations of SCN1A, encoding a neuronal sodium channel, in two families with GEFS+2. *Nat Genet*, Vol. 24, (2000/03/31), pp. 343-345, ISSN 1061-4036

Eunson, L.H., Rea, R., Zuberi, S.M., Youroukos, S., Panayiotopoulos, C.P., Liguori, R., Avoni, P., McWilliam, R.C., Stephenson, J.B., Hanna, M.G., Kullmann, D.M., & Spauschus, A. (2000). Clinical, genetic, and expression studies of mutations in the potassium channel gene KCNA1 reveal new phenotypic variability. *Ann Neurol*, Vol. 48, (2000/10/12), pp. 647-656, ISSN 0364-5134

Ficker, D.M., So, E.L., Shen, W.K., Annegers, J.F., O'Brien, P.C., Cascino, G.D., & Belau, P.G. (1998). Population-based study of the incidence of sudden unexplained death in epilepsy. *Neurology*, Vol. 51, (1998/11/18), pp. 1270-1274, ISSN 0028-3878

Goldman, A.M., Glasscock, E., Yoo, J., Chen, T.T., Klassen, T.L., & Noebels, J.L. (2009). Arrhythmia in heart and brain: KCNQ1 mutations link epilepsy and sudden unexplained death. *Sci Transl Med*, Vol. 1, (2010/04/07), pp. 2ra6, ISSN 1946-6242

Hartmann, H.A., Colom, L.V., Sutherland, M.L., & Noebels, J.L. (1999). Selective localization of cardiac SCN5A sodium channels in limbic regions of rat brain. *Nat Neurosci*, Vol. 2, pp. 593-595, ISSN 1097-6256

Henzi, V., & MacDermott, A.B. (1992). Characteristics and function of Ca(2+)- and inositol 1,4,5-trisphosphate-releasable stores of Ca2+ in neurons. *Neuroscience*, Vol. 46, (1992/01/01), pp. 251-273, ISSN 0306-4522

Heron, S.E., Crossland, K.M., Andermann, E., Phillips, H.A., Hall, A.J., Bleasel, A., Shevell, M., Mercho, S., Seni, M.H., Guiot, M.C., Mulley, J.C., Berkovic, S.F., & Scheffer, I.E. (2002). Sodium-channel defects in benign familial neonatal-infantile seizures. *Lancet*, Vol. 360, (2002/09/24), pp. 851-852, ISSN 0140-6736

Hitiris, N., Suratman, S., Kelly, K., Stephen, L.J., Sills, G.J., & Brodie, M.J. (2007). Sudden unexpected death in epilepsy: A search for risk factors. *Epilepsy Behav*, Vol. 10, pp. 138-141, ISSN 1525-5050

Hofman, N., Wilde, A.A., & Tan, H.L. (2007). Diagnostic criteria for congenital long QT syndrome in the era of molecular genetics: do we need a scoring system? *Eur Heart J*, Vol. 28, (2007/05/08), pp. 1399, ISSN 0195-668X

Hong, K., Bjerregaard, P., Gussak, I., & Brugada, R. (2005a). Short QT syndrome and atrial fibrillation caused by mutation in KCNH2. *J Cardiovasc Electrophysiol*, Vol. 16, pp. 394-396, ISSN 1045-3873

Hong, K., Piper, D.R., Diaz-Valdecantos, A., Brugada, J., Oliva, A., Burashnikov, E., Santos-de-Soto, J., Grueso-Montero, J., Diaz-Enfante, E., Brugada, P., Sachse, F., Sanguinetti, M.C., & Brugada, R. (2005b). De novo KCNQ1 mutation responsible for atrial fibrillation and short QT syndrome in utero. *Cardiovasc Res*, Vol. 68, pp. 433-440, ISSN 0008-6363

Imbrici, P., Jaffe, S.L., Eunson, L.H., Davies, N.P., Herd, C., Robertson, R., Kullmann, D.M., & Hanna, M.G. (2004). Dysfunction of the brain calcium channel CaV2.1 in absence epilepsy and episodic ataxia. *Brain*, Vol. 127, (2004/10/16), pp. 2682-2692, ISSN 1460-2156

Jehi, L., & Najm, I.M. (2008). Sudden unexpected death in epilepsy: impact, mechanisms, and prevention. *Cleve Clin J Med*, Vol. 75 Suppl 2, (2008/06/11), pp. S66-70, ISSN 0891-1150

Johnson, J.N., Hofman, N., Haglund, C.M., Cascino, G.D., Wilde, A.A., & Ackerman, M.J. (2009). Identification of a possible pathogenic link between congenital long QT syndrome and epilepsy. *Neurology*, Vol. 72, (2008/11/29), pp. 224-231, ISSN 1526-632X

Johnson, J.N., Tester, D.J., Bass, N.E., & Ackerman, M.J. Cardiac channel molecular autopsy for sudden unexpected death in epilepsy. *J Child Neurol*, Vol. 25, (2010/04/17), pp. 916-921, ISSN 1708-8283

Jouvenceau, A., Eunson, L.H., Spauschus, A., Ramesh, V., Zuberi, S.M., Kullmann, D.M., & Hanna, M.G. (2001). Human epilepsy associated with dysfunction of the brain P/Q-type calcium channel. *Lancet*, Vol. 358, (2001/09/21), pp. 801-807, ISSN 0140-6736

Kananura, C., Haug, K., Sander, T., Runge, U., Gu, W., Hallmann, K., Rebstock, J., Heils, A., & Steinlein, O.K. (2002). A splice-site mutation in GABRG2 associated with childhood absence epilepsy and febrile convulsions. *Arch Neurol*, Vol. 59, (2002/07/16), pp. 1137-1141, ISSN 0003-9942

Kostyuk, P., & Verkhratsky, A. (1994). Calcium stores in neurons and glia. *Neuroscience*, Vol. 63, (1994/11/01), pp. 381-404, ISSN 0306-4522

Kubisch, C., Schroeder, B.C., Friedrich, T., Lutjohann, B., El-Amraoui, A., Marlin, S., Petit, C., & Jentsch, T.J. (1999). KCNQ4, a novel potassium channel expressed in sensory outer hair cells, is mutated in dominant deafness. *Cell*, Vol. 96, (1999/02/20), pp. 437-446, ISSN 0092-8674

Lahat, H., Pras, E., Olender, T., Avidan, N., Ben-Asher, E., Man, O., Levy-Nissenbaum, E., Khoury, A., Lorber, A., Goldman, B., Lancet, D., & Eldar, M. (2001). A missense mutation in a highly conserved region of CASQ2 is associated with autosomal recessive catecholamine-induced polymorphic ventricular tachycardia in Bedouin families from Israel. *Am J Hum Genet*, Vol. 69, pp. 1378-1384, ISSN

Laitinen, P.J., Brown, K.M., Piippo, K., Swan, H., Devaney, J.M., Brahmbhatt, B., Donarum, E.A., Marino, M., Tiso, N., Viitasalo, M., Toivonen, L., Stephan, D.A., & Kontula, K. (2001). Mutations of the cardiac ryanodine receptor (RyR2) gene in familial polymorphic ventricular tachycardia. *Circulation*, Vol. 103, pp. 485-490, ISSN

Leenhardt, A., Lucet, V., Denjoy, I., Grau, F., Ngoc, D.D., & Coumel, P. (1995). Catecholaminergic polymorphic ventricular tachycardia in children. A 7-year follow-up of 21 patients. *Circulation*, Vol. 91, pp. 1512-1519, ISSN 0009-7322 (Print)

Lehnart, S.E. (2007). Novel targets for treating heart and muscle disease: stabilizing ryanodine receptors and preventing intracellular calcium leak. *Curr Opin Pharmacol*, Vol. 7, (2007/02/20), pp. 225-232, ISSN 1471-4892

Lehnart, S.E., Ackerman, M.J., Benson, D.W., Jr., Brugada, R., Clancy, C.E., Donahue, J.K., George, A.L., Jr., Grant, A.O., Groft, S.C., January, C.T., Lathrop, D.A., Lederer, W.J., Makielski, J.C., Mohler, P.J., Moss, A., Nerbonne, J.M., Olson, T.M., Przywara, D.A., Towbin, J.A., Wang, L.H., & Marks, A.R. (2007). Inherited arrhythmias: a National Heart, Lung, and Blood Institute and Office of Rare Diseases workshop consensus report about the diagnosis, phenotyping, molecular mechanisms, and therapeutic approaches for primary cardiomyopathies of gene mutations affecting ion channel function. *Circulation*, Vol. 116, (2007/11/14), pp. 2325-2345, ISSN 1524-4539

Lehnart, S.E., Mongillo, M., Bellinger, A., Lindegger, N., Chen, B.X., Hsueh, W., Reiken, S., Wronska, A., Drew, L.J., Ward, C.W., Lederer, W.J., Kass, R.S., Morley, G., & Marks,

A.R. (2008). Leaky Ca2+ release channel/ryanodine receptor 2 causes seizures and sudden cardiac death in mice. *J Clin Invest*, Vol. 118, (2008/05/17), pp. 2230-2245, ISSN 0021-9738

Lehnart, S.E., Wehrens, X.H., Laitinen, P.J., Reiken, S.R., Deng, S.X., Cheng, Z., Landry, D.W., Kontula, K., Swan, H., & Marks, A.R. (2004). Sudden death in familial polymorphic ventricular tachycardia associated with calcium release channel (ryanodine receptor) leak. *Circulation*, Vol. 109, pp. 3208-3214, ISSN

McKeon, A., Vaughan, C., & Delanty, N. (2006). Seizure versus syncope. *Lancet Neurol*, Vol. 5, (2006/01/24), pp. 171-180, ISSN 1474-4422

Medeiros-Domingo, A., Kaku, T., Tester, D.J., Torres, P.I., Itty, A., Ye, B., Valdivia, C., Quintero, A., Luna, M.T., Makielski, J.C., & Ackerman, M.J. (2007). Sodium channel β4 subunit (SCN4β) mutation causes congenital long QT syndrome. . *Circulation*, Vol. (*in press*), ISSN

Mignery, G.A., Sudhof, T.C., Takei, K., & De Camilli, P. (1989). Putative receptor for inositol 1,4,5-trisphosphate similar to ryanodine receptor. *Nature*, Vol. 342, pp. 192-195, ISSN 0028-0836

Mori, F., Okada, M., Tomiyama, M., Kaneko, S., & Wakabayashi, K. (2005). Effects of ryanodine receptor activation on neurotransmitter release and neuronal cell death following kainic acid-induced status epilepticus. *Epilepsy research*, Vol. 65, pp. 59-70, ISSN 0920-1211

Moss, A.J., & Schwartz, P.J. (2005). 25th anniversary of the International Long-QT Syndrome Registry: an ongoing quest to uncover the secrets of long-QT syndrome. *Circulation*, Vol. 111, (2005/03/09), pp. 1199-1201, ISSN 1524-4539

Moss, A.J., Shimizu, W., Wilde, A.A., Towbin, J.A., Zareba, W., Robinson, J.L., Qi, M., Vincent, G.M., Ackerman, M.J., Kaufman, E.S., Hofman, N., Seth, R., Kamakura, S., Miyamoto, Y., Goldenberg, I., Andrews, M.L., & McNitt, S. (2007). Clinical aspects of type-1 long-QT syndrome by location, coding type, and biophysical function of mutations involving the KCNQ1 gene. *Circulation*, Vol. 115, pp. 2481-2489, ISSN 1524-4539

Nabbout, R., Gennaro, E., Dalla Bernardina, B., Dulac, O., Madia, F., Bertini, E., Capovilla, G., Chiron, C., Cristofori, G., Elia, M., Fontana, E., Gaggero, R., Granata, T., Guerrini, R., Loi, M., La Selva, L., Lispi, M.L., Matricardi, A., Romeo, A., Tzolas, V., Valseriati, D., Veggiotti, P., Vigevano, F., Vallee, L., Dagna Bricarelli, F., Bianchi, A., & Zara, F. (2003). Spectrum of SCN1A mutations in severe myoclonic epilepsy of infancy. *Neurology*, Vol. 60, (2003/06/25), pp. 1961-1967, ISSN 1526-632X

Nagrani, T., Siyamwala, M., Vahid, G., & Bekheit, S. Ryanodine calcium channel: a novel channelopathy for seizures. *Neurologist*, Vol. 17, (2011/03/03), pp. 91-94, ISSN 1074-7931

Nashef, L., Hindocha, N., & Makoff, A. (2007). Risk factors in sudden death in epilepsy (SUDEP): the quest for mechanisms. *Epilepsia*, Vol. 48, pp. 859-871, ISSN 0013-9580

Nei, M., Ho, R.T., Abou-Khalil, B.W., Drislane, F.W., Liporace, J., Romeo, A., & Sperling, M.R. (2004). EEG and ECG in sudden unexplained death in epilepsy. *Epilepsia*, Vol. 45, (2004/03/20), pp. 338-345, ISSN 0013-9580

Nei, M., Ho, R.T., & Sperling, M.R. (2000). EKG abnormalities during partial seizures in refractory epilepsy. *Epilepsia*, Vol. 41, (2000/05/10), pp. 542-548, ISSN 0013-9580

Newton-Cheh, C., Eijgelsheim, M., Rice, K.M., de Bakker, P.I., Yin, X., Estrada, K., Bis, J.C., Marciante, K., Rivadeneira, F., Noseworthy, P.A., Sotoodehnia, N., Smith, N.L., Rotter, J.I., Kors, J.A., Witteman, J.C., Hofman, A., Heckbert, S.R., O'Donnell, C.J., Uitterlinden, A.G., Psaty, B.M., Lumley, T., Larson, M.G., & Stricker, B.H. (2009). Common variants at ten loci influence QT interval duration in the QTGEN Study. *Nat Genet*, Vol. 41, (2009/03/24), pp. 399-406, ISSN 1546-1718

Nichol, G., Thomas, E., Callaway, C.W., Hedges, J., Powell, J.L., Aufderheide, T.P., Rea, T., Lowe, R., Brown, T., Dreyer, J., Davis, D., Idris, A., & Stiell, I. (2008). Regional variation in out-of-hospital cardiac arrest incidence and outcome. *Jama*, Vol. 300, (2008/09/25), pp. 1423-1431, ISSN 1538-3598

Opherk, C., Coromilas, J., & Hirsch, L.J. (2002). Heart rate and EKG changes in 102 seizures: analysis of influencing factors. *Epilepsy research*, Vol. 52, (2002/11/30), pp. 117-127, ISSN 0920-1211

Osler, W. (1903). ON THE SO-CALLED STOKES-ADAMS DISEASE (SLOW PULSE WITH SYNCOPAL ATTACKS, &c.). *The Lancet*, Vol. 162, (2003/09/18), pp. 516-524, ISSN

Ottman, R., Hirose, S., Jain, S., Lerche, H., Lopes-Cendes, I., Noebels, J.L., Serratosa, J., Zara, F., & Scheffer, I.E. Genetic testing in the epilepsies--report of the ILAE Genetics Commission. *Epilepsia*, Vol. 51, (2010/01/27), pp. 655-670, ISSN 1528-1167

Plant, L.D., Bowers, P.N., Liu, Q., Morgan, T., Zhang, T., State, M.W., Chen, W., Kittles, R.A., & Goldstein, S.A. (2006). A common cardiac sodium channel variant associated with sudden infant death in African Americans, SCN5A S1103Y. *J Clin Invest*, Vol. 116, (2006/02/03), pp. 430-435, ISSN 0021-9738

Plaster, N.M., Tawil, R., Tristani-Firouzi, M., Canun, S., Bendahhou, S., Tsunoda, A., Donaldson, M.R., Iannaccone, S.T., Brunt, E., Barohn, R., Clark, J., Deymeer, F., George, A.L., Jr., Fish, F.A., Hahn, A., Nitu, A., Ozdemir, C., Serdaroglu, P., Subramony, S.H., Wolfe, G., Fu, Y.H., & Ptacek, L.J. (2001). Mutations in Kir2.1 cause the developmental and episodic electrical phenotypes of Andersen's syndrome. *Cell*, Vol. 105, pp. 511-519, ISSN 0092-8674

Postma, A.V., Denjoy, I., Hoorntje, T.M., Lupoglazoff, J.M., Da Costa, A., Sebillon, P., Mannens, M.M., Wilde, A.A., & Guicheney, P. (2002). Absence of calsequestrin 2 causes severe forms of catecholaminergic polymorphic ventricular tachycardia. *Circ Res*, Vol. 91, pp. e21-26, ISSN

Postma, A.V., Denjoy, I., Kamblock, J., Alders, M., Lupoglazoff, J.M., Vaksmann, G., Dubosq-Bidot, L., Sebillon, P., Mannens, M.M., Guicheney, P., & Wilde, A.A. (2005). Catecholaminergic polymorphic ventricular tachycardia: RYR2 mutations, bradycardia, and follow up of the patients. *J Med Genet*, Vol. 42, pp. 863-870, ISSN 1468-6244

Priori, S.G., Napolitano, C., Memmi, M., Colombi, B., Drago, F., Gasparini, M., DeSimone, L., Coltorti, F., Bloise, R., Keegan, R., Cruz Filho, F.E., Vignati, G., Benatar, A., & DeLogu, A. (2002). Clinical and molecular characterization of patients with catecholaminergic polymorphic ventricular tachycardia. *Circulation*, Vol. 106, pp. 69-74, ISSN

Priori, S.G., Napolitano, C., Tiso, N., Memmi, M., Vignati, G., Bloise, R., Sorrentino, V., & Danieli, G.A. (2001). Mutations in the cardiac ryanodine receptor gene (hRyR2) underlie catecholaminergic polymorphic ventricular tachycardia. *Circulation*, Vol. 103, pp. 196-200, ISSN

Priori, S.G., Pandit, S.V., Rivolta, I., Berenfeld, O., Ronchetti, E., Dhamoon, A., Napolitano, C., Anumonwo, J., di Barletta, M.R., Gudapakkam, S., Bosi, G., Stramba-Badiale, M., & Jalife, J. (2005). A novel form of short QT syndrome (SQT3) is caused by a mutation in the KCNJ2 gene. *Circ Res*, Vol. 96, pp. 800-807, ISSN 1524-4571

Roden, D.M. (2008). Clinical practice. Long-QT syndrome. *N Engl J Med*, Vol. 358, (2008/01/11), pp. 169-176, ISSN 1533-4406

Rugg-Gunn, F.J., Simister, R.J., Squirrell, M., Holdright, D.R., & Duncan, J.S. (2004). Cardiac arrhythmias in focal epilepsy: a prospective long-term study. *Lancet*, Vol. 364, (2004/12/22), pp. 2212-2219, ISSN 1474-547X

Sanguinetti, M.C., Curran, M.E., Zou, A., Shen, J., Spector, P.S., Atkinson, D.L., & Keating, M.T. (1996). Coassembly of K(V)LQT1 and minK (IsK) proteins to form cardiac I(Ks) potassium channel. *Nature*, Vol. 384, pp. 80-83, ISSN 0028-0836

Singh, N.A., Charlier, C., Stauffer, D., DuPont, B.R., Leach, R.J., Melis, R., Ronen, G.M., Bjerre, I., Quattlebaum, T., Murphy, J.V., McHarg, M.L., Gagnon, D., Rosales, T.O., Peiffer, A., Anderson, V.E., & Leppert, M. (1998). A novel potassium channel gene, KCNQ2, is mutated in an inherited epilepsy of newborns. *Nat Genet*, Vol. 18, (1998/01/13), pp. 25-29, ISSN 1061-4036

Spauschus, A., Eunson, L., Hanna, M.G., & Kullmann, D.M. (1999). Functional characterization of a novel mutation in KCNA1 in episodic ataxia type 1 associated with epilepsy. *Ann N Y Acad Sci*, Vol. 868, (1999/07/22), pp. 442-446, ISSN 0077-8923

Splawski, I., Timothy, K.W., Decher, N., Kumar, P., Sachse, F.B., Beggs, A.H., Sanguinetti, M.C., & Keating, M.T. (2005). Severe arrhythmia disorder caused by cardiac L-type calcium channel mutations. *Proc Natl Acad Sci U S A*, Vol. 102, pp. 8089-8096; discussion 8086-8088, ISSN 0027-8424

Splawski, I., Timothy, K.W., Sharpe, L.M., Decher, N., Kumar, P., Bloise, R., Napolitano, C., Schwartz, P.J., Joseph, R.M., Condouris, K., Tager-Flusberg, H., Priori, S.G., Sanguinetti, M.C., & Keating, M.T. (2004). Ca(V)1.2 calcium channel dysfunction causes a multisystem disorder including arrhythmia and autism. *Cell*, Vol. 119, pp. 19-31, ISSN 0092-8674

Splawski, I., Tristani-Firouzi, M., Lehmann, M.H., Sanguinetti, M.C., & Keating, M.T. (1997). Mutations in the hminK gene cause long QT syndrome and suppress IKs function. *Nat Genet*, Vol. 17, pp. 338-340, ISSN 1061-4036

Steinlein, O.K., Mulley, J.C., Propping, P., Wallace, R.H., Phillips, H.A., Sutherland, G.R., Scheffer, I.E., & Berkovic, S.F. (1995). A missense mutation in the neuronal nicotinic acetylcholine receptor alpha 4 subunit is associated with autosomal dominant nocturnal frontal lobe epilepsy. *Nat Genet*, Vol. 11, (1995/10/01), pp. 201-203, ISSN 1061-4036

Street, V.A., Bosma, M.M., Demas, V.P., Regan, M.R., Lin, D.D., Robinson, L.C., Agnew, W.S., & Tempel, B.L. (1997). The type 1 inositol 1,4,5-trisphosphate receptor gene is altered in the opisthotonos mouse. *J Neurosci*, Vol. 17, (1997/01/15), pp. 635-645, ISSN 0270-6474

Suls, A., Dedeken, P., Goffin, K., Van Esch, H., Dupont, P., Cassiman, D., Kempfle, J., Wuttke, T.V., Weber, Y., Lerche, H., Afawi, Z., Vandenberghe, W., Korczyn, A.D., Berkovic, S.F., Ekstein, D., Kivity, S., Ryvlin, P., Claes, L.R., Deprez, L., Maljevic, S., Vargas, A., Van Dyck, T., Goossens, D., Del-Favero, J., Van Laere, K., De Jonghe, P., & Van Paesschen, W. (2008). Paroxysmal exercise-induced dyskinesia and epilepsy is due to mutations in SLC2A1, encoding the glucose transporter GLUT1. *Brain*, Vol. 131, (2008/06/26), pp. 1831-1844, ISSN 1460-2156

Suls, A., Mullen, S.A., Weber, Y.G., Verhaert, K., Ceulemans, B., Guerrini, R., Wuttke, T.V., Salvo-Vargas, A., Deprez, L., Claes, L.R., Jordanova, A., Berkovic, S.F., Lerche, H., De Jonghe, P., & Scheffer, I.E. (2009). Early-onset absence epilepsy caused by mutations in the glucose transporter GLUT1. *Ann Neurol*, Vol. 66, (2009/10/03), pp. 415-419, ISSN 1531-8249

Surges, R., Thijs, R.D., Tan, H.L., & Sander, J.W. (2009). Sudden unexpected death in epilepsy: risk factors and potential pathomechanisms. *Nat Rev Neurol*, Vol. 5, (2009/08/12), pp. 492-504, ISSN 1759-4766

Suzuki, T., Delgado-Escueta, A.V., Aguan, K., Alonso, M.E., Shi, J., Hara, Y., Nishida, M., Numata, T., Medina, M.T., Takeuchi, T., Morita, R., Bai, D., Ganesh, S., Sugimoto, Y., Inazawa, J., Bailey, J.N., Ochoa, A., Jara-Prado, A., Rasmussen, A., Ramos-Peek, J., Cordova, S., Rubio-Donnadieu, F., Inoue, Y., Osawa, M., Kaneko, S., Oguni, H., Mori, Y., & Yamakawa, K. (2004). Mutations in EFHC1 cause juvenile myoclonic epilepsy. *Nat Genet*, Vol. 36, (2004/07/20), pp. 842-849, ISSN 1061-4036

Tester, D.J., Arya, P., Will, M., Haglund, C.M., Farley, A.L., Makielski, J.C., & Ackerman, M.J. (2006). Genotypic heterogeneity and phenotypic mimicry among unrelated patients referred for catecholaminergic polymorphic ventricular tachycardia genetic testing. *Heart Rhythm*, Vol. 3, pp. 800-805, ISSN 1547-5271

Tester, D.J., Kopplin, L.J., Will, M.L., & Ackerman, M.J. (2005). Spectrum and prevalence of cardiac ryanodine receptor (RyR2) mutations in a cohort of unrelated patients referred explicitly for long QT syndrome genetic testing. *Heart Rhythm*, Vol. 2, pp. 1099-1105, ISSN 1547-5271

Tian, G.F., Azmi, H., Takano, T., Xu, Q., Peng, W., Lin, J., Oberheim, N., Lou, N., Wang, X., Zielke, H.R., Kang, J., & Nedergaard, M. (2005). An astrocytic basis of epilepsy. *Nat Med*, Vol. 11, pp. 973-981, ISSN 1078-8956

Tomson, T., Nashef, L., & Ryvlin, P. (2008). Sudden unexpected death in epilepsy: current knowledge and future directions. *Lancet Neurol*, Vol. 7, (2008/09/23), pp. 1021-1031, ISSN 1474-4422

Van Norstrand, D.W., Tester, D.J., & Ackerman, M.J. (2008). Overrepresentation of the proarrhythmic, sudden death predisposing sodium channel polymorphism S1103Y in a population-based cohort of African-American sudden infant death syndrome. *Heart Rhythm*, Vol. 5, (2008/05/03), pp. 712-715, ISSN 1556-3871

Vanmolkot, K.R., Kors, E.E., Hottenga, J.J., Terwindt, G.M., Haan, J., Hoefnagels, W.A., Black, D.F., Sandkuijl, L.A., Frants, R.R., Ferrari, M.D., & van den Maagdenberg, A.M. (2003). Novel mutations in the Na+, K+-ATPase pump gene ATP1A2 associated with familial hemiplegic migraine and benign familial infantile convulsions. *Ann Neurol*, Vol. 54, (2003/09/04), pp. 360-366, ISSN 0364-5134

Wallace, R.H., Marini, C., Petrou, S., Harkin, L.A., Bowser, D.N., Panchal, R.G., Williams, D.A., Sutherland, G.R., Mulley, J.C., Scheffer, I.E., & Berkovic, S.F. (2001). Mutant GABA(A) receptor gamma2-subunit in childhood absence epilepsy and febrile seizures. *Nat Genet*, Vol. 28, (2001/04/28), pp. 49-52, ISSN 1061-4036

Wallace, R.H., Wang, D.W., Singh, R., Scheffer, I.E., George, A.L., Jr., Phillips, H.A., Saar, K., Reis, A., Johnson, E.W., Sutherland, G.R., Berkovic, S.F., & Mulley, J.C. (1998). Febrile seizures and generalized epilepsy associated with a mutation in the Na+-channel beta1 subunit gene SCN1B. *Nat Genet*, Vol. 19, (1998/08/11), pp. 366-370, ISSN 1061-4036

Wang, Q., Curran, M.E., Splawski, I., Burn, T.C., Millholland, J.M., VanRaay, T.J., Shen, J., Timothy, K.W., Vincent, G.M., de Jager, T., Schwartz, P.J., Toubin, J.A., Moss, A.J., Atkinson, D.L., Landes, G.M., Connors, T.D., & Keating, M.T. (1996). Positional cloning of a novel potassium channel gene: KVLQT1 mutations cause cardiac arrhythmias. *Nat Genet*, Vol. 12, pp. 17-23, ISSN 1061-4036

Wang, Q., Shen, J., Splawski, I., Atkinson, D., Li, Z., Robinson, J.L., Moss, A.J., Towbin, J.A., & Keating, M.T. (1995). SCN5A mutations associated with an inherited cardiac arrhythmia, long QT syndrome. *Cell*, Vol. 80, pp. 805-811, ISSN 0092-8674

Wang, Z., Tristani-Firouzi, M., Xu, Q., Lin, M., Keating, M.T., & Sanguinetti, M.C. (1999). Functional effects of mutations in KvLQT1 that cause long QT syndrome. *J Cardiovasc Electrophysiol*, Vol. 10, pp. 817-826, ISSN 1045-3873

Weber, Y.G., Storch, A., Wuttke, T.V., Brockmann, K., Kempfle, J., Maljevic, S., Margari, L., Kamm, C., Schneider, S.A., Huber, S.M., Pekrun, A., Roebling, R., Seebohm, G., Koka, S., Lang, C., Kraft, E., Blazevic, D., Salvo-Vargas, A., Fauler, M., Mottaghy, F.M., Munchau, A., Edwards, M.J., Presicci, A., Margari, F., Gasser, T., Lang, F., Bhatia, K.P., Lehmann-Horn, F., & Lerche, H. (2008). GLUT1 mutations are a cause of paroxysmal exertion-induced dyskinesias and induce hemolytic anemia by a cation leak. *J Clin Invest*, Vol. 118, (2008/05/03), pp. 2157-2168, ISSN 0021-9738

Westenskow, P., Splawski, I., Timothy, K.W., Keating, M.T., & Sanguinetti, M.C. (2004). Compound mutations: a common cause of severe long-QT syndrome. *Circulation*, Vol. 109, pp. 1834-1841, ISSN 1524-4539

Zhang, L., Vincent, G.M., Baralle, M., Baralle, F.E., Anson, B.D., Benson, D.W., Whiting, B., Timothy, K.W., Carlquist, J., January, C.T., Keating, M.T., & Splawski, I. (2004). An intronic mutation causes long QT syndrome. *J Am Coll Cardiol*, Vol. 44, (2004/09/15), pp. 1283-1291, ISSN 0735-1097

Zijlmans, M., Flanagan, D., & Gotman, J. (2002). Heart rate changes and ECG abnormalities during epileptic seizures: prevalence and definition of an objective clinical sign. *Epilepsia*, Vol. 43, (2002/08/16), pp. 847-854, ISSN 0013-9580

Zuberi, S.M., Eunson, L.H., Spauschus, A., De Silva, R., Tolmie, J., Wood, N.W., McWilliam, R.C., Stephenson, J.B., Kullmann, D.M., & Hanna, M.G. (1999). A novel mutation in the human voltage-gated potassium channel gene (Kv1.1) associates with episodic ataxia type 1 and sometimes with partial epilepsy. *Brain*, Vol. 122 (Pt 5), (1999/06/04), pp. 817-825, ISSN 0006-8950

Sudden Unexpected Death in Epilepsy: An Overview

Vera C. Terra[1], Américo C. Sakamoto[1],
Hélio R Machado[1] and Fulvio A. Scorza[2]
[1]*Centro de Cirurgia de Epilepsia (CIREP). Departamento de Neurociências e Ciências do Comportamento. Faculdade de Medicina de Ribeirão Preto, Universidade de São Paulo. Ribeirão Preto, São Paulo,*
[2]*Disciplina de Neurologia Experimental. Universidade Federal de São Paulo, Escola Paulista de Medicina (UNIFESP/EPM), São Paulo, Brasil*

1. Introduction

Epilepsy is one of the most frequent neurological disorders, both in children and adult persons. About 0.5-1% of general population suffer from epilepsy, which means that 50 million people in the world are affected. First years of life and very late adulthood are periods in human's life particularly predisposing to developing epilepsy. Patients with repetitive seizures may have a significantly lower quality of life, with frequent absences from work or school caused by seizures, difficulties in social life, frequent injuries, necessity of polytherapy and the risk of life-threatening situations, such as status epilepticus (Józwiak, 2007). People with epilepsy have also a two to three fold increased risk of death as compared to the age-matched general population and may die unexpectedly without a clear structural or pathologic identifiable cause. Increased risk of death primarily affects young adults mostly with drug resistant epilepsy and accounts for a large proportion of deaths among people with epilepsy. This condition is called sudden unexpected death in epilepsy (SUDEP).

SUDEP is defined as sudden, unexpected, witnessed or unwitnessed, non-traumatic and non-drowning death in patients with epilepsy, with or without the evidence of a seizure, excluding *status epilepticus*, and without a toxicological or anatomical cause of death in *post-mortem* examination (Tomson et al, 2008). Diagnosis of SUDEP is sometimes difficult since *post-mortem* examination is not always available. Annegers (1997) suggested six criteria to consider the etiology of death as being SUDEP: 1. The diagnosis of epilepsy; 2. Death in a victim in a reasonable state of health; 3. Death should occur suddenly; 4. During normal activities and in benign circumstances; 5. Without a medical cause; 6. Not directly caused by a seizure or *status epilepticus* (Annegers, 1997). In this way, definite SUDEP cases need to have a *post-mortem* examination to ensure patient did not have a concomitant disease that can justify death and probable cases are considered that with clinical findings suggestive of SUDEP but where necropsy is not available. These strict criteria may hamper the diagnosis of SUDEP in many cases and, in these lines, other authors suggest that a formal *post-mortem* examination may be replaced by a verbal autopsy, contributing to a more realistic assessment of SUDEP incidence (Lathers & Schraeder, 2009).

SUDEP incidence rates are variable depending on the cohort studied, being directly affected by seizure frequency. In this way, it range from 0.35 per 1,000 person-years of follow-up in population-based studies to 9.3 per 1,000 person-years in patients with refractory epilepsy (Asadi-Pooya & Sperling, 2009; Ryvlin et al, 2009), with an intermediate incidence of 1-2/1,000 person-years in patients with chronic epilepsy. The highest rates occur in patients with 20 to 40 years old (Tomson et al, 2005).

Interest in sudden unexpected and unexplained death in individuals with epilepsy was rekindled during the early 1980s and more recently by antiepileptic drug (AED) trials, medico legal issues and epidemiologic studies (Annegers, 1997). Although, if we search in PUBMED database the word SUDEP, approximately 250 articles are found and most of them reports small series of patients or describe single patient cases, with few articles reporting large controlled series (case-control or cohort studies). Moreover, most articles that tried to identify SUDEP risk factors report few cases, being observational studies. In this way, definition of potentially risk factors is essential. No single risk factor is common to all SUDEP cases, suggesting multiple mechanisms or trigger factors are involved (Tomson et al, 2005). Most deaths of SUDEP are unwitnessed and occur at home, usually in bed and presumably overnight, in association with a seizure (Opeskin & Berkovic, 2003; Kloster & Engelskjøn, 1999). Many victims have pulmonary oedema on *postmortem* examination, and some show ischemic damage of the heart despite normal coronary arteries. Nevertheless, the precise reason for a particular seizure being fatal in an otherwise healthy individual is as yet undetermined (McGugan, 2000).

Studies suggested that patients suffering of SUDEP had a significant longer mean duration of epilepsy compared with controls and that more people succumbing of SUDEP had had a seizure within the previous year (Hiritis et al, 2007). Interestingly, considering all deaths in epilepsy, patients that died of SUDEP are reported to die at younger ages than non-SUDEP deaths. Other possible related risk factors described in the literature are male sex, generalized tonic-clonic seizures, high seizure frequency, specific AEDs, polytherapy with several AEDs, mental retardation, psychiatric illness, psychotropic co-medication and an earlier epilepsy onset (Vlooswijk et al, 2007; Lear-Kaul et al, 2005). Summarizing all citations, main risk factors seems to be young age, high seizure frequency, frequent generalized tonic-clonic seizures, nocturnal seizures, poor drug compliance, medical refractory epilepsies, high number of antiepileptic drugs and long duration of epilepsy, but this still need confirmation with controlled studies (Téllez-Zenteno et al, 2005; Ryvlin et al, 2009).

A cohort study accompanied 3,688 subjects aged 15 to 49 years with more than four prescriptions for AED. Patients were followed since first AED prescription to one of the options: age 50 years, death, or last registration on system. In this group were observed 163 deaths and 153 death certificates were examined to identify potential SUDEP cases. There were 18 definite/probable SUDEPs and 21 possible SUDEPs, yielding a minimum incidence of 0.54 SUDEP per 1,000 person-years and a maximum of 1.35 SUDEP per 1,000 person-years. Main risk factors observed were male sex, number of AEDs ever prescribed, prescription of psychotropic drugs and in males with a history of treatment with three or more AEDs. Authors suggested that a 1.7 fold increased risk of SUDEP might be associated for each increment in maximum number of AED administered (Tennis et al, 1995). Although, this increase may simple reflect severity of epilepsy and not the directly effect of AED in increasing SUDEP risk. A causal relationship of SUDEP with antiepileptic drugs administration has not been proved, but the sudden decrease of antiepileptic drugs serum levels may cause cardiac arrhythmias potentially fatal (Garaizar, 2000). Although SUDEP has not been clearly associated with the use of any particular AED, some case-control studies have pointed to an association between SUDEP and polytherapy with AED and frequent dose changes independent of seizure frequency (Tomson et al, 2005). All currently available AED have been associated with SUDEP, but two specific drugs, carbamazepine and lamotrigine were considered by some authors as potentially increasing SUDEP risks. A review of Cardiff Epilepsy Unit data shows that carbamazepine was disproportionately represented in patients suffering SUDEP, achieving almost 85% of the cases described in some SUDEP series (Timmings, 1998).

Carbamazepine has a potential effect inducing lengthening of the ECG Q-T interval combined with a mild pro-arrhythmic action. This may cause transient cardiac instability leading to arrhythmic death (Timmings, 1998). Abrupt withdrawal of CBZ may lead to enhanced sympathetic activity in sleep as evidenced by heart frequency analysis and this increased activity in the setting of seizure-induced hypoxia could predispose to SUDEP (Hennessy et al, 2001). Isolated reports have described patients suffering of SUDEP or syncope associated with hyponatraemia generated by syndrome of inappropriate secretion of antidiuretic hormone (Kloster & Børresen, 1999; Ruiz et al, 2007). Interesting in all cases, patients were chronically using association of carbamazepine/oxcarbazepine and lamotrigine. Others authors have already suggested that current available studies do not support the hypothesis that CBZ is associated with a higher risk of SUDEP (Opeskin et al, 1999). In this way, it is unclear whether polytherapy, frequent dose changes, and high carbamazepine levels per se represent a risk factor or just reflect an unidentified aspect of an unstable, more severe form of epilepsy (Nilsson et al 2001). Anyway, a search for syndrome of inappropriate secretion of antidiuretic hormone in patients on carbamazepine and oxcarbazepine, and in cases of sudden death in epilepsy, is recommended.

With respect to lamotrigine, it has recently been shown that this DAE inhibit the cardiac rapid delayed rectifier potassium ion current and consequently increase the risk of cardiac arrhythmia and sudden unexpected death. Although Leestma et al (1997) suggested that the rate of SUDEP in patients using lamotrigine was unrelated to the drug, Aurlien et al (2007) registered in ten years, four consecutive cases of SUDEP in non-hospitalized patients that were all being treated with lamotrigine in monotherapy. However, as with other potential risk factors, there are no systematic studies that may confirm these suspicions.

In this way, to estimate the risk of SUDEP, Walczak et al (2001) determined SUDEP incidence and risk factors in a prevalence cohort of people with epilepsy enrolled prospectively. Most of the patients had been intensively evaluated and detailed information regarding possible risk factors for SUDEP was defined. In this study four thousand, five hundred seventy-eight patients were enrolled. One hundred eleven patients died during follow up, 28 of them of SUDEP. Three apparently independent risk factors for SUDEP were proposed: presence of tonic-clonic seizures, mental retardation and the number of anticonvulsant drugs used. Authors considered presence of tonic-clonic seizures as a major risk factor, since the great majority of patients that is in suspicion of SUDEP had history of experienced tonic-clonic seizure just before death, or circumstances of death when was carefully examined showed an evidence of tonic-clonic seizure preceding death. Also, death has been directly related to generalized convulsive seizures in an animal model of SUDEP (Faingold et al, 2010).

Based in this study, DeGiorgo et al (2010) validated a SUDEP-7 inventory. Inventory is composed by seven items which scores were based on the log of the odds ratio of the main risk factors reported previously (Walczak et al, 2001) (Table 1). Authors suggested that a high index will be correlated with a major risk of patient to have SUDEP and that this data could be correlated with others suspected risk factors. Although this inventory was the first attempt to stagger patients in a numeric way, it was not fully accepted and it is not being used in SUDEP literature. A validation with a larger cohort of patients is required to demonstrate if it can contribute to identify patients at major risk.

SUDEP RISK FACTOR	SCORES
1. More than three tonic clonic seizures in last year	0 or 2
2. One or more tonic-clonic seizures in last year	0 or 1
3. One or more seizures of any type over the last 12 months	0 or 1
3. More than 50 seizures of any type per month over the last 12 5. months	0 or 2
4. Duration of epilepsy of ≥ 30 years	0 or 3
5. Current use of three or more antiepileptic drugs	0 or 1
6. Mental retardation, intelligent coefficient < 70 or too impaired test	0 or 2

Table 1. SUDEP-7 inventory, from DeGiorgio et al, 2010.

2. Mechanisms of SUDEP

SUDEP is probable related to a set of risk factors that may involve structural, functional and genetic causes (Figure 1). As well as risk factors, the pathophysiology of SUDEP remains unclear, but a post-ictal central or obstructive apnea or a cardiac arrhythmia seems to represent the most likely mechanisms (Ryvlin et al, 2009). Experimental studies have suggested that damage to the central nucleus may be of functional significance in patients with SUDEP in particular with regard to their susceptibility to cardiac arrhythmias. In this way, neuronal loss was observed in the medial division of the lateral amygdaloid nucleus in SUDEP cases, but it seems not to be a specific finding since this pattern was present in patients that did not suffered SUDEP (Thom-M et al, 1999). Corroborating the hypotheses of neuronal loss, there are evidences of heat shock protein positive neurons in the hippocampus in SUDEP, suggesting an ante-mortem neuronal injury (Thom et al, 2003).

Physiologic studies in humans during seizures identified in some cases a central apnea, occasionally followed by asystole; in others patients, cardiac arrhythmia, of reflex neural origin, have been detected (Garaizar, 2000; Hennessy et al, 2001). The cardiac mechanism of greatest interest is the precipitation of arrhythmias by seizure discharges via the autonomic nervous system (Jehi & Najm, 2008). Studies assessing autonomic tone with functional tests as deep breathing, Valsalva maneuver, isometric exercise, cold pressor and tilt-table observed a higher vasomotor tone, higher sympathetic tone, lower parasympathetic tone, lower parasympathetic reactivity and more severe dysautonomia in the refractory epilepsy subjects. In this way, refractoriness may lead to an alteration in cardiovascular autonomic regulation, which might be a predisposing factor for SUDEP (Mukherjee et al, 2009).

There are few studies reporting genetic mutations in patients with SUDEP and most of them evaluated genes responsible for long QT syndrome. Recent studies demonstrated mutations in the SCN5A and KCNH2 genes coding for the cardiac sodium channel alpha subunit and raises the possibility that the mutation may explain both the epilepsy and the sudden death (Aurlien ET AL, 2009; Tu et al, 2010) and since, channelopaties may be another risk factor for SUDEP to be considered in patients with epilepsy.

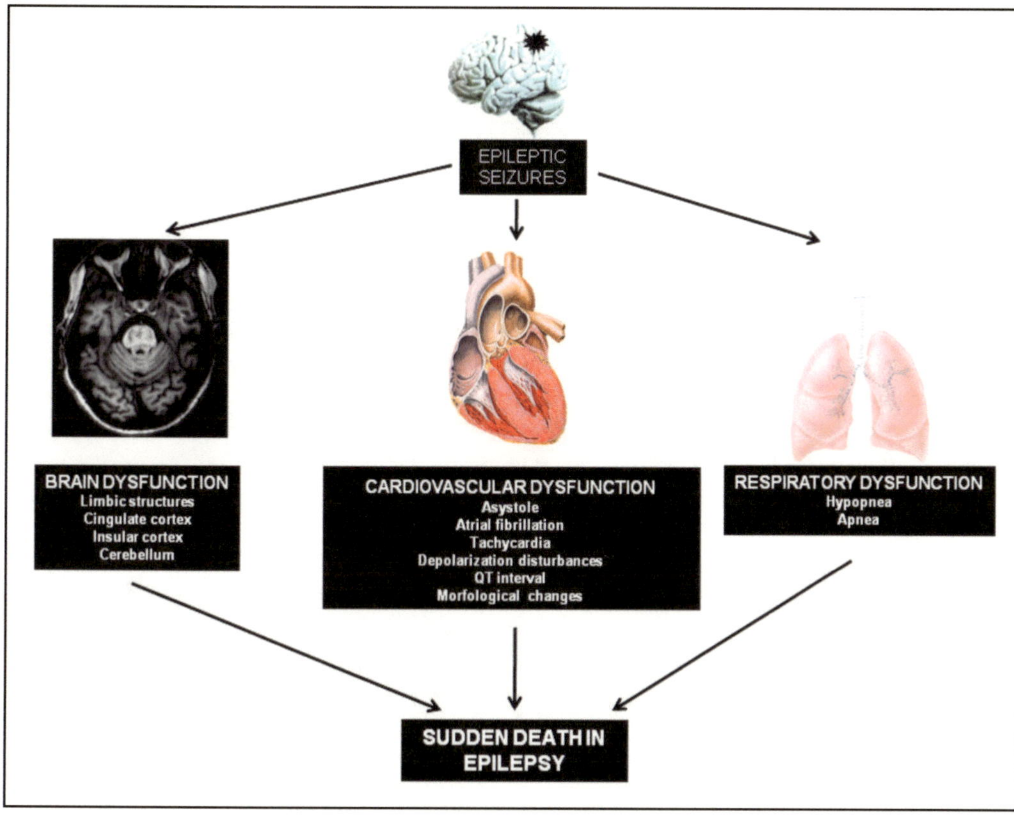

Fig. 1. Main possible mechanisms involved in SUDEP. Epileptic seizures act directly in lung, heart and brain, with multisystem dysfunction. In brain, repetitive epileptic seizures and antiepileptic drugs may act leading to brain volume loss and developing aberrant pathways. In heart, dysfunctions causing bradychardia or tachycardia *per se* could culminate in SUDEP, but this may be associated to morphological abnormalities. Considering respiration, mechanisms involved are related to decreased ventilation.

2.1 Respiratory mechanisms

Monitoring of seizures and respiratory function with pulse oximetry has shown that ictal respiratory changes accompany tonic-clonic seizures and even partial seizures, especially those of temporal lobe origin in both, children and adults. This changes diminished central drive that may be associated or not with peripheral airway obstruction (Blum, 2009). The finding of pulmonary edema in 86% of patients that suffered SUDEP at *postmortem* examination may support this obstructive theory (Salmo & Connolly, 2002).

Investigators have documented a range of respiratory parameters (respiratory effort, airflow, oxygen saturation) in conjunction with time-locked audio-video electroencephalograms and electrocardiograms to provide a more complete picture of the physiologic changes that occur during seizures. Apnea, mainly central, was present in all patients with generalized seizures and approximately one third of patients with complex partial seizures (Walker & Fisch, 1997). In other group of patients with partial seizures without secondary generalized convulsions, 34.8% of seizures had desaturations below 90%,

31.8% had desaturations below 80% and 12.5% had desaturations below 70%, which was significantly correlated with seizure duration and with electrographic evidence of seizure spread to the contralateral hemisphere. In this study, central apneas or hypopneas occurred in 50% of 100 seizures and mixed or obstructive apneas occurred in 9% of these seizures. Considering these findings, authors concluded that ictal hypoxemia occurs often in patients with localization-related epilepsy and may be pronounced and prolonged even with seizures that do not progress to generalized convulsions (Bateman et al, 2008).

Interestingly other study observed a close temporal relationship between spread of seizures to the contralateral hemisphere and the onset of seizure-associated apnea. Apnea onsets are more tightly linked to time of contralateral spread than to time of seizure onset, suggesting that contralateral seizure spread in patients with temporal lobe epilepsy may be a risk factor for ictal-related respiratory dysfunction (Seyal & Bateman, 2009). This finding did not alter the ability of postictal respiratory function, respiratory rate and amplitude that is even increased after the end of the seizures (Seyal et al, 2010).

Ictal/postictal hypoventilation may contribute to SUDEP with the resulting hypoxemia and acidosis leading to inadequate cortical function recovery and eventual cardiac failure (Bateman et al, 2010; Lhatoo et al, 2010). Alternatively, excessive post-seizure brainstem inhibition might result in blunting or transient abolition of central hypoxic and hypercarbic respiratory drive, with consequent post-ictal respiratory arrest, hypoxia exacerbation and death due to hypoxia/insufficient re-establishment of respiration and terminal cardiac arrhythmia (Timmings, 1998).

Corroborating this hypoventilation theory, studies of audiogenic seizure susceptible mice with generalized convulsive seizures demonstrated that electrocardiographic activity was detectable for four to six minutes after respiratory arrest and death was reversible with ventilation. If not reversed these animals die from respiratory arrest after generalized seizure, that is, die of SUDEP (Faingold et al, 2010).

2.2 Cardiac mechanisms

Cardiac arrhythmogenesis and cryptogenic epilepsy can be due to ion channel dysfunction and may coexist in the same patient, leaving them more susceptible for recurrent arrhythmias. In this way, epileptic survivors of near-sudden cardiac death may be at significantly greater risk of suffering of SUDEP (Badheka et al, 2010). Cardiac mechanisms involved in SUDEP may be associated with heart rate dysfunction, morphology of cardiac waves, anatomic disorders or what some authors refer as brain collapse. Considering this last hypothesis, recently there is a description of a patient submitted to ambulatory EEG that suffered a generalized tonic-clonic seizure that abruptly ended with cessation of all cerebral electrical activity and after a few seconds patient evolved to asystole and death. The circumstance was typical of SUDEP and in this case seems to be related to abrupt irreversible cerebral electrical shutdown during a seizure (McLean & Wimalaratna, 2007).

Also, the circadian heart-rate variability might be of relevance to SUDEP risk. Studies evaluating heart rate observed that patients with epilepsy may have one or more abnormalities of rhythm and/or repolarization during or immediately after seizures. Abnormalities included asystole, atrial fibrillation, marked or moderate sinus arrhythmia, supraventricular tachycardia (Figure 2), atrial premature depolarization, ventricular premature depolarization and bundle-branch block (Nei et al, 2000). Electrocardiogram

(ECG) abnormalities is more frequently observed in patients with refractory focal epilepsies (Surges et al, 2010), generalized tonic-clonic seizures and prolonged complex partial seizures (Nei et al, 2000). In this way, ictal or postictal dysregularion of the autonomic nervous system, affecting heart rate variability may contribute to SUDEP incidence.

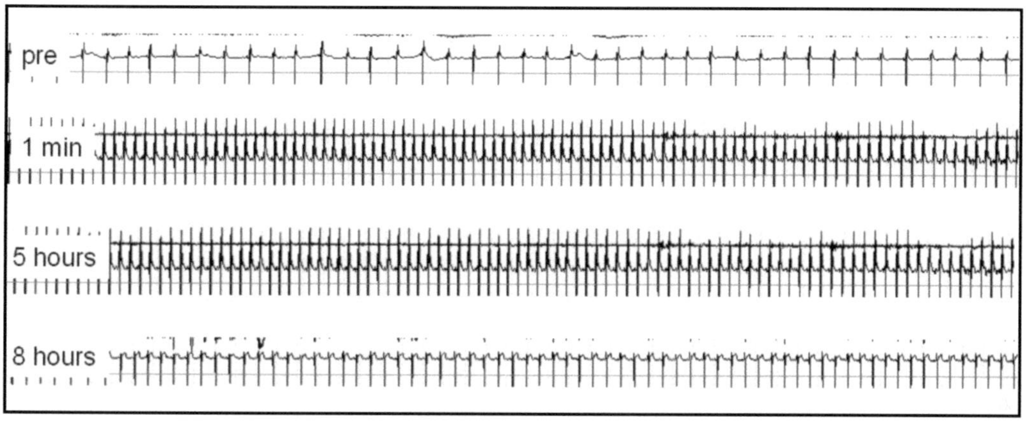

Fig. 2. Ictal tachycardia in a patient with temporal lobe epilepsy. Cardiac rate is illustrate one minute before seizure onset (pre), one minute after seizure onset (1 min), five hours after seizure end (5 hours) and 8 hours after seizure end (8 hours).

Heart rate abnormalities may be relative to tachycardia or asystole and heart rate variability reflects the integrity of vagus nerve-mediated autonomic control of the heart (DeGiorgio et al, 2010). Tachycardia is the main cardiac abnormality observed during seizures (Walker & Fisch, 1997) and fatal tachyarrhythmia as one plausible cause for SUDEP. This arrhythmia is more frequently observed during generalized tonic-clonic seizures, but tachycardia may be observed also in complex partial seizures (Surges et al, 2010). Evaluating the different studies, we observed interesting findings. Person et al (2007) observed that there was no major effect of epilepsy on heart rate variations in patients with untreated epilepsy, recently diagnosed. However, when patients were used as their own controls, heart rate variability was significantly lower after initiation of the treatment with AED and even more during the night, when the risk of SUDEP seems to be higher (Persson et al, 2007). Considering this hypothesis, Surges et al (2009) evaluated retrospectively the heart rate variability in 14 patients with chronic epilepsy (seven of them died from SUDEP). Authors could not determine a clear-cut ECG abnormality that may be considered as a predictor for SUDEP. However, in other studies, authors observed an elevation of heart rate immediately after seizures, which were maintained for 5-6 hours postically, indicating a long-term postictal disturbance of the autonomous nervous system, suggesting that seizures may cause prolonged heart dysfunction (Toth et al, 2010; Pinto et al, 2011).

Although seizure-induced asystole is a rare complication and tended to follow a period of apnea, epilepsy can be correlated to severe bradycardia or asystole (Walker & Fisch, 1997). The event appeared mainly in focal epilepsies and ictal bradycardia and asystole have been implicated in the etiology of SUDEP. Some authors suggested that this abnormality is most related to left side lateralization and that abnormally long postictal periods with altered consciousness might be associated with reduced cerebral perfusion because of ictal asystole. This could be related or not to central ictal apnea (Rocamora et al, 2003). In this way, Zubair et al (2009) described a patient with a history of complex partial seizures and drop attacks that presented during the video-monitoring a complex partial seizure with brady-arrhythmia followed by asystole. This patient was treated with a cardiac pacemaker and on follow-up, despite patient continued to present simple and complex partial seizures, drop attacks disappeared, confirming its cardiogenic origin.

Considering morphology of QRS complex, co-registered EEG and ECG showed a significant increase in the mean corrected QT (QTc) during interictal discharges, when compared retrospectively patients that died of SUDEP and patients that were still alive (Tavernor et al, 1996). Comparing patients with chronic epilepsy and normal matched control, the mean interictal QTc among epilepsy patients was significantly shorter than the QTc in the control group. Duration of the epilepsy, type of seizures and number of antiepileptic drugs were not significantly correlated to QTc. Nevertheless, patients with cryptogenic temporal lobe epilepsy had a mean QTc significantly shorter than patients with symptomatic epilepsy (Teh et al, 2007). Shortening of QTc also occurred in patients during the early postictal phase and significantly more often in secondarily generalized tonic-clonic seizures (Surges et al, 2010). Other authors reported the opposite, i.e. a significant lengthening of corrected QT cardiac repolarization time during some epileptic seizures considering this QT abnormality a potential risk factor for SUDEP (Brotherstone et al, 2010).

Anatomic examination of the heart of patients that died from SUDEP demonstrated an increased weight in some cases, suggesting that cardiac pathology including cardiac conduction pathology and coronary artery atheroma may contribute to SUDEP. In some of the epileptic deaths subtle abnormalities of the conduction system were identified and these may contribute to death by causing cardiac arrhythmia, when associated with apnoea, bradycardia or other cardiac arrhythmia related to an epileptic seizure (Opeskin et al, 2000). In patients with SUDEP, histological evaluation reveled foci of fibrotic changes that predominated in the deep and subendocardial myocardium of the SUDEP cases. Patient in this group were mainly young women with a mean late epilepsy onset, and infrequent seizures (P-Codrea et al, 2005). Authors suggested that fibrosis may be the consequence of myocardial ischemia as a direct result of repetitive epileptic seizures and these changes, when coupled with the ictal sympathetic storm, may lead to lethal arrhythmias (P-Codrea et al, 2005).

2.3 Brain mechanisms involved in SUDEP

The limbic system is often seen as a structure that ties together higher functions with autonomic and motor control to generate integrated behavior (Figure 3). This includes cortical control of the heart rate, particularly considering operculo-insulo-mesiotemporal-orbital pathway and the cingulate cortex (Devinsky *et al.* 1995). Simulation of the cingulate cortex may produce tachycardia or bradycardia (Pool *et al.* 1949). Asystole observed after cingulate cortex stimulation suggest a cortical control of heart rate on physiological basis. A parasympathetic-mediated pathway that involves the limbic system is possible the way bradyarrhythmia occur and may be implicated for the mechanism of SUDEP (Leung et al, 2007).

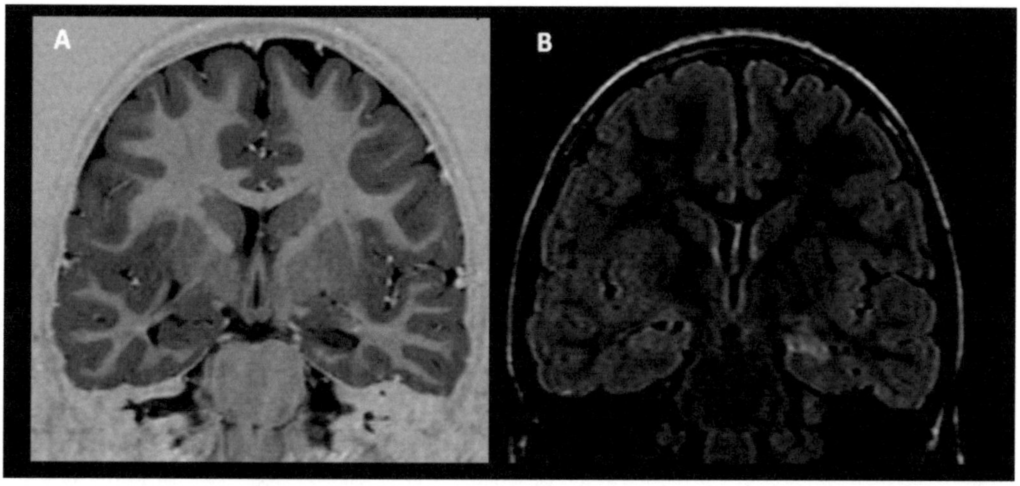

Fig. 3. Left mesial temporal sclerosis, a main cause of refractory epilepsy and observed in some patients that died from SUDEP.

Data from intracranial EEG records demonstrated that bradyarrhythmic episodes were mostly associated with temporal lobe seizures, nevertheless, seizure involvement of insular cortex or cingulated cortex could not be excluded (Altenmüller *et al.* 2004, Devinsky *et al.* 1997; Rossetti *et al.* 2005; Kahane *et al.* 1999). Also, some studies suggest amygdala central nucleus damage may contribute to SUDEP considering that his structure can play a role in respiratory timing (Nashef et al, 1996; Stollberger & Finsterer, 2004; Ryvlin et al, 2006; So, 2008; Surges et al, 2009.

Therefore, studies demonstrated a reduction of sympathetic cardiovascular modulation after temporal lobe epilepsy surgery that might result from decreased influences of interictal epileptogenic discharges on brain areas involved in cardiovascular autonomic control. Temporal lobe epilepsy surgery seems to stabilize the cardiovascular control in epilepsy patients by reducing the risk of sympathetically mediated tachyarrhythmias and excessive bradycardiac counter-regulation, and might contribute to reduce the risk of SUDEP (Hilz et al, 2002). Moreover, left temporal lobe epilepsy surgery is associated with a reduction (but not a normalization) of the overall mortality associated with chronic epilepsy. In patients with right-sided mesial temporal lobe sclerosis however, the postoperative mortality has remained similar to other groups with medically intractable seizures (Hennessy et al, 1999)

Interestingly, laterality of epileptic foci has been reported as related to ictal bradyarrhythmia, with left-side-onset being often observed, although the cerebral patient dominance may also need to be taken into account (Kahane *et al.* 1999; Tinuper et al. 2001). The laterality observed made researchers suspect parasympathetic system activation may be more influenced by the lef side or dominant hemisphere (Oppenheimer *et al,* 1992). The induction of bradyarrhythmia by direct stimulation of the left insular cortex but not the right insular cortex corroborates this hypothesis (Leung et al, 2007).

Others brain regions such as the cerebellum may be involved with breathing and cardiac control (Lutherer et al, 1983; Harper et al, 2000; Xu et al, 2001; Harper, 2002; Xu & Frazier, 2002; Harper et al, 2005.). Cerebellum has been correlated with regulation of blood pressure (limiting extreme changes in blood pressure with hypotension or hypertension) and breathing rhythm (Harper et al, 2005). Patients with epilepsy frequently have abnormalities of cerebellum, especially diffuse atrophy and this finding is probable related to chronic use of AEDs, age, presence of generalized tonic-clonic seizures, duration of epilepsy, or the seizure activity itself, causes also related to SUDEP occurrence (Engel, 1993; Specht et al, 1997; Sandok et al, 2000; Lawson et al, 2000; Hagemann et al, 2002). In respect to AED, it seems that prolonged use of phenytoin or phenytoin intoxication may induce severe irreversible cerebellum volume loss that chronically may predispose individuals to SUDEP (Masur et al, 1990; Ney et al, 1994). Cerebellum lesions or dysfunction is reported in patients with sudden infant death syndrome, a sleep-related syndrome suspected of resulting from a failure of enhanced respiratory efforts that compensate transient hypotension. This syndrome may also be related to an inability to recover from an excessive CO_2 challenge (Martin et al, 1996; Harper, 1998; Harper et al, 2000a; Harper et al, 2000b). Moreover, cerebellum injury was reported in patients with congenital central hypoventilation syndrome, a condition with deficient response to hypercapnia and hypoxia, with possible dysfunction of cerebellum, thalamic nuclei, basal ganglia and limbic structures (Harper et al, 2000b; 2005). In adults, a high incidence of obstructive apnea is observed in patients with olivopontocerebellar geneneration (Chokroverty et al, 1984). Considering all together, these evidences may suggest cerebellum lesion may directly affect the ability of central nervous system to react to acute respiratory and cardiac changes, such as apnea and hypopnea, or extreme hypotension or arrhythmia. These dysfunctions may be quite common in patients with epilepsy, especially during generalized tonic-clonic seizures, with a repetitive exposure to this risk in patients with refractory epilepsies. These dysfunctions seem also to be more evident during sleep, time when SUDEP is more common and, in this way, cerebellum lesion with consequent functional impairment may be a main risk factor for SUDEP occurrence and methods to prevent it, such as use of lower doses of AED should be considered.

Considering that parasympathetic activity is possible involved in SUDEP mechanisms, it is interesting to evaluate the effect of vagus nerve stimulation (VNS) on SUDEP incidence. VNS is a non-pharmacological therapy approved by the FDA for treatment of patients with epilepsy who are unsuitable candidates for epilepsy surgery. The precise mechanism of action of VNS remains unknown, but available evidence suggests that central autonomic nervous system pathways are involved, since vagus nerve influences many regions of central nervous system, through its extensive connectivity with nucleus of solitary tract which projects to reticular formation, hypothalamus, hippocampus, amygdale, dorsal raphe nucleus, locus ceruleus, thalamus and cerebral cortex. The most frequently VNS adverse effects typically occur during stimulation, but there are no apparent effects of VNS on vagally mediated visceral function (Schachter, 2006). In many series of patients chronically implanted with VNS, SUDEP cases are reported (Annegers et al, 1998; 2000; Ardesch et al, 2007; El Tahry et al, 2010). However, a cohort study of 791 implanted with VNS system (Annegers et al, 1998) and extended for 1,819 individuals (Anneger et al, 2000) showed a similar mortality and SUDEP rates to those reported from cohorts of severe epilepsy. Experimental models of epilepsy had demonstrated VNS-induced changes in hippocampal neurotransmitter levels, increasing hippocampal noradrenaline concentration. VNS also increased the latency between pilocarpine infusion and the onset of epileptiform discharges, and reduced the duration and severity of pilocarpine-induced limbic seizures (Klein & Ferrari, 2009). Other authors demonstrated an increase in the number of cells in the dentate gyrus, dentritic complexity and BDNF expression after acute or chronic VNS stimulation

(Raedt et al, 2011). However, although these morphological and functional changes have been described, there was not a significant impact on the incidence of SUDEP, suggesting that another factor, such as better seizure control might be involved.

2.4 Experimental models

Experimental models of epilepsy are fully studied in different research centers, but there are few models that can mimic SUDEP. Maybe the most related model in the literature is the one described by Szabó et al (2005) of genetic idiophatic epilepsy in baboons. Authors studied the occurrence of natural death in these animals and the pathological findings in necropsy (Szabó et al, 2009). Overall, animals with epilepsy died early than no epileptic animals and, considering group with epilepsy, animals that had a definite cause of death died significantly younger age than those epileptic animals whose cause of death could not be determined. Predominant causes of death in these animals with epilepsy were infection and trauma. Interestingly animals with unknown cause of death had a history of more frequent seizures and a longer duration of epilepsy. Autopsy of animals with unknown cause of death revealed pulmonary edema and chronic fibrotic changes in the myocardium and since animals were in a good health and died suddenly and unexpectedly the cause of death was considered SUDEP. This interesting model may be the best one available to study mechanisms and risk factors of SUDEP in human since clinical and pathological findings are very close in both species. In this way, authors suggested that phylogenetic similarities between species may permit transpose research information and contribute to elucidation of this devastating complication.

Other experimental models were described in the literature that confirms the suspicions of respiratory and cardiac mechanism involved in SUDEP genesis (Tupal et al, 2006; Scorza et al, 2009). In these models it was raised the possibility that an imbalance in neurotransmitter level, especially serotonin, may contribute to autonomic changes. Serotonin down regulation was observed in a model of epileptic mice that have respiratory changes and death following epileptic seizures. Pharmacological enhancement of serotonin in this model reduced significantly seizures related respiratory arrest. One other model of experimental epilepsy (epilepsy-prone rats - GEPR) with decreased hippocampus serotonin receptor shows an increase in seizure susceptibility, but it is not possible yet to exclude the role of other neurotransmitters in this model. Studies with positron emission tomography in patients with epilepsy have shown conflicting results about serotonin receptor expression, with reports of decreased, increased or unchanged binding (Theodore, 2003). In this way, although more studies are needed to elucidate this issue, it seems plausible to consider, at least with respect to serotonin levels in experimental epilepsy, that there is a cause effect relation between serotonin deficiency and respiratory abnormalities and seizure susceptibility and this may be considered as a possible factor influencing SUDEP risk.

3. Patient information and prevention

There is no consensus regarding the information if risk of SUDEP should be delivered to all patients with epilepsy, but it seems reasonable to individualize this information according to patient particularities (Ryvlin et al, 2009). Some authors recommend universal discussion of SUDEP considering that patients and their families have the right to know about the risks of epilepsy and the reasons for treatment, while others consider that SUDEP should be discussed only with patients at high risk (Brodie & Holmes, 2008). This controversial issue has greater weight due the reports of patients with idiopathic epilepsies, with rare seizures that suffered SUDEP and considering these patients are more susceptible to poor drug compliance and then tonic-clonic seizures, it should be advisable to discuss this matter with them.

A study conducted in England found that people with epilepsy wanted to know more information about the causes of epilepsy and other matters, such as SUDEP (Prinjha et al, 2005). However, a study conducted in Australia demonstrated that risk factors for SUDEP are not amenable to modification and in this way, discussion of SUDEP with patients could not alter outcome. Authors consider that information of SUDEP may adversely affect patients and families quality of life and suggested that an open and frank discussion of SUDEP risk should be reserved to those patients that seek the information (Beran et al, 2004).

The mechanisms underlying SUDEP are unclear, and there are no effective preventative therapies (Brodie & Holmes, 2008). However, even without precise knowledge of the underlying pathogenic mechanism(s), SUDEP prevention could start with the identification of the most prominent risk factors. SUDEP seems to occur more commonly during sleep and it preferentially affects young adults with medically intractable epilepsy (especially tonic-clonic seizures), individuals who also have neurologic comorbidity, and patients receiving antiepileptic drug polytherapy (Asadi-Pooya & Sperling, 2009). Considering SUDEP is probable a multifactorial event and not all risk factors are determined, now prevention should be centered on that most potential suspected risk factors, with effective seizure control, an optimal antiepileptic drug compliance, night supervision (since almost all deaths occur at night), control of tonic-clonic seizures, prevention of airway obstruction and postictally respiratory stimulation (Tao et al, 2010; Ryvlin et al, 2009; Langan et al, 2005; Langan et al, 2000). Also patients should routinely be investigated for the presence of ictal arrhythmias and whenever necessary the insertion of a pacemaker may be indicated, preventing life-threatening cardiac arrest, syncope and trauma (Strzelczyk et al, 2008). Ideally, caregivers should be able to deliver appropriate first aid after epileptic seizures with the guarantee of properly airway flow, stimulation to decreases the duration of postictal apnea and encourage epilepsy patients to sleep in the supine position. It is not clear whether these practices will prevent SUDEP, but they may be reasonable measures to suggest when discussing this issue with patients (Walczak et al, 2001). This prophylaxis orientation should be a routine during epilepsy patient attendance (Jehi & Najm, 2008).

Early identification of patients at risk of SUDEP would offer a unique opportunity for intervention to prevent this devastating condition (Jehi & Najm, 2008). Compliance with treatment clearly influences the frequency of tonic-clonic seizures, being of paramount importance in SUDEP prevention. Also compliance should be encouraged since it may prevent SUDEP in an epilepsy population with rare seizures, which is less closely followed. Physicians should make an effort to control tonic-clonic seizures with the fewest antiepileptic drugs as possible since politherapy has been also implicated as a risk factor for SUDEP (Walczak et al, 2001).

There are few studies that examined thoroughly brain of patients that suffered SUDEP especially that areas considered to have a main function on respiratory and cardiovascular regulation and these issues represent a specific line of research in the SUDEP field that should be investigated. Early and successful epilepsy surgery for drug-resistant epilepsy may significantly reduce the risk of SUDEP, thus patients with definite pharmacologic refractory epilepsies should be referred to an epilepsy surgery center (Shuele et al, 2007).

Confirming this statement studies involving epilepsy surgery programs clearly suggested that successful epilepsy surgery reduces the impending risks of SUDEP. In cohorts in whom the estimated risk of SUDEP is almost 1% per year without surgery, SUDEP incidence was significantly lower following epilepsy surgery (Schuele et al, 2007; Jehi & Najm, 2008). Although, not all refractory epilepsy patient is eligible for surgery and in this way, clarification of risk factors and establishment of the mechanisms of SUDEP are important so that as many people as possible can be saved from SUDEP (Bells & Sander, 2006). Further large-scale, multicenter, case-control or cohort prospective studies are needed to assess the role of AEDs and other potential risk factors in order to form a basis for treatment strategies aiming seizure control and prevention of SUDEP (Tomson et al, 2005). Postmortem examinations of all potential SUDEP patients are also essential, with a dedicated forensic protocol that will permit the correct differential diagnosis (So, 2006).

4. References

Altenmüller DM, Zehender M, Schulze-Bonhage A. (2004) High grade atrioventriular block triggered by spontaneous and stimulation induced epileptic activity in the left temporal lobe. *Epilepsia*; 45: 1640-1644.

Annegers JF, Coan SP, Hauser WA, Leestma J, Duffell W, Tarver B. (1998). Epilepsy, vagal nerve stimulation by the NCP system, mortality, and sudden,unexpected, unexplained death. *Epilepsia*; 39(2):206-212.

Annegers JF, Coan SP, Hauser WA, Leestma J. (2000). Epilepsy, vagal nerve stimulation by the NCP system, all-cause mortality, and sudden, unexpected, unexplained death. *Epilepsia*; 41(5):549-553.

Annegers JF. United States perspective on definitions and classifications. *Epilepsia*. (1997); 38(11 Suppl):S9-12.

Ardesch JJ, Buschman HP, Wagener-Schimmel LJ, van der Aa HE, Hageman G. (2007). Vagus nerve stimulation for medically refractory epilepsy: a long-term follow-up study. *Seizure*; 16(7):579-585.

Asadi-Pooya AA, Sperling MR. Clinical features of sudden unexpected death in epilepsy. *J Clin Neurophysiol*. (2009); 26(5):297-301.

Aurlien D, Leren TP, Taubøll E, Gjerstad L. (2009). New SCN5A mutation in a SUDEP victim with idiopathic epilepsy. Seizure. 2009 Mar;18(2):158-160.

Aurlien D, Taubøll E, Gjerstad L.(2007) Lamotrigine in idiopathic epilepsy - increased risk of cardiac death? *Acta Neurol Scand.*; 115(3):199-203.

Badheka A, Rathod A, Kizilbash MA, Lai Z, Mohamad T, Shah A, Afonso L, Jacob S. (2010) Epileptic patients who survived sudden cardiac death have increased risk of recurrent arrhythmias and death. *J Cardiovasc Med* (Hagerstown); 11(11):810-814.

Bateman LM, Li CS, Seyal M. (2008) Ictal hypoxemia in localization-related epilepsy: analysis of incidence, severity and risk factors. *Brain*; 131(Pt 12):3239-3245.

Bateman LM, Spitz M, Seyal M. (2010) Ictal hypoventilation contributes to cardiac arrhythmia and SUDEP: report on two deaths in video-EEG-monitored patients. *Epilepsia*; 51(5):916-920.

Bell GS, Sander JW. Sudden unexpected death in epilepsy. (2006) Risk factors, possible mechanisms and prevention: a reappraisal. *Acta Neurol Taiwan.*; 15(2):72-83.

Beran RG, Weber S, Sungaran R, Venn N, Hung A. (2004) Review of the legal obligations of the doctor to discuss Sudden Unexplained Death in Epilepsy (SUDEP)--a cohort controlled comparative cross-matched study in an outpatient epilepsy clinic. *Seizure*; 13(7):523-528.

Blum AS. (2009) Respiratory physiology of seizures. *J Clin Neurophysiol.*; 26(5):309-315.

Brodie MJ, Holmes GL. (2008) Should all patients be told about sudden unexpected death in epilepsy (SUDEP)? Pros and Cons. *Epilepsia*; 49 Suppl 9:99-101.

Brotherstone R, Blackhall B, McLellan A. (2010) Lengthening of corrected QT during epileptic seizures. *Epilepsia*; 51(2):221-232.

Chokroverty S, Sachdeo R, Masdeu J. (1984) Autonomic dysfunction and sleep apnea in olivopontocerebellar degeneration. *Arch Neurol*; 41:926-931.

DeGiorgio CM, Miller P, Meymandi S, Chin A, Epps J, Gordon S, Gornbein J, Harper RM. RMSSD, a measure of vagus-mediated heart rate variability, is associated with risk factors for SUDEP: the SUDEP-7 Inventory. Epilepsy Behav. 2010;19(1):78-81.

Devinsky O, Morrell MJ, Vogt BA. (1995) Contributions of anterior cingulate cortex to behaviour. *Brain*; 118: 279-306.

Devinsky O, Pacia S, Tatambhotla G. (1997) Bradycardia and asystole induced by partial seizures: A case report and literature review. *Neurology*; 48: 1712-1714.

El Tahry R, De Herdt V, Raedt R, Van Dycke A, Meurs A, Dewaele F, Boon P, Van Roost D, Vonck K. (2010). Evolution in VNS therapy for refractory epilepsy, experience with Demipulse devices at Ghent University Hospital. *Seizure*; 19(9):531-535.

Engel J. (1993) Clinical neurophysiology, neuroimaging, and the surgical treatment of epilepsy. *Curr Opin Neurol Neurosurg*; 6:240-249.

Faingold CL, Randall M, Tupal S. (2010). DBA/1 mice exhibit chronic susceptibility to audiogenic seizures followed by sudden death associated with respiratory arrest. *Epilepsy Behav.*; 17(4):436-440.

Garaizar C. (2000) Sudden unexpected and unexplained death in epilepsy. *Rev Neurol.* 1-15;31(5):436-41.

Hagemann G, Lemieux L, Free SL, Krakow K, Everitt AD, Kendall BE, et al. (2002) Cerebellar volumes in newly diagnosed and chronic epilepsy. *J Neurol*; 249:1651-1658.

Harper RM, Bandler R, Spriggs D, Alger JR. (2000) Lateralized and widespread brain activation during transient blood pressure elevation revealed by magnetic resonance imaging. *J Comp Neurol*; 417:195-204.a

Harper RM, Bandler R. (1998) Finding the failure mechanism in the sudden infant death syndrome. *Nat Med*; 4:157-158.

Harper RM, Kinney HC, Fleming PJ, Thach BT. (2000) Sleep influences on homeostatic functions: implications for sudden infant death syndrome. Respir Physiol; 119:123-132.b

Harper RM, Macey PM, Woo MA, Macey KE, Keens TG, Gozal D et al. (2005) Hypercapnic exposure in congenital central hypoventilation syndrome reveals CNS respiratory control mechanisms. *J Neurophysiol*; 93:1647-1658.

Harper RM. (2002) The cerebellum and respiratory control. *Cerebellum*; 1:1-2.

Hennessy MJ, Langan Y, Elwes RD, Binnie CD, Polkey CE, Nashef L. (1999) A study of mortality after temporal lobe epilepsy surgery. *Neurology*; 12;53(6):1276-1283.

Hennessy MJ, Tighe MG, Binnie CD, Nashef L. (2001) Sudden withdrawal of carbamazepine increases cardiac sympathetic activity in sleep. *Neurology*; 13;57(9):1650-1654.

Hilz MJ, Devinsky O, Doyle W, Mauerer A, Dütsch M. (2002(Decrease of sympathetic cardiovascular modulation after temporal lobe epilepsy surgery. *Brain*;125(Pt 5):985-995.

Hitiris N, Suratman S, Kelly K, Stephen LJ, Sills GJ, Brodie MJ. (2007) Sudden unexpected death in epilepsy: a search for risk factors. *Epilepsy Behav.*; 10(1):138-141.

Jehi L, Najm IM. (2008) Sudden unexpected death in epilepsy: impact, mechanisms, and prevention. *Cleve Clin J Med.*; 75 Suppl 2:S66-70.

Jóźwiak S. (2007) Contemporary opinions on classification, pathogenesis and treatment of drug-resistant epilepsy. *Wiad Lek.*; 60(5-6):258-264.

Kahane P, Di Leo M, Hoffmann D, *et al. (1999)* Ictal bradycardia in a patient with a hypothalamic hamartoma: a stereo-EEG study. *Epilepsia*; 40: 522-527.

Klein HU, Ferrari GM. (2010). Vagus nerve stimulation: A new approach to reduce heart failure. *Cardiol J.*; 17(6):638-644.

Kloster R, Børresen HC, Hoff-Olsen P. (1998) Sudden death in two patients with epilepsy and the syndrome of inappropriate antidiuretic hormone secretion (SIADH). *Seizure*; 7(5):419-420.

Kloster R, Engelskjøn T. (1999) Sudden unexpected death in epilepsy (SUDEP): a clinical perspective and a search for risk factors. *J Neurol Neurosurg Psychiatry.*; 67(4):439-444.

Langan Y, Nashef L, Sander JW. (2000) Sudden unexpected death in epilepsy: a series of witnessed deaths. *J Neurol Neurosurg Psychiatry.*; 68(2):211-213.

Langan Y, Nashef L, Sander JW. (2205) Case-control study of SUDEP. *Neurology;* 12;64(7):1131-1133.

Lathers CM, Schraeder PL. (2009) Verbal autopsies and SUDEP. *Epilepsy Behav.*; 14(4):573-576.

Lear-Kaul KC, Coughlin L, Dobersen MJ. (2005) Sudden unexpected death in epilepsy: a retrospective study. *Am J Forensic Med Pathol.*; 26(1):11-7.

Leestma JE, Annegers JF, Brodie MJ, Brown S, Schraeder P, Siscovick D, Wannamaker BB, Tennis PS, Cierpial MA, Earl NL. (1997) Sudden unexplained death in epilepsy: observations from a large clinical development program. *Epilepsia*; 38(1):47-55.

Leung H, Kwan P, Elger CE. (2006) Finding the missing link between ictal bradyarrhythmia, ictal asystole, and sudden unexpected death in epilepsy. *Epilepsy Behav*; 9:19–30.

Leung H, Schindler K, Kwan P, Elger C. (2007) Asystole induced by electrical stimulation of the left cingulate gyrus. *Epileptic Disord.*; 9(1):77-81.

Lhatoo SD, Faulkner HJ, Dembny K, Trippick K, Johnson C, Bird JM. (2010). An electroclinical case-control study of sudden unexpected death in epilepsy. *Ann Neurol.*; 68(6):787-796.

Lutherer LO, Lutherer BC, Dormer KJ, Janssen HF, Barnes CD. (1983). Bilateral lesions of the fastigial nucleus prevent the recovery of blood pressure following hypotension induced by hemorrhage or administration of endotoxin. *Brain Res*; 269:251-257.

Martin R, Roessmann U, Fanaroff A. (1996). Massive intracerebellar hemorrhage in low-birth-weight infants. J Pediatr; 89:290-293.

Masur H, Fahrendorf G, Oberwittler C, Reuther G. (1990). Cerebellar atrophy following acute intoxication with phenytoin. *Neurology*; 40:1800-1801.

McGugan EA. (1999). Sudden unexpected deaths in epileptics--a literature review. *Scott Med J.*; 44(5):137-139.

McLean BN, Wimalaratna S. (2007). Sudden death in epilepsy recorded in ambulatory EEG. *J Neurol Neurosurg Psychiatry.*; 78(12):1395-1397.

Mukherjee S, Tripathi M, Chandra PS, Yadav R, Choudhary N, Sagar R, Bhore R, Pandey RM, Deepak KK. (2009). Cardiovascular autonomic functions in well-controlled and intractable partial epilepsies. *Epilepsy Res.*; 85(2-3):261-269.

Nashef L, Walker F, Allen P, Sander JW, Shorvon SD, Fish R. (1996). Apnoea and bradycardia during epileptic seizures: relation to sudden death in epilepsy. *J Neurol Neurosurg Psychiatry*; 60:297-300.

Nei M, Ho RT, Sperling MR. (2000). EKG abnormalities during partial seizures in refractory epilepsy. *Epilepsia*; 41(5):542-548.

Ney GC, Lantos G, Barr WB, Schaul N. (1994). Cerebellar atrophy in patients with long-term phenytoin exposure and epilepsy. *Arch Neurol,*; 51:767-771.

Nilsson L, Bergman U, Diwan V, Farahmand BY, Persson PG, Tomson T. (2001). Antiepileptic drug therapy and its management in sudden unexpected death in epilepsy: a case-control study. *Epilepsia*; 42(5):667-673.

Opeskin K, Berkovic SF. (2003). Risk factors for sudden unexpected death in epilepsy: a controlled prospective study based on coroners cases. *Seizure*; 12(7): 456-464.

Opeskin K, Burke MP, Cordner SM, Berkovic SF. (1999). Comparison of antiepileptic drug levels in sudden unexpected deaths in epilepsy with deaths from other causes. *Epilepsia*; 40(12):1795-1798.

Opeskin K, Thomas A, Berkovic SF. (2000) Does cardiac conduction pathology contribute to sudden unexpected death in epilepsy? *Epilepsy Res.*; 40(1):17-24.

Oppenheimer SM, Gelb A, Girvin JP, *et al. (1992).* Cardiovascular effects of human insular cortex stimulation. *Neurology*; 42: 1727-1732.

P-Codrea Tigaran S, Dalager-Pedersen S, Baandrup U, Dam M, Vesterby-Charles A. (2005). Sudden unexpected death in epilepsy: is death by seizures a cardiac disease? *Am J Forensic Med Pathol.*; 26(2):99-105.

Persson H, Kumlien E, Ericson M, Tomson T. (2007). Circadian variation in heart-rate variability in localization-related epilepsy. *Epilepsia*; 48(5):917-922.

Pinto KG, Scorza FA, Arida RM, Cavalheiro EA, Martins LD, Machado HR, Sakamoto AC, Terra VC. (2011). Sudden unexpected death in an adolescent with epilepsy: All roads lead to the heart? *Cardiol J.*; 18(2):194-196.

Pool JL, Ransohoff J. (1949). Autonomic effects on stimulating the rostralportion of the cingulate gyri in man. *J Neurophysiol*; 12: 385-392.

Prinjha S, Chapple A, Herxheimer A, McPherson A. (2005). Many people with epilepsy want to know more: a qualitative study. *Fam Pract.*; 22(4):435-441.

Raedt R, Clinckers R, Mollet L, Vonck K, El Tahry R, Wyckhuys T, De Herdt V, Carrette E, Wadman W, Michotte Y, Smolders I, Boon P, Meurs A. (2011). Increased hippocampal noradrenaline is a biomarker for efficacy of vagus nerve stimulation in a limbic seizure model. *J Neurochem.*; Feb 16.

Rocamora R, Kurthen M, Lickfett L, Von Oertzen J, Elger CE. (2003). Cardiac asystole in epilepsy: clinical and neurophysiologic features. *Epilepsia*; 44(2):179-185.

Rossetti AO, Dworetzky BA, Madsen JR, *et al.* (2005). Ictal asystole with convulsive syncope mimicking secondary generalization: a depth electrode study. *J Neurol Neurosurg Psychiatry*; 76: 885-887.

Ruiz Ginés MA, García García S, Ruiz Ginés JA, Tze Kiong E, Fernández Rodríguez E. (2007). Symptomatic secondary hyponatraemia due to combined treatment anticonvulsant and antidepressant: risk of sudden death in epilepsy?. *An Med Interna*; 24(7):335-338.

Ryvlin P, Montavont A, Kahane P. (2006). Sudden unexpected death in epilepsy: from mechanisms to prevention. *Curr Opin Neurol,*; 19:194-199.

Ryvlin P, Tomson T, Montavont A. (2009). Excess mortality and sudden unexpected death in epilepsy. Presse Med.; 38(6):905-910.

Salmo EN, Connolly CE. (2002). Mortality in epilepsy in the west of Ireland: a 10-year review. *Ir J Med Sci.*; 171(4):199-201.

Sandok EK, O'Brien TJ, Jack CR, So EL. (2000). Significance of cerebellar atrophy in intractable temporal lobe epilepsy: a quantitative MRI study. *Epilepsia*; 41:1315-1320.

Schachter SC. (2006). Therapeutic effects of vagus nerve stimulation in epilepsy and implications for sudden unexpected death in epilepsy. *Clin Auton Res.*; 16(1):29-32.

Schuele SU, Widdess-Walsh P, Bermeo A, Lüders HO. (2007). Sudden unexplained death in epilepsy: the role of the heart. *Cleve Clin J Med.*; 74 Suppl 1:S121-127.

Scorza FA, de Albuquerque R, Arida RM, Schmidt B, de Almeida AC, Scorza CA, Cavalheiro EA. (2009). Could sudden death syndrome (SDS) in chickens (Gallus gallus) be a valid animal model for sudden unexpected death in epilepsy (SUDEP)? *Med Hypotheses*; 73(1):67-69.

Seyal M, Bateman LM, Albertson TE, Lin TC, Li CS. (2010). Respiratory changes with seizures in localization-related epilepsy: analysis ofperiictal hypercapnia and airflow patterns. *Epilepsia*; 51(8):1359-1364.

Seyal M, Bateman LM. (2009). Ictal apnea linked to contralateral spread of temporal lobe seizures: Intracranial EEG recordings in refractory temporal lobe epilepsy. *Epilepsia*; 50(12):2557-2562.

So EL. (2006). Demystifying Sudden Unesplainde Death in Epilepsy - Are We Close? *Epilepsia*; 47(Suppl. 1): 87-92.

So EL. (2008). What is known about the mechanisms underlying SUDEP? *Epilepsia*; 49:93-98.

Specht U, May T, Schulz R, Rohde M, Ebner A, Schmidt RC, et al. (1997). Cerebellar atrophy and prognosis after temporal lobe resection. *J Neurol Neurosurg Psychiatry*; 62:501-506.

Stollberger C, Finsterer J. (2004). Cardiorespiratory findings in sudden unexplained/unexpected death in epilepsy (SUDEP). *Epilepsy Res*; 59:51-60.

Strzelczyk A, Bauer S, Knake S, Oertel WH, Hamer HM, Rosenow F. (2008). Ictal asystole in temporal lobe epilepsy before and after pacemaker implantation. *Epileptic Disord.*; 10(1):39-44.

Surges R, Adjei P, Kallis C, Erhuero J, Scott CA, Bell GS, Sander JW, Walker MC. (2010). Pathologic cardiac repolarization in pharmacoresistant epilepsy and its potential role in sudden unexpected death in epilepsy: a case-control study. *Epilepsia*; 51(2):233-242.

Surges R, Henneberger C, Adjei P, Scott CA, Sander JW, Walker MC. (2009). Do alterations in inter-ictal heart rate variability predict sudden unexpected death in epilepsy? *Epilepsy Res.*; 87(2-3):277-280.

Surges R, Scott CA, Walker MC. (2010). Enhanced QT shortening and persistent tachycardia after generalized seizures. *Neurology*; 2;74(5):421-426.

Surges R, Thijs RD, Tan HL, Sander JW. (2009). Sudden unexpected death in epilepsy: risk factors and potential pathomechanisms. *Nat Rev Neurol.*; 5:492-504.

Szabó CA, Knape KD, Leland MM, Feldman J, McCoy KJ, Hubbard GB, Williams JT. (2009). Mortality in captive baboons with seizures: a new model for SUDEP? *Epilepsia*; 50(8):1995-1998.

Szabó CA, Leland MM, Knape K, Elliot JJ, Haines V, Williams JT. (2005). Clinical and EEG phenotypes of epilepsy in the baboon (Papio hamadryas spp). *Epilepsy Res*; 65:71–80.

Tao JX, Qian S, Baldwin M, Chen XJ, Rose S, Ebersole SH, Ebersole JS. (2010). SUDEP, suspected positional airway obstruction, and hypoventilation in postictal coma. *Epilepsia;* 51(11):2344-2347.

Tavernor SJ, Brown SW, Tavernor RM, Gifford C. (1996). Electrocardiograph QT lengthening associated with epileptiform EEG discharges--a role in sudden unexplained death in epilepsy? *Seizure;* 5(1):79-83.

Teh HS, Tan HJ, Loo CY, Raymond AA. (2007). Short QTc in epilepsy patients without cardiac symptoms. *Med J Malaysia;* 62(2):104-108.

Téllez-Zenteno JF, Ronquillo LH, Wiebe S. (2005). Sudden unexpected death in epilepsy: evidence-based analysis of incidence and risk factors. *Epilepsy Res.;* 65(1-2):101-115.

Tennis P, Cole TB, Annegers JF, Leestma JE, McNutt M, Rajput A. (1995). Cohort study of incidence of sudden unexplained death in persons with seizure disorder treated with antiepileptic drugs in Saskatchewan, Canada. *Epilepsia;* 36(1):29-36.

Theodore WH. (2003). Does serotonin play a role in epilepsy? *Epilepsy Curr.;* 3:173–177

Thom M, Griffin B, Sander JW, Scaravilli F. (1999). Amygdala sclerosis in sudden and unexpected death in epilepsy. *Epilepsy Res.;* 37(1):53-62.

Thom M, Seetah S, Sisodiya S, Koepp M, Scaravilli F. (2003). Sudden and unexpected death in epilepsy (SUDEP): evidence of acute neuronal injury using HSP-70 and c-Jun immunohistochemistry. *Neuropathol Appl Neurobiol.;* 29(2):132-143.

Timmings PL. (1998). Sudden unexpected death in epilepsy: is carbamazepine implicated? *Seizure;* 7(4):289-91.

Tomson T, Nashef L, Ryvlin P. (2008). Sudden unexpected death in epilepsy: current knowledge and future directions. *Lancet Neurol.;* 7:1021-1031.

Tomson T, Walczak T, Sillanpaa M, Sander JW. (2005). Sudden unexpected death in epilepsy: a review of incidence and risk factors. *Epilepsia;* 46 Suppl 11:54-61.

Toth V, Hejjel L, Fogarasi A, Gyimesi C, Orsi G, Szucs A, Kovacs N, Komoly S,Ebner A, Janszky J. (2010). Periictal heart rate variability analysis suggests long-term postictal autonomic disturbance in epilepsy. *Eur J Neurol.;* 1;17(6):780-787.

Tu E, Bagnall RD, Duflou J, Semsarian C. (20110. Post-mortem review and genetic analysis of sudden unexpected death in epilepsy (SUDEP) cases. *Brain Pathol.;* 21(2):201-208.

Tupal S, Faingold CL. (2006). Evidence supporting a role of serotonin in modulation of sudden death induced by seizures in DBA/2 mice. *Epilepsia;* 47(1):21-26.

Vlooswijk MC, Majoie HJ, De Krom MC, Tan IY, Aldenkamp AP. (2007). SUDEP in the Netherlands: a retrospective study in a tertiary referral center. *Seizure;* 16(2):153-159.

Walczak TS, Leppik IE, D'Amelio M, Rarick J, So E, Ahman P, Ruggles K, Cascino GD, Annegers JF, Hauser WA. (2001). Incidence and risk factors in sudden unexpected death in epilepsy A prospective cohort study. *Neurology;* 56:519–525.

Walker F, Fish DR. (1997). Recording respiratory parameters in patients with epilepsy. *Epilepsia;* 38(11 Suppl):S41-2.

Xu F, Frazier DT. (2002). Role of cerebellar deep nuclei in respiratory modulation. *Cerebellum;* 1:35-40.

Xu F, Zhang Z, Frazier DT. (*2001).* Microinjection of acetazolamide into the fatigial nucleus augments respiratory outoput in the rat. *J Appl Physiol.;* 91:2342-2350.

Zubair S, Arshad AB, Saeed B, Luqman S, Oommen KJ. (2009). Ictal asystole--late manifestation of partial epilepsy and importance of cardiac pacemaker. *Seizure;* 18(6):457-461.

8

Hallmarks in the History of Epilepsy: From Antiquity Till the Twentieth Century

Emmanouil Magiorkinis, Kalliopi Sidiropoulou and Aristidis Diamantis
Office for the Study of History of Hellenic Naval Medicine, Naval Hospital of Athens, Greece

1. Introduction

1.1 First reports on epilepsy

The history of epilepsy is intervened with the history of humanity. One of the first descriptions of epileptic seizures can be traced back to 2,000 B.C. in ancient Akkadian texts, a language widely used in the region of Mesopotamia. The author described a patient with symptoms resembling epilepsy:

his neck turns left, his hands and feet are tense and his eyes wide open, and from his mouth froth is flowing without having any conciousness.

The exorciser diagnosed the condition as *'antasubbû'* (the hand of Sin) brought about by the god of the moon (Labat, 1951).

Later reports on epilepsy can also be found in Ancient Egyptian medical texts. The Edwin Smith surgical papyrus (1700 B.C.) refers to epileptic convulsions in at least five cases (cases 4, 7, 29, 40, 42). Descriptions of epilepsy can also be found in ancient babylonian texts; epileptics are thought to be afflicted by evil spirits. (Longrigg, 2000). The *Sakikku,* one of the oldest Babylonian medical texts (1067-1046 B.C.), refers to epilepsy with the terms *'antasubba'* and *'miqtu'*[1]. The translated babylonian text describes unilateral and bilateral epileptic fits, the epileptic cry, the incontinence of feces, the description of simple and complex epileptic seizures, the epileptic aura and narcolepsy (Eadie & Bladin, 2001). The Hamurabbi code (1790 B.C.) also refers to epilepsy. The code states that a slave could be returned and the money refunded, if *bennu,* another word for epilepsy (Stol, 1993), appeared within the month after the purchase. In Indian medicine, Atreya attributed epilepsy to a brain dysfunction and not to divine intervention. In the *Caraka Saṃhitā Sutra* (6th century B.C.), he defines epilepsy as:

"paroxysmal loss of consciousness due to disturbance of memory and [of] understanding of mind attented with convulsive seizures" (Pirkner, 1929).

In the Indian text, four different kinds of epilepsy are descibed along with a description of premonitory symptoms and a type of epilepsy called *'Abasmara'*, in which the patients lose their memories.

---

[1] One can easily note the similarity between the Akkadian word *antasubbû* and the Babylonian *antasubba*

1.2 Epilepsy in ancient Greece: the era before Hippocrates

The nosological entity of epilepsy is found under many names in Ancient Greek texts: seliniasmos (*σεληνιασμός*), sacred disease, Herculian disease (because it affected the semi-god Hercules) or demonism. After all, the word 'epilepsy' (επιληψία) originates from the Greek verb "epilambanein" (*επιλαμβάνειν*), which means 'to seize, possess, or afflict'. The disease was initially called sacred, because of the belief for its divine origin. In his work *Lithica,* Orpheus describes eloquently the vengeance of Mene, goddess of the Moon, in the form of epilepsy (Gottfried et al., 1805):

".... to prove them sufferers from the sacred ill
For quickly will they bend and forwards tilt,
As to earth it draws them. Smeared by froth
From their own mouths, hither and tither will they turn,
And wallow on the ground. For filled with anger towards them
She laughs to see their woe, Mene, the horrid and swift"

Ancient Greeks considered epilepsy to be a *'miasma'*[2] (*μίασμα*) which was cast upon the soul. Considered a divine punishment for sinners, an aura of mysticism and superstition surrounded epilepsy; the disease was connected with *Selene* (*Σελήνη*), the goddess of the Moon, since people who offended her were afflicted with epilepsy. Depending on the special symptoms of the epileptic seizure, the Greeks would attribute the fits to a different deity such as Cybele, Poseidon, Mars, Hekate, Hermes or Apollo. According to the Hippocratic texts, for example, if the symptoms included teeth gnashing or convulsions on the right side, then epilepsy was attributed to Cybele, whereas if the patient screamed like a horse, then god Poseidon was to blame (Hippocrate, 1849c).

According to Plutarch (50-120 A.D.), all babies in ancient Sparta were examined by the *'Lesche'* (*Λέσχη*), a council of the elder of Sparta; epileptic babies were left to Apothetae, a short chasm of the mountain Taygetus (Plutarch, 1914). Heracletus of Ephesus (535–475 B.C) makes the first reference to the term 'sacred disease', however, not for describing epileptic seizures (Laertius, 1853). Alcmaeon of Croton (6th B.C.) was the first of the Greek physicians to ascertain that the brain was the organ where *'hegemonicon'* (*ηγεμονικόν*)[3] is founded, the source of memory and thoughts (Diels, 1906). Democritus of Abdera (5th B.C.) wrote a book on epilepsy (*Περί επιληψίας*) which now is extinct, suggesting that the brain is the center of the soul and that cognition and senses were one and the same, originating from the same force (Plutarch, 1888). Herodotus of Hallicarnassus (484 - 425 B.C.), the father of history, in the third book of his work *The Histories* (Thaleia) indirectly refers to epilepsy afflicting the Persian King Cambyses II, whose erratic behavior, according to Herodotus, could be attributed either to the retribution of an aggrieved god or to the so-called 'sacred disease'. Herodotus also noticed the hereditary nature of the disease (*εκ γενεής*) (Herodotus, 2000).

1.3 Epilepsy in the Hippocratic corpus

The first formal description of epilepsy as a disease should be attributed to the father of medicine, Hippocrates of Kos, in his classic treatise *On the sacred disease* (Περί ιερής νούσου). In this book, Hippocrates disputes the divine origin of epilepsy by saying:

"This disease is in my opinion no more divine than any other; it has the same nature as other diseases, and the cause that gives rise to individual diseases. It is also curable, no less than other illnesses,

---

[2] Miasma: a greek word for pollution, a noxious form of 'bad air'

[3] Hegemonicon comes from the word hegemon which means sovereign.

unless by long lapse of time it be so ingrained as to be more powerful than the remedies that are applied" (Hippocrate, 1849b)

Hippocrates was also the first who attempted a scientific approach toward the study of epilepsy by suggesting possible etiology and therapy for the disease. He was the first to attibute the etiology of epilepsy to brain disfunction (Hippocrate, 1849a), stressing the role of heredity in the disease. Among others, Hippocrates will describe the disease accurately, including its unilateral nature and the symptoms of aura (Hippocrate, 1849d). Hippocrates calls epilepsy the "great disease", the originator of the term 'grand mal.' He also describes symptoms reminiscent of psychomotor epilepsy and temporal lobe fits (Hippocrate, 1849e). The view of Hippocrates for the origin of epileptic convulsions and their association with life in utero is also interesting. He states unequivocally that "its birth begins in the embryo while it is still in the womb" (Hippocrate, 1849h). Among the predispositionary factors that can lead to a epileptic fit are: (a) the changes of the winds and of temperature, (b) the exposition of the head to sun, (c) crying, and (d) fear. Prognosis is also worse, when the disease is manifestated in early age (Hippocrate, 1849g), but, for older people, the prognosis is better (Hippocrate, 1849f). In his other treatise, *Injuries of the Head,* Hippocrates notes that head injuries often lead to convulsions, introducing the idea of traumatic epilepsy (Hippocrate, 1849i).

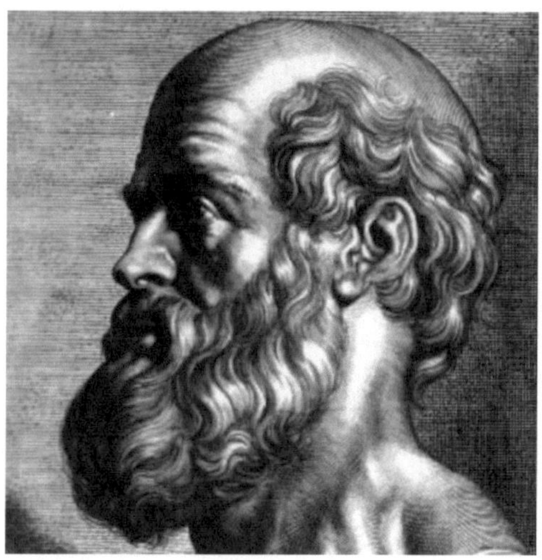

Fig. 1. Hippocrates of Kos (460 BC – ca. 370 BC)

1.4 Epilepsy in Alexandrian and Roman medicine

Medicine in the post-Hippocratic era did not make important achievements as far as the treatment of the disease is concerned. Diocles of Carystus employed the use of various remedies such as phlebotomy, whereas Praxagoras of Cos prescribed extreme remedies such as the cauterization (Drabkin, 1950).

On the other hand, Plato (428/427 BC - 348/347 BC), in his *Laws,* suggests specific punishment for people selling slaves with epilepsy, in parallel with the Hamurabi code of the Babylonians (Plato, 1871).During the Roman period, the proceedings of the Senate were interrupted or postponed, whenever a senator was struck by epilepsy during a session because epilepsy was considered a bad sign from the Gods. For that reason Romans called epilepsy *morbus comitialis,* since an epileptic attack tended to spoil the day of the *comitia,* the assembly of the people.

Various philosophers will refer to epilepsy such as the Pliny the Elder, in his *Naturalis Historia,* suggesting magical remedies such as the rubbing of patient's feet with menstrual blood (Pliny, 1856), Pedanius Dioscorides (40-90 A.D.) describing 45 different substances used as remedies for epilepsy (Temkin, 1971a) and Aurelius Cornelius Celsus who calls epilepsy, in his writings, *morbus comitialis* and suggests as a cure sexual intercourse for boys or the warm blood of slain gladiators in obstinate cases (Celsus, 1935).

One of the most important works of this period is that of Aelius Galenus or Claudius Galenus (131-201 AD) who systemized nosology and described epilepsy with accuracy in his classic treatise *Medical Definitions* (Galen, 1821c). He was able to discern three forms of epilepsy: (1) idiopathic, attributed to primary brain disorder (an analogue to grand mal epilepsies), (2) Secondary forms, attributed to disturbance of cardiac function transmitted through the flow of liquids secondarily to the brain (epilepsy by sympathy), and (3) a third type attributed to disturbance of another part of human body which is secondarily transmitted to the brain (probably Jacksonian epileptic seizures). Galen accurately sets the brain as the organ afflicted by the disease , and, most importantly, he described the aura, a greek word which originally means 'breeze', in his *De locis affectis* referring to the symptoms of a case of a 13-year-old boy (Galen, 1821a). Galen also differentiates epilepsy from tetanus because with epilepsy the whole body participates with a loss of consiousness (Galen, 1821b).

Aretaeus of Cappadocia (1st/2nd century AD) was the first to describe premonitionary symptoms of epilepsy, such as hallucinations that occasionally precede epileptic seizures; he noted that fetid odors, luminous circles of diverse color, noises from the ears, tremors and sensations in the hands or feet may occur before the seizure. He also noted the tendency of seizures to recur, once established, and the phenomenon of epileptic insanity (Aretaeus, 1856a). After the fall of the epileptic to the ground, Aretaeus, distinguished three main periods: manifestation, abatement, cessation. The manifestation is characterized by insensibility and tonic and clonic convulsions. At the end of the abatement stage, patients appear to suffocate, with its concomitant signs including erection of the genital. During the abatement stage, the patients unconsciously discharge urine, excrement, and semen, a hallmark symptom that discerns epilepsy from hysteria. Then, a flow of froth ends the suffocation. At the end of the abatement stage, they arise with the seizure having ended. During cessation period, patients still have various signs of physical and mental discomfort (Aretaeus, 1856c). Aretaeus gives an excellent description of 'grand mal' epilepsy in his text (Aretaeus, 1856c), as well as the first description of the so-called 'epileptic personality' (Aretaeus, 1856b).

Soranus of Ephesus (1st/2nd century AD) also referred to epilepsy without making any contribution to the understanding of the disease.

2. Epilepsy in the dark ages

2.1 Medieval times and medicine

The Medieval times is characterized by a domination of mysticism and dogmatism in all fields of science, including Medicine. Physicians tended to believe that diseases such epilepsy, hysteria and psychoses were the result of demonic possession; for that reason epileptics were treated as witches and warlocks. Many medieval mosaics, frescoes, miniatures and paintings depic the exorcism of a particular disease/devil by a particular saint. Beyerstein suggests that the curious behavior of the possessed people described in the classic *Malleus Maleficarum* (15th century AD) is likely symptoms of epilepsy or Tourette's syndrome (Beyerstein, 1988). Beginning at age 13, Joan d'Arc experienced moments of ecstasy with light, heard voices of saints, and claimed to see visions with angels, all probably symptoms of epileptic seizure (d'Orsi & Tinuper, 2006).

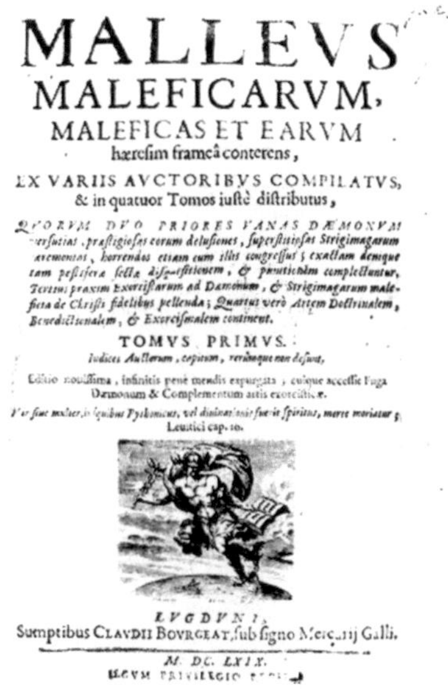

MALLEVS
MALEFICARVM,
MALEFICAS ET EARVM
hæresim frameâ conterens,
EX VARIIS AVCTORIBVS COMPILATVS,
& in quatuor Tomos iustè distributus,
QVORVM DVO PRIORES VANAS DÆMONVM versutias, præstigiosas eorum delusiones, superstitiosas Strigimagarum ceremonias, horrendos etiam cum illis congressus; exactam denique tam pestiferæ sectæ disquisitionem, & punitionem complectuntur. Tertius praxim Exorcistarum ad Dæmonum, & Strigimagarum maleficia de Christi fidelibus pellenda; Quartus verò Artem Doctrinalem, Benedictionalem, & Exorcismalem continent.
TOMVS PRIMVS.
Indices Auctorum, capitum, rerùmque non desunt.
Editio nouissima, infinitis penè mendis expurgata; cuique accessit Fuga Dæmonum & Complementum artis exorcisticæ.
Vir siue mulier, in quibus Pythonicus, vel diuinationis fuerit spiritus, morte moriatur; Leuitici cap. 10.
LVGDVNI,
Sumptibus CLAVDII BOVRGEAT, sub signo Merc..rij Galli.
M. DC. LXIX.
CVM PRIVILEGIO REGIS.

Fig. 2. Malleus Maleficarum (Lyon edition, 1669)

Another aspect on epilepsy during the Medieval times, was the theory that epilepsy was a contagious disease. The epileptics, considered to be possessed, were excused from oblation and Eucharist because they would desecrate the holy objects and would infect the common plate and cup (Dolger, 1933). Epilepsy was also included in the infectious diseases enumerated in the verse of the so-called *Schola Salernitana,* where it was named *pedicon* (Martin, 1922). Berthold of Regensburg, attributed the infection of the 'falling evil', as epilepsy was commonly called during this period, to the contagious character of the patient's evil breath. A connection of epilepsy with astrology was also a very popular theory in medieval times. Pagans believed that epilepsy was a vengeance of the goddess of the moon. The waxing moon supposedly heated the atmosphere surrounding the earth, which in turn melted the human brain and provoked the attack (Temkin, 1971c).

2.2 Epilepsy and the catholic church

Inevitably, many saints of the catholic church dealt with epilepsy. For example, St. Hildegard of Bingen (1098-1179 AD) distinguished between two kinds of epilepsy: a vengeful wrath sets the blood in motion causing one type of epilepsy while patients with unstable or low morals suffered the a second type (Hildegard, 1903). Saint Valentine, whose name in German originates from the phrase 'fall net hin' (Valentin) ('do not fall down'), was considered as patron of the epileptics (Kluger & Kudernatsch, 2009). Saint John the Baptist, was also connected with the disease, probably because his head fell to the ground after his decapitation by Herod (Budrys, 2007). St John was originally the patron of the dancing mania, and later, St. Vitus, a christian martyr of Sicily, became the specific saint of this neurosis and St. John of epilepsy. The three wise men from the biblical tale of Jesus' birth also had a reputation as patrons of epilepsy mainly because they fell down before the divine child and offered gifts (Kerler, 1905). On the other hand, the Greek Orthodox Church has the example of St. Tychonas of Cyprus who was considered to have cured many possessed people.

2.3 Byzantine and Arab physicians

Once should also note the views of famous byzantine physicians such as Oribasius of Pergamum, Aetius Amidenus, Alexander of Tralles and Paulus of Aegina on epilepsy. Overall, byzantine doctors recapitulate the theories of Ancient Greek physicians and further systemize the nosology of the disease by reporting interesting cases of epileptic patients. It is of note, though, that Alexander of Tralles (525-605 AD), in his treatise *Twelve books on Medicine*, takes an orthologic approach considering epilepsy a brain disturbance and reject extreme procedures such as trephinization (Tralles, 1878). Paulus of Aegina (7th century AD), according to Economou and Lascaratos, was the first Byzantine doctor who provided a clinical description of the epileptic fits, and also described a clinical condition that resembles *status epilepticus* (Economou & Lascaratos, 2005).

Arab doctors seem also to recapitulate the theories of Galen and Hippocrates without making any significant progress. Interesting descriptions of epileptic seizures can be found in the texts of Rhazes (Temkin, 1942) and those of Abulcasis (936 - 1013 AD) who also refers to cases of epilepsy due to daemonic possession (Abulcasim, 1519). He will also make important observations on traumatic epilepsy, correctly associating fractures of the skull and brain compression with the malady (Africanus, 1536-1539). Masoudi (late 10th century AD) refers to epilepsy of traumatic origin by noting that an obstruction of the brain may be the result of a compression from a fracture of the skull accompanied by severe pain (Abbas, 1523), whereas Avicenna (981-1037 AD), one of the most influential scientists in the Middle ages, supports the theory of blockage of humors as a possible mechanism of epileptic convulsions (Avicenna, 1999).

Constantinus the African (1020–1087 AD), a translator of Greek medical and Islamic texts, advises the parents of epileptics to take the patient to church during the second week following Whitsuntide (Pentecost) and expose them to the Friday or Saturday Mass (Temkin, 1971d).

2.4 Physicians of the Western Europe

Among the most influential physicans are Arnold of Villanova, famous physician, alchemist and magician, Bernard of Gordon, a teacher in Montpellier from 1285 to 1307, and John of Gaddesden, physician to Edward II of England. Arnold of Vilanova (1240 - 1311), perpetuates superstitious views emphasizing the depedence of the disease on the star constellations and especially the moon. (Vilanova, 1585b). He also notices that 'the true epilepsy is engendered with phleghm; spurious epilepsy by black bile mixed with phlegm' (Vilanova, 1585a). Bernard of Gordon (1303) suggested as therapy that a priest should recite a Gospel passage, which it should be written down to be carried by the patient as an amulet (Gordon, 1542). John of Gaddesden (1280-1361 AD) distinguishes three forms of epilepsy: minor, medium and major assigning the synonyms true, truer and truest. Minor epilepsy is attributed to the obstruction of arteries, medium epilepsy to the obstruction of the nerves and major to an obstruction of the ventricles of the brain (Gaddesden, 1595). Giovanni Michele Savonarola of Padova (1385 – 1466 AD) adopts a similar classification with different terms: primitive, antecedent and conjoint (Savonarola, 1547), as well as Matthaeus Platearius in his *Practica brevis* adding two clinical varieties that are distinguised as 'maior and 'minor' epilepsy (i.e., grand mal and petite mal) (Serapion, 1530).

3. Views on epilepsy in renaissance and enlightment

The end of the Medieval times and the beginning of the European Renaissance (14th-17th century) is marked with an exceptional production of literature regarding epilepsy. Science, emancipated from the restrains of the Catholic Church will undoubtly make important progress; in the field of epilepsy, almost all the prestigious and famous physicians of the era deal with the disease.

Various theories will be proposed regarding the mechanism that causes the epileptic fits as well as new classifications of the disease will come forth. For example, Petrus Forestus (1522-1597 AD), a Dutch physician, notes that the part of the body that epilepsy originates, leads to different manifestations. There is also a tedency to differentiate epilepsy and daemonism; in his *Daemonum investigatio peripatetica* (Peripatetic investigation of demons) Andreas Caesalpinus (1519-1603 AD), an Italian natural philosopher, tries to differ epileptic seizures and daemonic possesion (Caesalpinus, 1593).

One of the most famous physicians of this period, Paracelsus (1493–1541 AD), dealt with epilepsy. He agrees that epilepsy may originate from the brain or the liver, the heart, the intensines and the limbs. Paracelsus views about the human nature and the construction of the human body from mercury, sulfur and salt led him to a different model for the causes of epilepsy (Paracelsus, 1922-1933a). However, in his essay he clearly sets God above all, and stresses that the physician should ask for divine help in the treatment (Paracelsus, 1922-1933b). Ioannes Marcus Marci (1595-1667 AD), a Bohemian physician and scientist, broadened the definition of epilepsy 'to any affection of the body where the victims are disordered in their minds, while the members [of the body], be it all, or some, or only one, are moved against their will.' Thus, he tied cases of epileptic convulsions with mental manifestations (Marci a Kronland, 1678). Levinus Lemnius (1505-1568 AD), famous Dutch physician and student of Vesalius, all stressed the natural origin of the disease and rejected any theological superstitions (Lemnius, 1658).

Other physicians who also dealth with epilepsy include Charles Le Pois (1563-1636 AD), consultant physician to Charles III of France, who rejected previous theories such as those postulated by Petrus Forestus suggesting that peripheral organs led to epilepsy (Le Pois, 1733), Joannes Ambianus Fernelius (Jean François Fernel) (1497-1558), a French astrologist and physiologist, who supported the theory that poisonous vapors affected the brain and led to epileptic fits, and rejected the medieval belief about the contagious nature of epilepsy (Fernelius, 1577).

An important treatise of the period is that of Jean Taxil's *Traicté de l'épilepsie,* that summarize the knowledge around epilepsy, including its causes and various remedies; he was the first Renaissance doctor who seriously doubted demonic possession (Taxil, 1602).

William Harvey (1585-1657 AD) will be the first who will make important advances for the establishment of neurology as clinical speciality with his descriptions of various neurological disorders including epilepsy (Brain, 1959; R. Hunter & MacAlpine, 1957). An interesting theory on epileptic convulsions is that of Thomas Willis Thomas Willis (1621 - 1675) who assumed the existence of a '*spasmodic explosive copula*'. For Willis 'The convulsive disease for the most part, takes its origin from the head (Willis, 1684). In his *De morbus convulsivis* (Morbid convulsions) Willis places the cause of epilepsy in the brain, but differed with his predecessors who pointed to the middle of the brain itself or the meninges. His hypothesis suggested that since the brain is of a weak constitution, a strong *spasmodi copula* distills from the blood to the brain leading the animal spirits that lie in the middle of the brain to explode. The explosion of anial spirits cause all the mental symptoms of the epileptic attack, and a series of similar explosions occurr along the rest of the nervous system to bring about the convulsions of the body (Willis, 1682).

Interesting cases of epileptic patients appear during this period too. For example, Martinus Rulandus (1532-1602), German physician and alchemist, describes the case of a 40-year-old man suffering from epilepsy and mania. A woman considered to be a witch was accused of causing evil to this man, but during her confession she claimed that she could not cure him. So, Ruland was called and he managed to cure him by bloodletting, sternutatory and a strong cathartic (Rulandus, 1580). Thomas Erastus (1524-1583), a Swiss theologian, documents the case of a girl with characteristic psychomotor symptoms of epileptic convulsions. After convulsing, she wandered around the room for almost half an hour and the people who were around could not stop her. After the event should could not remember anything that happened (Erastus, 1581).Felix Plater (1536-1617), as referred by Tissot, describes a young man whose malady started with a headache, stubborn insomnia and deterioration of his faculties and ended with frequent convulsive attacks and emaciation. The post-mortem dissection revealed tumor in the anterior part of the brain (Tissot, 1770a).

Charles Drélincourt (1633-1694), finally, was the first to provoke epileptic convulsions experimentally by driving a needle into the fourth ventricle of a dog's brain (Drelincurtius, 1682).

4. Epilepsy during the 18th and 19th century

4.1 The work of 18th century physicians on epilepsy

The beginning of the 18th century is marked by the work of doctors of the Dutch medical school founded by Herman Boerhaave and his pupil Gerard van Swieten. Herman Boerhaave (1668–1738) provided a rather strict definition of epilepsy: 'Epilepsy is the sudden abolishment of all vital functions with accompanying increase of mobility and convulsions in all body muscles', whereas he adopts the Galenic classification of epilepsy (Boerhaave, 1761). The Dutch-Austrian Gerard Van Swieten (1700–1772) wrote a chapter on epilepsy in which he describes extensively the clinical characteristics of various forms of the disease and discusses epilepsy in comparison with apoplexy and hysteria. (Temkin, 1971b).

The first major treatise on epilepsy was written by the Swiss physician Simon August André David Tissot (1728–1787). Published in 1770, the *Traite de l' epilepsie* is considered to be a milestone in the scientific research on epilepsy. Tissot completely rejects the influence of the moon on epileptic seizures, accepts the hereditary forms of epilepsy, and states that it is the duty of the epileptic to remain unmarried (S. Tissot, 1770b). Among his extreme views about epilepsy is the belief that masturbation could cause epileptic seizures (S. Tissot, 1770b).

The French medical school of the 19th century took lead in the fields of neurology and psychiatry, and, therefore, were the main driving force on epilepsy research. Jacques-Louis Doussin Dubreuil (1762–1831) tried to explain the influence of various emotional states on epilepsy (Doussin-Dubreuil, 1825), whereas Louis Maisonneuve, a pupil of Philip Pinel (1745 - 1826), stated that 'epilepsy like all chronic diseases can be studied well only in hospital', stressing the variety of clinical manifestations of epilepsy (Maisonneuve, 1803).

Physicians of the British medical school also dealth with epilepsy such as Thomas Beddoes (1760–1808), who described accurately the premonitionary symptoms developing before the onset of an attack, (Maisonneuve, 1804) William Cullen (1712–1790), who included epilepsy as one of the spasmodic affections without fever, together with tetanus and chorea or St. Vitus dance (Cullen, 1778-1784). Finally, the first experimental provocation of convulsions was done in Italy. The Italian naturalist Felice Gaspar Ferdinand Fontana (1730–1803), in a series of experiments on stimulation of the cerbral cortex with electricity, demonstrated that convulsions could be produced by pressure on the brain, but not by irritation of the dura, as commonly believed (Garrison, 1935; Marchand & Hoff, 1955).

4.2 The 19th century: The "golden era" of French medicine and the contribution of the English school of physicians

4.2.1 The French medical school

The progress of the French medical school is marked by a peak during the 19th century. Marie-Jean-Pierre Flourens (1794–1867) established the basic rules regarding the irritability and sensibility of the central nervous system, noting that different functions can be attributed to different parts. His contribution is decisive for the research on epilepsy, since the loss of consciousness and the voluntary movements in epileptic attacks would imply the involvement of the cerebral lobes, were it not for the participation of the medulla that Flourens found (Flourens, 1823). The French psychiatrist Jean-Étienne Dominique Esquirol (1772–1840), distinguished severe from light epileptic seizures (grand mal and petit mal) and worked withh his pupils Bouchet and Cazauvieilh, on epilepsy and insanity. A later study by his students Bouchet and Cazauvieilh revealed a high frequency of epileptic attacks among patients considered to be insane (Esquirol, 1838). In 1827, Antoine Baron de Portal (1742-1832) published his clinical experience based on a large amount of clinical data and post-mortem reports, admitting that in many cases of epilepsy, dissection did not reveal any lesions either in the brain or other parts of the body (Portal, 1827b). He also makes important notes on the so-called *furor epilepticus*. He noticed this clinical status appeared before the onset of the epileptic seizure, as well as after; a patient in this condition could even commit murder (Portal, 1827a). Louis François Bravais (1801–1843) in his thesis defines epilepsy from a new basis, that of 'hemiplegic epilepsy', during which convulsions attack one side of the body followed by paralysis, whereas he is considered to be the first to describe of what was later called Jacksonian convulsions (Bravais, 1827). Francois-Emmanuel Foderé (1764–1835), denowed French physician and expert in forensic medicine, will discuss what he calls 'periodic delirium', which is clearly epileptic mania (Foderé, 1798). Charles-Édouard Brown-Séquard (1817–1894) managed to provoke epileptiform convulsions by transverse section of the lateral half of the spinal cord in animals (Brown-Séquard, 1857). Théodore Herpin (1799–1865) will publish 300 cases on epilepsy, providing insights on the symptoms preceding the onset of major seizures, the initial symptoms with which major attacks began and the minor attacks appearing in the intervals between complete attacks. Herpin also describes epilepsies with intellectual disturbances and with immediate loss of consciousness. (Herpin, 1867).

One should also note the important contibution of the French psychiatrists on the psychomotor symptoms of epilepsy. Bénédict Augustin Morel (1809–1879) noted that irritability and anger are the salient features of the epileptic personality (Morel, 1852-1853). Epileptic fury, according to Morel, appears in two forms: either before or after the epileptic attack or indepedently "like lightning and being condensed in terrible deeds" (Morel, 1852-1853). Jules Falret (1824–1902) will divide the mental disorders found in epileptics in three categories: premonitory symptoms, symptoms of the epileptic personality and epileptic insanity. Falret was also able to identify intellectual disturbances during the epileptic attack in cases where the patient did not lose consciousness, whereas he divided the mental disorders of the third type into *petit mal intellectuel* and *grand mal intellectuel*. (Falret, 1860).

4.2.2 The British medical school of the 19th century

The contribution of the British Medical school is equally important. James Cowles Prichard (1786–1848), notes that the 'epileptic delirium' appears when the patient revives from the comatose state consequent of a seizure, but it can also appear without any previous fit, whereas he describes the typical symptoms of epileptic mania (J. C. Prichard, 1822a). Prichard describes other states of mental confusion, suggesting they are like somnambulism or epileptic ecstasy:

'A more unusual circumstance in the history of epilepsy is the appearance of a species of somnambulism, or of a kind of ecstasis, during which the patient is in an undisturbed reverie, and walks about, fancying himself occupied in some of his customary amusements or avocations. This takes place during the waking as well as the sleeping hours'.

His observations are the forerunners of the concept of 'psychic equivalents of epilepsy' (James Cowles Prichard, 1822b). Prichard was also the first to establish the term 'partial epilepsy' in the literature, devoting to the topic an entire chapter in his treatise, called 'Of local convulsion or partial epilepsy'.

Richard Bright (1789–1858 attempted to combine anatomical data with clinical cases, and was able to show changes in the cortex of the cerebral hemispheres (R. Bright, 1831a). Bright supported the theory that the gray matter of the brain was the main functional part of the cerebral hemispheres, referring to the discoveries of Foville (Richard Bright, 1831b). Marshall Hall (1790–1857), on the other hand, suggested that epilepsy was due in part to anemia of the medulla and that paroxysmal discharges arose from the brain (M. Hall, 1851; Marshall Hall, 1852). Robert Bentley Todd (1809–1860), physician in King's College Hospital, in an experiment to determine the seat of epilepsy, observed discrete movements on the face of a rabbit upon stimulation of the cerebral hemispheres, but he did not appreciate the significance of his experiments, for he maintained that movement was the concern of structures from the corpora striatum rostrally. In 1836, Astley Cooper (1768–1841) reported his findings on provoking epileptic seizures by temporary anaemia, without the loss of blood.(Cooper, 1836).

John Russell Reynolds (1828–1896), was the first to identify 'epilepsy proper' with idiopathic epilepsy, to which, he believed, 'the name of epilepsy ought to be applied' (Reynolds, 1861b). His major account on epilepsy was published in 1861 entitled *Epilepsy: Its Symptoms, Treatment and Relation to Other Chronic Convulsive Diseases* (Reynolds, 1861a), which is considered to be a milestone in the English epileptology. Reynolds employs the terms 'epileptiform' or 'epileptoid' for seizures resembling epilepsy, rejecting, in that way, the existence of renal or uterine epilepsy and epilepsy from tumor of the brain; he claims that we 'find these confounded together with simple or idiopathic affection' (Reynolds, 1861a), adopting indirectly Delasiauve's theories about idiopathic epilepsy (Delasiauve, 1854) as epilepsy of cerebral origin with uknown pathology. Reynolds support also the theory about positive and negative symptoms arising from brain pathology (Pearce, 2004), earlier than his successor, Jackson; negative effects are associated with direct impact on structural pathology

that damaged or destroyed tissue, whereas positive symptoms are more remote effects of pathology arising from 'altered nutrition' that the pathology produced in surviving tissue. Reynolds also referrs to the epileptic aura without attempting to explain its pathogenesis.
William Richard Gowers (1845-1915), also contributed substantially into the understanding of the pathogenesis of the disease. During those lectures, Gowers presented and reviewed the clinical features of a series of 1,500 cases who observed and treated them in person. Those cases were published in some of the most prestigious contemporary medical journals (Gowers, 1880), and, then, he expanded further those findings in his monograph entitled *Epilepsy and other chronic convulsive disorders* (1881), including a series of 3,000 cases of epilepsy which covers every possible clinical feature of epilepsy (Gowers, 1881).

4.2.3 The Dutch and German medical school of the 19th century

Research into epilepsy was also advanced by the work of German and Dutch physicians of the era. Karl Friedrich Burdach (1776–1847), anatomist, physiologist and embryologist, published a series of 1,911 anatomical abnormalities observed in the brain. According to his data, the lateral ventricles were most frequently affected, with 86 out of 476 cases, of which 63 consisted of serous effusion (Burdach, 1826).
Friedrich Gustav Jacob Henle (1809–1895), writing in 1853, noted that epileptic convulsions are provoked by an increased turgor at the base of the brain, and that the loss of consciousness depends either on increase or decrease of blood flow in the hemispheres. (Henle, 1846). The same year, Adolf Kussmaul (1822–1902) along with Adolf Tenner published the classic treatise on epileptiform convulsions (Kussmaul & Tenner, 1859), whereas in 1859, Höring, a German physician, in his dissertation entitled *Über Epilepsie,* described a case of a young man who had grand mal attacks as well as many mild attacks during which he had complete lapses of memory (Horing, 1859). Wilhelm Griesinger (1817-1868), in 1868, will employ for the first time the term 'psycho-motor symptoms' in epileptoid conditions. (Griesinger, 1868-1869).

4.3 Therapies on epilepsy

The most important advance in anti-epileptic therapy of this period is the introduction of bromide potassium in the treatment of epilepsy by Edward Sieveking, in 1857 (Sieveking, 1857), a treatment further supported by Charles Locock (1799–1875) and especially Samuel Wilks (Richard Hunter, 1959-1960; Wilks, 1861). Locock described the anticonvulsant effect of bromides, although the earliest studies on the effects of various drugs as anticonvulsants were performed by Albertoni (1882), on animals with induced seizures (Albertoni, 1882). Extreme methods of therapy are still perpetuated such as trephining of the skull was supported by Charles-Édouard Brown-Séquard, Benjamin W. Dudley (1785–1870), John Saw Billings (1838–1913) and Paul Broca (1824–1880), most of whom had applied surgical therapy in various cases (Billings, 1861; Broca, 1867; Smith, 1852). Other surgical procedures suggested have been tracheoctomy, by Marsall Hall (M. Hall, 1841), and cauterization of the larynx with nitrate of silver, by Brown-Séquard (Brown-Séquard, 1853).

5. The age of John Hughlings Jackson

John Hughlings Jackson (1835-1911), is beyond any doubt the father of modern epileptology. His clinical observations from 1861 to 1870, which came well before the experimental reports of Eduard Hitzig (1839–1907) and David Ferrier (1843 –1928), were confirmed ultimately by Hitzig and Ferrier (Fritsch & Hitzig, 1870).

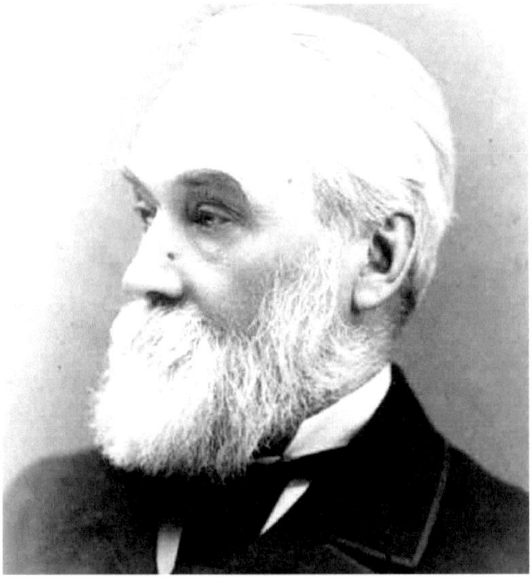

Fig. 3. John Hughlings Jackson (1835-1911), father of modern epileptology

Jackson studied epilepsy on a pathological and anatomical basis. He initially believed that focal convulsions were due to a discharging lesion from damage to nerve cells. He also believed, at first, that the part of the brain involved was the region of the corpus striatium or the convolutions near to it. In 1861, Jackson published his first paper containing reports from hospitals and from the medical literature (Jackson, 1861), whereas, in 1863, he observed about unilateral convulsions that 'in very many cases of epilepsy and especially in syphilitic epilepsy, the convulsions are limited to one side of the body; and, as autopsies of patients who have died after syphilitic epilepsy appear to show, the cause is obvious organic disease on the side of the brain, opposite to the side of the body convulsed, frequently on the surface of the hemisphere' (Jackson, 1863).

In 1864, Jackson published his an important in which he discusses the symptoms of aphasia (Jackson, 1864). Jackson thus offered an new explanation about epileptic seizures that differed that of his predecessors who claimed the seat of the disease lay in the medula oblongata.

In the following years, Jackson's views regarding the involvement of the corpus striatum in the genesis of seizures evolved rapidly. Jackson distinguishes four factors involved in the final cause of convulsions: the 'seat of the internal lesion', the functional cause of the change, the pathological process which brought about the functional change (embolus, tumor, syphilis or other cause) and the various circumstances that trigger the paroxysm (Jackson, 1931-1932a, 1931-1932b).

In 1866 Jackson discussed the mechanisms of various forms of epilepsy noting that 'in cases of sudden and temporary loss of conciousness in which convulsive movements were slight, or perhaps absent, the disorder of function was chiefly in the range of the anterior cerebral artery' (Jackson, 1866). For cases of loss of conciousness, he believed the disorder to be located 'in the very highest nervous centres of the cerebral hemisphere' (Jackson, 1931-1932b). As far as the mechanisms involved, genuine epilepsy was not different from unilateral epilepsy. He later refined his definition of epilepsy, suggesting an scientific and an empirical classification; in terms of anatomy and physiology epileptic vertigo, petit mal and grand mal were due to differences of a discharge 'beginning and spreading from the same parts of the brain' (Jackson, 1931-1932b). Empirically, he distinguished three classes of epilepsy proper from which the epileptiform or epileptoid group, including convulsions beginning unilaterally, unilateral dysaesthesia (migraine) and epileptiform amaurosis, had to be differentiated (Jackson, 1931-1932b).

In his lecture *On Convulsive Seizures* Jackson presented the most advanced form of his theory on epilepsy. According to Jackson, the central nervous system can be divided into three levels: (a) the lowest level, which consists of the spinal cord, the medula oblongata and the pons, representing the most rough and simple movements; (b) the 'motor province' consisting of the 'motor region of the cerebral cortex (Rolandic region) and of the ganglia of the corpus striatum representing complex movements of all parts of the body; and (c) the highest level formed by the centers of the prefrontal lobes ('the organ of mind') (Jackson, 1931-1932b). Fits beginning at the lower levels can spread to higher ones through interconnecting fibers as well as to neighboring cells of the same level. Jackson considered therefore middle level fits to correspond to *epileptiform* seizures and highest level fits to *epileptic* seizures. Jackson was careful to clarify his use of terms, however: 'I do not use the term cortical epilepsy because both epileptic and epileptiform seizures are, to my thinking, cortical fits… I formerly used the term epilepsy generically for all excessive discharges of the cortex and their consequences… I now use the term epilepsy for that neurosis which is often called "genuine" or "ordinary" epilepsy, and for that only' (Jackson, 1931-1932b). Epileptiform convulsions, according to Jackson, start from a definite place in the brain and always begin with a signal symptom which localizes the original discharging lession. The symptoms can be either be sensory or motor depending on the part of the brain where discharges take place, since according to Jackson all levels are sensorimotor. Discharging lesions are diseased because of 'morbid nutrition', and those cells who are discharged, lose their function and temporarily form a 'negative lession' (Jackson, 1931-1932b). Sensory or/and motor symptoms are present in each epileptic or epileptiform seizure; in epileptic seizures paralysis is generalized, whereas in epileptiform seizures it is located in certain parts of the body.

To explain post-epileptic states, Jackson suggests the four-layer theory of higher levels, though this theory was not supported by any anatomical data, as Jackson admits. He thought that discharges afflicting the first layer are responsible for impaired consciousness, the second for a single loss of consciousness, as in the case of epileptic mania, and the third for coma without affecting the vital operations (Jackson, 1931-1932b).

Jackson also refers to the 'dreamy state' some patients experience before the onset of the epileptic fits. He mentions, writing in 1876, a number of expressions used by patients to describe those symptoms of the so-called 'intellectual aura', some of which resemble states known in modern psychiatry and neurology as 'déjà vu': 'Old scenes revert, I fell in some strange place, a dreamy state, a panorama of something familiary and yet strange, if I were walking alone and had a fit, I should think "Oh, I saw that before" (Jackson, 1931-1932b).

6. Epilepsy in the twentieth century

Before the end of the 19th century, in 1898, William Letchworth (1823-1910) and Frederick Peterson (1859-1938) will organize the National Association for the Study of Epilepsy and the Care and Treatment of Epileptics in the US (Letchworth, 1901). At the beginning of the 20th century, William Spartling will be the first to use the term 'epileptologist' for a physician specializing in epilepsy. Cajal will describe neurons and synapses, a hallmark finding in the history of Neurology; in 1906, he will receive the Nobel prize for his discoveries.

In 1903, the first description of progressive myoclonic epilepsy by Herman Bernhard Lundborg (1868-1943) will be published (Lundborg, 1903), whereas Gowers will publish his famous book *The Borderlands of Epilepsy* (Gowers, 1903)

In 1912, Kaufmann will notice the electric changes in the brain during experimentally induced seizures (Kaufman, 1912), whereas in the same year Alfred Hauptmann (1881-1948) will synthesize phenobarbital, one of the first anti-epileptic drugs (Hauptmann, 1912). Two years later Napoleon Cybulski (1854 - 1919) and Jelenska-Macieszyna (Cybulski & Jelenska-Macieszyna, 1914) will publish the first fotographs of electroencephalography, whereas Walter Dandy (1886-1946) will describe in 1918 and 1919 pneumoventriculography and pneumoencephalography (Dandy, 1918, 1919a, 1919b). During the 1920's, William Gordon Lennox (1884–1960) and Cobb will focus on the effects of starvation, ketogenic diet and altered cerebral oxygen in seizures and they will publish their first monograph (Lennox & Cobb, 1928).

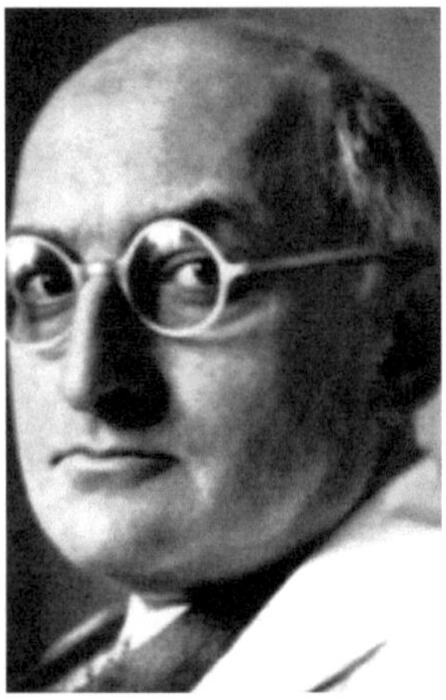

Fig. 4. Alfred Hauptmann (1881-1948)

In 1929, Hans Berger (1873-1941) will report human brain waves (Berger, 1929), confirmed later by Adrian and Matthews (Adrian & Mathews, 1934). In 1932, Berger reported sequential postictal EEG changes after a generalized tonicoclonic seizure, and in 1933 he published the first example of interictal changes and a minor epileptic seizure with 3/s rhytmic waves in the EEG (Berger, 1932, 1933). His work on epileptic EEG will be completed by Frederic Andrews Gibbs (1903–1992) and Erna Gibbs (1904-1987) who in collaboration with William G. Lennox will establish the correlation between EEG findings and epileptic convulsions (Gibbs et al., 1935; Gibbs et al., 1937; Gibbs et al., 1936). During the same period, H. Houston Merritt (1902 - 1979) and Tracy Putnam (1894-1975) will discover phenytoin and its effect on the control of epileptic seizures publishing their results in a series of papers (Merrit & Putnam, 1938a, 1938b, 1939, 1940). Phenytoin will become the first-line medication for the prevention of partial and tonic-clonic seizures and for acute cases of epilepsies or status epilepticus. Important advances will also be made on the fields of epileptic surgery by Wilder Penfield (1891-1976) who applied the Foerster method of removing epileptogenic lesions on an epilepsy patient (Penfield & Steelman, 1947). The concept of eugenics will become an issue in the control of epilepsy; in 1936, the American Neurological Association Committee for the Investigation of Eugenical Sterilization will publish a report (Myerson et al., 1936) stating that sterilization of epileptics should be voluntary, conducted under supervision and only with patient consent.

Kluver and Bucy will show, in 1939, that changes in behavior in monkeys may be associated with temporal lobe lessions (Kluver & Bucy, 1997), whereas in 1941 Jasper and Kershmann will prove that the temporal lobe is the site of origin of psychomotor seizures (Jasper & Kershmann, 1941). Percival Bailey (1892-1973) is the first to attempt temporal lobetomies for psychomotor seizures and the first to use electo-corticography for intra-operative localization (Bailey & Gibbs, 1951).

In 1946, a new anti-epileptic drug trimethadione was reported by Richards and Evertt to prevent pentylenetetrazol induced seizures (Richards & Everett, 1946). Other important advances in the field of epileptology were the development of a stereotactic human brain atlas by Talairach and Bancaud and the discovery of γ-aminobutiric acid (GABA) by Roberts and Frankel in 1949 (Roberts & Frankel, 1950).

The beginning of the 1950's is marked by the establishment of the National Institute of Neurological Diseases and Blindness (NINDB). William Penfield will perfect and establish his surgical procedures as a treatment of choice in intractable epilepsy, especially of neocortical regions (Penfield & Baldwin, 1952; Penfield & Flanigin, 1950; Penfield & Steelman, 1947), whereas one should also mention the method of hemispherectomy introduced by Roland Krynauw in 1950 (Krynauw, 1950). Bailey and Gibbs in 1951 will employ the EEG as a guide to perform temporal lobe surgery (Bailey & Gibbs, 1951), whereas in 1953, Murray Falconer in London introduced the en bloc anterior temporal lobe resection and the term mesial temporal sclerosis (Falconer et al., 1953). In 1954, Penfield will publish with Herbert Jasper, an eminent neurophysiologist, one of the great classics in neurology, *Epilepsy and the Functional Anatomy of the Human Brain* (Penfield & Jasper, 1954). An important and influential figure in the field of Epileptology who become active during this period was Henri Gastaut. He was the founder of International EEG Federation and, in 1953, became head of the Marseille Hospital Neurobiological laboratories. His contribution in the study of epileptology was monumental; he defined five major human EEG paterns (lambda waves, pi rhythm, mu rhythm, rolandic spikes and posterior theta rhythm) (Naquet, 1996a, 1996b). During this decade, new drugs will come up such as carbamazepine in 1953 (Schindler & Häfliger, 1954), ethosuximide in 1958 (Vossen, 1958), sodium valproate in 1963 (Meunier et al., 1963).

In 1961, the International Bureau for Epilepsy (IBE) was established. In 1966, Surgeon General William Stewart will create the Surgeon General's Public Health Service Advisory Committee on the Epilepsies, whereas, in 1969, the Society for Neuroscience was established. Important advances will be made in the field of neuroscience and in the physiology of synapses by Eccles, Kandel, Spencer, Speckman, Purpura, Meldrum and others. During this period important EEG studies will be conducted in animals mainly by Prince and his research team demonstrating the spikes and waves associated with synchronous paroxysmal depolarizing bursts occuring in cortical neurons (Matsumoto & Marsan, 1964a, 1964b; Prince, 1968a; Prince & Futamachi, 1968), and the spike-wave complex (Prince, 1968b). In 1968, Murray Alexander Falconer (1910-1977) will recognize the importance of hippocambal sclerosis in temporal lobe epilepsy (Falconer, 1968). James Kiffin

Penry (1929-1996), in 1969, will publish his treatise *Basic Mechanisms of the Epilpsies* and afterwards *Antiepileptic Drugs, Neurosurgical Management of the Epilepsis, Complex Partial Seizures and their Treatment* and *Antiepileptic Drugs Mechanisms of Action.* Although carbamazepine and valproate were available in Europe during the 60s, no other drug was licensed in the US.

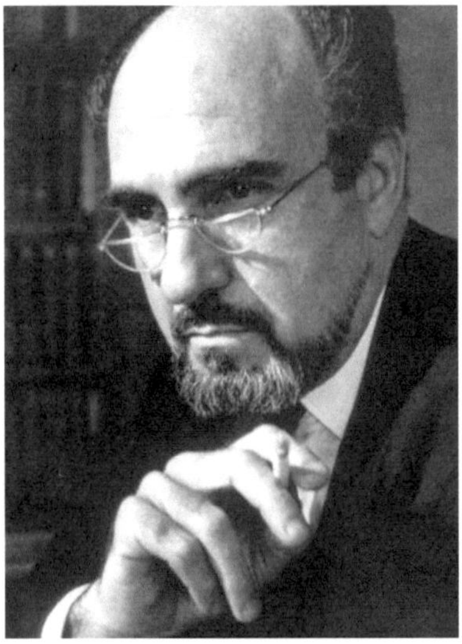

Fig. 5. Henri Gastaut (1915 -1995)

In 1970, Penry and Cereghino were employed in designing clinical trials for anti-epileptic drugs (AEDs). Carbamazepine was the first drug to be licensed by the FDA based on the results of clinical trials. Charles Pippenger (1939-) developed methods for measuring blood levels of AEDs (Painter et al., 1978), whereas Fritz Dreifuss (1926-1997) worked on video-monitoring of absence seizures and helped in the classification of various epileptic conditions (Penry et al., 1975). An important development in the field of neuroscience was that of Erwin Neher (1944-), who invented the patch clamp method to measure the flow of current through single-ion channels (Neher et al., 1978). Prince *et al* will make the first studies of cellular phenomena of epileptic events in the human cortex (Schwartzkroin & Prince, 1978; Wong & Prince, 1978, 1981). Meldrum will prove that the assumption connecting brain damage from seizures as a result of hypoxia, is wrong (Meldrum & Horton, 1973a, 1973b; Meldrum et al., 1973); he demonstrated that the excessive excitatory activity is responsible for the brain cellular loss.

The advent of the new decade, the 1908s, was marked by huge advances in the fields of neuro-imaging techniques, such as the CT, MRI, PET-scanning, and video-EEG monitoring. Epileptics are being evaluated psychologically and socially and before 1990, Quality of Life tools were developed. During the 1990s, the decade of the brain, the Global Campaign Against Epilepsy, launched in 1997 by the WHO, ILAE and IBE brought epilepsy out of the Shadows improving diagnosis, treatment, prevention and social acceptability. Various changes regarding the epileptic brain damage will also be studied, such as the mossy fiber sprouting and synaptic reorganization (Houser et al., 1990; Sutula et al., 1989; Sutula et al., 1988) (Tauck & Nadler, 1985). In 1993, Gabapentin (Neurontin) marketed in the US as the first AED which is not metabolized in the liver.

The most important evolution, however, in the field of epileptology during the last twenty years was the connection between genetic factors and epilepsy; in 1989 Leppert was the first to identify the link between chromosome 20 and idiopathic human epilepsy syndrome in a family with benign familial neonatal convulsions (Leppert et al., 1989). The growing evidence on the connection between various genes and epilepsies is the cutting edge of modern epilepsy research, and in the next decades new exciting discoveries are going to change epileptology (Baulac & Baulac, 2010).

7. Conclusions

The fascinating history of epilepsy is connected with the history of humanity; early reports on epilepsy go back to the ancient assyrian and babylonian texts, scanning a period of almost 4,000 years. The first hallmark in the history of epilepsy are the Hippocratic texts which set in doubt the divine origin of the disease. Major advances in the understanding of epilepsy will come much later, during the 18th and 19th century; theories on epilepsy during this period are formulated on a solid scientific basis and epileptics are for the first time treated as patients and not as lunatics or possessed. During this period, experimental studies were conducted as well as advances made in the pathology of the disease and the connection of epilepsy with various psychiatric symptoms. The work of John Hughlings Jackson was preceded by a plethora of studies by Dutch, German, English and French physicians who evolved scientific thought and performed thorough studies on epilepsy. The advent of the 20th century led to the in-depth understanding of the mechanisms of the disease, the development of effective drugs and neuro-imaging methods. Last but not least, one should mention the important advances in the molecular biology of the disease and the connection of various genes with various forms of epilepsy.

8. References

Abbas, Ali Ibn. (1523). Theorica, In: *Liber totius medicine necessaria continens quem sapientissimus haly filius abbas .... Edidit, regique inscripsit, unde et regalis, dispositionis nomen assumpsit*, IX, 6, fol 103, Lyon.

Abulcasim (1519). *Liber theoricae nec non practicae alsaharavii, qui vulgo acararius dicitur*, fol. 34, Augsburg.

Adrian, E.D., & Mathews, B.H.C. (1934). The berger rhythm: Potential changes from the occipital lobes in man. *Brain*, Vol. *57*, No. 4, (December 1934), pp 355-385, ISSN 1460-2156

Africanus, C. (1536-1539). De communibus medico etc. Ix, 7 vol. 2, In: *Opera omnia*, p. 247, Basel.

Albertoni, P. (1882). Untersuchungen über die wirkung einiger arzneimittel auf die erregbarkeit des grosshirns nebst beitragen zur therapie der epilepsie, . *Arc Exp Path Pharm*, Vol. *15*, No. 3-4, pp 248-288,

Aretaeus (1856a). Cure of the paroxysm of the epileptics, chapter v, on acute diseases book i, In: F. Adams (Ed.), *The extant work of aretaeus*, p. 399-400, The Sydenham Society, London.

Aretaeus (1856b). On epilepsy, chapter iv, on chronic diseases, book i., In: F. Adams (Ed.), *The extant works of aretaeus, the cappadocian.*, p. 297, The Sydenham society, London.

Aretaeus (1856c). On epilepsy, chapter v, on the causes and symptoms of acute diseases, book i. , In: F. Adams (Ed.), *The extant work of aretaeus the cappadocian*, pp. 244-246, The Sydenham society, London.

Avicenna (1999). *The canon of medicine*, Kazi Publications, Chicago, ISBN: 1871031672.

Bailey, P., & Gibbs, F.A. (1951). The surgical treatment of psychomotor epilepsy. *JAMA*, Vol. *145*, No. 6, (February 1951), pp 365-370, ISSN 0002-9955

Baulac, S., & Baulac, M. (2010). Advances on the genetics of mendelian idiopathic epilepsies. *Clin Lab Med*, Vol. *30*, No. 4, (December 2010), pp 911-929, ISSN 1557-9832

Berger, H. (1929). Über das elektroenkephalogramm des menschen. *Archiv für Psychiatrie und Nervenkrankheiten*, Vol. *87*, pp 527-570.

Berger, H. (1932). Uber das elektroenzephalogram des menschen. *Arch Psychiatr Nervenkr*, Vol. *97*, pp 6-26.

Berger, H. (1933). Uber das elektroenzephalogram des menschen. *Arch Psychiatr Nervenkr*, Vol. *100*, No. pp 301-320,

Beyerstein, B. L. (1988). Neuropathology and the legacy of spiritual possession. *Skeptical Inquirer*, Vol. *12.3*, pp 248-262.

Billings, J. S. (1861). The surgical treatment of epilepsy. *Cincinnati Lancet and Observer*, Vol. *4*, pp 334-341.

Boerhaave, H. (1761). *Praelectiones academicae de morbis nervorum, t. Ii*, Lugduni Batavorum : Petrum vander Eyk et Cornelium de Pecker, Leiden.

Brain, Sir R. (1959). William harvey, neurologist. *Brit Med J*, Vol. *2*, No. 5157, (November 1959), pp 899, ISSN 0959-8138.

Bravais, L. F. (1827). *Recherches sur les symptômes et le traitement de l'épilepsie hémiplégique. [these de paris no. 118]*, Paris.

Bright, R. (1831a). *Reports of medical cases, vol. Ii, part ii*, p. 644, Richard Taylor for Longman, Rees, Orme, Brown, and Green, London.

Bright, R. (1831b). *Reports of medical cases, vol. Ii, part ii*, p. 514, Richard Taylor for Longman, Rees, Orme, Brown, and Green, London.

Broca, P. (1867). Trépanation du crâne pratiquée avec succès dans un cas de fracture avec enfoncement et enclavement. *Bull Soc Chir Paris*, Vol. *7*, No. pp 508-512,

Brown-Séquard, E. (1853). *Experimental researches applied to physiology and pathology*, pp. 80-84, H. Bailliere, New York.

Brown-Séquard, E. (1857). Experimental and clinical researches applied to physiology and pathology. *Boston Medical and Surgical Journal*, Vol. *56*, pp 216-220.

Budrys, V. (2007). Neurology in holy scripture. *Eur J Neurol*, Vol. *14*, No. 7, (July 2007), pp e1-6, ISSN 1468-1331.

Burdach, K. F. (1826). *Vom baue und leben des gehirns, vol. 3*, p. 297, Erster Band, Leipzig.

Caesalpinus, A. (1593). Daemonum investigation peripatetica, In: *Quastionum peripateticarum lib. V.. Daemonum investigatio peripatetica, quaestionum medicarum libri ii, de medicament. Facultatibus lib. Ii*, c. 1, fol. 145 C.

Celsus, A. C. (1935). Liber iii, In: F. Marx, Spencer, W. G. (transl) (Ed.), *On medicine, vol i*, p. 338, par. 323 Harvard University Press/Loeb Classical Library, Cambridge, MA/London.

Cooper, Sir Astley. (1836). Some experiments and observations on tying the carotid and vertebral arteries, and the pneumnogastric, phrenic and sympathetic nerves. *Guy's Hospital Reports*, Vol. *1*, pp 457-475.

Cullen, W. (1778-1784). Of neuroses, or nervous diseases part ii, In: *First lines of the practice of physic*, William Creech, Edinburgh.
Cybulski, N, & Jelenska-Macieszyna, X. (1914). Action currents of the cerebral cortex *Bull Acad Sci Cracov*, Vol. *B*, pp 776-781.
d'Orsi, G., & Tinuper, P. (2006). "I heard voices...": From semiology, a historical review, and a new hypothesis on the presumed epilepsy of joan of arc. *Epilepsy Behav*, Vol. *9*, No. 1, (August 2006), pp 152-157, ISSN 1525-5050.
Dandy, W. E. (1918). Ventriculography following the injection of air into the cerebral ventricles. *Ann Surg*, Vol. *68*, No. 1, (January 1918), pp 5-11, ISSN 0003-4932.
Dandy, W. E. (1919a). Rontgenography of the brain after the injection of air into the spinal canal. *Ann Surg*, Vol. *70*, No. 4, (October 1919), pp 397-403, ISSN 0003-4932.
Dandy, W. E. (1919b). Ventriculography following the injection of air into the cerebral ventricles. *Amer J Roentgenol*, Vol. *6*, No. pp 26-36, ISSN 1546-3141.
Delasiauve, L. J. F. (1854). *Traité de l'épilepsie*, Victor Masson, Paris.
Diels, H. (1906). Alcmeon, no 13 aët. V 17, 3 (d. 427), In: *Die fragmente der vorsokratiker*, Weidmannsche Buchhandlung, Berlin.
Dolger, F. J. (1933). Der ausschluss der besessenen (epileptiker) von oblation und kommunion nach der synode von elvira. *Antike und Christentum* Vol. *4*, pp 110-129, ISSN 0066-4790.
Doussin-Dubreuil, J. L. (1825). *De l' epilepsie en général, et particulièrement de celle qui'est déterminée par des causes morale*, p. 144, Roret, Paris.
Drabkin, I. E. (1950). *Caelius aurelianus. On acute diseases and on chronic diseases*, par. 131-133, The University of Chicago Press, Chicago.
Drelincurtius, C. (1682). *Experimenta anatomica*, canicid. 3, p. 8, Ernestum Gottfried Heyseum, Leiden.
Eadie, M. J., & Bladin, B. F. (2001). *A disease once called sacred. A history of the medical understanding of epilepsy.*, pp 17-20, John Libbey, ISBN 0-86196-607-4, Eastleigh.
Economou, N. T., & Lascaratos, J. (2005). The byzantine physicians on epilepsy. *J Hist Neurosciences*, Vol. *14*, No. (December 2005), pp 346-352, ISSN 1744-5213.
Erastus, Thomas. (1581). *Comitis montani vincentini novi medicorum censoris quinque librorum de morbis nuper editorum viva anatome*, p. 195, Petri Pernae, Basel.
Esquirol, J-E. D. (1838). *Des maladies mentales: Considérées sous les rapports médical, hygiénique et médico-légal. [vol. 1]*, p. 284, J-B Baillière, Paris.
Falconer, M. A. (1968). The significance of mesial temporal sclerosis (ammon's horn sclerosis) in epilepsy. *Guys Hosp Rep*, Vol. *117*, No. 1, (January 1968), pp 1-12, ISSN 0017-5889.
Falconer, M. A., Pond, D. A., Meyer, A., & Woolf, A. L. (1953). Temporal lobe epilepsy with personality and behaviour disorders caused by an unusual calcifying lesion; report of two cases in children relieved by temporal lobectomy. *J Neurol Neurosurg Psychiatry*, Vol. *16*, No. 4, (November 1953), pp 234-244, ISSN 0022-3050.
Falret, J. (1860). De l'état mental des épileptiques. *Archives Générales de Médecine* Vol. *Ve* serie 16, pp 661-679.
Fernelius, Joannes. (1577). De abditis rerum causis, In: *Universa medicina*, II, c. 15, p. 87, a. M., Frankfurt.
Flourens, P. (1823). *Recherches expérimentales sur les propriétés et les fonctions du système nerveux, dans les animaux vertébrés*, Chez Crevot, Paris.

Foderé, F. (1798). *Les lois éclairées par les sciences physiques ou traité de médecine légale et d'hygiène publique,* p. 93, chez Croullebois et chez Deterville, Paris.

Fritsch, G., & Hitzig, E. (1870). Ueber die elektrische erregbarkeit des grosshirns. *Arch Anat Physiol wiss Med,* Vol. *37,* pp 300-332.

Gaddesden, J. (1595). Rosa anglica, In: *Ioannis anglici praxis medica, rosa anglica dicta, recens edita opera ac studio clar. V. Doct. Philippi schopffi, medici physici durlacensis, 2 vol.S,* p. 40, Typis Michaëlis Mangeri, Augsburg.

Galen. (1821a). De locis affectis, vol. 8, In: C. G Kuhn (Ed.), *Opera omnia,* p. 194, Cnobloch, Leipzig.

Galen. (1821b). De simplicium medicamentorum temperamentis ac facultatibus vol. 12, In: C. G Kuhn (Ed.), *Opera omnia,* III, 9; p. 336, Cnobloch, Leipzig.

Galen. (1821c). Definitiones medicae, vol. 19, In: C. G Kuhn (Ed.), *Opera omnia,* p. 414, Cnobloch, Leipzig.

Garrison, F. H. (1935). Felice fontana, a forgotten physiologist of the trentino. *Bull N Y Acad Med,* Vol. *11,* No. 3, (March 1935), pp 117-122, ISSN 1099-3460.

Gibbs, F. A., Davis, H., & Lennox, W.G. (1935). The electroencephalogram in epilepsy and in conditions of impaired consciousness. *Arch Neurol Psychiatry,* Vol. *34,* No. 6, (December 1935), pp 1133-1148, ISSN 0096-6886.

Gibbs, F.A., Gibbs, E.L., & Lennox, W.G.. (1937). Epilepsy: A paroxysmal cerebral dysrythmia. *Brain,* Vol. *60,* No. 4, (December 1937), pp 377-388, ISSN 1460-2156.

Gibbs, F.A., Lennox, W.G., & Gibbs, E.L. (1936). The electroencephalogram in diagnosis and in localization of epileptic seizures. *Arch Neurol Psychiatry,* Vol. *36,* No. 6, (December 1936), pp 1225-1235, ISSN 0096-6886.

Gordon, B. (1542). Lilium medicinae, In: *Omnium aegritudinum a vertice ad calcem, opus praeclariss. Quod lilium medicinae appellatur,* fol. 119, Joannem Foucherium, Paris.

Gottfried, H., Eschenbach, A.C., Etsienne, H., Gesner, J. M., & Tyrwhitt, T. (1805). Lithica, v. 474-484, In: *Orphica,* pp. 412-413, Fritsch, Lipsiae.

Gowers, W. R. (1880). Goulstonian lectures on epilepsy. *Lancet,* Vol. *1,* No. pp 315-318, 353-355, 391-393, 433-436, 473-475, 513-517, 552-554, ISSN 0140-6736.

Gowers, W. R. (1881). *Epilepsy and other chronic convulsive disorders: Their causes, symptoms and treatment,* Churchill, London.

Gowers, W. R. (1903). *The border-land of epilepsy. Faints, vagal attacks, vertigo, migraine, sleep symptoms, and their treatment* P. Blakiston's son & Co, Philadelphia.

Griesinger, W. (1868-1869). Über einige epileptoide zustände. *Archiv fur Psychiatrie und Nervekrankheiten,* Vol. *1,* pp 320-333.

Hall, M. (1841). *On the diseases and derangement of the nervous system,* p. 279, H. Baillière, London.

Hall, M. (1851). *Synopsis of cerbral and spinal seizures of inorganic origin and of paroxysmal form as a class; and of their pathology as involved in the structures and actions of the neck,* J. Mallet, London.

Hall, M. (1852). *Synopsis of apoplexy and epilepsy; with observations on the trachelismus, laryngismus and tracheotomy; and the proposal for a hospital for epileptics.,* J. Mallett, London.

Hauptmann, A. (1912). Luminal bei epilepsie. *Munchen Med Wochenschr,* Vol. *59,* pp 1907-1909.

Henle, J. (1846). *Hanbuch der rationellen pathologie, 2. Band 2. Abtheilung,* Vieweg, Braunschweig.

Herodotus. (2000). Thaleia, book three, In: G. Rawilnson (Ed.), *The histories of Herodotus of Hallicarnasus,* pp. 36-37, Omphaloskepsis, Ames, Iowa.

Herpin, T. (1867). *Des accès incomplets d'épilepsie,* p. 111, J-B. Baillère, Paris.

Hildegard, St. (1903). Causae et cureae, 13-16, In: P. Kaiser (Ed.), *Hildegardis causae et cureae,* p. 156, Teubner, Leipzig.

Hippocrate. (1849a). De la maladie sacree, livre 6, In: E. Littre (Ed.), *Oeuvres completes d' hippocrate,* p. 366, J-B. Baillère, Paris.

Hippocrate. (1849b). De la maladie sacree, livre 6, In: E. Littre (Ed.), *Oeuvres completes d' hippocrate,* p. 364, J-B. Baillère, Paris.

Hippocrate. (1849c). De la maladie sacree, livre 6, In: E. Littre (Ed.), *Oeuvres completes d' hippocrate,* pp. 360-362, J-B. Baillère, Paris.

Hippocrate. (1849d). De la maladie sacree, livre 6, In: E. Littre (Ed.), *Oeuvres completes d' hippocrate,* p. 382, J-B. Baillère, Paris.

Hippocrate. (1849e). De la maladie sacree, livre 6, In: E. Littre (Ed.), *Oeuvres completes d' hippocrate,* p. 354, J-B. Baillère, Paris.

Hippocrate. (1849f). De la maladie sacrée, livre 6, In: E. Littré (Ed.), *Oeuvres complètes d' hippocrate,* p. 382, J-B. Baillère, Paris.

Hippocrate. (1849g). De la maladie sacrée, livre 6, In: E Littré (Ed.), *Oeuvres complètes d' hippocrate,* pp. 380-382, J-B. Baillère, Paris.

Hippocrate. (1849h). De la maladie sacrée, livre 6, In: E. Littré (Ed.), *Oeuvres complètes d' hippocrate,* p. 368, J-B. Baillère, Paris.

Hippocrate. (1849i). Des plaies de tête, livre 3, In: E. Littre (Ed.), *Oeuvres complètes d' hippocrate,* p. 254, J-B. Baillère, Paris.

Horing, C. F. F. (1859). *Uber epilepsie, eine inaugural-disseration unter dem praesidium von dr. W. Griesinger [diss. Tubingen].*

Houser, C. R., Miyashiro, J. E., Swartz, B. E., Walsh, G. O., Rich, J. R., & Delgado-Escueta, A. V. (1990). Altered patterns of dynorphin immunoreactivity suggest mossy fiber reorganization in human hippocampal epilepsy. *J Neurosci,* Vol. *10,* No. 1, (January 1990), pp 267-282, ISSN 0270-6474.

Hunter, R., & MacAlpine, I. (1957). William harvey: His neurological and psychiatric observation. *J Hist Med Allied Sci,* Vol. *12,* No. 4, p. 126, ISSN 0022-5045

Hunter, R. (1959-1960). Status epilepticus: History, incidence and problems. *Epilepsia 4th series,* Vol. *1,* pp 162-188, ISSN 0013-9580.

Jackson, J.H. (1861). Cases of epilepsy associated with syphilis. *Medical Times and Gazette,* Vol. *1,* pp 648-652; 642: 659-660.

Jackson, J. H. (1863). Convulsive spasms of the right hand and arm preceding epileptic seizures. *Medical Times and Gazette,* Vol. *1,* pp 110-111.

Jackson, J. H. (1864). Epileptic aphemia with epileptic seizures on the right side. *Medical Times and Gazette,* Vol. *2,* p. 167.

Jackson, J. H. (1866). Clinical remarks on the occasional occurence of subjective sensations of smell in patients who are liable to epileptiform seizures, or who have symptoms of mental derangement, and in others. *Lancet,* Vol. *1,* pp 659-660.

Jackson, J. H. (1931-1932a). *Selected writings, vol. 1,* p. 23, Hodder and Stoughton, London.

Jackson, J. H. (1931-1932b). *Selected writings, vol. 1,* p. 35, Hodder and Stoughton, London.

Jasper, H., & Kershmann, J. (1941). Electroencepahlografic classification of the epilepsies. *Arch Neurol Psychiatry,* Vol. *45,* No. 6, (June 1941), pp 903-943.

Kaufman, P.Y. (1912). Electric phenomena in cerebral cortex. *Obz Psichiatr Nev Eksp Psikhol,* Vol. *7-9,* pp 403.

Kerler, D. H. (1905). *Die patronate der heiligen,* Kerler, Ulm.

Kluger, G., & Kudernatsch, V. (2009). St. Valentine--patron saint of epilepsy: Illustrating the semiology of seizures over the course of six centuries. *Epilepsy Behav,* Vol. *14,* No. 1, (Janurary 2009), pp 219-225, ISSN 1525-5069.

Kluver, H., & Bucy, P. C. (1997). Preliminary analysis of functions of the temporal lobes in monkeys. 1939. *J Neuropsychiatry Clin Neurosci,* Vol. *9,* No. 4, (September 1997), pp 606-620, ISSN 0895-0172.

Krynauw, R.W. (1950). Infantile hemiplegia treated by removal of one cerebral hemisphere. *J Neurol Neurosurg Psychiatry,* Vol. *13,* No. 4, (November 1950), pp 243-267, ISSN 1468-330X.

Kussmaul, A., & Tenner, A. (1859). *On the nature and origin of epileptiform convulsions caused by profuse bleeding, and also those of true epilepsy.,* pp. 57, 89-90 The New Sydenham Society, London.

Labat, R. (1951). *Traité akkadien de diagnostics et pronostics médicaux,* pp. 80-81, 188-199, Académie internationale d'histoire des sciences, Brill, Paris-Leiden.

Laertius, D. (1853). Life of heraclitus, vi, In: C. D. Yonge (transl) (Ed.), *Lives of philosophers,* Henry G. Bohn, London.

Le Pois, C. (1733). De epilepsia, consilium [chapter 7]. , In: Herman Boerhaave (Ed.), *Caroli pisonis....Selectiorum observationum et consiliorum... Liber singularis,* p. 115, Leiden.

Lemnius, L. (1658). The secret miracles of nature, ii, 3, In: *The secret miracles of nature,* p. 93, London.

Lennox, W.G., & Cobb, S. (1928). *Epilepsy from the standpoint of physiology and treatment. Medicine monograph xiv,* Williams and Wilkins, Baltimore.

Leppert, M., Anderson, V.E., Quattlebaum, T., Stauffer, D., O' Connel, P., Nakamura, Y., White, R. (1989). Benign familial neonatal convulsions linked to genetic markers on chromosome 20. *Nature,* Vol. *337,* No. 6208, (February 1989), pp 647-648, ISSN 0028-0836

Letchworth, W.P. (1901). *Transactions of the national association for the study for the of epilepsy at the annual meeting held in washington d.C., may 14th and 15th, 1901,* CE Brinkworth Buffalo, New York.

Longrigg, J. (2000). Epilepsy in ancient greek medicine--the vital step. *Seizure,* Vol. *9,* No. 1, (January 2000), pp 12-21, ISSN 1059-1311

Lundborg, H. (1903). *Die progressive myoklonus-epilepsy (unverricht's myoklonie),* Almquvist und Wiskell, Uppsala.

Maisonneuve, J. G. F. (1803). *Recherches et observations sur l'épilepsie, presentées a l'école de médecine de paris,* p. 8, Paris.

Maisonneuve, J. G. F. (1804). *Recherches et observations sur l'épilepsie, presentées a l'école de médecine de paris,* p. 187, Paris.

Marchand, J. F., & Hoff, H. E. (1955). Felice fontana: The laws of irritability. *J Hist Med Allied Sci,* Vol. *10,* No. 2, (April 1955), pp 197-206, ISSN 1468-4373

Marci a Kronland, M. (1678). *Liturgia mentis seu disceptatio medica, philosophica et optica de natura epilepsiae illius ortu et causis,* Jacobo Joanne Wenceslao Dobrzensky, Regensburg.

Martin, A. (1922). Warum galten epilepsie und geisteskrankheit (frenesis) als ansteckend? *Deutsche Zeitschrift fur Nervenheilkunde,* Vol. *75,* No. pp 103-110,

Matsumoto, H., & Marsan, C. A. (1964a). Cortical cellular phenomena in experimental epilepsy: Ictal manifestations. *Exp Neurol,* Vol. *9,* (April 1946), pp 305-326, ISSN 0014-4886.

Matsumoto, H., & Marsan, C. A. (1964b). Cortical cellular phenomena in experimental epilepsy: Interictal manifestations. *Exp Neurol,* Vol. *9,* No. 4, (April 1964), pp 286-304, ISSN 0014-4886.

Meldrum, B. S., & Horton, R. W. (1973a). Cerebral functional effects of 2-deoxy-d-glucose and 3-o-methylglucose in rhesus monkeys. *Electroencephalogr Clin Neurophysiol,* Vol. *35,* No. 1, (July 1973), pp 59-66, ISSN 0013-4694.

Meldrum, B. S., & Horton, R. W. (1973b). Physiology of status epilepticus in primates. *Arch Neurol,* Vol. *28,* No. 1, (January 1973), pp 1-9, ISSN 0003-9942.

Meldrum, B. S., Vigouroux, R. A., & Brierley, J. B. (1973). Systemic factors and epileptic brain damage. Prolonged seizures in paralyzed, artificially ventilated baboons. *Arch Neurol,* Vol. *29,* No. 2, (August 1973), pp 82-87, ISSN 0003-9942.

Merrit, H.H., & Putnam, T.J. (1938a). A new series of anticonvulsant drugs tested by experiments in animals. *Arch Neurol Psychiatry,* Vol. *39,* No. 5, (May 1938), pp 1003-1015, ISSN 0096-688.

Merrit, H.H., & Putnam, T.J. (1938b). Sodium diphenyl hydantoinate in the treatment of convulsive disorders. *JAMA,* Vol. *111,* No. 12, (September 1938), pp 1068-1073, ISSN 0098-7484.

Merrit, H.H., & Putnam, T.J. (1939). Sodium diphenyl hydantoinate in the treatment of convulsive seizures. Toxic symptoms and their prevention. *Arch Neurol Psychiatry,* Vol. *42,* No. 6, (December 1939), pp 1053-1058, ISSN 0096-688.

Merrit, H.H., & Putnam, T.J. (1940). Further experiences with the use of sodium diphenyl hydantoinate in the treatment of convulsive disorders. *Am J Psychiatry,* Vol. *96,* No. 5, (March 1940), pp 1023-1027, ISSN 0002-953X.

Meunier, H., Carraz, G., Meunier, Y., Eymard, P., & Aimard, M. (1963). Propriétés pharmacodynamiques de l'acide n-dipropylacetique. *Therapie,* Vol. *18,* No. pp 435-438, ISSN 0040-5957.

Morel, B.A. (1852-1853). *Etudes cliniques.Traité théorique et pratique des maladies mentales considérées dans leur nature, leur traitement et dans leur rapport avec la médecine légale des aliénés, vol. 2,* p. 321, J-B Baillière, Nancy-Paris.

Myerson, A., Ayer, J.B., Putnam, T.J., Keeler, C.E., & Alexander, L. (1936). *Eugenical sterilization- a reorientation of the problem. By the committee of the american neurological association for the investigation of eugenical sterilization,* Macmillan, New York.

Naquet, R. (1996a). Henri gastaut (1915-1995). *Electroencephalogr Clin Neurophysiol,* Vol. *98,* No. 4, (April 1996), pp 231-235, ISSN 0013-4694.

Naquet, R. (1996b). Tribute to henri gastaut (1915-1995). *Neurophysiol Clin,* Vol. *26,* No. 3, (January 1996), pp 170-176, ISSN 0987-7053.

Neher, E., Sakman, B., & Steinbach, J.H. (1978). The extracellular patch clamp: A method for resolving currents through individual open channels in biological membranes. *Pflügers Archiv* Vol. *375*, No. 2, (February 1978), pp 219-228, ISSN 0031-676.

Painter, M.J., Pippenger, C. E., MacDonald, H., & Pitlick, W. (1978). Phenobarbital and diphenylhydantoin levels in neonates with seizures. *J Pediatr*, Vol. *92*, No. 2, (February 1978), pp 315-319, ISSN 0022-3476.

Paracelsus. (1922-1933a). Von den hinfallenden siechtagen, vol. 8, In: *Samtliche werke, 1. Abteilung, medizinische naturwissenschaftlische und philosophische schriften, herausgegebn von k. Sudfhoff 14 vols.*, p. 280, Oldenbourg, Munich-Berlin.

Paracelsus. (1922-1933b). Von den hinfallenden siechtagen, vol. 8. , In: *Samtliche werke, 1. Abteilung, medizinische naturwissenschaftlische und philosophische schriften, herausgegebn von k. Sudfhoff 14 vols*, p. 281-284, Oldenbourg, Munich-Berlin.

Pearce, J. M. S. (2004). Positive and negative cerbral symptoms: The roles of russel reynolds and hughlings jackson. *J Neurol Neurosurg Psychiatry*, Vol. *75*, No. 8, (August 2004), pp 1148, ISSN 0022-3050.

Penfield, W., & Baldwin, M. (1952). Temporal lobe seizures and the technic of subtotal temporal lobectomy. *Ann Surg*, Vol. *136*, No. 4, (April 1952), pp 625-634, ISSN 1528-1140.

Penfield, W., & Flanigin, H. (1950). Surgical therapy of temporal lobe seizures. *AMA Arch Neurol Psychiatry*, Vol. *64*, No. 4, (October 1950), pp 491-500, ISSN 0096-6886.

Penfield, W., & Jasper, H. (1954). *Epilepsy and the functional anatomy of the human brain*, W. Little, Brown and Co, Boston.

Penfield, W., & Steelman, H. (1947). The treatment of focal epilepsy with cortical excision. *Ann Surg*, Vol. *126*, No. 5, (November 1947), pp 740-762, ISSN 0003-4932.

Penry, J.K., Porter, R.J., & Dreifuss, R.E. (1975). Simultaneous recording of absence seizures with video tape and electroencephalography. A study of 374 seizures in 48 patients. *Brain*, Vol. *98*, No. 3, (June 1975), pp 427-440, ISSN 0006-8950.

Pirkner, E. H. (1929). Epilepsy in the light of history. *Ann Med Hist*, Vol. *1*, No. pp 453-480, ISSN 0743-3131.

Plato (1871). Book xi In: B. Jowett (Ed.), *Laws*, Charles Scribner and Company, New York.

Pliny (1856). Book xxvii, chapter 2, remedies derived from man, In: J. Bostock & H.T. Rilly (Eds.), *The natural history of pliny, vol. V*, p. 277, Henry G. Bohn, York Street, Covent Garden, London.

Plutarch (1888). How one may be aware of one's progres in virtue, In: AR Shilleto (trans) (Ed.), *Plutarch's morals*, George Bell and Sons, York Street, Covent Garden, London.

Plutarch (1914). The life of lycurgus, par. 16, In: *The parallel lives*, Loeb Classical Library edition,

Portal, Le Baron. (1827a). *Observations sur la nature et le traitement de l'épilepsie*, pp. 11, 55, J-B Baillière, Paris.

Portal, Le Baron. (1827b). *Observations sur la nature et le traitement de l'épilepsie*, pp. 47-48, J-B Baillière, Paris.

Prichard, J. C. (1822a). *A treatise on diseases of the nervous system, part the first*, p. 99, Thomas and George Underwood, London.

Prichard, J. C. (1822b). *A treatise on diseases of the nervous system, part the first*, p. 100, Thomas and George Underwood, London.

Prince, D. A. (1968a). The depolarization shift in "epileptic" neurons. *Exp Neurol,* Vol. *21,* No. 4, (August 1968), pp 467-485, ISSN 0014-4886.

Prince, D. A. (1968b). Inhibition in "epileptic" neurons. *Exp Neurol,* Vol. *21,* No. 3, (July 1968), pp 307-321, ISSN 0014-4886.

Prince, D. A., & Futamachi, K. J. (1968). Intracellular recordings in chronic focal epilepsy. *Brain Res,* Vol. *11,* No. 3, (December 1968), pp 681-684, ISSN 0006-8993.

Reynolds, J. R. (1861a). *Epilepsy: Its symptoms, treatment, and relation to other chronic convulsive diseases,* John Churchill, New Burlington Street, London.

Reynolds, J. R. (1861b). *Epilepsy: Its symptoms, treatment, and relation to other chronic convulsive diseases.,* p. 27, John Churchill, New Burlington Street, London.

Richards, R.K., & Everett, G.M. (1946). Tridione: A new anticonvulsant drug. *J Lab Clin Med,* Vol. *31,* No. 6, pp 1330-1336, ISSN 0022-3018.

Roberts, E., & Frankel, S. (1950). Gamma-aminobutyric acid in the brain: Its formation from glutamic acid. *J Biol Chem,* Vol. *187,* No. 1, pp 55-63, ISSN 0021-9258.

Rulandus, M. (1580). Curatinum etc centuria sexta, curatio 100, In: *Curationum empiricarum et historicarum in certis locis et notis personis optime expertarum, et rite probatarum, centuria prima (secunda) emendatius impressa.,* pp. 132-133, Henricpetrina, Basel.

Savonarola, J. M. (1547). Practica maior, In: *Practica maior,* tract. 6, c. 1, rubrica 20; fol. 71, apud Vincentium Valgrifium, Venice.

Schindler, W., & Häfliger, F. (1954). Über derivate des iminodibenzyls. *Helvetica Chimica Acta,* Vol. *37,* No. 2, pp 472-483, ISSN 0018-019X.

Schwartzkroin, P. A., & Prince, D. A. (1978). Cellular and field potential properties of epileptogenic hippocampal slices. *Brain Res,* Vol. *147,* No. 1, (May 1978), pp 117-130, ISSN 0006-8993.

Serapion, J. (1530). Platearii practica brevis, In: *Necessarium ac perutile opus totius medicine practice profundissimi ac antiquissimi arabis domini joannis filii serapionis... Practica etiam brevis domini joannis plateari j salernitani ultisiima* fol. 172, Impressum mandato & expensis heredum Octaviani Scoti ac sociorum, Venice.

Sieveking, E. H. (1857). Analysis of fifty-two cases of epilepsy. *Med Chir Trans,* Vol. *40,* pp 527-528.

Smith, S. (1852). The surgical treatment of epilepsy, with statistical tables, comprising all the recorded cases of ligature of the carotid artery: And also of trephining the cranium by american surgeons. *New York Journal of Medicine,* Vol. *8,* pp 220-242.

Stol, M. (1993). *Epilepsy in babylonia,* Brill Publishers, Amsterdam.

Sutula, T., Cascino, G., Cavazos, J., Parada, I., & Ramirez, L. (1989). Mossy fiber synaptic reorganization in the epileptic human temporal lobe. *Ann Neurol,* Vol. *26,* No. 3, (September 1989), pp 321-330, ISSN 0364-5134.

Sutula, T., He, X. X., Cavazos, J., & Scott, G. (1988). Synaptic reorganization in the hippocampus induced by abnormal functional activity. *Science,* Vol. *239,* No. 4844, (March 1988), pp 1147-1150, ISSN 0036-8075 .

Tauck, D. L., & Nadler, J. V. (1985). Evidence of functional mossy fiber sprouting in hippocampal formation of kainic acid-treated rats. *J Neurosci,* Vol. *5,* No. 4, (April 1985), pp 1016-1022, ISSN 0270-6474.

Taxil, Jean. (1602). *Traicte de l' epilepsie, maladie vulgairement appellee au pays de provence, la gouttete aux petits enfans* c. 17, R. Reunaud, Tournon.

Temkin, O. (1942). A medieval translation of rhaze's clinical observations. *Bull Hist Med,* Vol. *12,* No. pp 102-117,

Temkin, O. (1971a). Ancient origins, In: *The falling sickness: A history of epilepsy from the greeks to the beginnings of modern neurology,* 79, The John Hopkins University Press, Ltd, London.

Temkin, O. (1971b). Great systems and period of enlightenment, In: *The falling sickness: A history of epilepsy from the greeks to the beginnings of modern neurology,* 218, The John Hopkins University Press Ltd, London.

Temkin, O. (1971c). The middle ages, In: O. Temkin (Ed.), *The falling sickness: A history of epilepsy from the greeks to the beginnings of modern neurology.,* 95, The John Hopkins University Press Ltd, London.

Temkin, O. (1971d). The middle ages, In: O. Temkin (Ed.), *The falling sickness: A history of epilepsy from the greeks to the beginnings of modern neurology,* 105, The John Hopkins University Press, Ltd, London.

Tissot. (1770a). *Traité de l'épilepsie, faisant le tome troisième du traité des nerfs et de leurs maladies,* p. 117, Didot, P.F., Paris.

Tissot, SA. (1770b). *Traité de l'épilepsie, faisant le tome troisième du traité des nerfs et de leurs maladies,* Didot, P.F., Paris.

Tralles, Alexander of. (1878). Alexander von tralles, vol. I, In: T. von Puschmann (Ed.), *Alexander von tralles, original-text und ubersetzung,* I, 15, p. 575, Braumuller, Vienna.

Vilanova, Arnald of. (1585a). Breviarium, In: *Opera omnia,* I, 22, col. 1071, Basel.

Vilanova, Arnald of. (1585b). De epilepsia, In: *Opera omnia,* c. 1; col. 1603, Basel.

Vossen, R. (1958). Uber die antikonvulsive wirking von succinimiden. *Dtsch Med Wochenschr,* Vol. *83,* No. pp 1227-1230,

Wilks, S. (1861). Bromide and iodide of potassium in epilepsy. *Medical Times and Gazette,* Vol. *2,* No. pp 635-636,

Willis, T. (1682). De morbis convulsivis, In: *Opera omnia,* c. 1, pp. 13-14, Henricum Wetstenium, Amsterdam.

Willis, T. (1684). Of convulsive diseases, chapter 1., In: *Dr. Willi's practice of physick, being the whole works of that.... Physician,* p. 5, Fletcher, London.

Wong, R. K., & Prince, D. A. (1978). Participation of calcium spikes during intrinsic burst firing in hippocampal neurons. *Brain Res,* Vol. *159,* No. 2, (December 1978), pp 385-390, ISSN 0006-8993.

Wong, R. K., & Prince, D. A. (1981). Afterpotential generation in hippocampal pyramidal cells. *J Neurophysiol,* Vol. *45,* No. 1, (January 1981), pp 86-97, ISSN 0022-3077.

9

Epilepsy and Oral Health

Taskin Gurbuz
Department of Pedodontics, Faculty of Dentistry,
Atatürk University, Erzurum
Turkey

1. Introduction

Epilepsy is the most common chronic neurologic disorder in paediatric neurology and the predominant aetiologies are birth injury and congenital abnormalities. Epilepsy has a tendency to recurrent seizures. Most of these will have primary or idiopathic epilepsy (i.e., no underlying cause will be evident), but some will have secondary epilepsy due to a cause such as head injury, meningitis, or birth asphyxia. The international classification of epileptic seizures divides the epilepsies into those that are generalized, where the whole brain is involved, and the partial seizures, where the aberrant activity involves only a part of the brain (Koch & Poulsen, 2009). In infants, birth injuries and congenital defects are the primary causes of epilepsy. Birth injuries, genetic factors, infections, and trauma are major contributing factors in children and adolescents from 2 to 20 years of age. For individuals between 20 and 30 years of age, brain tumors and other structural lesions are the foremost contributing causes. In those older than 50 years of age, cerebral vascular accidents and metastatic tumors are significant causes of seizure activity (Aragon & Burneo, 2007).

Epilepsy is the most common neurological problem of childhood, and its incidence is the highest in the first decade of life, a period during which children begin and complete a critical part of their social and educational development. Epilepsy is a common chronic neurologic disorder that affects 1-3% of the population, and almost 10% of the population will have one or more seizures at some time in their lives (Hauser et al., 1996). The epilepsies form an array of more or less discrete epilepsy syndromes, characterized by age of onset, hereditary factors, seizure types, electroencephalogram (EEG) abnormalities, and prognosis (Roger, 2005).

A seizure is classified as "partial" when the electrical discharge causing it to occur in a specific area of the brain or "generalized" when the discharge affects the entire brain cortex. When there is loss of awareness, seizures are termed complex. The classification of epilepsy is similar. Epilepsy can be partial or generalized. Based on the cause, it can be symptomatic (caused by a developmental malformation), idiopathic (when a genetic condition is responsible) or cryptogenic (when the cause is unknown) (Aragon & Burneo, 2007). Epilepsy is the most common disorder in paediatric neurology and the predominant aetiologies are birth injury and congenital abnormalities.

2. Classification of seizures

There are five types of epilepsy, they are:
Grand mal seizures

Petit mal seizures
Psychomotor seizures
Focal seizure (Jacksonian seizures)
Self induced seizures (Rao, 2008).

2.1 Grand mal seizures

Onset is rapid and preceded by momentary aura. Associated with tonic and clonic phases of muscular spasm, patient losses consciousness and becomes pale. Pupils dilate, eyeballs roll upwards or to one side, the face becomes distorted and there is often rapid contraction of the jaw muscles. Micturition and defecation may occur.
Patient may experience cyanosis during the tonic phase (continuous tension or contraction) lasting for 20-40 seconds. Clonic phase (alternating series of contractions and partial relaxation) may last for several minutes. Patient wakes up from seizure with severe headache and in a general state of confusion. A patient who experiences a grand mal seizure in the dental office should be handled conservatively and be put in a position in which he cannot harm himself possibly on the floor away from the dental equipment. If the seizure is prolonged, administration of oxygen may be necessary. A rubber or plastic mouth prop has to be inserted to prevent the patient from biting his tongue. A tongue blade wrapped with gauze and adhesive may be utilized. It is usually sufficient that the dentist wait until the seizure stops and then evaluate him. If the seizure is prolonged, administration of oxygen may be necessary. Recovery may be quick or patient may be irritable.

2.2 Petit mal seizures

It appears between 3 years of age and puberty. More common in girls. It consists of transient loss of consciousness. It may occur once or twice a month or very frequently at less intervals and lasting for less than 30 seconds. Other features are upward rolling of eyes, moving of the lids, drooling or rhythmic nodding of the head or slight quivering of the trunk and limb muscles. They may also go unnoticed.

2.3 Psychomotor seizures

They are difficult to recognize and control. Slight aura is manifested as a shrill of cry or an attempt to run for help. Child is often drowsy or sleeps for a short time after the spell. Seizure consists of loss of postural tone. 1-5 minutes of unconsciousness is followed by normal sleep or activity. No tonic or clonic movements present.

2.4 Focal seizure (Jacksonian seizures)

It is produced by injury to the brain. Seizures are clonic in nature. Muscles involved are the ones most specialized for voluntary movements in the hand, face and tongue.

2.5 Self induced seizures

It is possible for some children to induce petit mal or grand mal seizures by over breathing, watching a blinking light or by performing some other form of learned behavior. In such cases drug therapy alone is usually unsatisfactory. Patient by doing so tries to draw attention to himself and is usually associated with complex family problems and psychiatric consultation is indicated.

3. Diagnosis and treatment

3.1 Diagnosis

The diagnosis of epilepsy requires the presence of recurrent, unprovoked seizures. Patients presenting with seizures should have a general and neurologic examination, looking for other causes of loss of consciousness (eg, cardiac abnormalities, evidence of infection), contributing factors or secondary causes of epilepsy, and focal neurologic signs. Some of the important clinical findings include alterations in consciousness, sensation, motor abilities, and reflexes. Detailed accounts of the seizures from either the patient or eyewitnesses can be important in making a correct diagnosis.

Diagnostic tools, such as electroencephalography (EEG) and magnetic resonance imaging (MRI), are required to classify epilepsy. EEG records waves generated by the brain cortex. These waves have characteristics that allow the differentiation of normal from abnormal electrical discharges and provide information about localization. EEG amplifies the waves and transfers them to a computer for interpretation (Aragon & Burneo, 2007).

When diagnosing epilepsy, the underlying disease must be identified. The signs and symptoms of the patient before, during, and after the seizure are vital for determining the cause. The patient and any witnesses should be questioned, and a physical examination for trauma, infections, and other conditions should be completed. Electroencephalography studies will often reveal an abnormality, especially when additional stimuli are recorded, such as flashing lights, music or rhythmic sounds, sleep deprivation, or hyperventilation. The use of blood tests, magnetic resonance imaging, or computed tomography may also yield helpful information leading to a diagnosis. Primary epilepsy is often diagnosed by exclusion of all other causes (Hupp, 2001).

3.2 Treatment

Seizure disorders are generally more severe in people who have mental retardation. Patients who have developmental disabilities and epilepsy are treated for their seizure type or types and syndrome just like any other person who has epilepsy. Several options exist for the treatment of epileptic seizures, including antiseizure medications, vagal nerve stimulation, ketogenic diet, and surgery. These options are may be used concurrently in the same individual if needed (Robbins, 2009). The choice of medication is related to the type of seizure (Table). In some cases, a trial of anti-seizure medication may be used in a patient with strong evidence of more than one seizure, whereas a patient with a single seizure is usually monitored but not given medication. Long-term therapy using one anticonvulsant medication is most desirable, although some patients need a combination to achieve efficacy with limited toxicity (Hupp, 2001). The most common oral side effect of antiepileptic drugs seen in the dental office is gingival hyperplasia (Fig. 1). Gingival hyperplasia is characterized by unusual growth of the gingival subepithelial connective tissue and epithelium, for unknown reasons; it is reversed once the drug is discontinued. Anticonvulsant drugs such as phenytoin, carbamazepine, valproic acid, and others have been used individually and in combinations. They act to reduce the frequency of seizures, elevate the seizure threshold of the motor cortex, and limit the spread of the excitation from the focus of the seizure (Hupp, 2001). In an epilepsy program, the objective is to find out whether the patient is a surgical candidate by using special tests, such as prolonged monitoring video-electroencephalography (VEEG) and structural MRI. VEEG allows confirmation of epilepsy syndrome and location of the epileptogenic focus. The behavioural changes captured by video and the focal epileptiform abnormalities in the EEG are the most important pieces of information in the presurgical evaluation.

Drug	Type of seizure	Most common oral side effects and dental considerations
Phenytoin	GTCS, partial	Gingival hyperplasia, delayed healing, gingival bleeding, osteoporosis
Carbamazepine	GTCS, partial	Agranulocytosis, aplastic anemia, xerostomia, delayed healing, gingival bleeding (thrombocytopenia), osteoporosis
Valproic acid	Absence, any type	Excessive bleeding, decreased platelet aggregation, delayed healing, osteoporosis, xerostomia, stomatitis, gingivitis, drug interactions with aspirin and nonsteroidal anti-inflammatory drugs
Phenobarbital	Any type	Drowsiness, drug interactions, xerostomia, stomatitis, osteoporosis
Ethosuximide	Absence	Leukopenia, Stevens-Johnson syndrome, orofacial edema, dysgeusia
Primidone	Partial (psychomotor)	Ataxia, vertigo, stomatitis, osteoporosis
Gabapentin	Partial	Xerostomia, stomatitis, gingivitis, glossitis, orofacial edema, dysgeusia

Table 1. Adverse effects of antiepileptic drugs commonly used in children.

Temporal lobectomy is perhaps the most common type of surgery for epilepsy. In the only randomized controlled trial of surgery versus medical treatment, the success rate was 64%. However, patients can experience a significant decline in verbal memory (McKhann et al., 2002). Which can be partly predicted through a detailed neuropsychologic evaluation (Loring, 1997).

4. Treating dental patients with epilepsy

4.1 General situation

The medical literature contains little information on the influence of epilepsy in dental care. Most existing studies focus on phenytoin-induced gingival hyperplasia. These individuals often have worse oral health status than the general population. They tend to have a higher incidence of dental caries and difficulty in accessing dental care (Chikte et al., 1991). The main reason for higher prevalence of dental caries in disabled individuals is the inadequate plaque removal. Visually impaired cannot visualize the plaque on the teeth surfaces so even

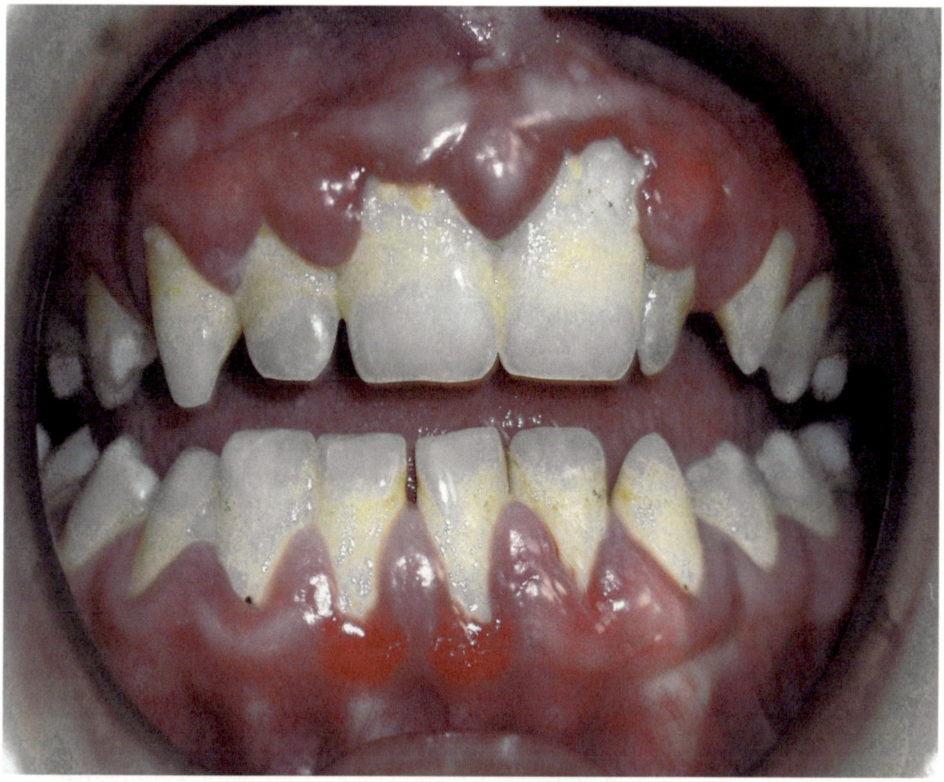

Fig. 1. Severe gingival enlargement in a child with epilepsy.

understanding the importance of oral hygiene is difficult for them, which results in the progression of dental caries as well as inflammatory disease of the periodontium (Mann et al., 1984). Patients living with epilepsy have special needs during dental treatment. In almost all aspects of oral health and dental status, the condition of patients with epilepsy is significantly worse than age-matched groups in the general (nonepileptic) population (Karolyhazy et al., 2003). Furthermore, patients who have poorly controlled epilepsy and experience frequent generalized tonic-clonic seizures exhibit worse oral health in comparison with patients who are better controlled or only have seizures that do not involve the masticatory apparatus (Karolyhazy, et al., 2003).
The number of decayed and missing teeth, the degree of abrasion and periodontal indexes are significantly worse in patients with epilepsy. Those with epilepsy also have significantly fewer restored and replaced teeth than the general population (Karolyhazy et al., 2005).

4.2 Dental status and oral health

4.2.1 Trauma

Dentofacial trauma occurring during seizures has been reported to include injuries to the tongue, buccal mucosa, facial fractures, avulsion, luxation or fractures of teeth, and subluxation of the temporomandibular joint (Ogunbodede et al., 1998).
Generalized tonic-clonic seizures often cause minor oral injuries, such as tongue biting, (Pick & Bauer, 2001) but also frequently lead to tooth injuries (Buck et al., 1997), and in some cases to maxillofacial trauma (Aragon et al., 2001).

Gurbuz et al. (Gurbuz & Tan, 2010) found a traumatic anterior dental injury rate of 68.8% in children with epilepsy in Erzurum, Turkey. This probably resulted from insufficient seizure control or from placing hard objects between the teeth of patients during seizures. According to O'Sullivan, the prevalence of traumatic anterior dental injury was 11–30% in children without epilepsy (Curzon, 2001). Generalized tonic–clonic seizures often cause minor oral injuries, such as tongue biting, but also frequently lead to tooth injuries (Buck, et al., 1997) and in some cases to maxillofacial trauma (Aragon, et al., 2001).
Patients with epilepsy can be at increased risk of fracture because enzyme-inducing antiepileptic drugs (e.g., phenytoin, phenobarbital, carbamazepine) alter the metabolism and clearance of vitamin D and have been associated with osteopenia and osteomalacia. Of interest, increased fracture risk has also been associated with the use of benzodiazepines, antidepressants and antipsychotics, suggesting that underlying brain disease or adverse effects of the medication are responsible for falls and injuries (Mattson & Gidal, 2004).
Fractures can have catastrophic effects on the lives of patients with epilepsy, and measures are available to minimize the risk of fractures, such as ensuring adequate calcium and vitamin D supplementation (a minimum of 1,000 mg and 400 IU daily, respectively) especially in patients taking phenobarbital, phenytoin or primidone (Sato et al., 2001).

4.2.2 Periodontal problems

Children younger than 15 years constitute a large group among epileptic individuals, and a considerable proportion of them also have mental and motor deficits (Bourgeois, 1995; Brodie & Dichter, 1996). These patients are at risk for oral health due to their poor self-care and the side-effects of anticonvulsant treatment: in particular, the use of phenytoin and phenobarbital can be associated with gingival enlargement (Delasnerie-Laupretre & Turpin, 1991; Thomason et al., 1992). Patients with epilepsy can be at increased risk of fracture because enzyme-inducing anti-epileptic drugs (AED; e.g., phenytoin, phenobarbital, carbamazepine) alter the metabolism and clearance of vitamin D and have been associated with osteopenia and osteomalacia (Mattson & Gidal, 2004). The association of phenytoin with gingival enlargement was first described by Kimball in 1939 (Kimball, 1939); subsequently, many articles have reported on its incidence or severity in different populations. The literature reveals a wide variation in its incidence, ranging from 3 to 93%. The variability is primarily due to differences in criteria for assessing the severity of the hyperplasia, the different sizes and ages of studied groups, and variations in the duration and dosage of phenytoin treatment. However, it is now widely accepted that clinically significant hyperplasia is seen in about 50% of patients taking phenytoin (Majola et al., 2000; Ogunbodede, et al., 1998; Perlik et al., 1995; Thomason, et al., 1992).
The logical approach in drug-induced gingival enlargement is a reduction of the dose or replacement with another drug (Dahllof et al., 1991; Lundstrom et al., 1982; R. A. Seymour et al., 1985).
Because gingival enlargement has not been reported with carbamazepine so far and appears to be extremely rare with valproate, these drugs have been proposed as alternatives in the treatment of patients who develop or are at risk of phenytoin-induced gingival enlargement (R. A. Seymour, et al., 1985).
Gingival enlargement as a complication of phenytoin use has been well studied (Angelopoulos, 1975a, 1975b). About 50% of patients taking this medication will develop gingival hyperplasia within 12–24 months of initiation of treatment. Despite the existence of

newer medications that are equally effective and have fewer side effects, phenytoin remains one of the most commonly used drugs. Evidence regarding best treatment for gingival hyperplasia is lacking. Some clinicians advocate the use of chlorhexidine, folic acid rinses or both, but excellent oral hygiene will probably prevent or significantly decrease the severity of the condition. In severe cases, surgical reduction is needed (Stoopler et al., 2003).

The newer antiepileptic drugs produce oral manifestations only infrequently. Xerostomia and stomatitis have been reported rarely as side effects of carbamazepine, (Ogunbodede, et al., 1998) and rash that may involve the oral cavity has been associated with lamotrigine and can be exacerbated by the concomitant use of valproic acid (Li et al., 1996).

Although phenytoin-induced gingival enlargement has been better studied, its pathogenesis is still unclear. Several mechanisms related to an interaction between phenytoin and the gingival fibroblasts have been hypothesized. Phenytoin decreases cellular folate uptake possibly by inhibiting cation currents, leading to local folate deficiency. This results in insufficient synthesis of collagenase activator proteins, which play a role in connective tissue catabolism. As connective tissue catabolism is limited, gingival enlargement develops (Brown et al., 1991). The sensitivity of gingival fibroblasts to phenytoin is different in each individual and is genetically determined. This might, in some degree, explain why not all phenytoin-treated individuals develop gingival enlargement. Recently, several reports revealed that the pathogenesis of phenytoin-induced gingival enlargement might be related to certain cytokines, including interleukin-1, -6, and -8; platelet-derived growth factor BB; and basic fibroblast growth factor (Hong & Trackman, 2002; Modeer et al., 2000; Sasaki & Maita, 1998). Whether similar mechanisms play a role in valproate-induced gingival enlargement is unclear.

Valproic acid can cause direct bone marrow suppression, which can impair wound healing and increase post-operative bleeding and infections. Decreased platelet count is the most common and best-recognized hematologic effect of valproic acid; the incidence varies from 5% to 40%. Clinically significant bleeding is uncommon because the thrombocytopenia is usually not severe. For elective surgery, laboratory evaluation – including bleeding time, fibrinogen level, prothrombin time, partial thromboplastin time and von Willebrand factor level – is needed to assess the risk of peri- and postoperative bleeding. Bleeding as a potential side effect should be discussed with patients and their families in preparation for surgery (Acharya & Bussel, 2000).

According to Tan et al., VPA can be associated with side-effects in gingival tissue in children by a mechanism attributable to the drug rather than oral hygiene or inflammation (Tan et al., 2004).

Those findings are consistent with the present results. Seymour reported that the most important determinant of phenytoin-induced gingival enlargement was poor oral hygiene (R.A. Seymour, 1992).

The pathogenesis of phenytoin-induced gingival enlargement is still not well known but several mechanisms, all related to an interaction between phenytoin and the gingival fibroblast, have been hypothesized. Valproic acid can cause direct bone marrow suppression, which can impair wound healing and increase postoperative bleeding and infections (Aragon & Burneo, 2007). The reaction begins as a diffuse swelling of the interdental papillae, which enlarge and coalesce. Clinically significant overgrowth occurs in approximately 50% of patients (Cameron & Widmer, 2008). The incidence and severity of overgrowth are the greatest on the labial surfaces on maxillary and mandibular anterior teeth (Fig. 1).

4.2.3 Prosthodontic problems

Epilepsy is a chronic disease that can affect oral health and prosthodontic status in different ways. However, epilepsy is a condition of various etiologies and seizure types, and different patients may have differing needs in prosthodontic care (Karolyhazy, et al., 2005).

In a recent analysis of the prosthodontic status of patients with epilepsy, it was found out that compared with age-matched controls, patients with epilepsy have a tendency to become edentulous earlier. It was also found that prosthodontic treatment is suboptimal, as significantly fewer teeth are replaced, despite the fact that epileptic patients tend to have more missing teeth. Based on these findings, the authors suggested a classification for patients with epilepsy according to dental risk factors and dental manageability and provided recommendations for dental treatment (Aragon & Burneo, 2007).

Friedlander and Cummings (Friedlander & Cummings, 1989) mentioned that in patients with epilepsy replacement of missing teeth is important to prevent the tongue from being caught in the edentulous spaces during seizures.

Specific guidelines were also provided, such as discouragement of incisal restorations, use of fixed rather than removable prostheses and inclusion of additional abutments if fixed partial dentures are to be used (Karolyhazy, et al., 2005). In addition, the use of metal base for complete dentures and telescopic retention with denture bases made of metal or reinforced with metal for nearly edentulous patients was recommended for those with frequent partial seizures involving the masticatory apparatus, frequent generalized tonic-clonic seizures and other seizures associated with falls. Patients with epilepsy have an increased risk for loosing teeth, and the prosthodontic status of epilepsy patients is not optimal. This may unfavorably affect quality of life.

4.2.4 Orthodontic problems

Anti-epileptic drugs related to oral findings include recurrent aphthous-like ulcerations, gingival bleeding, hypercementosis, root shortening, anomalous tooth development, delayed eruption, and cervical lymphadenopathy (Johnstone et al., 1999).

Of particular interest to the orthodontist is a recent report of facial and body asymmetries affecting 41% of patients with partial seizures in the population studied; asymmetries included both hemihypertrophy and atrophy (Fong et al., 2003).

Gingival enlargement may cause delays in permanent teeth eruption and malocclusions in children with mixed dentition (Fig. 2). The hypertonicity of the oral musculature has caused the protrusion of the anterior teeth and the orthopaedic compression of the maxilla.

5. Dental management

Understanding of epilepsy and seizures raises awareness of the disorder's impact on patients' general medical and psychological health. Dental treatment of patients with epilepsy and seizures should be carried out by dentists who are knowledgeable about these disorders (Aragon & Burneo, 2007). The medical literature contains little information on the influence of epilepsy in dental care.

Patients who have epilepsy have been shown to have significantly worse dental condition than the general population (Karolyhazy, et al., 2003). The disease may affect the dental status and oral health of patients in several ways. Patients who have seizure disorders tend to have less'than ideal oral health, with higher numbers of decayed and missing teeth. They tend to receive less dental treatment, with significantly fewer restored and replaced teeth

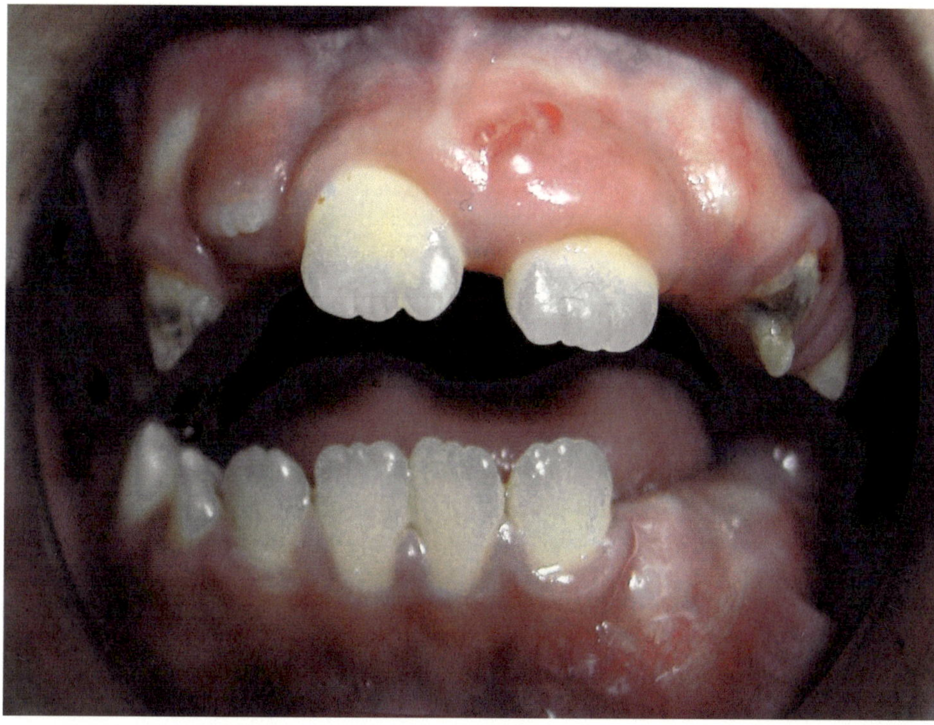

Fig. 2. Tooth eruption problem in a child with epilepsy.

than the general population. This situation can be especially true in patients who have development disabilities, who may have trouble accessing dental care anyway. The seizures themselves can cause injuries to the teeth and dental prostheses. Some of the drugs can cause periodontal disease. Specific considerationsfor epileptic patients include the treatment of oral soft tissue side effects of medications and damage to the hard and soft tissue of the orofacial region secondary to seizure trauma, especially in patients who suffer from poorly controlled generalized tonic-clonic seizures (Robbins, 2009).

Dentists with a thorough knowledge of seizure disorders and the medications used to treat them can provide necessary dental and oral health care for those patients. Patients with seizure disorders may report a history of fainting or dizzy spells, seizures, or epilepsy, as well as medications to treat the seizures. A thorough evaluation of a patient's seizure disorder is necessary before initiation of any dental treatment. Important aspects to evaluate include the type of seizures, any known cause, frequency, duration, known triggers such as stress or bright lights, presence of aura before seizure activity, and history of injuries related to effects or drug interactions noted. The drug history can give some indication as to the degree of seizure seizures. Drug history should be carefully reviewed and updated at each visit, and any potential drug side severity or control (Robbins, 2009). The general goal of dental management is the avoidance of a seizure. It is important to know the type of epilepsy and any precipitating factors, medications and dosage, compliance and degree of seizure control before commencing treatment. In addition, drug interactions with anticonvulsants are common and their half-life and blood levels can be increased substantially. Consultation with the child's neurologist is essential before commencement of treatment (Cameron & Widmer, 2008). Unfortunately, even if the patient has been compliant with the medication, breakthrough seizures can occur. These may be related to fatigue or lack of sleep, menstrual cycle, decreased overall health, a missed meal, alcohol use, physical or emotional stress, or pain. If the patient typically has an aura, it should be noted so that the dentist or staff members can notice any changes and move to protect the patient (Hupp, 2001).

Other conditions can lead to seizures in the dental office. The most common nonepileptic cause is an overdose of local anesthetic. In addition, hypoglycaemia or insulin overdose, hypoxia secondary to syncope, cerebrovascular accident or transient ischemic attack, and hyperventilation can occur in the dental office. If a patient has a convulsive seizure while undergoing dental treatment, stop the procedure and protect the patient from injury. This may involve removing any sharp objects from the area, such as handpieces, placing a soft mouth-prop, and cushioning the patient's head. It may also be necessary to control or gently restrain their arms and legs, keep them from falling out of the dental chair, and loosen any tight clothing. As the patient progresses to the postictal phase, maintain the airway because the muscles may become flaccid. Check for level of awareness, reassure them, and determine whether medical assistance is needed. Patients with partial or absence seizures usually are not at significant risk of loss of consciousness; nevertheless, they must be protected from injury. In some patients, the dental staff may be unaware that an episode has even occurred. Status epilepticus of a convulsive seizure must be treated urgently. Intravenous administration of diazepam or midazolam is needed before permanent brain injury occurs. Either drug should be titrated to the point at which seizure activity ceases. Basic life support (ie, airway, breathing, circulation) should be performed as required, and fluid in the mouth should be suctioned from the buccal aspect of the clenched teeth. Nothing should be forced between the teeth at any time, because temporomandibular joint injury or fractured teeth could result. Notification of emergency medical personnel is needed (Hupp, 2001).

It is advisable to check that the patient has taken his/her routine medications, has eaten normally, is not excessively tired, and has not been recently ill before starting dental treatment. Stress and fatigue are factors that can trigger a seizure. If the patient is not feeling well or is overly tired, it may be prudent to reschedule the appointment. Appointments should be scheduled during a time of day when seizures are less likely to occur, if predictable, and stress and anxiety should be minimized. Explaining the dental procedures to the patient before starting, and offering assurance during the procedure may be helpful. The use of nitrous oxide or conscious sedation may be necessary to provide dental care safely and effectively. In patients whose seizure disorder is poorly controlled and whose developmental disabilities make the delivery of dental care difficult, general anesthesia may need to be considered. General anaesthesia is preferable in children with poor seizure control as the abnormal neural activity is completely ablated during the procedure. Dental trauma is an obvious consequence in the child with frequent, poorly controlled seizures. Removable appliances are contraindicated in an epileptic child due to potential airway obstruction (Cameron & Widmer, 2008). Light can be a trigger in inducing an epileptic seizure. Dark glasses used as eye protection and careful positioning of the dental light so that it is directed into the mouth and not flashed in the patient's eyes can minimize any problems (Robbins, 2009).

It is well known that phenytoin causes gingival hyperplasia in a majority of patients. Studies have reported that the drug induces fibroblasts and osteoblasts, that there is an excessive deposition of extracellular matrix, and that normal tissue turnover and wound healing are altered. The most common sites for hyperplasia are the labial aspects of the maxillary and mandibular ridges. The tissue has normal color and surface texture, with lobular shape of the interdental papillae and a firm, resilient feel, often without inflammation. Local irritants make the response more exuberant in some patients, with the typical erythema, edema, and easy bleeding of common gingivitis. If significant hyperplasia leads to discomfort, inability to function, or esthetic concerns, surgical reduction is necessary. The anterior labial surfaces of the maxillary and mandibular gingiva are the most commonly affected (Fig. 1) and it is strongly correlated with poor plaque control. It is believed that excellent oral hygiene will prevent or reduce the gingival response to phenytoin.

Most convulsive disorders are controlled through medication and pose few problems in dental treatment. It should be made sure that the child has taken the daily dose of medicines. Since anxiety is a frequent precipitation factor, premedication with minor tranquilizers will be effective. These children often arrive at the dental office in a slightly sedated state due to the CNS depressed activity of anticonvulsant medications. Use of mouth props is mandatory during treatment because once the seizure begins; it is difficult to insert any device to prevent intraoral injury due to clenching of the jaws. If appliances are indicated for tooth movement or tooth replacement purposes, fixed appliance is preferred because there is less chance of dislodgement (Rao, 2008). Generalized tonic-clonic seizures often cause minor oral injuries such as tongue biting and tooth injuries. Traumatic injury to anterior teeth should be evaluated in the standard way. Fractures of the anterior teeth can be repaired with composite restorations. A chest radiograph may be indicated if a tooth is avulsed and cannot be accounted for. Soft tissue wounds should be explored for tooth fragments when incisal fractures occur. Patients who have epilepsy can also be at increased risk for maxillofacial fractures caused by drugs-induced osteoporosis (Turner & Glickman, 2005).

The coarsening of facial features in patients on phenytoin is related to the increased activity of osteoblasts. Other intraoral side effects are seen with anticonvulsant medications, especially in the first few weeks of therapy. A rash or erythema multiforme may develop that can manifest in the mouth as erosions and ulcerations. Phenytoin has been associated with aphthous ulcers. Some of the medications (ie, carbamazepine, phenytoin, phenobarbital) affect bone marrow function, which can lead to altered immune response, thrombocytopenia, and bleeding. Valproic acid inhibits platelet aggregation. Others affect liver function (ethosuximide, carbamazepine), which impairs coagulation. If signs of petechial hemorrhage or abnormal bleeding are noted, hemostasis should be evaluated before surgical treatment. Drug interactions should also be considered for patients on anticonvulsants. A patient taking barbiturates (eg, primidone, phenobarbital) should avoid any other central nervous system depressants such as narcotics or nitrous oxide. Anti-epileptic drugs can cause xerostomia, which can put patients at increased risk for developing caries, especially in the cervical region and candidiasis. In children, increased dental caries can also be seen if drugs are delivered in a syrup form. Carbamazepine can cause ulcerations, xerostomia, glossitis, and stomatitis. The frequency of dental check-ups and prophylaxis appointments should be based on the patient's needs. The recall and hygiene interval may be more frequent for epileptic patients because of increased risk for gingival hyperplasia secondary to use of an anti-epileptic drug. Patients who are xerostomic should be put on supplemental topical fluoride to prevent dental decay and monitored regularly for candidal infections. The importance of good oral hygiene should be stressed to the patient and caregivers (if appropriate) (Robbins, 2009). Aspirin carbamazepine increase liver microsomal enzyme activity, decreasing the activity of concurrent, nonsteroidal anti-inflammatory medications, and the antifungal fluconazole will increase the blood level of phenytoin and add to the platelet effects of valproic acid. Propoxyphene and erythromycin interfere with the metabolism of carbamazepine, which can lead to toxic levels of the anticonvulsant (Hupp, 2001). Thereafter, patients on VPA should be educated on oral hygiene and their oral health should carefully be followed. Gingivectomy is the treatment of choice in case of gingival hyperplasia that usually occurs with phenytoin therapy. They usually tend to reccur. Hence the drug or the dose can be modified upon consultation with the paediatrician.

The presence of a seizure disorder can influence prosthodontic treatment decisions. Missing teeth should be replaced to prevent the tongue from being caught in the edentulous space and injured. Treatment planning considerations must consider fabrication of dental prostheses designed to minimize the risk for displacement of teeth or further damage. Fixed prostheses or implants are preferable to removable appliances because the latter can dislodge during a seizure and cause oral injury or airway obstruction. Large posterior restorations are prone to fracture in someone who may have jaw spasms during a tonic-clonic seizure. All-metal units should be considered whenever aesthetically possible, to minimize the chance of porcelain fracture. In the anterior, metal crowns with acrylic or composite facings can be used to facilitate repair as needed. For fixed partial dentures, the use of additional abutments may be advisable for more stability. If removable partial prostheses are unavoidable, they should be constructed with metallic palates and bases instead of acrylic and metal backings to anterior denture teeth (Robbins, 2009).

The danger of injury to the teeth and prostheses during this type of seizure is the highest and should be considered when designing dental prostheses. For occlusal restorations, the use of ceramic inlays is best avoided; complete metal-ceramic crowns are recommended instead. Generally, fixed rather than removable prostheses are preferred. For fixed partial dentures, the use of additional abutments may be advisable for more stability. If removable partial dentures are unavoidable, the dentures should be designed with a large metal base. As more teeth are lost, telescopic retention may be advised with a base made of metal or reinforced with metal. The base of complete dentures should also be metal or reinforced with metal, because an acrylic base may fracture, increasing the risk of aspiration or dislodgement into the esophagus. A small number of patients with epilepsy, primarily those where the disease is associated with inborn or perinatal encephalopathy, have a severe mental handicap that precludes cooperation. In these patients, general anesthesia is usually necessary to perform dental treatment, and prosthodontic rehabilitation is usually not performed. Seizure-related injuries to prostheses are also an issue, but only for those who are refractory to treatment and suffer from frequent generalized tonic-clonic seizures. Therefore, the large majority of patients can and should receive prosthodontic treatment without restrictions. In a smaller portion of patients, however, certain restrictions apply to prevent potentially dangerous seizure-related complications (Karolyhazy, et al., 2005).

Patients with epilepsy and a malocclusion should have a comprehensive orthodontic evaluation. It is important for the orthodontist to be alert to dental or facial trauma that may have previously occurred during seizures. The level of orthodontic intervention must take into account the type of seizure disorder and efficacy of control. History related by the patient should be confirmed during a discussion with the patient's physician. Adverse side effects of drugs and past dental trauma should be researched by the orthodontist and reviewed as part of patient informed consent. Mechanical challenges such as closing interdental spaces in the presence of gingival hypertrophy should be considered when estimating treatment time. One patient did have a tonic-clonic seizure during fixed orthodontic treatment and suffered laceration of the lip mucosa and luxation of maxillary incisors; the patient's mother believed that the orthodontic appliance prevented incisor avulsion during the seizure. Accepting such risks should be decision of the patient and/or the guardian after careful discussion with the orthodontist. The metal in a fixed orthodontic appliance may distort images obtained by magnetic resonance imaging (MRI). Any metal portions of the orthodontic appliance close to the area being scanned decreases MRI quality. In some patients, an acceptable MRI may be obtained if arch wires and other removable components are removed before the scan; others will require the removal of the entire orthodontic appliance. This author treated one patient who required yearly MRI brain imaging. The patient's orthodontic treatment was impacted in the following way: fixed appliances were placed the day after MRI scan; 12 months into treatment, all appliances were removed; the MRI was obtained, and appliances were replaced. The fixed appliance was removed after 23 months of therapy, just before the next scheduled MRI scan (Sheller, 2004).

5.1 Management of the epileptic patient in the dental office

It is the responsibility of every dentist to have emergency procedures planned and rehearsed with their office staff on a regular basis. The dentist should reduce stress of the child by behavioral management and conscious sedation techniques. Reduce direct overhead lighting, particularly for the photosensitive form of epilepsy. Avoid seizure-promoting medications such as CNS stimulants and local anaesthetics containing adrenaline (epinephrine). Emergency drugs such as oxygen, intravenous or rectal diazepam (Valium) and intravenous phenobarbital sodium should be readily available. Take a complete health history and a complete seizure history. List all medications, including side effects and potential drug interactions (Gingival hyperplasia and bleeding tendencies in patients taking drug). Minimize risk for damaging or displacing restorations or prostheses during seizure.
The dentist should be careful while positioning of dental light and avoide of known precipitating factors. Consider use of mouth prop at the beginning of procedure. If a seizure occurs while a patient is in the dental chair. Firstly, clear all instruments away from the patient. Place the dental chair in a supported, supine position as near to the floor as possible. Place the patient on his or her side (to decrease the chance of aspiration of secretions or dental materials in the patient's mouth). If possible, remove any foreign material from mouth. If possible, turn patient onto his/her side. Passively restrain only to prevent patient from falling out of chair or hitting nearby objects. After the seizure, it is better to discontinue the therapy. If a cavity is already prepared, either temporize or complete the final restoration. Time the seizure (the duration of the event may seem longer than it actually is). After seizure, turn patient to the side to avoid aspiration and examine for traumatic injuries. If seizure last more than 3 minutes or patient become cyanotic. Administer oxygen at a rate of 6–8 L/minute. If the seizure lasts longer than 1 minute or for repeated seizures, administer a 10-mg dose of diazepam intramuscularly (IM) or intravenously (IV), or 2 mg of ativan, IV or IM, or 5 mg of midazolam, IM or IV. Be aware of the possibility of compromised airway or uncontrollable seizure. Also, contact the patient's family, if he or she is alone (Aragon & Burneo, 2007; Rao, 2008; Robbins, 2009).

6. Conclusion

The oral conditions observed demonstrate the need for dentists to follow up and treat these children. In addition, there is an ongoing need to improve the oral hygiene of these individuals to prevent the development of periodontal and dental disease in later life. Advances in diagnostic technology, pharmacotherapy and understanding of neurologic processes allow dentists to understand and manage patients with epilepsy better. People with epilepsy can be safely treated in a general dental practice. A thorough medical history should be taken and updated at each visit. Seizure history must be taken into account when planning treatment. Dentists with a comprehension of seizure disorders can provide an invaluable service to their patients, providing not only oral health, but also maintaining and promoting the systemic health of these patients. Patients who have developmental disabilities and epilepsy can be safely treated in a general dental practice. Most patients who have epilepsy can and should receive functionally and esthetically adequate dental care.

7. References

Acharya, S. & Bussel, J. B. (2000). *Hematologic toxicity of sodium valproate.* Journal Of Pediatric Hematology/Oncology: Official Journal Of The American Society Of Pediatric Hematology/Oncology, Vol.22, No.1, pp.62-65.

Angelopoulos, A. P. (1975a). *A clinicopathological review. Diphenylhydantoin gingival hyperplasia: 2. Aetiology, pathogenesis, differential diagnosis and treatment.* Dental Journal, Vol.41, No.5, pp.275-277, 283.

Angelopoulos, A. P. (1975b). *Diphenylhydantoin gingival hyperplasia. A clinicopathological review. 1. Incidence, clinical features and histopathology.* Dental Journal, Vol.41, No.2, pp.103-106.

Aragon, C. E.; Burneo, J. G. & Helman, J. (2001). *Occult maxillofacial trauma in epilepsy.* The Journal Of Contemporary Dental Practice, Vol.2, No.4, pp.26-32.

Aragon, C. E. & Burneo, J. G. (2007). Understanding the patient with epilepsy and seizures in the dental practice. J Can Dent Assoc, Vol.73, No.1, pp.71-76.

Bourgeois, B. F. (1995). *Antiepileptic drugs in pediatric practice.* Epilepsia, Vol.36 Suppl 2, pp.S34-45.

Brodie, M. J. & Dichter, M. A. (1996). *Antiepileptic drugs.* N Engl J Med, Vol.334, No.3, pp.168-175.

Brown, R. S.; Beaver, W. T. & Bottomley, W. K. (1991). *On the mechanism of drug-induced gingival hyperplasia.* J Oral Pathol Med, Vol.20, No.5, pp.201-209.

Buck, D.; Baker, G. A.; Jacoby, A.; Smith, D. F. & Chadwick, D. W. (1997). *Patients' experiences of injury as a result of epilepsy.* Epilepsia, Vol.38, No.4, pp.439-444.

Cameron, A. C. & Widmer, R. P. (2008). *Handbook of pediatric dentistry*, Mosby/Elsevier, 0-7234-3452-2, Edinburgh ; New York.

Chikte, U. M.; Pochee, E.; Rudolph, M. J. & Reinach, S. G. (1991). *Evaluation of stannous fluoride and chlorhexidine sprays on plaque and gingivitis in handicapped children.* Journal Of Clinical Periodontology, Vol.18, No.5, pp.281-286.

Curzon, M. E. J. (2001). Injuries to the primary dentition: diagnosis and treatment modalities. In: *Handbook of dental trauma : a practical guide to the treatment of trauma to the teeth* (E. A. O'Sullivan (Ed.), pp.1100-1121). Butterworth-Heinemann, 0-7236-1741-4, Oxford.

Dahllof, G.; Axio, E. & Modeer, T. (1991). *Regression of phenytoin-induced gingival overgrowth after withdrawal of medication.* Swedish Dental Journal, Vol.15, No.3, pp.139-143.

Delasnerie-Laupretre, N. & Turpin, J. C. (1991). *[Evaluation of the prevalence of side effects of phenobarbital in patients in the Champagne-Ardenne region]*. Pathol Biol (Paris), Vol.39, No.8, pp.780-784.

Fong, G. C.; Mak, Y. F.; Swartz, B. E.; Walsh, G. O. & Delgado-Escueta, A. V. (2003). *Body part asymmetry in partial seizure.* Seizure, Vol.12, No.8, pp.606-612.

Friedlander, A. H. & Cummings, J. L. (1989). *Temporal lobe epilepsy: its association with psychiatric impairment and appropriate dental management.* Oral Surgery, Oral Medicine, And Oral Pathology, Vol.68, No.3, pp.288-292.

Gurbuz, T. & Tan, H. (2010). *Oral health status in epileptic children.* Pediatrics International: Official Journal Of The Japan Pediatric Society, Vol.52, No.2, pp.279-283.

Hauser, W. A.; Annegers, J. F. & Rocca, W. A. (1996). *Descriptive epidemiology of epilepsy: contributions of population-based studies from Rochester, Minnesota.* Mayo Clinic Proceedings Mayo Clinic, Vol.71, No.6, pp.576-586.

Hong, H. H. & Trackman, P. C. (2002). *Cytokine regulation of gingival fibroblast lysyl oxidase, collagen, and elastin.* Journal Of Periodontology, Vol.73, No.2, pp.145-152.

Hupp, W. S. (2001). *Seizure disorders.* Oral Surg Oral Med Oral Pathol Oral Radiol Endod, Vol.92, No.6, pp.593-596.

Johnstone, S. C.; Barnard, K. M. & Harrison, V. E. (1999). *Recognizing and caring for the medically compromised child: 4. Children with other chronic medical conditions.* Dent Update, Vol.26, No.1, pp.21-26.

Karolyhazy, K.; Kovacs, E.; Kivovics, P.; Fejerdy, P. & Aranyi, Z. (2003). *Dental status and oral health of patients with epilepsy: an epidemiologic study.* Epilepsia, Vol.44, No.8, pp.1103-1108.

Karolyhazy, K.; Kivovics, P.; Fejerdy, P. & Aranyi, Z. (2005). Prosthodontic status and recommended care of patients with epilepsy. J Prosthet Dent, Vol.93, No.2, pp.177-182.

Kimball, O. P. (1939). *The Treatment of Epilepsy by Sodium Diphenylhydantoinate.* JAMA, No.112, pp.1244-1241.

Koch, G. & Poulsen, S. (2009). Children with chronic health conditions: implications for oral health. In: *Pediatric dentistry : a clinical approach* (M. L. Dadllöf Göran (Ed.), pp.315-330). Wiley-Blackwell, 1-4051-6100-0, Chichester, UK ; Ames, Iowa

Li, L. M.; Russo, M.; O'Donoghue, M. F.; Duncan, J. S. & Sander, J. W. (1996). *Allergic skin rash with lamotrigine and concomitant valproate therapy: evidence for an increased risk.* Arquivos De Neuro-Psiquiatria, Vol.54, No.1, pp.47-49.

Loring, D. W. (1997). *Neuropsychological evaluation in epilepsy surgery.* Epilepsia, Vol.38 Suppl 4, pp.S18-23.

Lundstrom, A.; Eegolofsson, O. & Hamp, S. E. (1982). *Effects of Anti-Epileptic Drug-Treatment with Carbamazepine or Phenytoin on the Oral State of Children and Adolescents.* Journal Of Clinical Periodontology, Vol.9, No.6, pp.482-488.

Majola, M. P.; McFadyen, M. L.; Connolly, C.; Nair, Y. P.; Govender, M. & Laher, M. H. (2000). *Factors influencing phenytoin-induced gingival enlargement.* Journal Of Clinical Periodontology, Vol.27, No.7, pp.506-512.

Mann, J.; Wolnerman, J. S.; Lavie, G.; Carlin, Y. & Garfunkel, A. A. (1984). *Periodontal treatment needs and oral hygiene for institutionalized individuals with handicapping conditions.* Spec Care Dentist, Vol.4, No.4, pp.173-176.

Mattson, R. H. & Gidal, B. E. (2004). *Fractures, epilepsy, and antiepileptic drugs.* Epilepsy & Behavior: E&B, Vol.5 Suppl 2, pp.S36-40.

McKhann, G. M., 2nd; Bourgeois, B. F. & Goodman, R. R. (2002). *Epilepsy surgery: indications, approaches, and results.* Seminars In Neurology, Vol.22, No.3, pp.269-278.

Modeer, T.; Domeij, H.; Anduren, I.; Mustafa, M. & Brunius, G. (2000). *Effect of phenytoin on the production of interleukin-6 and interleukin-8 in human gingival fibroblasts.* Journal Of Oral Pathology & Medicine: Official Publication Of The International Association Of Oral Pathologists And The American Academy Of Oral Pathology, Vol.29, No.10, pp.491-499.

Ogunbodede, E. O.; Adamolekun, B. & Akintomide, A. O. (1998). *Oral health and dental treatment needs in Nigerian patients with epilepsy.* Epilepsia, Vol.39, No.6, pp.590-594.

Perlik, F.; Kolinova, M.; Zvarova, J. & Patzelova, V. (1995). *Phenytoin as a risk factor in gingival hyperplasia.* Therapeutic Drug Monitoring, Vol.17, No.5, pp.445-448.

Pick, L. & Bauer, J. (2001). [Dentistry and epilepsy]. Der Nervenarzt, Vol.72, No.12, pp.946-949.

Rao, A. (2008). Dental Management of Handicapped Children. In: *Principles and practice of pedodontics* (pp.348-350). Jaypee Brothers Medical Publishers, 8184483457, New Delhi.

Robbins, M. R. (2009). *Dental management of special needs patients who have epilepsy.* Dental Clinics Of North America, Vol.53, No.2, pp.295-309, ix.

Roger, J. (2005). Epileptic Syndromes, In: *Infancy, Childhood And Adolescence* (3 ed.), 0-86196-320-2, John Libbey Eurotext Ltd, 2005.

Sasaki, T. & Maita, E. (1998). *Increased bFGF level in the serum of patients with phenytoin-induced gingival overgrowth.* Journal Of Clinical Periodontology, Vol.25, No.1, pp.42-47.

Sato, Y.; Kondo, I.; Ishida, S.; Motooka, H.; Takayama, K.; Tomita, Y., et al. (2001). *Decreased bone mass and increased bone turnover with valproate therapy in adults with epilepsy.* Neurology, Vol.57, No.3, pp.445-449.

Seymour, R. A.; Smith, D. G. & Turnbull, D. N. (1985). *The effects of phenytoin and sodium valproate on the periodontal health of adult epileptic patients.* Journal Of Clinical Periodontology, Vol.12, No.6, pp.413-419.

Seymour, R. A. (1992). Selected side effects: 7. Phenytoin and gingival overgrowth. Prescr. J., No.32, pp.124-126.

Sheller, B. (2004). *Orthodontic Management of Patients with Seizure Disorders.* Semin Orthod, Vol.10, pp.247-251.

Stoopler, E. T.; Sollecito, T. P. & Greenberg, M. S. (2003). *Seizure disorders: update of medical and dental considerations.* General Dentistry, Vol.51, No.4, pp.361-366; quiz 367.

Tan, H.; Gurbuz, T. & Dagsuyu, I. M. (2004). *Gingival enlargement in children treated with antiepileptics.* J Child Neurol, Vol.19, No.12, pp.958-963.

Thomason, J. M.; Seymour, R. A. & Rawlins, M. D. (1992). *Incidence and severity of phenytoin-induced gingival overgrowth in epileptic patients in general medical practice.* Community Dentistry And Oral Epidemiology, Vol.20, No.5, pp.288-291.

Turner, M. D. & Glickman, R. S. (2005). *Epilepsy in the oral and maxillofacial patient: current therapy.* J Oral Maxillofac Surg, Vol.63, No.7, pp.996-1005.

10

Clinical Features of Epilepsy Secondary to Neurocysticercosis at the Insular Lobe

Humberto Foyaca-Sibat and Lourdes de Fátima Ibañez Valdés
Division of Neurology, Nelson Mandela Academic Hospital,
School of Medicine, Faculty of Health Sciences,
Walter Sisulu University, Mthatha,
South Africa

1. Introduction

1.1 Background

Neurocysticercosis is eradicable parasitic zoonoses of the brain if it is manages by public health sector and agricultural sector with the dedicated support of veterinarian doctors. Neurocysticercosis is the only zoonotic infection which has been considered as eradicable by the World Health Assembly. Therefore, we will focus on that, and other parasitic zoonoses causing epilepsy will be discussed in another chapter. In this chapter new aspect about insular epilepsy secondary to NC will be introduced as well.

Like other pathological disorders, early diagnosis and treatment can significantly decrease morbidity and mortality rates of parasitic infections. Diseases that have their origins in infected animals, such as H1N1 influenza or SARS have highlighted the need for a better understanding of their origin on an affected animal.

The ease and speed of modern travel facilitates the spread of diseases once confined to specific geographic areas, as recently occurred with the widely publicized H1N1 influenza. Animal migration and trade pose a similar threat, as was shown by the outbreaks in the United States of West Nile fever, and monkey-pox, two diseases haven't previously known in the Western Hemisphere. Each of these examples highlights the need for accurate, up-to-date information and ongoing research on those public health problems. (Carabin, personal communication, 2010)

Pig farming has increased considerably during the past decade in Eastern and Southern Africa (ESA); especially in rural, resource-poor, smallholder communities where sanitation is poor. Hence, it is highly suspected that the frequency of epilepsy secondary to NC in the region may further increase in the foreseeable future. We see a lot of pigs affected by cysticercosis free of neurological signs but when there is a sign it can indicate the etiology of human's disease. Let us to address it in a better way, for example pigs with NC do not suffer of epilepsy, however presence of cysticercosis of pigs (intermediate host) indicates that NC is the most likely cause of epilepsy of peoples living around, being yet another reason to support that health worker and agriculture worker should work together in this field. In places where there are not clinical health laboratory facilities and CT/MR images or simply patients have not free to these investigations and the prevalence of epilepsy is considerably high we do suggest to confirm diagnosis of cysticercosis on pig's population by physical inspection of the tongue (Figure 1).

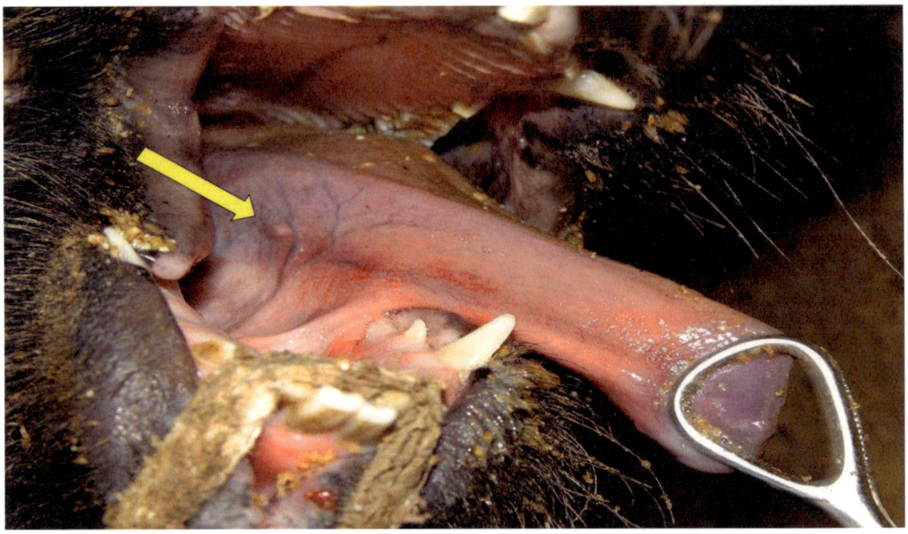

Fig. 1. A cystic lesion on the tongue in a pig affected by cysticercosis is pointed by the yellow arrow. Photo taken by Prof. RC Krecek (CWGESA)

The other choice is to take blood samples from jugular veins (Figure 2) and request ELISA for cysticercosis at the nearest veterinarian laboratory. It may help suspecting the etiological diagnosis of epilepsy in these patients and to support their treatment.

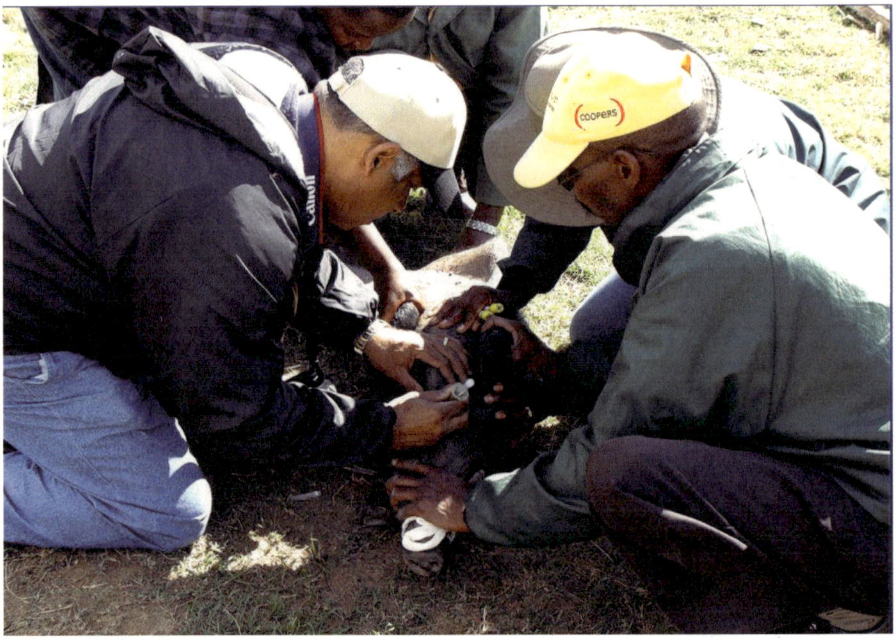

Fig. 2. Shows agricultural workers and Prof. Foyaca taken a blood sample from the jugular veins in infected pig. (Photo taken by Prof RC Krecek)

Taenia solium cysticercosis' life cycle starts when humans become infected by eating undercooked pork containing cysticerci (See figure 3) and later they develop taeniosis. People with taeniosis pass eggs with their faeces which are ingested by humans and pigs.

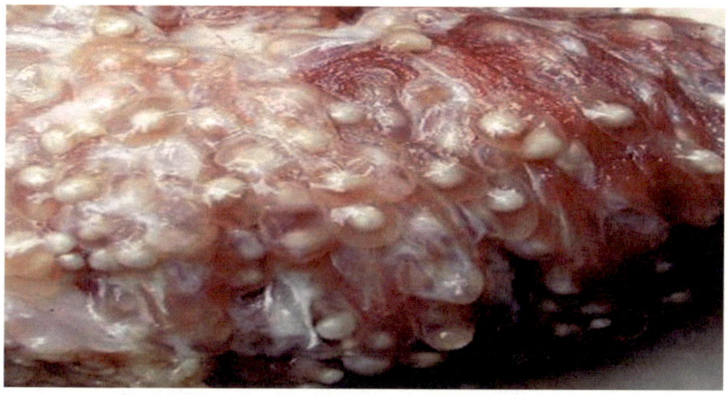

Fig. 3. Shows a maseter muscle from infected pig containing numerous cysticerci. Photo taken by Prof. A Lee (CWGESA).

Seems to be that measly pork meat has been described long ago according to this sentence found in ancient documents:

In 384-323 BC, Aristotle said:
When only a few measles are found the meat is sweet, but when numerous, the meat becomes watery and unpalatable."

Eggs develop into larval cysts causing human and porcine cysticercosis. Risk factors for taeniosis include the consumption of undercooked infected pork meat and inadequate meat inspection. Risk factors of cysticercosis include free-range pig farming, poor sanitation, close contact of humans and pigs and inadequate hygiene of food handlers. (See graphic 1)

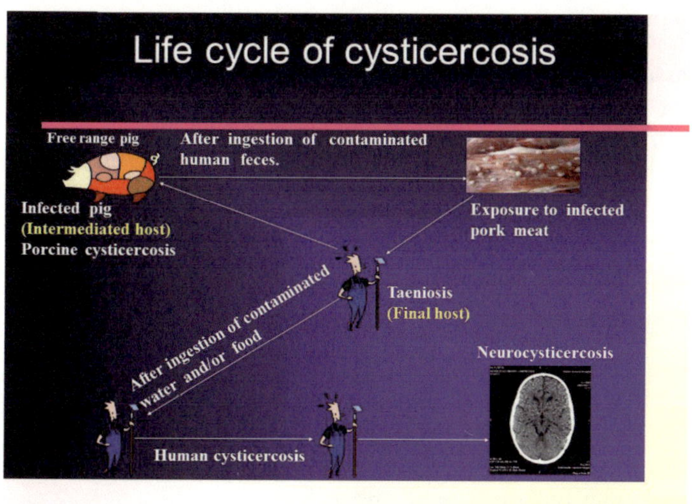

Graphic 1. Shows the life cycle of T Solium cysticercosis and the path toward to NC. Graphic modified from by Prof. Carabin. (CWGESA)

Cysticercosis is thus strongly associated with poverty and other socio-economic-cultural problems (Del Rio & Foyaca-Sibat, 2005, 2005a, 2007, 20008; Foyaca-Sibat & Del Rio, 2004, 2005, 2005a). In both humans and pigs, cysts migrate mostly to the subcutaneous tissue, skeletal muscle, the eye, and the central nervous system (CNS). Currently, NC is not only the major cause of acquired epilepsy in many developing countries, but is also of growing concern in northern/western countries due to globalization and immigration of infected people as before-cited.

In South Africa, epilepsy secondary to NC is quite common in ECP particularly in the poor, former black homeland, rural areas of the former Transkei, where pigs are allowed to roam freely and sanitation facilities are inadequate or nonexistent. Pig keeping and pork consumption have increased significantly during the past decade especially in rural smallholder communities, primarily due to the lack of grazing land for ruminants and the recognition of farmers of a quicker and more impressive return on their investment from raising pigs contact of humans and pigs and inadequate hygiene of food handlers.

Consumption of uninspected pork meat is undoubtedly a major source of human taeniasis. The transmission of *T. solium* to pigs, the essential partner in the pig-man-pig cycle, requires that pigs have access to human feces and that people consume improperly cooked pork.

The major risk factors related to transmission of eggs to pigs can be summarized as follows:

Extensive or free-range pig rearing
Outdoor human defecation near or in pig rearing areas
Use of pigs to scavenge and eat human feces ("sanitary policeman")
Deliberate use of human feces as pig feed
Connection of pig pens to human latrines ("pig sty privies");
Use of sewage effluent, sludge or "night soil" to irrigate and/or fertilize pig pastures and food crops
Involvement of humans' carriers in pig rearing and care.

The diagnostic assessment for NC was proposed by Del Brutto et al., (2001), and we used an abbreviated set of these criteria for the definition of NC in our studies.

Absolute criteria include:

cystic lesions showing the scolex on CT or MRI (See figure 4)
visualization of *T solium* on fundoscopy
demonstration of T solium from biopsied specimens

Other criteria are:

Major criteria:

cystic lesions without scolex, enhancing lesions
typical parenchyma brain calcifications
positive serum Ag-ELISA for cysticercosis

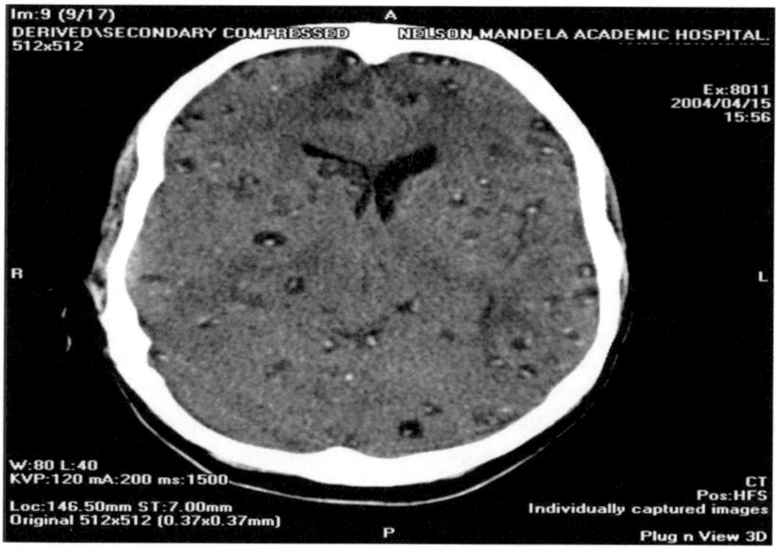

Fig. 4. CT scan of the brain showing multiple active cystic lesions and their scolex inside. Patient presenting tonic-clonic generalize and recurrent frontal lobe seizures.

Minor criteria:

lesions compatible with NC on neuroimaging studies
clinical manifestations of NC
cysticercosis outside the CNS

Epidemiological criteria:

evidence of household contact with peoples with cysticercosis
residence in a cysticercosis endemic area
visiting an endemic area for cysticercosis

For the present study, definite NC will be defined as: 1 absolute criteria or 2 major criteria or 1 major, 2 minor and 1 epidemiologic criterion; probable NC as: 1 major and 2 minor criteria or 1 major, 1 minor and 1 epidemiologic criterion or three minor and one epidemiologic criterion; and possible NC as: 1 major criteria or 2 minor criteria or 1 minor and 1 epidemiologic criterion.

The pilot study conducted by us at the Nelson Mandela Academic Hospital consisted of asking 57 epilepsy patients with confirmed NC, 52 epileptic patients without NC and 61 patients from the dermatology and ophthalmology clinics to answer a questionnaire interview about epilepsy and pig raising and management. A very preliminary analysis suggests that, using dermatology and ophthalmology clinic patients as the reference group, the POR of owning pigs and having NC was 6.8 (95% CI: 2.1-21.7) and the POR for consuming pork compared to never consume pork and having NC was 2.1 (0.7-6.2). Using the epilepsy patients without NC as the reference group, the POR of consuming pork in those with NC was 14.2 (5.1-39.5) and of owning pigs was 17.5 (5.4-56.2). Why the association between owning pigs and NC was stronger when the epilepsy patients were used as a reference group needs further investigation, but it is possible that the NC and 2the non-epilepsy groups came from rural areas whereas the epilepsy non-NC group came from more urban areas with less exposure to infected pigs. Further analyses will determine whether these results are confounded by the age of the patients or where they live (i.e. Persons who only had epilepsy may be more likely to live in more urbanized areas). We also participated in the pilot study conducted at the St-Elisabeth hospital from ECP in SA. We studied 433 consecutive patients consulting the outpatient clinic for suspected new-onset seizures or existing epilepsy cases. (Foyaca-Sibat et al., 2009)

Of these, 281 were diagnosed as recurrent focal or generalized motor seizures due to secondary epilepsy. Each consenting participant was administered the questionnaire and asked to provide a blood sample for a serological analysis of antibodies to and antigens of the larval stage of *T. solium*. Additionally, each week for consenting, randomly selected patients with the confirmed diagnosis of seizures disorder were transported to Mthatha for a CT scan of the brain and EEG. Among these 281 patients, the prevalence of seropositivity of antibodies to the larval stage of *T. solium* was 33% (95% CI: 27%-38%) in the 273 tested. Serological antigens were available for 189 patients with confirmed seizures or epilepsy. In this group the prevalence of seropositivity to antigens to *T. solium* was 8% (95%CI: 4.5%-13%). Modified from the original one done by Prof. Carabin. A total of 92 patients with recurrent seizures and who also completed a questionnaire were referred to Mthatha for a CT-scan. Of these, 34 (37.0%, 95%CI: 27.1%-47.7%) had a definite diagnosis of NC, 14 of whom had active lesions visible on CT, 39 (42%) had no CT abnormality, and 19 (21%) had other, undefined non-NC calcifications. The age of the NC cases ranged from 5 to 67 years old whereas the epilepsy cases ranged from 5 to 76 years old. Antibody ELISA results were available for 33 of the 34 patients classified as probable NC and for all 39 without NC. The predictive value of a positive antibody test in identifying NC in persons with epilepsy was 60% (95% CI: 41%-77%)._Serological results for antigen ELISA were available for 23 confirmed NC cases and 22 non-NC cases. The predictive value of a positive antigen test in identifying NC in persons with epilepsy was 67% (95% CI: 22%-96%). Thus, it is clear that serology alone cannot be used to diagnose NC in this population. HIV status was available from 50 patients with epilepsy. Among the 47 patients with antibody ELISA results available, the antibody seroprevalence of T. solium was 30.0% among HIV positive patients and 48.1% among HIV negative patients. Interestingly, among the 33 patients with antigen ELISA results, the antigen seroprevalence of *T. solium* was 16.7% among the HIV positive patients but only 9.5% among the HIV negative patients. Even though these results are based on a very small sample, it does suggest that HIV patients may be less able to mount a detectable antibody response to cysticercosis but might be more likely to be infected with active cysts. A total of 22 of these patients (13 HIV negative and 9 HIV positive) were referred for a CT-scan. Of these, five HIV negative and seven HIV positive patients had CT evidence of NC with two HIV negative and five HIV positive patients harboring active cysts. These very preliminary and imprecise results do suggest that there may be an association between NC and HIV infection. (Foyaca-Sibat et al., 2009)

2. Other types of epilepsy secondary to neurocysticercosis

2.1 Occipital lobe epilepsy secondary to neurocysticercosis

In our series patients presenting occipital lobe epilepsy usually is reporting

Structured visual hallucinations and moving colored shapes
Flashes light and transitory cortical blindness
Forced blinking and eyelid flutter follow by horizontal gaze deviation.

Calcified NC with or without perilesional edema is the most common cause. This presentation is uncommon despite it has been underestimated importantly. It can be associated to insula epilepsy or other types of epilepsy mainly in multiple calcified NC. Seems to be that measly pork meat has been described long ago according to this sentence. The medication of choice is carbamazepine.

Menon (2007) reported two young patients with symptomatic occipital lobe epilepsy due to discrete lesions of cysticercosis were misdiagnosed and treated for 2 years as migraine with visual aura. The patients suffered from frequent visual seizures often followed by migraine-like headache. Seizures manifested with colored and mainly circular elementary visual hallucinations of up to 1 minute duration. Headache, often severe and of long duration, was frequently associated with nausea, photophobia, and phonophobia. Both patients became seizure-free with appropriate treatment of the underlying disease and epileptic seizures.

2.2 Frontal lobe epilepsy secondary to neurocysticercosis

Clinical features of epileptic seizures may help to identify the specific frontal region of onset. (So, 1998; Kotagal & Arunkumar, 1998) as follow:

Dominant hemisphere involvement= Prominent speech disturbances
Supplementary motor area= Unilateral or asymmetric bilateral tonic posturing and facial grimacing, vocalization, or speech arrest; somatosensory aura; and complex automatisms such as kicking, laughing, or pelvic thrusting
Primary motor cortex= focal simple motor seizures with clonic or myoclonic movements
Medial frontal, cingulate gyrus, orbitofrontal, or frontopolar regions=Complex behavioural events (motor agitation and gestural automatisms) ; viscerosensory symptoms and strong emotional feelings; pelvic thrusting, pedalling, or thrashing, vocalizations, laughter, or crying.
Dorsolateral cortex=- Tonic posturing or clonic movements often associated with either contralateral head and eye deviation, or less commonly, ipsilateral head turn
Operculum= Swallowing, salivation, mastication, epigastric aura, fear, and speech arrest often associated with clonic facial movements and gustatory hallucinations.

This modality of seizures often bizarre and diagnosed incorrectly as psychogenic and can be associated to insular seizures. Despite calcified NC is the commonest cause no always locations of the lesions cause same clinical manifestations and quite often some lesions remain silent for years.

2.2.1 Nocturnal frontal lobe epilepsy

Patients presenting nocturnal occipital lobe epilepsy (NFLE) usually report

Seizure clusters occurring only during sleep
The history of similar events with other family members (Autosomal dominant)
The frenetic or agitated appearance of onset and normal intelligent
Dystonic posturing, jerking, bending, and rocking; difficult to distinguish from parasomnias

With nocturnal frontal lobe epilepsy, seizures begin shortly after falling asleep or in the early hours before awakening with a gasp, grunt, hums, moan or word, and are followed by sudden thrashing movements. Patients remain conscious but can neither control the movements nor speak. Thrashing can be vigorous enough to throw the patient out of bed, which can result in possible injury. Nocturnal frontal lobe epilepsy is typically treated with carbamazepine and, in some cases, surgery. We did not identify this type of seizures in our series. If there is evidence of NC on imagenology then a diagnosis of NFLE is ruled out.

2.3 Parietal lobe epilepsy

Parietal lobe epilepsy is the least common of syndromes defined by the area of brain affected. Parietal seizures spread rapidly, producing a range of symptoms that are also seen with other syndromes. A few signs are typical but appear in less than half of children who have this syndrome. Among the symptoms are:

Tingling, pricking or crawling sensations upon the skin
The feeling of burning, itching or pain
Pain occurs in the extremities and sometimes in the abdomen

Patients can present an acute confusional state (delirium) and the commonest affected parts of the body are: upper limbs and face. Partial seizures are divided into two major categories, simple and complex. Simple partial seizures occur in full consciousness; complex partial seizures occur with impaired awareness that ranges from slight to complete unconsciousness. (Epileptic Foundation)

2.4 Mesial temporal lobe epilepsy

Seizures often begin with auras or conscious feelings of a rising sensation from the stomach and of fear
One of the sensory perceptions may also be triggered
Impaired awareness follows, typically with staring and movements of the lips, tongue or jaw
Fumbling, picking or gesturing may also occur

3. Insular lobe

Remembering the lost island of Atlantis, this lobe remains hidden and lies submerged beneath the parietal, frontal, and temporal opercular cortices, buried under a tangled web of middle cerebral artery branches. The insula is not visible from the surface of the brain, it's the best protected region of the whole cerebral cortex, and the poorest studied region all over the brain; IL represents a remarkable challenge for further researchers among new generations of neurologists, neurophysiologists, neuroinmunologists, and neuropathologist among others. Some functions of the right insular lobe are a little bit known such as its role in taste perception its intensity and recognition for the ipsilateral tongue (rostrodorsal insula) and some functions of the left insular cortex for the intensity of the stimulus ipsilateral to the tongue and taste recognition bilaterally, gustatory mechanism, movements of the mouth, and oropharyngeal swallowing (anterior insular) are not well known neither, and almost nothing has been demonstrated about the role of the insular lobe over the amygdala complex and emotional behavior. The human IL is also considered as paralimbic cortex, because of its connections with limbic and sensorimotor cortices, the IL is believed to play a role in affective and attention aspects of human behavior as well. Paralimbic insular regions have functional specialization for behaviors requiring integration between extra personal stimuli and the internal milieu. Based on these connections, one might expect that lesions of the insular cortex may result in disorders of neglect (Foyaca-Sibat & Ibañez-Valdés, 2006).

3.1 Insula lobe epilepsy

3.1.1 Background

Insular lobe epilepsy (ILE) and insular lobe seizures (ILS) are still not included in the current classification for epileptic seizures, epilepsy or epileptic syndromes belong to "The International League Against Epilepsy" therefore most of neurologists, epileptologists, clinician pediatrician, and general practitioner do not include this entity in their list of differential diagnosis in patients presenting "aberrant" types of temporal lobe epilepsy (TLE), "stereotype" simple focal seizures and others. Insular seizures may mimic temporal, parietal or frontal lobe seizures and may coexist with seizures from other lobes.

The electroencephalographic (EEG) studies of the insula lobe (IL) are not confident because it is the only cortical part of the brain that is not accessible at the surface of the cerebral hemisphere, because it is totally covered by the fronto-parietal and temporal opercula, therefore accuracy of EEG made by surface electrode is uncertain.

The insula is one of the five cerebral lobes and its cortex is situated deep within each hemisphere. It is overlayed by the frontal and temporal neocortex and this explains how difficult it should be to get a reliable EEG sampling from the insular cortex and to define an "insular epileptic syndrome" as has been done with temporal lobe epilepsy. Adequate sampling from the insula can only be obtained by depth or subdural electrodes' implantation or acute intraoperative electrocorticography. Depth or subdural electrodes implantation of the insular faces some technical problems. There is substantial evidence that the insula is involved as a somesthetic area, including a major role in the process of nociceptive input. The role of the insula in some epileptic patients was recently investigated by means of depth electrode recordings made following Talairach's stereoelectroencephalography (SEEG) methodology. It appears that ictal signs associated with an insular discharge is very similar to those usually attributed to mesial temporal lobe seizures (Robles et al, 2009]) others authors reported: sensation of laryngeal constriction and paresthesiae, often unpleasant, affecting large cutaneous territories, most often at the onset of a complex partial seizure (five of the six patients) as a common presentation [Isnard J, et al., 2004] while other said: the most common clinical feature associated with damage to the insula is the complex partial seizures with involvement of the visceral sensations (Duffau H, et al., 2002). Different authors reported ictal symptoms associated with insular discharges mainly made up of respiratory, viscerosensitive (chest or abdominal constriction), or oroalimentary (chewing or swallowing) manifestations. Unpleasant somatosensory manifestation always opposite the discharging side, are also frequent and they concluded that Ictal signs arising from the insula occur in full consciousness; these are always simple partial seizures. Seizures arising from the temporal lobe always invade the insular region, but in approximately 10% of cases, the seizures originate in the insular cortex itself (Isnard, 2004; Guenot, 2008). In 2005, Isnard studied 50 patients using intrainsular electrodes and found that the clinical presentation of insular lobe seizures was a simple partial seizures occurring in full consciousness patient, beginning with a sensation of laryngeal constriction followed by paresthesiae that were often unpleasant affecting large cutaneous territories. These initial symptoms were eventually followed by dysarthric speech and/or elementary auditory hallucinations, and seizures often ended with focal dystonic postures. Four years later he studied 164 patients in whom 472 insular electrodes were implanted, he again found that clinical presentation of insular lobe seizures are that of simple partial seizures occurring in full consciousness, beginning with a sensation of laryngeal constriction followed by paresthesia that were often unpleasant on extensive cutaneous territories. These initial symptoms were eventually followed by dysarthric speech and/or elementary auditory hallucinations, and seizures often ended with focal dystonic postures. He was able to reproduce several of the spontaneous ictal symptoms in the six patients with insular seizures. (Isnard, 2009). Looking into other ways to check clinical features of IL due to focal lesions, we reviewed what happen in patients presenting NC on the IL.

According to the publications made in the last decade, very little is known about NC on the IL (Foyaca-Sibat & Ibañez-Valdés, 2006). It is important to highlight that it is a dangerous location of NC because apart from epilepsy other complications such as: autonomic dysfunction (Oppenheimer et al., 2001), neurogenic heart (Tamayo & Hachinski, 2003), electrocardiographic changes (Blumhardt et al., 1986) and sudden unexpected death in epilepsy [SUDEP] (Leestma, 1984; Mc Gugan, 1999; Langan Y, 2000) can occur

The main aim of our study was to identify ictal manifestations in patients presenting focal lesions (NC) on the IL proved by imagenology. To our knowledge, it is the first time that results from ILE secondary to focal NC in a case-control study are reported in the medical literature.

3.2 Material and method

3.2.1 Participants and study area

This is an epidemiological descriptive study of patients diagnosed as NC from Umtata General Hospital and Nelson Mandela Academic Hospital (South Africa) from January 2004 to January 2010 who were selected for a case control study in the project Neurocysticercosis protocol. (Database, n=3015). All selected patients were included in group A or group B.

3.2.2 Inclusion criteria:

Group A: fulfilled the following selected criteria:

1.-Positive serology ELISA test for cysticercosis
2.-CT/MRI images of the brain with intravenous contrast or gadolinium enhancement, consistent with definitive evidence of active and calcified NC on the insula lobe suitable to evaluate: ictal manifestations.
3.-Positive serology ELISA test for cysticercosis
4.-ELISA test for HIV/AIDS

Group B:

1.-NC on the temporal lobe and similar age group
2.-CT/MRI images of the brain with intravenous contrast or gadolinium enhancement, consistent with definitive evidence of active and calcified NCC on the temporal lobe suitable to evaluate: ictal manifestation.
3.-Positive serology ELISA test for cysticercosis
4.-ELISA test for HIV/AIDS

Demographic and clinical data were obtained through interviews with the patients and their relatives.

The differences between groups A and B were evaluated for statistical significance with the use of Statistical Package for the Social Sciences version 16.0 for windows (SPSS Inc., Chicago, Ill)

All patients received 800 mg of albendazole and 40 mg of prednisone per os daily for a week as part of treatment for NC and 200mg of carbamazepine orally every 8 hour to control epileptic seizures.

All images were acquired on the same CT scan and MR images using a three-dimensional T1-fast field echo sequence providing an isotropic voxel size of 1 mm^3. Images underwent correction for no uniform intensity and were linearly registered into a standardized stereotaxic space. The interval between the first and last scan was 31 ± 21 months (range = 10 to 52).

3.2.3 Exclusion criteria

Epilepsy due to other causes
Terminal diseases, serious psychological illnesses, active addictions to psychoactive substances
Patients younger than 13 years old, pregnant ladies, patients on HAART
No written consent.

3.2.4 Withdrawal criteria

Any event that may lead to a situation that discourages the intervention or that may prevent communication with the healthcare professional.

3.2.5 Ethical aspects

Written informed consent was obtained in the first assessment of eligible patients for participation. All patients received information on the study's objective and procedures in addition to ethical considerations, including and the participant's right to intimacy, anonymity, confidentiality, withdrawal, and information. Both investigators completed CITI training-course on the Protection of Human Research and sworn to the Hippocratic Oath and committed to respecting the norms of good clinical practice, as well as the requirements of the Helsinki Declaration.

Methods for patient selection and information processing was accepted by clinical governance at Mthatha General Complex, and approval From the University of Transkei, and Walter Sisulu University IRB and the respective Ethical Committees (UNITRA:0018/05, and WSU:0068/009) were obtained.

3.3 Results and comments

The total number of patients with ILE due to unilateral calcified and active NC on the IL in our database is 21 and its prevalence is 0.69%. Four patients (19%) from this group presented an associated ischemic stroke due to infectious vasculitis. Three of them were HIV-positive (See figure 5)

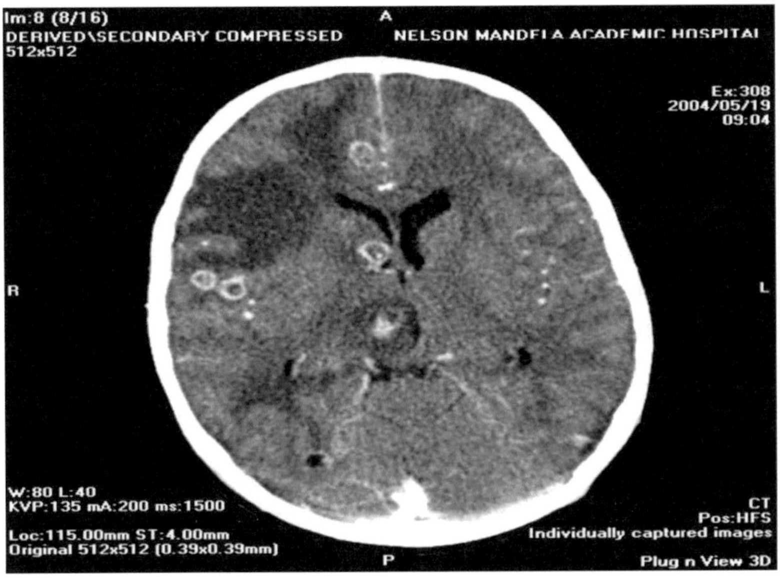

Fig. 5. CT scan of the brain shows calcified and active NC, some ring enhancing lesion is seen. Hypodensity lesion secondary to ischemic stroke on the right frontal and insular lobes with partial compression of the right lateral ventricle is also observed.

Demographic features are summarized in Table 1 and no remarkable differences among both groups including HIV status were found.

Groups	Age	Gender (%)		HIV (%)		
	Mean (Std)	Male	Female	+	-	Unknown
A (n=21)	32.2 (16.9)	49.1	50.9	13.9	31.2	54.9
B (n=22)	31.9 (15.3)	47.9	52.1	15.7	28.8	55.6

Table 1. Demographics characteristics

Commonest ictal manifestations with statistical significance (p>0.0001) were: sensation of laryngeal constriction (n=16) and unpleasant paresthesia (n=9) in fully conscious patients. See Table 2 and Graphic 1.

Less common problems without statistical value were: dysphagia, levitation and mild chest oppression.

Group	A	B	Fisher test X^2	OR (CI=95.0 %)
Laryngeal constriction	**76%** (n=16)	18.4% (n=3)	***P*< 0.0001** 21.390	**20.26**(Wolf=4.18)
Unpleasant paresthesia	**42.8%** (n=9)	4.54% (n=1)	***P*< 0.0001** 8.836	**15.75**(Wolf=1.77)
Dysphagia	38.09% (n=8)	9.09% (n=2)	*P*= 0.0281 5.064	6.15 (Wolf=1.12)
Levitation	23.80% (n=5)	4.54% (n=1)	*P*= 0.0918 3.321	6.25 (Wolf=0.61)

Table 2. Clinical features commonest found

Patients with NC on the temporal lobe presented TLE or partial secondary to generalized motor seizures except one who complained of a sensation of laryngeal constriction, perioral parentheses and sense of levitation and later loss of consciousness and tonic-clonic secondary generalized seizures.

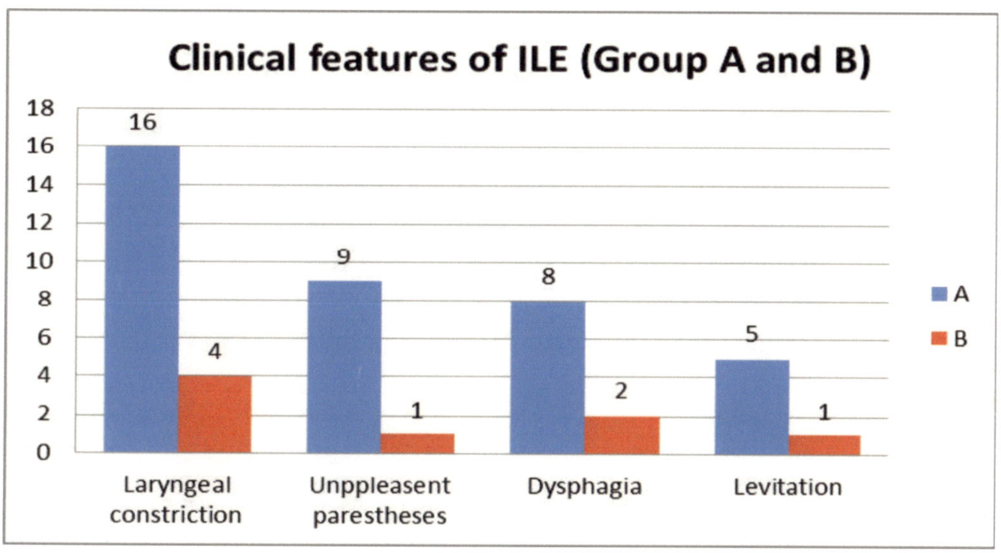

Source: Table 2

Graphic 1. Clinical features of insula lobe epilepsy

We tried to correlate the location of the lesion and ictal manifestation considering NC lesion small enough to produce non additional damage on surrounding tissue avoiding situations reported by Roper et al. in 1993 and Duffau in 2003. They described insular epilepsy in patients presenting seizures involved visceral sensory hallucinations followed by motor automatism and motor seizures with somatic sensory hallucinations and then produced visceral motor effects. Unfortunately, they studied patients with mass lesion (low-grade astrocytoma) big enough to involve the temporal lobe region. In our series, lesions of NC active or calcified measured less than 15 mm in both groups to assure that no surrounding tissue was affected. Fortunately, we also had previous information about insular NC from a pilot study made five years back (Foyaca-Sibat & Ibañez-Valdés, 2006) and based on those results we refined our selecting criteria. Our prevalence of ILE is low because it is an uncommon epileptic disorder.

Previous studies based on video ictal recordings, and direct electric insular stimulation of the insular cortex for presurgical evaluation of temporal lobe epilepsy described clinical features of ictal manifestation on IL eventually followed by dysarthric speech and focal motor convulsive symptoms no present in our series. Other clinical manifestation in our series including speech problems, neurogenic heart and sudden unexpected death were not included for statistical analysis at this time because were not considered in our objectives.

Some patients became a little bit surprised when we asked for some symptoms that they did not expressed before because these symptoms did not recall attention from patients and relatives which may contribute to an underestimate prevalence of this type of seizures mainly in patients presenting it sporadically . A fully conscious patient with laryngeal discomfort, dyspnea, unpleasant perioral or somatic paresthesia, and dysarthric speech, followed by somatomotor symptoms, implies an insular onset and a good respond to antiepileptic treatment can help to confirm it.

Antiparasitic treatment for NC at the IL should be prescribed with caution because the risk of developing complications such as: the neurogenic heart and/or SUDEP. One patient from this series died because subendocardic hemorrhage probable due to active and calcified NC on the right insula cortex documented by postmortem examination (See figure 6)

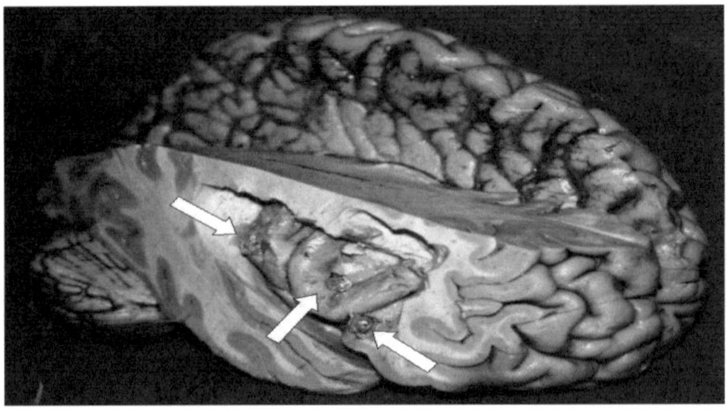

Fig. 6. Lateral view of the right insular lobe fixed in formalin. One cyst with the scolex inside (in vesicualr stage) on anterior insula is seen, another cyst without scolex with turbid fluid-filled oval cysts and local inflammatory reaction on the middle-anterior (agranular) insula is observed. Left insula was normal and no other cysts were found all over the brain. Cause of death: SUDEP/Neurogenic heart (subendocardial hemorrhage)

3.3.1 Sudden unexpected death in epilepsy secondary to neurocysticercosis

Although largely neglected in earlier literature, sudden unexpected death in epilepsy (SUDEP) is the most important epilepsy-related mode of death, and is the leading cause of death in people with chronic uncontrolled epilepsy. Research during the past two to three decades has shown that incidence varies substantially depending on the epilepsy population studied, ranging from 0–09 per 1000 patients-years in newly diagnosed patients to 9 per 1000 patient-years in candidates for epilepsy surgery.(Tomson et al., 2008)

By definition, the cause of death in SUDEP is currently unknown, but it is very probable that cardiac arrhythmia during and between seizures plays a potential role. It has been suggested on postmortem studies and interictal cardiac abnormalities observed (Falconer & Rajs, 1976; Leestma, 1989; Ryvlin et al., 2006; Stollberger & Finsterer, 2004). Several suggestions have been made concerning the mechanisms behind SUDEP, most involving speculations on the possible role of autonomic effects such as cardiorespiratory disturbances. Clinical and experimental studies have shown that physical activity can decrease seizure frequency, as well as lead to improved cardiovascular and psychological health in patients with epilepsy (Arida et al., 2007). Information concerning risk factors for SUDEP is conflicting, but potential risk factors include: cold temperatures (Scorza et al., 2007), certain seizure types (Foyaca-Sibat &Ibañez-Valdés, 2006; Kloster & Engelskojon,1999), early adulthood (Lesstma,1997) early onset of epilepsy (Nilsson, 1999), long duration of epilepsy (Walczak et al., 2001), uncontrolled TLE (Walczak et al., 2001; Speling et al.,1999), high seizure frequency(Lagan & Nashef, 2005), and higher numbers of AED (Nilsson et al.,2001) and. Additionally, potential pathomechanisms for SUDEP are unknown, but it is very probable that cardiac arrhythmias during and between seizures, electrolyte disturbances, arrhythmogenic drugs or transmission of epileptic activity to the heart via the autonomic nervous system potentially play a role (Stollberger & Finsterer, 2004). An increasing number of reports about SUDEP secondary to NC are seen on the medical literature gradually (Holmes, 2010) more details about SUDEP can be found in the other chapters of this book.

Mortality due to epilepsy is a significant concern._Patients with epilepsy have a mortality rate significantly higher compared with the general population. The standardized mortality rate (SMR) is shown to be 1.6-9.3 times higher in this group (Nouri, 2011). Based on our observations we consider that ILE can be differentiated from TLE if patients remain fully conscious during the attack. When epileptic activity spread from IL to temporal lobe or vice versa then clinical differentiation can be almost impossible to perform.

If the above-cited features are not keeping in mind, diagnosis of ILE never going to be made and cardiac complications or SUDEP may happen.

We have hypothesized that NC on the temporal lobe can cause ictal manifestations which can be spread to the IL leading to a combination of TLE and ILE but most symptoms from IL are masked by those from TLE even before patients become unconscious. Further investigation should be made to reach final conclusions. In our experience, this sequence of ictal symptoms: laryngeal constriction, perioral paresthesia, dysphagia, and sense of levitation look reliable enough to characterize insular lobe epileptic seizures secondary to NC. To our knowledge, it is the first time that results from ILE secondary to focal NC in a case-control studies are reported.

4. Acknowledgment

We like to express our gratitude to all veterinarian doctors working in this field particularly: Professors Rosina Tammi Krecek, Albert Lee Willingham, Linda Cowan, Samson Mukaratiwua and other members of the Cysticercosis Working Group for Eastern and Southern Africa (CWGESA) for their dedications and commitment.

Special thanks to Professor Helen Carabin from the Department of Biostatistics and Epidemiology College of Public Health University of Oklahoma Health Sciences Center for her invaluable enthusiasm, persistence, and leadership in our research team.

We want to thanks to all radiologists and radiographers from Nelson Mandela Academic Hospital and Inkhosi Albert Luthuli Central Hospital in South Africa for their contribution to this study.
Special thanks are due to the Cuban Ministry of Health, the Institute of Tropical Medicine Pedro Kouri, authorities of Faculty of Health Sciences and Directorate: Research Development from Walter Sisulu University and Nelson Mandela Academic Hospital for their unconditional support.
We also acknowledge financial support from, Directorate of Research Development from Walter Sisulu University in South Africa, and South African Medical Research Council.
The founder had no role in study design, data collection and analysis, decision to publish, or the preparation of manuscript.
Finally, we wish to declare our eternal and deepest gratitude to our family, relatives, and colleagues for their unconditional and permanent support.
Finally, we wish to declare our eternal, deepest love and gratitude to Lorna María Foyaca García, Thabo Humberto Jorge Foyaca Ibañez and Fátima Susana Adolfina Foyaca Ibañez, because without their love and unconditional support this chapter would not have been written.

5. References

Arida RM, Cavalheiro EA, Silva AC, Colugnati DB, Pansani AP, Albuquerque M, Scorza FA. Sudden unexpected death in epilepsy: sudden death risk decreased by physical activity. Einstein. 2007; 5(3):281-286

Carabin H, Krecek RC, Cowan LD, Michael L, Foyaca-Sibat H, Nash T, Willingham AL "Estimation of the monetary burden of Taenia solium cysticercosis in the Eastern Cape, South Africa". Trop. Med. Int. Health.(ISSN: 1360-2276). 2006;11: 906-916.

Del Rio A, Foyaca-Sibat H, Ibañez-Valdés LdeF: Epidemiological Survey About Socio-Economic Characteristic Of Mpindweni Location, South Africa . The Internet Journal of Neurology. 2005 Volume 4 Number 2 http://www.ispub.com/journal/the_internet_journal_of_neurology/volume_4_number_2_27/article/epidemiological_survey_about_socio_economic_characteristic_of_mpindweni_location_south_africa.html

Del Rio-Romero AH, Foyaca-Sibat H, Ibañez-Valdés LdeF, Vega-Novoa E. Prevalence Of Epilepsy And General Knowledge About Neurocysticercosis At Nkalukeni Village, South Africa The Internet Journal of Neurology.2005 3(2) http://www.ispub.com/journal/the_internet_journal_of_neurology/volume_3_number_2_31/article/prevalence_of_epilepsy_and_general_knowledge_about_neurocysticiercosis_at_nkalukeni_village_south_africa.html

Del Rio-Romero A, Foyaca-Sibat H, Ibañez-Valdés LdeF: :Neuroepidemiological Survey For Epilepsy, Knowledge About Epilepsy, Neurocysticercosis And HIV/Aids At The Makaula Village In South Africa". The Internet Journal of Neurology.(ISSN: 1531-295X). 2007;7(3):41-49 http://www.ispub.com/journal/the_internet_journal_of_neurology/volume_7_number_2_5/article/neuroepidemiological_survey_for_epilepsy_knowledge_about_epilepsy_neurocysticercosis_and_hiv_aids_at_the_makaula_village_in_south_africa.html

Del Rio- Romero AI, Foyaca-Sibat H, Ibañez-Valdés LdeF: "Neuroepidemiology Findings As Contributors For Epilepsy Due To Neurocysticercosis At Mngceleni Location, South Africa". The Internet Journal of Neurology.(ISSN: 1531-295X). 2008;9(1):33-40 http://www.ispub.com/journal/the_internet_journal_of_neurology/volume_9_number_1_6/article/neuroepidemiology_findings_as_contributors_for_epilepsy_due_to_neurocysticercosis_at_mngceleni_location_south_africa.html

Dobesberger J, Ortler M, Unterberger I, Walser G, Falkenstetter T, Bodner T, Benke T, Bale R, Fiegele T, Donnemiller E, Gotwald T, Trinka E. Successful surgical treatment of insular epilepsy with nocturnal hypermotor seizures. *Epilepsia,* 49(1):159–162, 2008

Duffau H, Capelle L, Lopes M, Bitar A, Sichez AP, van Effenterre R. Medically intractable epilepsy from insular low-grade gliomas: improvement after an extended lesionectomy Acta Neurochir. 2002;144(6):563-573

Epileptic Foundation. Full free article available at the URL: http://www.epilepsyfoundation.org/infants/partialepilepsy.html (last review on Mach 09, 2011)

Falconer B, Rajs J. Post-mortem findings of cardiac lesions in epileptics: a preliminary report. Forensic Sci. 1976;8:63-71.

Foyaca-Sibat H, Ibañez-Valdés LdeF."Clinical trial of praziquantel and prednisone in rural patients with neurocysticercosis presenting recurrent epileptic attacks" The Internet Journal of Neurology 2002;2):41-50 http://www.ispub.com/journal/the_internet_journal_of_neurology/volume_1_number_2_39/article/clinical_trial_of_praziquantel_and_prednisone_in_rural_patients_with_neurocysticercosis_presenting_with_recurrent_epileptic_attacks.html

Foyaca-Sibat H, "Tapeworm and the brain" Journal of Sciences of Africa 2002;1:5-12 http://www.scienceofafrica.co.za/2002/june.worn.htm

Foyaca-Sibat H, Ibañez-Valdés LdeF, Awotedu A, Fernandez-Mena C,"Neurocysticercosis in the former Transkei" 7th Internet World Congress for Biomedical Sciences. Inabis2002 Conference Proceeding IBSN 2002-WX54-4689 http://www.inabis2002.org/poster-congress/area-01/01011/010117.pdf

Foyaca-Sibat H, Ibañez-Valdés LdeF."Intraventricular neurocysticercosis in HIV patients. Should be approaching surgically?" II International Congress of Neurosurgery on Internet. 2003 Conference Proceeding http://www.neuroc.sld.cu/paper/TL-neurocys.htm

Foyaca-Sibat H , Ibañez-Valdés LdeF & A. A. Awotedu : Effect Of Prednisone On Guillain-Barré Syndrome In HIV Positive Patients . The Internet Journal of Neurology. 2003 Volume 2 Number 1 http://www.ispub.com/journal/the_internet_journal_of_neurology/volume_2_number_1_37/article/effect_of_prednisone_on_guillain_barre_syndrome_in_hiv_positive_patients.html

Foyaca-Sibat H, Ibañez-Valdés LdeF "Enfermedad de Binswanger en pacientes con neurocysticercosis" III International Congress of Psychiatry on Internet. Conference Proceeding. http://www.psiquiatria.com/interpsiquis2003/9638

Foyaca-Sibat H, Ibañez-Valdés LdeF "Neuro-Behçet syndrome treated with herbal medication" Electron J Biomed 2003;1:1-9 http://www.ispub.com/journal/the_internet_journal_of_neurology/volume_2_number_2_34/article/neuro_behcet_s_syndrome_a_case_report.html

Foyaca-Sibat H, Ibañez-Valdés LdeF "Intraventricular neurocysticercosis in HIV patients" The Internet Journal of Neurology 2003;2(1):23-31 http://www.ispub.com/journal/the_internet_journal_of_neurology/volume_2_number_1_37/article/intraventricular_neurocysticercosis_in_hiv_positive_patients.html

Foyaca-Sibat H, Ibañez-Valdés LdeF."Pseudoseizures and Epilepsy in neurocysticercosis" Electron J Biomed 2003;2(2):20-29

http://www.uninet.edu/reb/2003/n2/2foyaca.html
Foyaca-Sibat H, Ibañez-Valdés LdeF "Neurocysticercosis in HIV-positive patients" The Internet Journal of Infectious Diseases 2003:2(2):15-23 http://www.ispub.com/ostia/index.php?xmlFilePath=journals/ijn/current.xml
Foyaca-Sibat H, Ibañez-Valdés LdeF: "Binswanger's disease and neurocysticercosis" The Internet Journal of Neurology 2003;2(1):11-21 http://www.ispub.com/journal/the_internet_journal_of_neurology/volume_2_number_1_37/article/binswanger_s_disease_and_neurocysticercosis.html
Foyaca- Sibat H, Ibañez-Valdés LdeF. Vascular demential type binswager's disease in patients with active neurocysticerocis. Electron Biomed / Electron J Biomed 2003;1(1):32-42 http://biomed.uninet.edu/2003/n1/foyaca.html
Foyaca-Sibat H, Ibañez-Valdés LdeF. "Pseudoseizures and Epilepsy in neurocysticercosis: some advices to Family Doctors" The Internet Journal of Neurology 2004:2(2):4-17 http://www.ispub.com/journal/the_internet_journal_of_neurology/volume_2_number_2_34/article/pseudoseizures_and_epilepsy_in_neurocysiticercosis_some_advice_for_family_doctors.html
Foyaca-Sibat H, Del Rio AR, Ibañez-Valdés LdeF, Vega-Novoa EC, Awotedu A. "Neuroepidemiological survey for Epilepsy and knowledge about neurocysticercosis at the Sidwadweni location, South Africa" Electron J Biomed 2004;2(1):40-48 http://www.biomed.edu/2004/n1/foyaca.html
Foyaca-Sibat H, Del Rio-Romero AH, Ibañez-Valdés LdeF, Vega-Novoa E. Neuroepidemiological Survey For Epilepsy And Knowledge About Neurocysticiercosis At the Ngqwala Location, South Africa. The Internet Journal of Neurology 2005 3(2) http://www.ispub.com/journal/the_internet_journal_of_neurology/volume_3_number_2_31/article/neuroepidemiological_survey_for_epilepsy_and_knowledge_about_neurocysticiercosis_at_ngqwala_location_south_africa.html
Foyaca-Sibat H, Del Rio-Romero A, Ibañez-Valdés LdeF : Prevalence Of Epilepsy And General Knowledge About Neurocysticercosis At the Ngangelizwe Location, South Africa . The Internet Journal of Neurology. 2005 Volume 4 Number 1 http://www.ispub.com/journal/the_internet_journal_of_neurology/volume_4_number_1_30/article/prevalence_of_epilepsy_and_general_knowledge_about_neurocysticercosis_at_ngangelizwe_location_south_africa.html
Foyaca-Sibat H. Ibañez-Valdés LdeF. Insular Neurocysticercosis: Our Finding and Review of the Medical Literature. The Internet Journal of Neurology 2006 vol 5 Number 2 http://www.ispub.com/journal/the_internet_journal_of_neurology/volume_5_number_2_19/article/insular_neurocysticercosis_our_findings_and_review_of_the_medical_literature.html
Foyaca-Sibat H, Ibañez-Valdés LdeF : Occipital Lobe Syndrome Due To Giant Intraparenchymal Neurocysticercosis . The Internet Journal of Neurology. 2006 Volume 5 Number 2 http://www.ispub.com/journal/the_internet_journal_of_neurology/volume_5_number_2_19/article/occipital_lobe_syndrome_due_to_giant_intraparenchymal_neurocysticercosis.html
Foyaca-Sibat H, RIA Del Rio: "Epilepsy, Neurocysticercosis and, Poverty at Mphumaze and Marhambeni Locations, in South Africa". The Internet Journal of Neurology (ISSN: 1531-295X). 2007;7(1):8-14

http://www.ispub.com/journal/the_internet_journal_of_neurology/volume_7_number_1_7/article/epilepsy_neurocysticercosis_and_poverty_at_mphumaze_and_marhambeni_locations_in_south_africa.html
Foyaca-Sibat H, Ibañez-Valdés LdeF: "Generalized Cysticercosis With Cardiac Involvement". The Internet Journal of Neurology.(ISSN: 1531-295X). 2007;7(2):6-11 http://www.ispub.com/journal/the_internet_journal_of_neurology/volume_7_number_2_5/article/generalized_cysticercosis_with_cardiac_involvement.html
Foyaca-Sibat H, Ibañez-Valdés LdeF, Del Rio IA: "Prevalence of Epilepsy and General Knowledge about Neurocysticercosis at Ngangelizwe Location, South Africa". The Internet Journal of Neurology.(ISSN: 1531-295X). 2005; 4(1):23-37 http://www.ispub.com/journal/the_internet_journal_of_neurology/volume_4_number_1_30/article/prevalence_of_epilepsy_and_general_knowledge_about_neurocysticercosis_at_ngangelizwe_location_south_africa.html
Foyaca-Sibat H, Ibañez-Valdés LdeF: "Co-morbidity of Spinal Cord Neurocysticercosis And Tuberculosis In A HIV-Positive Patient". The Internet Journal of Neurology. (ISSN: 1531-295X). 2007;7(3):5-10 http://www.ispub.com/journal/the_internet_journal_of_neurology/volume_7_number_2_5/article/comorbidity_of_spinal_cord_neurocysticercosis_and_tuberculosis_in_a_hiv_positive_patient.html
Foyaca-Sibat H, Del Rio- Romero AI: "Prevalence Of Epilepsy In An Endemic Area For Neurocysticercosis In South Africa". The Internet Journal of Neurology.(ISSN: 1531-295X). 2008;9(1):8-18 http://www.ispub.com/journal/the_internet_journal_of_neurology/volume_9_number_1_6/article/prevalence_of_epilepsy_in_an_endemic_area_for_neurocysticercosis_in_south_africa.html
Foyaca-Sibat H Cowan LD, Carabin H, Serrano-Ocaña G, , Krecek RC, Willingham A. "Accuracy of the serological exam for the diagnosis of neurocysticercosis in outpatients with epilepsy, Eastern Cape Province, South Africa" PLOS Negleted Trop.Dis.Dec.2009;3(3):1-7
Foyaca-Sibat H, Ibañez-Valdés LdeF & J. Moré-Rodríguez : Parasitic Zoonoses Of The Brain: Another Challenger?. The Internet Journal of Neurology. 2010 Volume 12 Number 2 http://www.ispub.com/journal/the_internet_journal_of_neurology/volume_12_number_2_4/article/parasitic-zoonoses-of-the-brain-another-challenger.html
Geier S, Bancaud J, Talairach J, Bonis A, Szikla G, Enjelvin M. The seizures of frontal lobe epilepsy. A study of clinical manifestations. *Neurology1997;* 27:951–958.
Guenot M, Isnard J. Epilepsy and insula. Neurochirugie. 2008;54(3):374-378
Holmes N, Iles L, Andrew D, Korman T Neurocysticercosis Causing Sudden Death. Amer J Forensic Med & Pathology. 2010;31(2):117-119
Ibañez-Valdés LdeF & Foyaca-Sibat H. Refractory epilepsy in neurocysticercosis. The Internet Journal of Neurology. 2006;5(2):34-41 http://www.ispub.com/journal/the_internet_journal_of_neurology/volume_5_number_2_19/article/refractory_epilepsy_in_neurocysticercosis.html
Ibañez-Valdés LdeF & Foyaca-Sibat H. "Neurogenic heart secondary to insular stroke and neurocysticercosis" International Journal of Stroke (ISSN 1747-4949). 2006;1(1):68.
Isnard J, Guenot M, Sindou M, Mauguiere F. Clinical Manifestations of Insular Lobe Seizures: A Stereo-electroencephalographic Study. Epilepsia. 2004;45:1079–1090.
Isnard J, Mauquiere F. The insula in partial epilepsy. Rev Neurol (Paris). 2005;16(1):17-26
Isnard J. Insular epilepsy: A model of cryptic epilepsy. The Lyon experience. Rev Neurol (Paris). 2009;165(10):746-749

Kloster R, Engelskjon T. Sudden unexpected death in epilepsy (SUDEP): a clinical perspective and a search for risk factors. J Neurol Neurosurg Psychiatr. 1999;67:439-44.

Kotagal P, Arunkumar GS. Lateral frontal lobe seizures. *Epilepsia*. 1998;39(4):62-68

Langan Y, Nashef L, Sander JW. Case-control study of SUDEP. Neurology. 2005;64:1131-1133.

Leestma JE, Walczak T, Hughes JR, Kalelkar MB, Teas SS. A prospective study on sudden unexpected death in epilepsy. Ann Neurol. 1989;26:195-203.

Leestma JE, Annegers JF, Brodie MJ, Brown S, Schraeder P, Siscovick D, Wannamaker BB, Tennis PS, Cierpial MA, Earl NL. Sudden unexplained death in epilepsy: observations from a large clinical development program. Epilepsia. 1997;38:47-55.

Menon B. Symptomatic occipital epilepsy misdiagnosed as migraine. Headache 2007;47(2):287-289

Nilsson L, Farahmand BY, Persson PG, Thiblin I, Tomson T. Risk factors for sudden unexpected death in epilepsy: a case-control study. Lancet. 1999;353:888-93.

Nilsson L, Bergman U, Diwan V, Farahmand BY, Persson PG, Tomson T. Antiepileptic drug therapy and its management in sudden unexpected death in epilepsy: a case-control study. Epilepsia. 2001;42:667-73.

Nouri S. Sudden Unexpected Death in Epilepsy. eMedicine Specialties Jan 2011. Full text available at the URL: http://emedicine.medscape.com/article/1187111-overview

Provini F, Plazzi G, Tinuper P, Vandi S, Lugaresi E, Montagna P. Nocturnal frontal lobe epilepsy. A clinical and polygraphic overview of 100 consecutive cases. *Brain 1999;*122:1017–1031.

Ryvlin P, Montavont A, Kahane P. Sudden unexpected death in epilepsy: from mechanisms to prevention. Curr Opin Neurol. 2006;19:194-99.]

Robles SG, Gelisse P, El Fertit H, Tancy C, Duffau H, Crespel A Coubes P. Parasagital transinsular electrodes for stereo-EEG in temporal and insular lobe epilepsies. Stereotact Funct Neurosurg. 2009;87(6):368-372

Roper SN, Lévesque MF, Sutherling WW, Engel J Jr.Surgical treatment of partial epilepsy arising from the insular cortex. Report of two cases Neurosurg. 1993 ;79(2):266-269.

Scheffer IE, Bhatia KP, Lopes-Cendes I, Fish DR, Marsden CD, Andermann E, Andermann F, Desbiens R, Keene D, Cendes F, Manson JI, Constantinou JEC, McIntosh A, Berkovic SF. Autosomal dominant nocturnal frontal lobe epilepsy. A distinctive clinical disorder.*Brain1995;* 118:61–73.

Scorza FA, de Albuquerque M, Arida RM, Cavalheiro EA,. Sudden unexpected death in epilepsy: Are winter temperatures a new potential risk factor? Epilepsy Behav. 2007;10:509-10.

Scorza F, Cysneiros R, Arida R, Terra-Bustamante V, Albuquerque M, Cavalheiro A. The other side of the coin: Beneficiary effect of omega-3 fatty acids in sudden unexpected death in epilepsy. Epilepsy & Behavior.2008;13(20:279-283.

So NK. Mesial frontal epilepsy. *Epilepsia*. 1998;39(4):49-61.

Sperling MR, Feldman H, Kinman J, Liporace JD, O'Connor MJ. Seizure control and mortality in epilepsy. Ann Neurol. 1999;46:45-50.

Stollberger C, Finsterer J. Cardiorespiratory findings in sudden unexplained/unexpected death in epilepsy (SUDEP). Epilepsy Res. 2004;59:51-60.

Tamayo A, Hachinski V. Central nervous system the neurogenic heart. CAR 2003;3:1-8

Tomson T, Nashef L, Ryvlin P. Sudden unexpected death in epilepsy: current knowledge and future directions. The Lancet Neurology 2008;7(1):1021-1031.

Walczak TS, Leppik IE, D'Amelio M, Rarick J, So E, Ahman P, Ruggles K, Cascino GD, Annegers JF, Hauser WA. Incidence and risk factors in sudden unexpected death in epilepsy: a prospective cohort study. Neurology. 2001;56:519-25.

11

Epileptic Channelopathies and Dysfunctional Excitability - From Gene Mutations to Novel Treatments

Sigrid Marie Blom[1] and Henrik Sindal Jensen[2]
[1]*Department of Physiology, University of Bern*
[2]*Neuroscience Drug Discovery, H. Lundbeck A/S*
[1]*Switzerland*
[2]*Denmark*

1. Introduction

Epilepsy is not a single disorder, but a collection of disorders that all are characterized by episodic abnormal synchronous electrical activity in the brain. This abnormal activity represents a disturbance of the balance between excitatory and inhibitory neurotransmission. The majority (50%) of epilepsies are cryptogenic, meaning there is a presumptive but no identifiable underlying etiology. Approximately 20% of epilepsies have an identifiable cause (i.e. they are symptomatic) and are usually a result of trauma to the head, stroke, brain tumours, or infections. The remaining 30% are idiopathic, meaning there is no apparent underlying cause (Berg et al., 1999). However, as they are usually associated with a family history of similar seizures, they are mostly considered to be genetic. Mutations in over 70 genes have been found to cause epilepsy (Noebels, 2003). Given the dependence of seizures on synaptic transmission and neuronal excitability, it is not surprising that many of these mutations affect the function of ion channels. Since the identification of the first epilepsy-causing ion channel mutation, scientists have come a long way in the understanding of the pathogenesis of the disease. This chapter deals with some of the main questions that have been asked, and looks at some of the proposed answers to the questions. How do mutations in certain ion channels lead to hyperexcitability and seizures? Why do mutations in one ion channel cause a particular epilepsy syndrome? Why are the seizures often initiated during specific physiological events? And why do most of the childhood epilepsies remit with age? Furthermore, ion channels as targets for antiepileptic drugs will be discussed.

2. Idiopathic epilepsies

In most cases genetic epilepsy syndromes have a complex rather than a simple inheritance pattern. Although the epilepsies described here are thought to be monogenic, not even those considered inherited in a dominant fashion have a penetrance of 100%. Mutations within the same gene can result in clinically distinct phenotypes. Variable expressivity is also a common feature of inherited epilepsy demonstrated by family members with the same mutation that exhibit differences in the clinical severity of the disease (Hayman et al., 1997).

On the other hand, some of the disorders display locus heterogeneity where mutations in distinct genes result in the same syndrome. This indicates that other factors beside the primary mutation influence the clinical manifestation of the epilepsy, e.g. environmental factors, developmental events, or differences in inheritance of genetic susceptibility alleles. The latter is supported by mouse models where differences between the genetic backgrounds of two mouse strains influence the severity of a disease caused by the same sodium channel mutation (Bergren et al., 2005).

Unfortunately, discovery of the responsible gene for an epilepsy syndrome have not led to a prompt understanding of the pathogenesis of the disease. Many of the mutated channels have been characterized in expression systems, but only in some cases have this led to a better understanding of the disease. In other cases this have led to more confusion, as some mutations in a particular channel are found to enhance channel function while others appear to cause a loss of function, even though the clinical manifestation are similar. There are also large discrepancies between results depending on the expression system used to characterize the channels. The mutated channel can e.g. show enhanced function when expressed in *Xenopus laevis* oocytes, while the opposite is shown when expressed in mammalian cells (Meadows et al., 2002). To make it even more difficult, it has been demonstrated that depending on the type of neuron in which a mutated channel is expressed, it can have strikingly different effects on the excitability of the cell (Waxman, 2007). While a mutation can make one type of neuron hyperexcitable, the same mutation can make another neuron hypoexcitable. So changes in neuronal fuction are not necessarily predictable solely from the change in the behaviour of the mutated channel itself, but have to be considered in the cell background in which the mutated channel is expressed. Further, depending on whether a mutated channel mainly is expressed in excitatory or inhibitory neurons, it can have completely opposite effects on the excitability status of the neuronal network (Yu et al., 2006).

The ion channel mutations are bound to cause relative subtle changes in neuronal function. Mutations that cause dramatic changes would likely result in a more severe phenotypes or lethality. The mutations apparently allow normal behaviour under most circumstances, but disturb the equilibrium between excitatory and inhibitory neuronal networks, so that small external perturbations such as fever are sufficient to break the homeostasis and induce seizures.

3. Mutations in sodium channel subunit genes

3.1 Voltage-gated sodium channels

Voltage-gated sodium channels play an essential role in the initiation and propagation of action potentials. These channels open as the membrane depolarizes and inactivate within a few milliseconds of opening. As the membrane polarizes again, the inactivation is removed and a second depolarizing stimulus is able to reopen the channel.

Sodium channels are large, multimeric complexes composed of an α subunit and one or more auxiliary β subunits. The α subunit has four homologous domains, each consisting of six transmembrane helices. The β subunit has one transmembrane segment and an extracellular domain with an immunoglobulin-like fold and belongs to the Ig superfamily of cell adhesion molecules (CAMs) (Catterall, 2000). The association with β subunits modulate cell surface expression and localization, voltage-dependence and kinetics of activation and inactivation, as well as cell adhesion and association with signalling and cytoskeletal molecules (Patino and Isom, 2010). Nine α subunits ($Na_V1.1$ - $Na_V1.9$ encoded by SCN1A-SCN11A) and four β subunits (encoded by SCN1B-SCN4B) have been characterized so far. In addition, the enigmatic NaX channel, which appears not to be gated by voltage but rather by sodium, is encoded by the SCN7A gene (previously assigned as SCN6A) (Hiyama et al., 2002). $Na_V1.1$, $Na_V1.2$, $Na_V1.3$ and $Na_V1.6$ are the sodium channel α subunits most abundantly expressed in the brain (Yu and Catterall, 2003).

3.2 GEFS+ and SMEI

Febrile seizures, i. e. seizures induced by elevated body temperature, affect approximately 3% of children under 6 years of age and are by far the most common seizure disorder. Generalized Epilepsy with Febrile Seizures Plus (GEFS+) is an autosomal dominant epileptic syndrome where the febrile seizures may persist beyond 6 years of age and which may be associated with afebrile generalized seizures (Scheffer and Berkovic, 1997). The disease has a penetrance of approximately 60%. In 1998, GEFS+ was linked to mutation in SCN1B, the voltage-gated sodium channel β1 subunit gene (Wallace et al., 1998). GEFS+ can also result from mutations in the sodium channel α subunit genes SCN1A (Escayg et al., 2000) and SCN2A (Sugawara et al., 2001), and from mutations in the GABRG2 gene which encodes the γ2 subunit of the $GABA_A$ receptor (Baulac et al., 2001). Heterozygous mutations in SCN1A can also result in Severe Myoclonic Epilepsy of Infancy (SMEI), also known as Dravet syndrome (Claes et al., 2001). This rare form of epilepsy is characterized by generalized tonic, clonic, and tonic-clonic seizures that are initially induced by fever, light, sound, or physical activity and typically begin around 6-9 months of age. Later, SMEI patients also manifest other seizure types including absence, myoclonic, and simple and complex partial seizures. Psychomotor development stagnates around the second year of life and the patients often respond poorly to antiepileptic drugs. The disorder usually occurs in isolated patients as a result of *de novo* mutations (Claes et al., 2003; Ohmori et al., 2002).

3.3 How mutations in sodium channels can cause seizures

As sodium channels are responsible for the upstroke of the action potential one might expect that epilepsy-causing mutations in sodium channel genes increase the activity of the channel, thereby allowing increased influx of sodium ions and consequently neuronal hyperexcitability. Indeed, biophysical analyses of the mutant channels have shown that several of the mutations are gain-of-function mutations that increase sodium currents, e. g. by impairing inactivation or by causing a hyperpolarizing shift in the voltage-dependence of the channel (Lossin et al., 2002; Spampanato et al., 2003; Spampanato et al., 2004). The first identified GEFS+ mutation, a C121W missense mutation that disrupts a conserved disulphide bridge in the extracellular Ig domain of the β1 subunit, causes subtle changes in modulation of sodium channel function and alter the ability of β1 to mediate protein-protein interactions that are critical for channel localization (Meadows et al., 2002; Wallace et al., 1998). Electrophysiological and biochemical studies on the mutant C121W β1 subunit co-expressed with $Na_V1.2$ or $Na_V1.3$ have shown that the C121W mutation causes a reduction in current rundown during high-frequency channel activation and increases the fraction of sodium channels that are available to open at subthreshold membrane potentials (Meadows et al., 2002). The mutation is therefore thought to enhance sodium channel function, thereby increasing neuronal excitability and predisposing to seizures.

On the other hand, many of the characterized sodium channel mutations are found to cause attenuation of sodium current (Barela et al., 2006; Lossin et al., 2003; Sugawara et al., 2001).

While it seems like the mild phenotype of GEFS+ mostly is associated with missense mutations that alter the biophysical properties of the channels, the more severe SMEI phenotype is usually caused by nonsense or frameshift mutations that prevent production of functional channels (Claes et al., 2003; Claes et al., 2001; Nabbout et al., 2003; Ohmori et al., 2002). But how can loss-of-function mutations in a sodium channel cause epilepsy when reduced sodium current should lead to hypoexcitability rather than hyperexcitability? The answer seems to be related to the expression pattern of the channels. $Na_V1.1$ is predominantly found in inhibitory interneurons and is thought to conduct most of the sodium current in these cells, whereas excitatory pyramidal neurons express only negligible levels of $Na_V1.1$ (Ogiwara et al., 2007). Catterall and co-workers showed that haploinsufficiency of $Na_V1.1$ channels in heterozygous knock-out mice led to a phenotype resembling that of SMEI (Oakley et al., 2009; Yu et al., 2006). In these mice, sodium currents in GABAergic interneurons in the hippocampus were substantially reduced, whilst the effect in pyramidal cells was much less severe. Loss of one SCN1A copy led to a reduction in action potential number, frequency and amplitude in the interneurons (Yu et al., 2006). Similarly, studies in several animal models carrying nonsense or missense mutations in SCN1A show impaired interneuron function (Martin et al., 2010; Mashimo et al., 2010; Ogiwara et al., 2007; Tang et al., 2009). These studies indicate that functional loss of one copy of SCN1A reduces the inhibitory function of GABAergic interneurons and enhances the excitability of downstream synaptic targets, thereby predisposing to epileptic seizures.

But if this is true, how does the predicted changed $Na_V1.1$ function in many of the patients lead to hyperexcitability when the consequence should be increased GABA action? One possibility is that enhanced sodium current in the interneurons causes too much inhibition, and that this leads to synchronization of the downstream synaptic targets, as has been suggested in the pathogenesis of autosomal dominant nocturnal frontal lobe epilepsy (ADNFL) (Klaassen et al., 2006) (discussed later). Another possibility is that the functional consequences of the mutations in vivo are different from that predicted after in vitro characterization of the mutant channels, and that all of the mutations actually cause a reduction of sodium current in inhibitory neurons. This is supported by studies on knock-out mice lacking the β1 subunit (Chen et al., 2004). These mice show downregulated $Na_V1.1$ expression, indicating that β1 function might be necessary for normal expression of $Na_V1.1$. As the inhibitory interneurons seem to be most affected by a reduction in $Na_V1.1$, the consequences of the β1 mutations might be reduced sodium current in interneurons rather than, or in addition to, increased $Na_V1.2$ and $Na_V1.3$ function.

As mutations in SCN1A most often are associated with febrile seizures the mutations seem not to be sufficient to cause spontaneous seizure themselves. Why are the seizures triggered by fever? Why are the seizures most prevalent in young children? And what is the reason for the age-specific onset of SMEI? It is known that an increase in body temperature leads to an increase in the rate of respiration, especially in young children (Gadomski et al., 1994). This increased respiration can cause respiratory alkalosis in the immature brain, and alkalosis of brain tissue can lead to enhanced neuronal activity and to epileptoform activity (Lee et al., 1996). Studies on rat pups showed that seizure activity induced by hyperthermia had a well-defined pH threshold and that a rise in brain pH to the threshold level by injection of bicarbonate could provoke seizures (Schuchmann et al., 2006). By suppressing the alkalosis with a moderate elevation of ambient CO_2 to 5%, seizures could be abolished within 20 seconds without affecting body temperature. Bicarbonate-induced pH changes and seizures could also be blocked by elevation of ambient CO_2. In older rats, hyperthermia only led to a moderate increase in the respiration rate and did not cause respiratory alkalosis and seizures (Schuchmann et al., 2006). Fever and the accompanying elevated pH and enhanced neuronal activity seem therefore to be the drop that makes the barrel overflow and induce the seizures. As several ion channels are sensitive to changes in pH (Jensen et al., 2005; Prole et al., 2003), it will be interesting to see whether some mutations in sodium channel genes render the channels pH-sensitive, which could make the affected individuals specifically susceptible to febrile seizures.

SMEI patients are normal until their first seizure that typically occurs around 6-9 months of age. This age-specificity may to be related to the time-specific expression of sodium channels. $Na_V1.1$ is undetectable during prenatal and early postnatal development, a stage where $Na_V1.3$ is preferentially expressed. $Na_V1.3$ expression declines at the expression of $Na_V1.1$ increases. An animal model of SMEI has shown that loss of inhibition and seizure onset correlates in time with an increase in $Na_V1.1$ levels and decline in $Na_V1.3$ levels (Oakley et al., 2009).

4. Mutations in $GABA_A$ receptor subunit genes

4.1 GABA receptors

GABA is the major inhibitory neurotransmitter in the central nervous system. There are three types of GABA receptors: $GABA_A$, $GABA_B$, and $GABA_C$. $GABA_A$ and $GABA_C$ receptors are ionotropic while $GABA_B$ receptors are G-protein coupled and often act by activating potassium channels. Most of the cortical inhibitory effects of GABA are mediated by $GABA_A$ receptors (Chebib and Johnston, 1999).

The $GABA_A$ receptors are pentameric chloride channels formed by various combinations of different types of α ($\alpha1$ to $\alpha6$), β ($\beta1$ to $\beta3$), γ ($\gamma1$ to $\gamma3$), δ, ε, π, θ, and ρ ($\rho1$ to $\rho3$) subunits, that each have four transmembrane segments, M1 to M4 (Benarroch, 2007). The most prevalent subunit combination consists of $\alpha1\beta2\gamma2$ (McKernan and Whiting, 1996). The subunit composition determines the functional and pharmacological characteristics of the receptors (Meldrum and Rogawski, 2007; Sieghart and Sperk, 2002). Binding of GABA to the receptor triggers opening of the chloride channel, allowing rapid influx of chloride that hyperpolarizes the neuron and thereby decreases the probability of generation of an action potential.

4.2 GEFS+ and ADJME

As mentioned, GEFS+ can also result from mutation in the GABRG2 gene encoding the $\gamma2$ subunit of the $GABA_A$ receptor (Baulac et al., 2001). Mutations in the $\alpha1$ subunit gene (GABRA1) have been linked to Autosomal Dominant Juvenile Myoclonic Epilepsy (ADJME) (Cossette et al., 2002), an idiopathic epilepsy that is not associated with febrile seizures. This disorder typically manifests itself between the ages of 12 and 18 with myoclonic seizures occurring early in the morning and with additional tonic-clonic and absence seizures in some patients.

4.3 How mutant $GABA_A$ receptor subunits can cause seizures

It has been shown that mutations in the $\gamma2$ subunit of the $GABA_A$ receptor cause retention of the receptor in the endoplasmatic reticulum (ER) (Harkin et al., 2002; Kang and Macdonald, 2004). Similarly, the A322D mutation in the $\alpha1$ subunit causes rapid ER associated degradation of the subunit through the ubiquitin-proteasome system (Gallagher et al., 2007).

This reduced cell surface expression would result in decreased inhibitory $GABA_A$ receptor current, and consequently an increase in neuronal excitability and seizure susceptibility. But why are γ2 mutations associated with febrile seizures? And why are mutations in α1 not? Variations in temperature have effects on most cellular events. For example, synaptic vesicle recycling has been shown to be temperature dependent with increased temperature speeding both endo- and exocytosis, and there is evidence that inhibitory synaptic strength can be modulated within 10 min through recruitment of more functional $GABA_A$ receptors to the postsynaptic plasma membrane (Wan et al., 1997). Studies on cultured hippocamplal neurons showed that while trafficking of wild-type α1β2γ2 receptors is slightly temperature dependent with a small decrease in surface expression after incubation at 40°C for 2h, trafficking of receptors with mutations in the γ2 subunit is highly temperature dependent (Kang et al., 2006). Increases in temperature from 37°C to 40°C impaired trafficking and/or accelerated endocytosis of the mutant receptors within 10 min, suggesting that the febrile seizures may be a result of a temperature-induced reduction in GABA-mediated inhibition. The study also showed that the A322D mutation in the α1 subunit did not cause a temperature-dependent reduction in surface expression, consistent with a resulting epilepsy syndrome not associated with febrile seizures (Kang et al., 2006).

5. Mutations in potassium channel genes

5.1 Kv7 channels and the M-current

The Kv7 family of voltage-gated potassium channels consists of five members, Kv7.1 -5 (also termed KCNQ1-5). All five members share the general structure of voltage-gated potassium channels with four subunits that assemble to form functional tetramers. Each subunit consists of six transmembrane helices, S1-S6, and has a pore forming domain, which is formed by a P-loop between the fifth and the sixth helix. The P-loop contains the GYG (glycine-tyrosine-glycine) sequence, which is highly conserved among potassium channels and confers K^+ selectivity. The fourth helix forms the voltage sensor; it contains several arginine residues and is therefore strongly positive. A S4-S5 linker in one subunit couples the voltage sensor to the intracellular activation gate in S6 of the adjacent subunit (Laine et al., 2003). Although heavily debated, it is believed that when the membrane potential depolarize, the voltage sensor is pushed out leading to bending of the S6 so potassium can enter the channel pore (Long et al., 2005).

All Kv7 channels are strongly inhibited upon activation of muscarinic receptors and are hence called M-channels (Schroeder et al., 2000; Selyanko et al., 2000). The current conducted by these channels, the M-current, was first described in bullfrog sympathetic ganglia as a slowly activating, slowly deactivating, sub-threshold voltage-dependent K^+ current that showed no inactivation (Brown and Adams, 1980). The Kv7 channels have slow activation and deactivation kinetics, and in line with other voltage-gated potassium channels they open upon membrane depolarization. However, the threshold for activation is low compared to most other channels, approximately -60 mV. Since the channels open at voltages that are around or below the threshold for generation of an action potential they allow potassium flow that opposes the depolarization required to generate action potentials, and hence make the neuron less excitable. If the M-channels remain open during excitation of the nerve, the spike frequency is dampened, whiles inhibition of the M-current by activation of muscarinic acetylcholine receptors enables repetitive firing (Hille, 2001).

Kv7 channels are primarily localized at the axon initial segment, the site where synaptic inputs are integrated and action potentials are generated (Pan et al., 2006; Rasmussen et al., 2007). Additionally, immunohistochemical studies have demonstrated a widespread pre-synaptic distribution of some Kv7 channel subunits (Cooper et al., 2000), where they may play a role in depolarization-induced neurotransmitter release (Martire et al., 2004; Martire et al., 2007). Activation of pre-synaptic M-current may hyperpolarize the nerve endings, thus reducing Ca^{2+} influx through voltage-gated Ca^{2+} channels and limiting the amount of neurotransmitter released.

5.2 Benign neonatal familial convulsions

Benign Neonatal Familial Convulsions (BNFC) is a rare autosomal dominant idiopathic form of epilepsy. It is characterized by tonic-clonic seizures that typically begin around three days after birth and remit after 3-4 months. Yet ~16% of patients also experience seizures later in life (Ronen et al., 1993). BNFC is caused by mutations in the genes encoding Kv7.2 (Biervert et al., 1998; Singh et al., 1998) or Kv7.3 (Charlier et al., 1998).

5.3 How mutations in Kv7.2 and Kv7.3 can cause BNFC

All characterized mutations in Kv7.2 and Kv7.3 cause a reduction in M-current, either by changing the channel kinetics (Dedek et al., 2001), by altering the trafficking of the channel to the cell membrane (Schwake et al., 2000), or by decreasing the subunit stability (Soldovieri et al., 2006). The mutations usually cause a reduction in M-current of about 25% (Schroeder et al., 1998). Considering the role of Kv7 channels in controlling neuronal excitability, it is not surprising that a reduction in M-current can cause hyperexcitability and predispose to seizures. Several transgenic strategies have been employed to examine how Kv7.2 and Kv7.3 malfunction lead to BNFC. The traditional knock-out approach resulted in mice that died within a few hours after birth due to pulmonary atelectasis (collapse of the lung) (Watanabe et al., 2000). Even though BNFC often results from Kv7.2 haploinsufficiency, heterozygous KCNQ2$^{+/-}$ mice did not experience neonatal seizures and appeared normal. They did, however, have increased susceptibility to chemically induced seizures (Watanabe et al., 2000). To overcome the postnatal lethality Dirk Isbrandt and colleagues developed mice conditionally expressing dominant-negative Kv7.2 subunits (Kv7.2-G279S) where expression of the transgene could be turned on after birth (Peters et al., 2005). These mice showed spontaneous seizures, exhibited behavioural hyperactivity and had morphological changes in the hippocampus. Mark Leppert and co-workers developed orthologous mouse models carrying disease-causing mutations in the *KCNQ2* (A306T) or *KCNQ3* (G311V) gene (Singh et al., 2008). Mice heterozygous or homozygous for either mutation had reduced seizure threshold, but only mice homozygous for the mutations exhibited spontaneous seizures. The epileptic phenotype was dependent on the specific mutation, the genetic background, sex, and seizure model (Otto et al., 2009). Hence, none of these transgenic strategies have fully recapitulated the human condition but nevertheless provide us with important clues regarding the pathophysiology of BNFC.

It can be questioned why the disease usually only is clinically manifested in neonates when mutations in the channels cause general hyperexcitability. One possible explanation for the age-dependent remission of seizures is related to the expression of Kv7 channels. There is evidence for a developmental upregulation of Kv7 channels (Weber et al., 2006), suggesting that a reduction in M-current of 25% might have a more prominent effect in the fetal brain and that this reduction is not sufficient to cause seizures later in life when expression levels of Kv7 channels are higher.

Another possible mechanism is related to developmental changes in GABA function. During the first weeks of life, GABA, the main inhibitory neurotransmitter in the adult brain, provides the main excitatory drive to immature hippocampal neurons (Ben-Ari, 2002). Due to delayed expression of a chloride exporter there is a high intracellular concentration of chloride that leads to a negative shift in the reversal potential for chloride ions, so opening of ionotropic GABA receptors leads to an efflux of negative chloride ions and therefore depolarization. When the chloride-extruding system becomes operative, chloride is efficiently transported out of the cell, and GABA begins to exert its conventional inhibitory action (Ben-Ari, 2002). Because of this, the inhibition in neonatal circuits appears mainly to be mediated through presynaptic control of neurotransmitter release. As Kv7 channels are involved in the release of neurotransmitters (Martire et al., 2004; Martire et al., 2007), it was proposed that these channels serve as the main inhibitor in neonates, and that attenuation of M-current due to mutations in Kv7.2 and Kv7.3 causes reduced inhibition that is sufficient to cause epilepsy (Peters et al., 2005). If Kv7 channels are expressed in GABAergic neurons, the reduced M-current would possibly also cause increased GABA release which further would increase excitability at this point of development. It is also important to note that the neonatal brain is particularly prone to seizures (Holmes and Ben-Ari, 1998). As development continues and overall excitability decreases, reduced M-current apparently becomes less problematic and the seizures abate.

Yet, if this is the fact, why do ~16% of the patients experience seizures later in life after GABA has gained its inhibitory function? There is evidence to indicate that suppression of M-current within the first postnatal week can cause developmental defects, and that the resulting morphological changes in the brain, rather than reduced M-current causes the seizures in adulthood (Peters et al., 2005). In other words, it appears to become a symptomatic epilepsy with an idiopathic aetiology.

6. Mutations in nAChR subunit genes

6.1 Nicotinic acetylcholine receptors

Nicotinic acetylcholine receptors (nAChRs) consist of five subunits that assemble to form functional pentamers. Each subunit consists of a long extracellular N-terminal domain, four transmembrane helices (TM1-TM4), and a short extracellular C-terminal end. The second transmembrane segment (TM2) from each subunit lines the channel pore. The amino acids that compose the TM2 are arranged in such a way that three rings of negatively charged amino acids are oriented toward the central pore of the channel. These provide a selectivity filter that ensures that only cations can pass through the pore. Brief exposure to high concentrations of Ach causes opening of the water-filled pore and permits an influx of Na^+ and Ca^{2+} and an efflux of K^+ (Waxham, 2003). After a few milliseconds, the receptor closes to a nonconducting state. Prolonged exposure to agonist causes desensitization of the channel, which stabilizes the receptor in an unresponsive, closed state (Dani and Bertrand, 2007).

The neuronal nAChRs can be either homomeric, consisting of five α subunits, or heteromeric with two α subunits and three β subunits. So far, 12 nAChR subunits expressed in the brain have been identified (α2-α10 and β2-β4). The most widely distributed nAChRs in the human brain are the homomeric α7 and the heteromeric α4β2. The biochemical, pharmacological and biophysical characteristic of the channels are dependent on the subunit composition (Dani and Bertrand, 2007).

6.2 Autosomal Dominant Nocturnal Frontal Lobe Epilepsy

Autosomal Dominant Nocturnal Frontal Lobe Epilepsy (ADNFLE) is a focal epilepsy characterized by clusters of brief nocturnal motor seizures with hyperkinetic or tonic manifestations. Seizures typically occur very soon after falling asleep or during the early morning hours, initiated during stage 2 non-rapid-eye-movement (NREM) sleep. Onset usually occurs around age 10 and the seizures often persist through adult life. However, in most patients the seizures tend to peter out in adulthood.

In 1995, a missense mutation (S248F) in the nAChR α4 subunit gene (CHRNA4) was found to underlie ADNFLE (Steinlein et al., 1995). Additional disease causing mutations in this gene (Hirose et al., 1999; Steinlein et al., 1997), and mutations in the β2 subunit gene (CHRNB2) (Phillips et al., 2001) have later been identified. Because α4 and β2 subunits combine, it is not strange that mutations in either subunit produce comparable epileptic symptoms. Almost every known mutation is found in the TM2 region of the two subunits. A common finding among the mutations is that the sensitivity to ACh is increased (Bertrand et al., 2002).

6.3 How mutations in nAChRs can cause ADNFLE

Stage 2 NREM sleep is characterized by the appearance of sleep spindles and slow waves, transient physiological rhythmic oscillations that are produced by synchronized synaptic potentials in cortical neurons. It appears that the seizure often arise from a sleep spindle that transforms into epileptic discharges (Picard et al., 2007). Thalamocortical circuits are thought to play a role in the generation of these sleep spindles.

Thalamic relay neurons are reciprocally connected to cortical neurons by excitatory synapses. Both thalamic and cortical neurons also excite GABAergic interneurons of the nucleus reticularis, which in turn inhibit thalamic relay neurons thus forming a feedback-loop (Kandel et al., 2000). The thalamic relay neurons have two different modes of signalling activity: a transmission mode during wakefulness and rapid eye movement (REM) sleep and a burst mode during NREM sleep. In the transmission mode, the resting membrane potential of the thalamic relay neurons is near the firing threshold and incoming excitatory synaptic potentials drive the neuron to fire in a pattern that reflects the sensory stimuli. During the burst mode the thalamic relay neurons are hyperpolarized and respond to brief depolarization with a burst of action potentials, which indicates that the thalamus is unable to relay sensory information to the cortex (Kandel et al., 2000). The thalamic relay neurons can be in different modes because they possess special Ca^{2+} channels named T-type channels. These channels are inactivated at the resting membrane potential but become available for activation when the cell is hyperpolarized, and can then be transiently opened by depolarization (Contreras, 2006). The interneurons of the nucleus reticularis that form synapses at the relay neurons hyperpolarize the relay neurons upon activation of $GABA_A$ receptors, thus removing the inactivation of the T-type Ca^{2+} channels. Incoming excitatory synaptic potentials can then trigger transient opening of the T-type Ca^{2+} channels and the resulting influx of Ca^{2+} brings the neuron's membrane potential above threshold. The cell now fires a burst of action potentials that produces the synchronized postsynaptic potentials in cortical neurons that cause the spindle waves seen on the electroencephalogram. When sufficient Ca^{2+} has entered the cell a Ca^{2+}-activated K^+ current is triggered that hyperpolarizes the relay neurons and terminate the spindle (Contreras, 2006). Because of the feedback loops from the relay neurons and cortical neurons that innervate the interneurons of the nucleus reticularis, these are again activated, which allows for another round of burst firing.

There is a high expression of the α4β2 nAChR subtype in the thalamus and the subtype can be found diffusely distributed onto pyramidal cells and GABAergic interneurons in the cortex. The thalamic relay neurons and the nucleus reticularis receive input from two groups of cholinergic neurons in the upper brain stem: the pedunculopontine and laterodorsal tegmental nuclei (LDT). These are critical for keeping the thalamic relay neurons in transmission mode during wakefulness and REM sleep. The LDT releases Ach during NREM sleep at the time of an arousal that interrupts the sleep spindle oscillations through depolarization of thalamic relay neurons (Lee and McCormick, 1997). The cortex receives cholinergic input from neurons in the nucleus basalis of Meynert that enhance cortical response to incoming sensory stimuli (Kandel et al., 2000).

After studying transgenic ADNFLE mice with heterozygous expression of an ADNFLE mutation ($Chrna4^{S252F}$ or $Chrna4^{+264}$), Boulter and colleagues suggested that an Ach-dependent sudden increase in the response of GABAergic cortical interneurons contributes to the epileptogenesis in ADNFLE patients (Klaassen et al., 2006). They showed that asynchronously firing cortical pyramidal cells got synchronized when relived from a large GABAergic inhibition triggered by cholinergic over-activation of mutant nAChRs in the cortical interneurons.

Dani and Bertrand suggested that this, together with an increased positive response of cortical pyramidal cells through cholinergic stimulation of their hypersensitive α4β2 nAChRs, contributes to induction of the seizures (Dani and Bertrand, 2007). As the cortical pyramidal cells project back to the thalamus, excitatory stimuli will be boosted on to the interneurons of the nucleus reticularis and the relay neurons and induce synchronous activity and seizures (Dani and Bertrand, 2007).

In addition, PET studies using a high affinity α4β2 agonist have showed a clear difference in the pattern of the nAChR density in the brains of ADNFLE patients compared to control subjects (Picard et al., 2006). The studies showed that patients had increased α4β2 density in the epithalamus, the interpeduncular nucleus (IPN) of the ventral mesencephalon and in the cerebellum, while the density in the right dorsolateral prefrontal region was decreased. As the IPN projects to the LDT, the authors proposed that prolonged depolarizations in IPN neurons, because of both increased density of α4β2 and hypersensitive receptors, could result in over-activation of the LDT and consequently the thalamic relay neurons (Picard et al., 2006). At the time of arousals, ACh acting on sensitized thalamic relay neurons could prevent the normal arousal-induced interruption of the sleep spindle oscillations and transform them into pathological Thalamocortical oscillations, triggering epileptic seizures (Picard et al., 2006).

Neither of these mechanisms excludes the others. In fact, they might work together yielding even stronger possibilities for induction of seizures.

7. Ion channel modulators as antiepileptic drugs

Many of the antiepileptic drugs on the market today exert strong effects on ionic currents. Sodium channel blockers were used in the treatment of epilepsy as early as in 1940, and since then several other sodium channel blockers have been developed. Carbamazepine, first introduced in 1968, stabilizes the inactive conformation of sodium channels and is widely used in the treatment of partial and generalized tonic-clonic seizures. Lamotrigine blocks sodium channels in a voltage- and use-dependent manner and is efficient for partial, absence, myoclonic and tonic-clonic seizures (Kwan et al., 2001). Drugs that potentiate GABA receptor function, such as benzodiazepines, have also been used as anticonvulsants for several years. These act by binding to the interface between the α and γ subunits of the $GABA_A$ receptor, resulting in allosteric activation of the receptor (Kwan et al., 2001). Several established and novel antiepileptic drugs have been reported to act on various K^+ currents, but none of them exert their main effect on potassium channels (Meldrum and Rogawski, 2007). Carbamazepine also exerts an effect on nAChRs by blocking the open conformation of the channel and is very effective in treatment of patients with ADNFLE. This effect might be related to the fact that several of the disease causing mutations in CHRNA4 and CHRNA2 increase the sensitivity to the drug (Ortells and Barrantes, 2002).

The knowledge of how mutations in ion channels cause neuronal hyperexcitability and epilepsy has led to new therapeutic strategies for prevention of seizures. The mutated proteins serve as mechanistic proof of concept that pharmacological antagonization of the epilepsy causing mechanisms could have desirable effects on neuronal excitability. These mechanisms are not necessarily targeted for treatment of the respective epilepsy syndrome, but as they are showed to cause hyperexcitability in the affected patients, antagonizing drugs may reduce excitability in patients with other types of epilepsy. An excellent example of this is Retigabine (other names are Trobalt, Potiga, or Ezogabine), which was approved by both the European Medicines Agency and the U.S. Food and Drug Administration in 2011 as adjunctive treatment for partial onset seizures. It was originally synthesized as a GABA modulator, but it was later shown that its main molecular target is the neuronal Kv7 channels (Main et al., 2000; Rundfeldt and Netzer, 2000; Wickenden et al., 2000). Retigabine induces a large hyperpolarizing shift in the voltage-dependence of activation of Kv7 channels, accelerates the activation kinetics and slows deactivation kinetics. Enhancement of M-current would clearly be effective in prevention of seizures in BNFC patients, but mutations in the Kv7 channels might render them insensitive to such drugs, which hampers the use of Kv7 channel openers in the treatment of BNFC. The hypothesis of reduced $Na_V1.1$ current in the pathogenesis of GEFS+ and SMEI, together with its primary expression in inhibitory interneurons, indicates that this sodium channel subtype plays a role in reducing neuronal excitability (Ogiwara et al., 2007; Yu et al., 2006). This opens the intriguing possibility that selective $Na_V1.1$ openers can function as anticonvulsants, even though sodium channel openers generally are known as epileptogenic substances.

An understanding of the etiology of the epilepsy syndromes and the causal factors in individual patients are also critical for selection of the right medication. Sodium channel blockers, which normally would exhibit anticonvulsant properties, would clearly not be the right choice to treat patients with SMEI, where a lack of sodium current seems to be the underlying cause. Similarly, as too much inhibition seems to play a role in the pathogenesis of ADNFLE, GABA receptor agonist might have a negative effect in these patients. In fact, Boulter and co-workers showed that the $GABA_A$ receptor antagonist picrotoxin, which normally exhibits convulsive properties, was efficient in preventing seizures in the ADNFLE mice (Klaassen et al., 2006).

8. Conclusion

As about 30% of all patients with epilepsy respond poorly to antiepileptic drugs, there is clearly a need for development of new therapies. The growing understanding of the epileptic channelopathies and the structural and functional characterization of the mutated channels provide several opportunities for creation of novel and improved drugs.

9. References

Barela, A.J., Waddy, S.P., Lickfett, J.G., Hunter, J., Anido, A., Helmers, S.L., Goldin, A.L., & Escayg, A. (2006). An Epilepsy Mutation in the Sodium Channel SCN1A That Decreases Channel Excitability. *Journal of Neuroscience* Vol. 26, No. 10, pp. 2714-2723, ISSN 0270-6474

Baulac, S., Huberfeld, G., Gourfinkel-An, I., Mitropoulou, G., Beranger, A., Prud'homme, J.F., Baulac, M., Brice, A., Bruzzone, R., & LeGuern, E. (2001). First genetic evidence of GABAA receptor dysfunction in epilepsy: a mutation in the [gamma]2-subunit gene. *Nature Genetics* Vol. 28, No. 1, pp. 46-48, ISSN 1061-4036

Ben-Ari, Y. (2002). Excitatory actions of gaba during development: the nature of the nurture. *Nature Reviews Neuroscience* Vol. 3, No. 9, pp. 728-739, ISSN 1471-003X

Benarroch, E.E. (2007). GABAA receptor heterogeneity, function, and implications for epilepsy. *Neurology* Vol. 68, No. 8, pp. 612-614, ISSN 0028-3878

Berg, A.T., Shinnar, S., Levy, S.R., & Testa, F.M. (1999). Newly Diagnosed Epilepsy in Children: Presentation at Diagnosis. *Epilepsia* Vol. 40, No. 4, pp. 445-452, ISSN 0013-9580

Bergren, S., Chen, S., Galecki, A., & Kearney, J. (2005). Genetic modifiers affecting severity of epilepsy caused by mutation of sodium channelScn2a. *Mammalian Genome* Vol. 16, No. 9, pp. 683-690, ISSN 0938-8990

Bertrand, D., Picard, F., Le Hellard, S., Weiland, S., Favre, I., Phillips, H., Bertrand, S., Berkovic, S.F., Malafosse, A., & Mulley, J. (2002). How Mutations in the nAChRs Can Cause ADNFLE Epilepsy. *Epilepsia* Vol. 43, No. s5, pp. 112-122, ISSN 0013-9580

Biervert, C., Schroeder, B.C., Kubisch, C., Berkovic, S.F., Propping, P., Jentsch, T.J., & Steinlein, O.K. (1998). A Potassium Channel Mutation in Neonatal Human Epilepsy. *Science* Vol. 279, No. 5349, pp. 403-406, ISSN 0036-8075

Brown, D.A., & Adams, P.R. (1980). Muscarinic suppression of a novel voltage-sensitive K+ current in a vertebrate neurone. *Nature* Vol. 283, No. 5748, pp. 673-676, ISSN 0028-0836

Catterall, W.A. (2000). From Ionic Currents to Molecular Mechanisms: The Structure and Function of Voltage-Gated Sodium Channels. *Neuron* Vol. 26, No. 1, pp. 13-25, ISSN 0896-6273

Charlier, C., Singh, N.A., Ryan, S.G., Lewis, T.B., Reus, B.E., Robin, J., & Leppert, M. (1998). A pore mutation in a novel KQT-like potassium channel gene in an idiopathic epilepsy family. *Nature Genetics* Vol. 18, No. 1, pp. 53-55, ISSN 1061-4036

Chebib, M., & Johnston, G.A.R. (1999). THE 'ABC' OF GABA RECEPTORS: A BRIEF REVIEW. *Clinical and Experimental Pharmacology and Physiology* Vol. 26, No. 11, pp. 937-940, ISSN 0305-1870

Chen, C., Westenbroek, R.E., Xu, X., Edwards, C.A., Sorenson, D.R., Chen, Y., McEwen, D.P., O'Malley, H.A., Bharucha, V., Meadows, L.S., Knudsen, G.A., Vilaythong, A., Noebels, J.L., Saunders, T.L., Scheuer, T., Shrager, P., Catterall, W.A., & Isom, L.L. (2004). Mice Lacking Sodium Channel {beta}1 Subunits Display Defects in Neuronal Excitability, Sodium Channel Expression, and Nodal Architecture. *Journal of Neuroscience* Vol. 24, No. 16, pp. 4030-4042, ISSN 0270-6474

Claes, L., Ceulemans, B., Audenaert, D., Smets, K., Lofgren, A., Del-Favero, J., Ala-Mello, S., Basel-Vanagaite, L., Plecko, B., Raskin, S., Thiry, P., Wolf, N.I., Van Broeckhoven, C., & De Jonghe, P. (2003). De Novo SCN1A mutations are a major cause of severe myoclonic epilepsy of infancy. *Human Mutation* Vol. 21, No. 6, pp. 615-621, ISSN 1059-7794

Claes, L., Del-Favero, J., Ceulemans, B., Lagae, L., Van Broeckhoven, C., & De Jonghe, P. (2001). De novo mutations in the sodium-channel gene SCN1A cause severe myoclonic epilepsy of infancy. *American Journal of Human Genetics* Vol. 68, No. 6, pp. 1327-1332, ISSN 0002-9297

Contreras, D. (2006). The Role of T-Channels in the Generation of Thalamocortical Rhythms. *CNS & Neurological Disorders - Drug Targets* Vol. 5, pp. 571-585, ISSN 1871-5273

Cooper, E.C., Aldape, K.D., Abosch, A., Barbaro, N.M., Berger, M.S., Peacock, W.S., Jan, Y.N., & Jan, L.Y. (2000). Colocalization and coassembly of two human brain M-type potassium channel subunits that are mutated in epilepsy. *Proceedings of the National Academy of Sciences of the USA* Vol. 97, No. 9, pp. 4914-4919, ISSN 0027-8424

Cossette, P., Liu, L., Brisebois, K., Dong, H., Lortie, A., Vanasse, M., Saint-Hilaire, J.M., Carmant, L., Verner, A., Lu, W.Y., Tian Wang, Y., & Rouleau, G.A. (2002). Mutation of GABRA1 in an autosomal dominant form of juvenile myoclonic epilepsy. *Nature Genetics* Vol. 31, No. 2, pp. 184-189, ISSN 1061-4036

Dani, J.A., & Bertrand, D. (2007). Nicotinic Acetylcholine Receptors and Nicotinic Cholinergic Mechanisms of the Central Nervous System. *Annual Review of Pharmacology and Toxicology* Vol. 47, No. 1, pp. 699-729, ISSN 0362-1642

Dedek, K., Kunath, B., Kananura, C., Reuner, U., Jentsch, T.J., & Steinlein, O.K. (2001). Myokymia and neonatal epilepsy caused by a mutation in the voltage sensor of the KCNQ2 K+ channel. *Proceedings of the National Academy of Sciences of the USA* Vol. 98, No. 21, pp. 12272-12277, ISSN 0027-8424

Escayg, A., MacDonald, B.T., Meisler, M.H., Baulac, S., Huberfeld, G., An-Gourfinkel, I., Brice, A., LeGuern, E., Moulard, B., Chaigne, D., Buresi, C., & Malafosse, A. (2000). Mutations of SCN1A, encoding a neuronal sodium channel, in two families with GEFS+2. *Nature Genetics* Vol. 24, No. 4, pp. 343-345, ISSN 1061-4036

Gadomski, A.M., Permutt, T., & Stanton, B. (1994). Correcting respiratory rate for the presence of fever. *Journal of Clinical Epidemiology* Vol. 47, No. 9, pp. 1043-1049, ISSN 0895-4356

Gallagher, M.J., Ding, L., Maheshwari, A., & Macdonald, R.L. (2007). The GABAA receptor {alpha}1 subunit epilepsy mutation A322D inhibits transmembrane helix formation and causes proteasomal degradation. *Proceedings of the National Academy of Sciences of the USA* Vol. 104, No. 32, pp. 12999-13004, ISSN 0027-8424

Harkin, L.A., David, N.B., Leanne, M.D., Rita, S., Fiona, P., Robyn, H.W., Michaella, C.R., David, A.W., John, C.M., Samuel, F.B., Ingrid, E.S., & Steven, P. (2002). Truncation of the GABAA-Receptor g2 Subunit in a Family with Generalized Epilepsy with Febrile Seizures Plus. *American Journal of Human Genetics* Vol. 70, pp. 530-536, ISSN 0002-9297

Hayman, M., Scheffer, I.E., Chinvarun, Y., Berlangieri, S.U., & Berkovic, S.F. (1997). Autosomal dominant nocturnal frontal lobe epilepsy: Demonstration of focal frontal onset and intrafamilial variation. *Neurology* Vol. 49, No. 4, pp. 969-975, ISSN 0028-3878

Hille, B. (2001). *Ion channels of excitable membranes,* (3. edn.) Sinauer Associates Inc., ISBN 0-87893-321-2, Sunderland, USA.

Hirose, S., Iwata, H., Akiyoshi, H., Kobayashi, K., Ito, M., Wada, K., Kaneko, S., & Mitsudome, A. (1999). A novel mutation of CHRNA4 responsible for autosomal dominant nocturnal frontal lobe epilepsy. *Neurology* Vol. 53, No. 8, pp. 1749, ISSN 0028-3878

Hiyama, T.Y., Watanabe, E., Ono, K., Inenaga, K., Tamkun, M.M., Yoshida, S., & Noda, M. (2002). Nax channel involved in CNS sodium-level sensing. *Nature Neuroscience* Vol. 5, No. 6, pp. 511-512, ISSN 1097-6256

Holmes, G.L., & Ben-Ari, Y. (1998). Seizures in the Developing Brain: Perhaps Not So Benign after All. *Neuron* Vol. 21, No. 6, pp. 1231-1234, ISSN 0896-6273

Jensen, H.S., Callo, K., Jespersen, T., Jensen, B.S., & Olesen, S.P. (2005). The KCNQ5 potassium channel from mouse: A broadly expressed M-current like potassium channel modulated by zinc, pH, and volume changes. *Molecular Brain Research* Vol. 139, No. 1, pp. 52-62, ISSN 0169-328X

Kandel, E.R., Schwartz, J.H., & Jessell, T.M. (eds.) (2000). *Principles of Neural Science,* (4. edn.) McGraw-Hill, ISBN 0-8385-7701-6, New York, USA.

Kang, J., & Macdonald, R.L. (2004). The GABAA Receptor γ2 Subunit R43Q Mutation Linked to Childhood Absence Epilepsy and Febrile Seizures Causes Retention of α1β2γ2S Receptors in the Endoplasmic Reticulum. *Journal of Neuroscience* Vol. 24, No. 40, pp. 8672-8677, ISSN 0270-6474

Kang, J.Q., Shen, W., & Macdonald, R.L. (2006). Why Does Fever Trigger Febrile Seizures? GABAA Receptor γ2 Subunit Mutations Associated with Idiopathic Generalized Epilepsies Have Temperature-Dependent Trafficking Deficiencies. *Journal of Neuroscience* Vol. 26, No. 9, pp. 2590-2597, ISSN 0270-6474

Klaassen, A., Glykys, J., Maguire, J., Labarca, C., Mody, I., & Boulter, J. (2006). Seizures and enhanced cortical GABAergic inhibition in two mouse models of human autosomal dominant nocturnal frontal lobe epilepsy. *Proceedings of the National Academy of Sciences of the USA* Vol. 103, No. 50, pp. 19152-19157, ISSN 0027-8424

Kwan, P., Sills, G.J., & Brodie, M.J. (2001). The mechanisms of action of commonly used antiepileptic drugs. *Pharmacology & Therapeutics* Vol. 90, No. 1, pp. 21-34, ISSN 0163-7258

Laine, M., Lin, M.c., Bannister, J.P.A., Silverman, W.R., Mock, A.F., Roux, B., & Papazian, D.M. (2003). Atomic Proximity between S4 Segment and Pore Domain in Shaker Potassium Channels. *Neuron* Vol. 39, No. 3, pp. 467-481, ISSN 0896-6273

Lee, J., Taira, T., Pihlaja, P., Ransom, B.R., & Kaila, K. (1996). Effects of C02 on excitatory transmission apparently caused by changes in intracellular pH in the rat hippocampal slice. *Brain Research* Vol. 706, No. 2, pp. 210-216, ISSN 0006-8993

Lee, K.H., & McCormick, D.A. (1997). Modulation of spindle oscillations by acetylcholine, cholecystokinin and 1S,3R-ACPD in the ferret lateral geniculate and perigeniculate nuclei in vitro. *Neuroscience* Vol. 77, No. 2, pp. 335-350, ISSN 0306-4522

Long, S.B., Campbell, E.B., & MacKinnon, R. (2005). Voltage Sensor of Kv1.2: Structural Basis of Electromechanical Coupling. *Science* Vol. 309, No. 5736, pp. 903-908, ISSN 0036-8075

Lossin, C., Rhodes, T.H., Desai, R.R., Vanoye, C.G., Wang, D., Carniciu, S., Devinsky, O., & George, A.L., Jr. (2003). Epilepsy-Associated Dysfunction in the Voltage-Gated Neuronal Sodium Channel SCN1A. *Journal of Neuroscience* Vol. 23, No. 36, pp. 11289-11295, ISSN 0270-6474

Lossin, C., Wang, D.W., Rhodes, T.H., Vanoye, C.G., & George, A.L. (2002). Molecular basis of an inherited epilepsy. *Neuron* Vol. 34, No. 6, pp. 877-884, ISSN 0896-6273

Main, M.J., Cryan, J.E., Dupere, J.R.B., Cox, B., Clare, J.J., & Burbidge, S.A. (2000). Modulation of KCNQ2/3 Potassium Channels by the Novel Anticonvulsant Retigabine. *Molecular Pharmacology* Vol. 58, No. 2, pp. 253-262, ISSN 0026-895X

Martin, M.S., Dutt, K., Papale, L.A., Dube, C.M., Dutton, S.B., de Haan, G., Shankar, A., Tufik, S., Meisler, M.H., Baram, T.Z., Goldin, A.L., & Escayg, A. (2010). Altered Function of the SCN1A Voltage-gated Sodium Channel Leads to gamma-Aminobutyric Acid-ergic (GABAergic) Interneuron Abnormalities. *Journal of Biological Chemistry* Vol. 285, No. 13, pp. 9823-9834, ISSN 0021-9258

Martire, M., Castaldo, P., D'Amico, M., Preziosi, P., Annunziato, L., & Taglialatela, M. (2004). M Channels Containing KCNQ2 Subunits Modulate Norepinephrine, Aspartate, and GABA Release from Hippocampal Nerve Terminals. *Journal of Neuroscience* Vol. 24, No. 3, pp. 592-597, ISSN 0270-6474

Martire, M., D'Amico, M., Panza, E., Miceli, F., Viggiano, D., Lavergata, F., Iannotti, F.A., Barrese, V., Preziosi, P., Annunziato, L., & Taglialatela, M. (2007). Involvement of KCNQ2 subunits in [3H]dopamine release triggered by depolarization and pre-synaptic muscarinic receptor activation from rat striatal synaptosomes. *Journal of Neurochemistry* Vol. 102, No. 1, pp. 179-193, ISSN 0022-3042

Mashimo, T., Ohmori, I., Ouchida, M., Ohno, Y., Tsurumi, T., Miki, T., Wakamori, M., Ishihara, S., Yoshida, T., Takizawa, A., Kato, M., Hirabayashi, M., Sasa, M., Mori,

Y., & Serikawa, T. (2010). A Missense Mutation of the Gene Encoding Voltage-Dependent Sodium Channel (Na(v)1.1) Confers Susceptibility to Febrile Seizures in Rats. *Journal of Neuroscience* Vol. 30, No. 16, pp. 5744-5753, ISSN 0270-6474

McKernan, R.M., & Whiting, P.J. (1996). Which GABAA-receptor subtypes really occur in the brain? *Trends in Neurosciences* Vol. 19, No. 4, pp. 139-143, ISSN 0166-2236

Meadows, L.S., Malhotra, J., Loukas, A., Thyagarajan, V., Kazen-Gillespie, K.A., Koopman, M.C., Kriegler, S., Isom, L.L., & Ragsdale, D.S. (2002). Functional and Biochemical Analysis of a Sodium Channel beta 1 Subunit Mutation Responsible for Generalized Epilepsy with Febrile Seizures Plus Type 1. *Journal of Neuroscience* Vol. 22, No. 24, pp. 10699-10709, ISSN 0270-6474

Meldrum, B.S., & Rogawski, M.A. (2007). Molecular Targets for Antiepileptic Drug Development. *Neurotherapeutics* Vol. 4, No. 1, pp. 18-61, ISSN 1933-7213

Nabbout, R., Gennaro, E., Dalla Bernardina, B., Dulac, O., Madia, F., Bertini, E., Capovilla, G., Chiron, C., Cristofori, G., Elia, M., Fontana, E., Gaggero, R., Granata, T., Guerrini, R., Loi, M., La Selva, L., Lispi, M.L., Matricardi, A., Romeo, A., Tzolas, V., Valseriati, D., Veggiotti, P., Vigevano, F., Vallee, L., Bricarelli, F.D., Bianchi, A., & Zara, F. (2003). Spectrum of SCN1A mutations in severe myoclonic epilepsy of infancy. *Neurology* Vol. 60, No. 12, pp. 1961-1967, ISSN 0028-3878

Noebels, J.L. (2003). THE BIOLOGY OF EPILEPSY GENES. *Annual Review of Neuroscience* Vol. 26, No. 1, pp. 599-625, ISSN 0147-006X

Oakley, J.C., Kalume, F., Yu, F.H., Scheuer, T., & Catterall, W.A. (2009). Temperature- and age-dependent seizures in a mouse model of severe myoclonic epilepsy in infancy. *Proceedings of the National Academy of Sciences of the USA* Vol. 106, No. 10, pp. 3994-3999, ISSN 0027-8424

Ogiwara, I., Miyamoto, H., Morita, N., Atapour, N., Mazaki, E., Inoue, I., Takeuchi, T., Itohara, S., Yanagawa, Y., Obata, K., Furuichi, T., Hensch, T.K., & Yamakawa, K. (2007). Nav1.1 Localizes to Axons of Parvalbumin-Positive Inhibitory Interneurons: A Circuit Basis for Epileptic Seizures in Mice Carrying an Scn1a Gene Mutation. *Journal of Neuroscience* Vol. 27, No. 22, pp. 5903-5914, ISSN 0270-6474

Ohmori, I., Ouchida, M., Ohtsuka, Y., Oka, E., & Shimizu, K. (2002). Significant correlation of the SCN1A mutations and severe myoclonic epilepsy in infancy. *Biochemical and Biophysical Research Communications* Vol. 295, No. 1, pp. 17-23, ISSN 0006-291X

Ortells, M.O., & Barrantes, G.E. (2002). Molecular modelling of the interactions of carbamazepine and a nicotinic receptor involved in the autosomal dominant nocturnal frontal lobe epilepsy. *British Journal of Pharmacology* Vol. 136, No. 6, pp. 883-895, ISSN 0007-1188

Otto, J.F., Singh, N.A., Dahle, E.J., Leppert, M.F., Pappas, C.M., Pruess, T.H., Wilcox, K.S., & White, H.S. (2009). Electroconvulsive seizure thresholds and kindling acquisition rates are altered in mouse models of human Kcnq2 and Kcnq3 mutations for benign familial neonatal convulsions. *Epilepsia* Vol. 50, No. 7, pp. 1752-1759, ISSN 0013-9580

Pan, Z., Kao, T., Horvath, Z., Lemos, J., Sul, J.Y., Cranstoun, S.D., Bennett, V., Scherer, S.S., & Cooper, E.C. (2006). A Common Ankyrin-G-Based Mechanism Retains KCNQ and NaV Channels at Electrically Active Domains of the Axon. *Journal of Neuroscience* Vol. 26, No. 10, pp. 2599-2613, ISSN 0270-6474

Patino, G.A., & Isom, L.L. (2010). Electrophysiology and beyond: Multiple roles of Na+ channel beta subunits in development and disease. *Neuroscience Letters* Vol. 486, No. 2, pp. 53-59, ISSN 0304-3940

Peters, H.C., Hu, H., Pongs, O., Storm, J.F., & Isbrandt, D. (2005). Conditional transgenic suppression of M channels in mouse brain reveals functions in neuronal excitability, resonance and behavior. *Nature Neuroscience* Vol. 8, No. 1, pp. 51-60, ISSN 1097-6256

Phillips, H.A., Favre, I., & Kirkpatrick, M. (2001). CHRNB2 is the second acetylcholine receptor subunit associated with autosomal dominant nocturnal frontal lobe epilepsy. *American Journal of Human Genetics* Vol. 68, pp. 225-231, ISSN 0002-9297

Picard, F., Bruel, D., Servent, D., Saba, W., Fruchart-Gaillard, C., Schollhorn-Peyronneau, M.A., Roumenov, D., Brodtkorb, E., Zuberi, S., Gambardella, A., Steinborn, B., Hufnagel, A., Valette, H., & Bottlaender, M. (2006). Alteration of the in vivo nicotinic receptor density in ADNFLE patients: a PET study. *Brain* Vol. 129, No. 8, pp. 2047-2060, ISSN 0006-8950

Picard, F., Megevand, P., Minotti, L., Kahane, P., Ryvlin, P., Seeck, M., Michel, C.M., & Lantz, G. (2007). Intracerebral recordings of nocturnal hyperkinetic seizures: Demonstration of a longer duration of the pre-seizure sleep spindle. *Clinical Neurophysiology* Vol. 118, No. 4, pp. 928-939, ISSN 1388-2457

Prole, D.L., Lima, P.A., & Marrion, N.V. (2003). Mechanisms Underlying Modulation of Neuronal KCNQ2/KCNQ3 Potassium Channels by Extracellular Protons. *The Journal of General Physiology* Vol. 122, No. 6, pp. 775-793, ISSN 0022-1295

Rasmussen, H.B., Frokjaer-Jensen, C., Jensen, C.S., Jensen, H.S., Jorgensen, N.K., Misonou, H., Trimmer, J.S., Olesen, S.P., & Schmitt, N. (2007). Requirement of subunit co-assembly and ankyrin-G for M-channel localization at the axon initial segment. *Journal of Cell Science* Vol. 120, No. 6, pp. 953-963, ISSN 0021-9533

Ronen, G.M., Rosales, T.O., Connolly, M., Anderson, V.E., & Leppert, M. (1993). Seizure characteristics in chromosome 20 benign familial neonatal convulsions. *Neurology* Vol. 43, No. 7, pp. 1355-1360, ISSN 0028-3878

Rundfeldt, C., & Netzer, R. (2000). The novel anticonvulsant retigabine activates M-currents in Chinese hamster ovary-cells tranfected with human KCNQ2/3 subunits. *Neuroscience Letters* Vol. 282, No. 1-2, pp. 73-76, ISSN 0304-3940

Scheffer, I.E., & Berkovic, S.F. (1997). Generalized epilepsy with febrile seizures plus. A genetic disorder with heterogeneous clinical phenotypes. *Brain* Vol. 120, No. 3, pp. 479-490, ISSN 0006-8950

Schroeder, B.C., Hechenberger, M., Weinreich, F., Kubisch, C., & Jentsch, T.J. (2000). KCNQ5, a Novel Potassium Channel Broadly Expressed in Brain, Mediates M-type Currents. *Journal of Biological Chemistry* Vol. 275, No. 31, pp. 24089-24095, ISSN 0021-9258

Schroeder, B.C., Kubisch, C., Stein, V., & Jentsch, T.J. (1998). Moderate loss of function of cyclic-AMP-modulated KCNQ2/KCNQ3 K+ channels causes epilepsy. *Nature* Vol. 396, No. 6712, pp. 687-690, ISSN 0028-0836

Schuchmann, S., Schmitz, D., Rivera, C., Vanhatalo, S., Salmen, B., Mackie, K., Sipila, S.T., Voipio, J., & Kaila, K. (2006). Experimental febrile seizures are precipitated by a hyperthermia-induced respiratory alkalosis. *Nature Medicine* Vol. 12, No. 7, pp. 817-823, ISSN 1078-8956

Schwake, M., Pusch, M., Kharkovets, T., & Jentsch, T.J. (2000). Surface Expression and Single Channel Properties of KCNQ2/KCNQ3, M-type K+ Channels Involved in Epilepsy. *Journal of Biological Chemistry* Vol. 275, No. 18, pp. 13343-13348, ISSN 0021-9258

Selyanko, A.A., Hadley, J.K., Wood, I.C., Abogadie, F.C., Jentsch, T.J., & Brown, D.A. (2000). Inhibition of KCNQ1-4 potassium channels expressed in mammalian cells via M1 muscarinic acetylcholine receptors. *The Journal of Physiology* Vol. 522, No. 3, pp. 349-355, ISSN 0022-3751

Sieghart, W., & Sperk, G. (2002). Subunit Composition, Distribution and Function of GABA-A Receptor Subtypes. *Current Topics in Medicinal Chemistry* Vol. 2, No. 8, pp. 795-816, ISSN 1568-0266

Singh, N.A., Charlier, C., Stauffer, D., DuPont, B.R., Leach, R.J., Melis, R., Ronen, G.M., Bjerre, I., Quattlebaum, T., Murphy, J.V., McHarg, M.L., Gagnon, D., Rosales, T.O., Peiffer, A., Anderson, V.E., & Leppert, M. (1998). A novel potassium channel gene, KCNQ2, is mutated in an inherited epilepsy of newborns. *Nature Genetics* Vol. 18, No. 1, pp. 25-29, ISSN 1061-4036

Singh, N.A., Otto, J.F., Dahle, E.J., Pappas, C., Leslie, J.D., Vilaythong, A., Noebels, J.L., White, H.S., Wilcox, K.S., & Leppert, M.F. (2008). Mouse models of human KCNQ2 and KCNQ3 mutations for benign familial neonatal convulsions show seizures and neuronal plasticity without synaptic reorganization. *The Journal of Physiology* Vol. 586, No. 14, pp. 3405-3423, ISSN 0022-3751

Soldovieri, M.V., Castaldo, P., Iodice, L., Miceli, F., Barrese, V., Bellini, G., del Giudice, E.M., Pascotto, A., Bonatti, S., Annunziato, L., & Taglialatela, M. (2006). Decreased Subunit Stability as a Novel Mechanism for Potassium Current Impairment by a KCNQ2 C Terminus Mutation Causing Benign Familial Neonatal Convulsions. *Journal of Biological Chemistry* Vol. 281, No. 1, pp. 418-428, ISSN 0021-9258

Spampanato, J., Escayg, A., Meisler, M.H., & Goldin, A.L. (2003). Generalized epilepsy with febrile seizures plus type 2 mutation W1204R alters voltage-dependent gating of Na(v)1.1 sodium channels. *Neuroscience* Vol. 116, No. 1, pp. 37-48, ISSN 0306-4522

Spampanato, J., Kearney, J.A., de Haan, G., McEwen, D.P., Escayg, A., Aradi, I., MacDonald, B.T., Levin, S.I., Soltesz, I., Benna, P., Montalenti, E., Isom, L.L., Goldin, A.L., & Meisler, M.H. (2004). A novel epilepsy mutation in the sodium channel SCN1A identifies a cytoplasmic domain for beta subunit interaction. *Journal of Neuroscience* Vol. 24, No. 44, pp. 10022-10034, ISSN 0270-6474

Steinlein, O.K., Magnusson, A., Stoodt, J., Bertrand, S., Weiland, S., Berkovic, S.F., Nakken, K.O., Propping, P., & Bertrand, D. (1997). An insertion mutation of the CHRNA4 gene in a family with autosomal dominant nocturnal frontal lobe epilepsy. *Human Molecular Genetics* Vol. 6, No. 6, pp. 943-947, ISSN 0964-6906

Steinlein, O.K., Mulley, J.C., Propping, P., Wallace, R.H., Phillips, H.A., Sutherland, G.R., Scheffer, I.E., & Berkovic, S.F. (1995). A missense mutation in the neuronal nicotinic acetylcholine receptor [alpha]4 subunit is associated with autosomal dominant nocturnal frontal lobe epilepsy. *Nature Genetics* Vol. 11, No. 2, pp. 201-203, ISSN 1061-4036

Sugawara, T., Tsurubuchi, Y., Agarwala, K.L., Ito, M., Fukuma, G., Mazaki-Miyazaki, E., Nagafuji, H., Noda, M., Imoto, K., Wada, K., Mitsudome, A., Kaneko, S., Montal, M., Nagata, K., Hirose, S., & Yamakawa, K. (2001). A missense mutation of the Na+ channel alpha II subunit gene Nav1.2 in a patient with febrile and afebrile seizures causes channel dysfunction. *Proceedings of the National Academy of Sciences of the USA* Vol. 98, No. 11, pp. 6384-6389, ISSN 0027-8424

Tang, B., Dutt, K., Papale, L., Rusconi, R., Shankar, A., Hunter, J., Tufik, S., Yu, F.H., Catterall, W.A., Mantegazza, M., Goldin, A.L., & Escayg, A. (2009). A BAC transgenic mouse model reveals neuron subtype-specific effects of a Generalized Epilepsy with Febrile Seizures Plus (GEFS plus) mutation. *Neurobiology of Disease* Vol. 35, No. 1, pp. 91-102, ISSN 0969-9961

Wallace, R.H., Wang, D.W., Singh, R., Scheffer, I.E., George, A.L., Phillips, H.A., Saar, K., Reis, A., Johnson, E.W., Sutherland, G.R., Berkovic, S.F., & Mulley, J.C. (1998). Febrile seizures and generalized epilepsy associated with a mutation in the Na+-channel sz1 subunit gene SCN1B. *Nature Genetics* Vol. 19, No. 4, pp. 366-370, ISSN 1061-4036

Wan, Q., Xiong, Z.G., Man, H.Y., Ackerley, C.A., Braunton, J., Lu, W.Y., Becker, L.E., MacDonald, J.F., & Wang, Y.T. (1997). Recruitment of functional GABAA receptors to postsynaptic domains by insulin. *Nature* Vol. 388, No. 6643, pp. 686-690, ISSN 0028-0836

Watanabe, H., Nagata, E., Kosakai, A., Nakamura, M., Yokoyama, M., Tanaka, K., & Sasai, H. (2000). Disruption of the epilepsy KCNQ2 gene results in neural hyperexcitability. *Journal of Neurochemistry* Vol. 75, No. 1, pp. 28-33, ISSN 0022-3042

Waxham, M.N. (2003). Neurotransmitter receptors. In: *Fundamentle Neuroscience*, Squire, L.R., Bloom, F.E., McConnel, S.K., Roberts, J.L., Spitzer, N.C., & Zigmond, M.J., (Eds.) pp. 225-258, Academic Press, ISBN 0-12-660303-0, California, USA.

Waxman, S.G. (2007). Channel, neuronal and clinical function in sodium channelopathies: from genotype to phenotype. *Nature Neuroscience* Vol. 10, No. 4, pp. 405-409, ISSN 1097-6256

Weber, Y.G., Geiger, J., Kampchen, K., Landwehrmeyer, B., Sommer, C., & Lerche, H. (2006). Immunohistochemical analysis of KCNQ2 potassium channels in adult and developing mouse brain. *Brain Research* Vol. 1077, No. 1, pp. 1-6, ISSN 0006-8993

Wickenden, A.D., Yu, W., Zou, A., Jegla, T., & Wagoner, P.K. (2000). Retigabine, A Novel Anti-Convulsant, Enhances Activation of KCNQ2/Q3 Potassium Channels. *Molecular Pharmacology* Vol. 58, No. 3, pp. 591-600, ISSN 0026-895X

Yu, F.H., & Catterall, W.A. (2003). Overview of the voltage-gated sodium channel family. *Genome Biology* Vol. 4, No. 3, pp. 207, ISSN 1465-6906

Yu, F.H., Mantegazza, M., Westenbroek, R.E., Robbins, C.A., Kalume, F., Burton, K.A., Spain, W.J., McKnight, G.S., Scheuer, T., & Catterall, W.A. (2006). Reduced sodium current in GABAergic interneurons in a mouse model of severe myoclonic epilepsy in infancy. *Nature Neuroscience* Vol. 9, No. 9, pp. 1142-1149, ISSN 1097-6256

12

Educating People Participating in the Pig Industry to Reduce Epilepsy due to Taenia Solium

Cate E. Dewey[1], Florence K. Mutua[2],
Mike Levy[1] and Jared M. Wohlgemut[1]
[1]*University of Guelph, Canada;*
[2]*University of Nairobi,*
Kenya

1. Introduction

In the developing countries of Africa, Asia and Latin America, neurocysticercosis is the major cause of adult-onset epilepsy (Garcia et al., 2004; Roman et al., 2000; Garcia et al., 2005; Sarti et al., 1994; Sciutto et al., 2000; Mahajan RC, 1982). In 1992, this form of epilepsy, and the *Taenia solium* tapeworm was declared a potentially eradicable disease by the International Task Force for Disease Eradication (Aarata et al., 1992; Shantz et al., 1993). However, there are several barriers to eradication such as lack of knowledge, lack of resources, poor hygiene and the fundamental implications of the management of pigs as a source of banking and income generation for the poorest of the poor. This chapter will discuss promising results of an educational program, the fact that the education should include the various actors in the swine industry, and illustrate the need for a broader geographic focus to promote the eradication of epilepsy due to neurocysticercosis.

2. Life cycle of the *Taenia solium* parasite

T. solium, called the pork tapeworm, has people as its definitive host. The adult tapeworm grows in the intestine of the infected person, shedding proglotids which are mature segments of the worm. These proglotids, that contain approximately 50,000 eggs, are shed each day in the stool of the infected person. Pigs, as the intermediate host, are infected by *Cysticercus cellulosae.* When a pig ingests the eggs that have been shed in the stool of the human, the egg crosses the intestinal wall. Next, the egg enters the blood stream and migrates to the muscle tissue. There the egg develops into a larval cyst. The tapeworm is transmitted to another person when this second person eats infected, undercooked pork. However, people can also act as an intermediate host. If a person ingests a tapeworm egg, it crosses from the intestine to the blood stream and preferentially migrates to nervous tissue. There it develops into a larval cyst. Epilepsy is caused by the space occupying lesions of the cysts in the brain of the infected person. This form of the disease is called neurocysticercosis (Serpa et al., 2007).

Epilepsy is a devastating clinical problem in rural areas where there is little education, high rates of poverty, and poor access to health care. People suffering from epilepsy are often misunderstood, ostracised, and limited in their participation in society. The family members experience shame and may choose to keep the person suffering from epilepsy confined to the home. Often the affected person will not receive a proper diagnosis or appropriate medication. Epilepsy left unmedicated may advance significantly to increase the frequency and severity of seizures and may result in secondary trauma such as severe lacerations or burns. The eradication of the epilepsy due to this parasite requires the disruption of its life cycle (Mafojane et al., 2003; Phiri et al., 2003).

3. Situation in Sub Saharan East Africa

Pig rearing in Sub Saharan East Africa has been increasing by 10% per year over the past decade and in Uganda pork production increased by ten times between 1985 and 2005. Many people living in rural areas of East Africa depend for their livelihood on smallholder pig farming. The advantage of keeping pigs over cattle or sheep are that pigs grow faster and have more offspring in a short time period, eat leftover food, and are very easy to sell (Lekule & Kyvsgaard 2003; Mutua *et al.* 2010). Smallholder farmers typically live in extended family compounds on an average of one to two acres of land (Kagira *et al* 2010; Mutua *et al.* 2010). Some family members may not use a latrine because of cultural norms or they may not have a functional latrine in the family compound (Githigia et al., 2005; Mutua et al., 2007). When one or more family members does not use the latrine, the life cycle of *T. solium* is enhanced because pigs gain access to human stool. Smallholder farmers who live in poverty grow their own food and therefore have insufficient land for other livestock. Therefore, *T. solium* tends to be a problem of the poorest of the poor. If there is a competition between the food resources between people and pigs, the pigs are kept in the traditional manner in a mixture of free range and tethered management style, largely because the inputs are much lower than under intensive management (Kagira *et al.* 2010; Lekule & Kyvsgaard 2003). Pigs are purchased when the family has some extra money to buy a weaned piglet. Then the pigs are kept to bank small amounts of money, for income generation, and to source money in a hurry when there is a family emergency such as medical needs, school fees, or for food between harvest seasons (Kagira *et al.* 2010; Lekule & Kyvsgaard 2003; Mutua *et al.* 2010).

In areas where *T. solium* is endemic, eradication is only possible by eliminating the reservoirs of the parasite. However, it is difficult to find live infected pigs because the test that is used, an examination of tongue for evidence of cysts, has a very low sensitivity of approximately 50%. Therefore, the only method of keeping infected pigs from the food chain is to ensure that all pigs are inspected by a government official after slaughter. In many developing countries the inspection system is poor and often people in the villages use home slaughter after which they sell meat from the family's farm (Roman et al., 2000).

4. Education

One study indicates that community behavioural and environmental practices must be modified to prevent continued transmission of cysticercosis and taeniasis (Sarti et al., 1992). This is perhaps best accomplished through education. Researchers have found that education in conjunction with community involvement reduces opportunities for transmission of *T. solium* in the human-pig cycle Sarti et al., 1997. A successful long-term change will only occur if the intervention program is associated with community participation and health education programs (Sarti et al., 1997; Cao et al., 1997; Sanchez et al., 1999; Carrique-Mas et al., 2001).

Education of farmers, butchers and government extension workers is likely the best method to prevent the lifecycle of *T. solium*. The government workers should include public health, adult education, veterinary and livestock specialist and social workers who are responsible for facilitating farmer groups. Ideally the education will also include key community leaders such as teachers, village elders and village chiefs (or the equivalent depending on the societal structure) whose opinion will be valued. It is important that the education includes the pig butchers as well because they are often responsible for slaughtering the pigs and selling raw and cooked pork. The farmers are in the most opportune position to interrupt the life cycle of the parasite by keeping the pig tied and away from human stool and the pig butchers and government veterinary inspectors can identify infected pigs to reduce the number of positive pigs in the food chain.

5. Education model

Although there are many education models that are likely successful, one such model that was used in Western Kenya will be described in this chapter (Wohlgemut et al., 2010). Regardless of the education model used, the long-term success of the program must be evaluated.

5.1 Farmer education

This four-part study included baseline data collection using individual farmer interviews followed by a workshop. Approximately half of any group of farmers is expected to attend one-day workshops. The farmers included in the data collection were randomly chosen within each selected village whereas the workshops were open to all pig farmers, village elders and village chiefs who wished to attend. Two subsequent farm visits followed the workshop, each 5 months apart. During these farm visits, a questionnaire was completed followed by one-on-one training. Farmers were asked if they attended the workshop and if not, they were given the education about the lifecycle of *T. solium* and prevention of the disease in people and in pigs. All farmers were encouraged to ask questions about *T. solium*, pig management or disease. The farmer was not limited in the number of questions they could ask or the time the researchers spent answering questions. During each visit, the farmer was interviewed in their native tongue by a local person who was hired by the research team and trained to conduct the interview. These research assistants translated for the English speaking researchers who were experts in pig production and disease. Phase 3 of the program was to provide a 2nd set of workshops for the farmers two years after the first farm visit. The workshop was based on the research results obtained during the longitudinal project and provided an opportunity to discuss *T. solium*. The final phase was to return to the community four years after the start of the study, which was two years after the phase 3. During this phase the researchers conducted one-on-one interviews to determine what behaviours the farmers adopted in response to the education (Wohlgemut et al., 2010).

5.2 Government staff education

A Training of the Trainers model was used in this project. The advantage of this model is that the government staff are taught the material that the researchers hope to spread to the entire community. The education program is longer term and more widespread because the staff can continue to disseminate the information for years after the project has ended. It is also important that the staff are given the same information that the farmers receive. Finally, the staff are able to converse with the farmers in their own local language. The researchers provided three, one-day workshops for government staff and local community leaders including teachers and village chiefs. The workshops occurred at the start of the project and then two and four years later. At each workshop, the staff were given 20 to 30 page booklets that summarized the information taught and gave the background scientific information to justify the content. Staff who attended the workshops included veterinary, livestock, public health, and adult education specialists, veterinarians and social workers. The workshops included sections of the lifecycle of T solium, the cause of neurocysticercosis and pig management, housing, breeding, feeding, diseases, and care. Each participant was required to participate in at least 3 workshops for the farmers in the local villages. At the end of the government workshop, the researchers assisted the staff in the preparation and planning for the farmer workshops (Wohlgemut et al., 2010).

5.3 Butcher education

The workshops for the pig butchers were facilitated directly by the researchers (Levy et al., 2009). The workshops focused on a study of the fixed and variable costs of a pig butcher business, income and profit calculation. The workshop also included a section on enhancing pork safety that included the life cycle of *T. solium,* the recognition of larval cysts in pig muscle, the importance of having every carcass inspected, and personal and butchershop hygiene. Finally, each butcher determined the cost of slaughtering the pig at a slaughter slab and government inspection based on the required kilogram of pork sales per pig to cover the cost. Many butchers were not able to leave their work to attend the workshops. One-on-one training was given to these butchermen. This format was not likely as valuable because during the workshops, the butchers discussed many of the issues presented and shared information with one another.

6. Knowledge acquisition

The educational opportunities enabled the farmers to learn about the life cycle of *T. solium.* However, the life cycle is complicated and the one-on-one training was more effective than the workshops in the longterm retention of the knowledge. One-on-one training enabled the farmer to ask the researcher questions as she explained the lifecycle of *T. solium.* Further, the farmer was able to hold a picture of the life cycle during the training rather than relying on following a poster at the front of the classroom. One-on-one training was also associated with having heard of the tapeworm in people and having seen the proglotids in a person's stool. This may have been because the researcher showed a picture of the proglotids during the training. Although one-on-one training is expensive, it is worth the cost if it results in long-term behaviour changes in a community that then reduce the incidence of *T. solium* due to epilepsy. That too has a high societal cost (Wohlgemut et al., 2010).

All farmers who had some education were more likely to correctly describe how pigs and people became infected and how people developed epilepsy from *T. solium* than before the study began (Wohlgemut et al., 2010). However, farmers who had been taught one-on-one were more able to correctly describe how people and pigs became infected than farmers who had only attended the workshop. Farmers who had completed primary school were also more likely to retain this information than farmers with less formal education. Leonard (1977) found that the level of education and prior knowledge of Swahili impacted the Kenyan farmers' capacity to understand complex messages. This puts an extra responsibility on the educators who must first be well educated to understand, and subsequently convey clear and accurate messages (Flisser & Lightowlers, 2001). The connection between former education and knowledge acquisition illustrates the potential advantage of introducing this information into the late primary school education curriculum. If people who are used to learn in a classroom are more likely to understand and retain this material, a large number of families can be accessed through the educational system. This may be the most appropriate educational model in countries with a high uptake of primary school education among the poor.

Understanding the lifecycle of the tapeworm enables the farmer to determine how to interrupt the transmission through regular use of a pit latrine, improved personal hygiene and confining the pig. It is important that farmers understand the connection between the tapeworm and epilepsy so that they have a reason to make management changes to the pig rearing operation. Pigs that are tethered or housed must be fed on a daily basis. This takes time and money. Farmers who are not used to feeding their pig must also be taught about the locally available foods that can be used in combination to provide a complete ration for the pigs (Mutua et al., 2011). By using waste food stuff such as fruits that are spoiled, weeds, kitchen waste, and inexpensive sources of protein, farmers are able to reduce the costs of feeding the pig. All famers, from the beginning of the study knew that they should seek medical treatment if they saw worms in their stool. The educators should encourage whole families to use anti-parasiticides if one family member has proglotids in their stool.

7. Extension of knowledge to the community

The information about the life cycle of T. solium was rarely conveyed from one family member who attended the workshop to another family member who was interviewed five months later. This fact was frustrating for the researchers. One report from the United States Agency for International Development noted that it is of special importance to ensure access of education and training to women, as they are key contributors to the agricultural workforce, and could further contribute if recognized as a priority audience.[23] However, when looking at the long-term behaviour changes from the educational program, four years after the project began, farm families had adopted preventative management changes. Regardless of whether it was a man or woman who attended the training, four years after the start of the study, women were boiling the pork for 20 minutes prior to frying. Also, all the pigs were either in barns or tethered. A few farmers also mentioned either repairing or building pit latrines for the family to use. One study found that the prevalence of porcine cysticercosis was higher in pigs reared in households lacking latrines than pigs raised in households that had latrines (Ngowi et al., 2004). Similarly, the decline in *T. solium* infections in parts of Europe over the past century was due to improved public sanitation, rather than any specifically targeted control measures (Mahajan, 1982). Approximately 18% of families that did not participate in the educational project adopted behaviour changes because their neighbours had shared the information.

8. Confining pigs

After the initial farmer training workshop, the number of farmers that tethered their pigs increased from 32% to 51%. This rate increased to 62% after the one-on-one training. Four years after the study began, 100% of the farmers who had either participated in the research program or attended one of the workshops were either housing or tethering their pigs. This illustrates the long-term behaviour changes that results from these educational opportunities.

9. Safe pork

Four years after the study began, farmers and butchers were boiling the pork for 20 minutes before they fried the meat. The larval cyst will be killed if it is cooked at a boiling temperature for 10 minutes. Farmers said they purchased pork from butchers rather than from backyard operations because they wanted to buy meat that was inspected. Butchers regularly took the pigs to the slaughter slab to have them inspected prior to sale. The business education was important to the butchers because they kept track of their expenses and were sure to save enough money from each pig to pay for the inspection of the next pig. In a World Bank project in Kenya found that over 80% of farmers who are taught recommended practices choose to adopt them (Gautam 2000). This education had both a positive short- and long-term impact (Gautam 2000).

10. Conclusions

Reducing the prevalence of epilepsy due to neurocysticercosis requires people working in the pig industry to make substantial behaviour changes. To interrupt the lifecycle of the *T. solium* parasite, pigs must be confined so that they cannot gain access to human stool; pork must be inspected to keep infected carcasses out of the human food chain; pork must be well cooked to ensure that cysts not observed by inspectors are killed; people who carry the tapeworm must be treated; and people must be encouraged to improve personal hygiene by using a pit latrine and washing their hands after defecating. Knowledge is power. People will be motivated to make behaviour changes when they understand the link between the pork tapeworm, pigs, pork, hygiene and epilepsy. There are financial implications to preventing epilepsy due to *T. solium* and interrupting the lifecycle. Farmers who keep their pigs confined must source feed for the pig. There is a cost to purchase some of the food and other food, such as weeds, will require the farmer to spend time collecting. The butchers must spend additional money to transport the pig to and from the slaughter slab, to use the slab and to have the government staff person inspect the carcass. If the carcass is condemned due to cysts, the butcher assumes the entire purchase price of the pig.

Workshops using a Training of the Trainers model by teaching the government staff and local community leaders who then teach the farmers are an effective way to increase knowledge and elicit long-term behaviour changes by the farmers. One-on-one training of the farmers increases the level of knowledge, in particular, for difficult concepts such as the lifecycle of the tapeworm. It is important that workshops are followed up by individual training sessions between farmers and researchers so that the material is presented more than once, in more than one training method and those farmers have an opportunity to ask questions in a safe and private environment. Workshops for the pork butchers in which the education is linked to business practice were particularly important. The butchers acquired useful information about how to track and understand the costs, income, and profits of their business. They learned about their role in preventing epilepsy due to neurocysticercosis and felt responsible for ensuring the safety of the pork they sell. The butchers did change their behaviour by having a higher proportion or all of the pork carcasses inspected prior to sale. Both farmers and butchers changed how they cooked the pork by boiling it for 20 minutes prior to consumption or sale. Together, the systematic changes across the entire pig industry are expected to reduce the prevalence of epilepsy in these communities. This model needs to be repeated around the world, wherever pigs are kept in a free range manner and neurocysticercosis occurs.

11. References

Aarata, A.A.; Hopkins, D.R.; Ruiz-Tiben E. & Pawlowski ZS. (1992). International task force for disease eradication. *Journal of the American Medical Association 268:* 1841. *ISSN*: 00987484.

Cao W.; van der Ploeg C.P.; Xu, J.; Gao, C.; Ge, L. & Habbema JD. (1997) Risk factors for human cysticercosis morbidity: a population-based case-control study. *Epidemiology and Infection 119:* 231-235. ISSN: 0950-2688

Carrique-Mas, J.; Iihoshi, N.; Widdowson, MA.; Roca, Y.; Morales, G.; Quiroga, J.; Cejas, F.; Caihuara, M.; Ibarra, R. & Edelsten M. (2001). An epidemiological study of *Taenia solium* cysticercosis in a rural population in the Bolivian Chaco. *Acta Tropica 21:* 229-235. *ISSN*: 0001-706X

Flisser, A. & Lightowlers, M.W. (2001). Vaccination against *Taenia solium* cysticercosis. *Memorias do* Instituto Oswaldo Cruz, *96:* 353-356. *ISSN* 0074-0276

Garcia, H.H., Pretell, E.J., Gilman, R.H., Martinez, S.M., Moulton, L.H., Del Brutto, O.H., Herrera, G., Evans, C.A. & Gonzalez, A.E. (2004). A trial of antiparasitic treatment to reduce the rate of seizures due to cerebral cysticercosis. *New England Journal of Medicine* 350: 249-258. *ISSN* 0028-4793

Garcia, H.H. & Del Brutto, O.H. (2005). Neurocysticercosis: updated concepts about an old disease. *Lancet Neurology 4:* 653-661. *ISSN*: 1474-4422

Gautam, M. (2000). Agricultural Extension: The Kenya Experience: An Impact Evaluation. Washington, DC: *World Bank, Operations Evaluation Department,* 1-34. lnweb90.worldbank.org/oed/oeddoclib.nsf/0/.../$FILE/ARDE_2000.pdf

Githigia, S.M.; Murekefu, A. & Otieno, RO. (2005). Prevalence of porcine cysticercosis and risk factors for *Taenia solium* taeniosis in Funyula Division of Busia District, Kenya. *The Kenya Veterinarian 29:* 37-39. *ISSN*: 0256-5161.

Kagira. J.M.; Kanyari.; P.W.N.; Ndicho Maingi, N.; Githigia, S.M.; Ng'ang'a, J.C. & Karuga, J.W. (2010) 'Characteristics of the smallholder free-range pig production system in western Kenya'. *Tropical Animal Health and Production* 42:865–873 *ISSN*: 0049-4747

Lekule, F.P. & N.C. Kyvsgaard. (2003). 'Improving pig husbandry in tropical resource-poor communities and its potential to reduce risk of porcine cysticercosis', *Acta Tropica* 87, 1: 111-7. *ISSN*: 0001-706X

Leonard, D.K. (1977). Researching the Peasant Farmer- Organization Theory and Practice in Kenya. Chicago, IL: University of Chicago Press, 140-147. *ISBN* 0 226 10390 0

Levy, M.; Dewey. C.; Weersink, A. & Mutua, F.K. (2009). 'Comparative profitability of pig butcher businesses in western Kenya', *Proceedings 12th International Society for Veterinary Epidemiology and Economics* Durban, South Africa, August, 2009. 12:544 *ISSN*: 0754-2186

Lightowlers, M.W. (1999). Eradication of *Taenia solium* cysticercosis: a role for vaccination of pigs. *International Journal of Parasitology 29:* 811-817. ISSN: 0020-7519

Mafojane, N.A.; Appleton, C.C.; Krecek, R.C.; Michael, L.M. & Willingham III A.L. (2003). The current status of neurocysticercosis in Eastern and Southern Africa. *Acta Tropica 87:* 25-33. *ISSN*: 0001-706X

Mahajan, R.C. (1982). Geographical distribution of human cysticercosis. In:Flisser A, Willms K.; Laclette JP.; Larralde C.; Ridaura C, BeltraÂn F, eds. *Cysticercosis: present state of knowledge and perspectives.* New York, NY: Academic Press, 39-46. ISBN: 0122607406

Mutua, F.K.; Randolph, T.F.; Arimi, S.M.; Kitala, P.M.; Githigia, S.M.; Willingham, A.L. & Njeruh, F.M. (2007). Palpable lingual cysts, a possible indicator of porcine cysticercosis, in Teso District, Western Kenya. *J Swine Health Prod 15:* 206-212. *ISSN* 1537-209X

Mutua, F.K .; Arimi, S., Ogara, W.; Dewey, C.E. & Schelling, E. (2010). Farmer Perceptions on Indigenous Pig Farming in Kakamega District, Western Kenya. *Nordic Journal of African Studies* 19(1): 43–57. *ISSN* 1459-9465

Mutua, F.K.; Dewey, C.E.; Arimi, S.M.; Schelling, E. & Ogara, W.O. (2011). Prediction of live body weight using length and girth measurements for pigs in rural Western Kenya. *Journal of Swine Health and Production*. 19(1):26-33. *ISSN* 1537-209X

Ngowi, H.A.; Kassuku, A.A.; Maeda, G.E.M.; Boa, M.E.; Carabin, H. & Willingham III, A.L. (2004). Risk factors for prevalence of porcine cysticercosis in Mbulu District, Tanzania. *Veterinary Parasitology 120:* 275-283. *ISSN*: 0304-4017

Phiri, I.K.; Ngowi, H.; Afonso, S.; Matenga, E.; Boa, M.; Mukaratirwa, S.; Githigia, S.; Saimo, M.; Sikasunge, C.; Maingi, N.; Lubega, G.W.; Kassuku, A.; Michael, L.; Siziya, S.; Krecek, R.C.; Noormahomed, E.; Vilhena M.; Dorny, P. & Willingham III, A.L. (2003). The emergence of *Taenia solium* cysticercosis in Eastern and Southern Africa as a serious agricultural problem and public health risk. *Acta Tropica*, 87(1), pp. 13-23. *ISSN*: 0001-706X

Roman, G.; Sotelo, J.; Del Brutto, O.; Flisser, A.; Dumas, M.; Wadia, N.; Botero D.; Cruz, M.; Garcia, H.; de Bittencourt, PR.; Trelles, L.; Arriagada, C.; Lorenzana, P.; Nash, T.E. & Spina-França, A. (2000). A proposal to declare neurocysticercosis an international reportable disease. *Bull World Health Organ 78:* 399-406. *ISSN*:1564-0604

Sanchez, A.L.; Lindback, J.; Schantz, P.M.; Sone, M.; Sakai, H.; Medina, M.T. & Ljungstrom I. (1999). A population based, case-control study of *Taenia solium* taeniosis and cysticercosis. *Ann Tropical Medical Parasitology 93:* 247-258. *ISSN* (printed): 0003-4983

Sarti, E., Schantz, P.M.; Plancarte, A.; Wilson, M.; Gutierrez, I.O.; Lopez, A.S.; Roberts, J. & Flisser, A. (1992). Prevalence and risk factors for *Taenia solium* taeniasis/cysticercosis in humans and pigs in a village in Morelos, Mexico. *American Journal of Tropical Medicine and Hygiene 46:* 677-684. *ISSN* 0002-9637

Sarti, E.; Schantz, P.M.; Plancarte, A.; Wilson, M.; Gutierrez, O.I.; Aguilera, J.; Roberts, J. & Flisser, A. (1994). Epidemiological investigation of *Taenia solium* taeniasis and cysticercosis in a rural village of Michoacan state, Mexico. *Transactions Royal Society of Tropical Medicine and Hygiene 88:* 49-52. *ISSN*:0035-9203

Sarti, E.; Flisser, A.; Schantz, PM.; Gleizer, M.; Loya, M.; Plancarte, A.; Avila, G.; Allan ,J.; Craig, P.; Bronfman, M. & Wijeyaratne, P. (1997). Development and Evaluation of a Health Education Intervention against *Taenia solium* in a Rural Community in Mexico. *American Journal of Tropical Medicine and Hygiene 56:* 127-132. *ISSN* 0002-9637

Schantz, P.M.; Cruz, M.; Sarti, E. & Pawlowski, Z. (1993). Potential eradicability of taeniasis and cysticercosis. *Bulliten Pan American Health Organization 27:* 397-403. *ISSN*: 0085-4638

Sciutto, E.; Fragoso, G.; Fleury, A.; Laclette, J.P.; Sotelo, J.; Aluja, A.; Vargas, L. & Larralde, C. (2000). *Taenia solium* disease in humans and pigs: an ancient parasitosis disease rooted in developing countries and emerging as a major health problem of global dimensions. *Microbes and Infection 2:* 1875-1890. *ISSN*: 1286-4579

Serpa, J,A,; Moran, A.; Goodman, J,C.; Giordano, T,P. & White, A.C. Jr. (2007). Neurocysticercosis in the HIV Era: A case report and review of the literature. *American Journal of Tropical Medicine and Hygiene 77:* 113-117. *ISSN* 0002-9637

Wohlgemut, J.; Dewey, C.E.; Levy, M.A. & Mutua, F.K. (2010). Evaluating the efficacy of teaching methods used to convey information to farmers in Western Kenya about the prevention of neurocysticercosis due to Taenia solium. *American Journal of Tropical Medicine & Hygiene.* 2010;82:634-642 *ISSN* 0002-9637

13

Myoclonic Epilepsy in Lysosomal Storage Disorders

Andrea Dardis and Bruno Bembi
Regional Coorddinator Centre for Rare Diseases
University Hospital "Santa Maria della Misericordia" of Udine Piazzale, Santa Maria della Misericordia, Udine, Italy

1. Introduction

Progressive myoclonic epilepsy (PME) constitutes an heterogeneous group of diseases, usually of genetic origin, which begins in childhood and adolescence and presents a variable evolution, ranging from slowly to rapidly progressive forms with refractory seizures and dead within few years (Marseille Consensus Group, 1990). Despite its broad spectrum of manifestations, patients affected with PME share some common specific clinical and electrophysiological features, such as: myoclonus, multiple type of seizures, delay or regression of psychomotor development, cerebellar ataxia, slow background activity on electroencephalogram (EEG), spikes and waves induced by intermittent photo-stimulation and sensory evoked giant potentials (Marseille Consensus Group, 1990).

From the genetic point of view, PME occurs in disorders presenting different genetic inheritance, including: the dentatorubralpallidolusyian atrophy (DRPLA), a disease of trinucleotide repeats, the myoclonic epilepsy with ragged red fibers (MERRF), a mitochondrial disease and autosomal recessive disorders, which may be divided in two main categories: non-lysosomal-related diseases such as Lafora disease and lysosomal-related-disease such as lysosomal storage disorders (LSDs).

Lysosomal storage disorders are severe genetic diseases caused by the defective activity of lysosomal proteins, cofactors or integral membrane proteins, which result in the intra-lysosomal accumulation of undegraded metabolites such as sphingolipids, cholesterol, glycoproteins, mucopolysaccharides or glycogen. Even if they are individually rare, the combined frequency of LSDs is estimated to be approximately 1 in 8000 live births (Meilke et al., 1999; Poorthuis et al., 1999; Applegarth et al., 2000; Dionisi-Vici et al., 2002; Pinto et al., 2004; Poupetova et al., 2010).

More than 50 LSDs have been described to date (Staretz-Chacham et al., 2009). Although they are characterized by a wide spectrum of clinical phenotypes, many of these disorders present with severe progressive neurological impairment. Among the neurological symptoms, the presence of PME has been reported in different LSDs, including Gaucher disease, action myoclonus-renal failure syndrome, neuronal ceroid lipofuscinoses, sialidosis, Niemann Pick type C disease, and GM2 gangliosidosis. Each of these LSDs is characterized by a series of specific sings and symptoms. However, many of them share some clinical and biochemical features, such as the presence of signs of neurological impairments other than PME or organ disorders, which may be useful in the diagnosis of patients presenting with PME due to LSD.

Although LSDs are the main cause of the inherited form of PME, lysosomal defects are poorly known as a cause of PME and the differential diagnosis might be challenging, particularly in adult patients who may present a milder form of the diseases.
Therefore, the aim of this review is to overview the clinical and molecular findings in patients with PME affected with LSDs and their therapeutic options.

2. Gaucher disease (GD)

GD, the most frequent LSD, is an autosomal recessive inherited disease due to the deficiency in the lysosomal hydrolase, acid β-glucosidase (GBA). The enzyme is present in the lysosomes of all nucleated cells and cleaves the β−glucosidic linkage of glucosylceramide (GlcCer) yielding glucose and ceramide. GBA deficiency leads to the progressive lysosomal accumulation of GlcCer and other glycosphingolipids (GSLs) and subsequent multi-organ dysfunction. The storage predominantly occurs in cells of the monocyte-macrophage lineage, but an increase in GlcCer concentration is detectable in most of the body tissues (Beutler & Grabowski, 2001).
GD is panethnic (Beutler & Grabowski, 2001; Zimran et al., 1992; Cox & Shofield, 1997; Erikson, 1986) and presents an incidence of one case per 60,000 live births in the general population (Meikle et al., 1999). However, it is the most frequent genetic disease in the Ashkenazi Jewish population where it shows a incidence of one case per 850 live births (Beutler et al., 1993).

2.1 Clinical aspects

The disease has been classically classified in three major clinical variants based on the presence and progression of central nervous system involvement. Type 1 GD (MIM# 230800), the most common phenotype, is characterized by enlargement and dysfunction of liver and spleen, displacement of normal bone marrow by storage cells and bone damage leading to infarctions and fractures. Although type 1 GD is considered a non-neuropathic form, there is increasing evidence that neurological involvement (i.e. Parkinson syndrome, seizures, oligophrenia, perceptive deafness) can occur. Type 2 GD (MIM# 230900) is a rare phenotype associated with an acute neurodegenerative course and death at a very early age. These patients commonly present during the first month of life with evidence of brainstem dysfunction consisting in supranuclear gaze palsy and hepatosplenomegaly followed by progressive deterioration, opisthotonus dysphagia, pyramidal signs, failure to thrive and cachexia. They may also have intersititial lung disease and repeated respiratory infections. Type 3, the chronic neuronopathic GD (MIM# 231000), comprises an extremely heterogeneous group of patients who present with either mild or severe systemic disease associated with some form of neurological involvement and with an onset of symptoms that might range from childhood to early adulthood (Beutler & Grabowski, 2001). A most consistent finding in patients affected with this form of GD is an abnormality of the horizontal gaze. Among GD3 patients it has been widely demonstrated the existence of a subgroup of patients sharing the rare finding of PME (Rapin et al., 1986; Seeman et al., 1996; Garvey et al., 2001; Park et al., 2003; Kraoua et al., 2010, Tylki-Szymanska et al., 2010). Published data from the International Collaborative Gaucher Group showed the presence of myoclonic epilepsy in 3 out of 121 patients who had suffered from seizures when first assessed. However, a study performed in a French cohort of 10 patients affected with GD3

showed the presence of PME in 2 (Kraoua et al., 2010). Similarly, unpublished data collected from GD3 patients followed in our Center showed that 3 out of 13 developed PME.
The analysis of the clinical phenotype in a group of 16 GD3 patients presenting with PME , showed that this is not an homogeneous phenotype. In fact, many clinical features found among this group were quite variable including age, sex, ethnic background, degree of visceral, skeletal, cognitive and cerebellar involvement and MRI findings. However, a clinical finding shared by all patients was the slowing of the horizontal saccadic eye movements, a feature present in GD3 patients that was independent of the extent of non-neurological manifestations. In addition, another finding shared among these patients was the abnormal EEG, often with generalized seizures. As disease progressed many of them developed ataxia, dementia and spasticity (Park et al., 2003).

2.2 Molecular aspects

Human GBA is a peripheral membrane glycoprotein. The mature non-glycosylated polypeptide is composed of 497 aminoacids with a molecular weight of about 56 kD while the glycosylated enzyme has a molecular weight of 63 kD (Leonova and Grabowski, 2000).
The human *GBA1* gene (GBA; MIM# 606463; GenBank accession no. J03059.1) of approximately 7.5 kb is located on chromosome 1q21 and contains 11 exons. A highly homologous 5.5 kb-pseudogene (GBAP; MIM# 606463; GenBank accession no. J03060.1) is located 16 kb downstream from the active gene (Horowitz et al.,1989). The *GBA* mRNA has two in-frame ATG translational sites located in exons 1 and 2 (Sorge et al., 1985). Both are efficiently translated and produce two polypeptides with signal peptides of 39 and 19 residues, respectively (Sorge et al., 1987; Pasmanik-Chor et al., 1996).
More than 300 mutations in the *GBA* gene have been reported to date, including all kinds of defects such as single base changes, splicing alterations, insertions, partial and total deletions, gene-pseudogene rearrangements (www.hgmd.org; Stenson et al., 2003).
Mutations N370S, 84GG, L444P, IVS2+1G>A account for 90% of mutant alleles in the Jewish population while they represent fewer than 75% of alleles among non-Jewish Caucasian patients with some differences in defined subpopulations (Beutler & Gelbart, 1993; Grabowski & Horowitz, 1997). In any case N370S and L444P alleles are the most prevalent throughout most population.
Although, no consistent correlation between the genotype and phenotype has been found, some general conclusions can be drawn regarding the neuroprotective nature of the N370S mutation and the association between the L444P allele and the severe phenotype.
The molecular study of the *GBA1* gene in a cohort of 16 GD3 patients with PME showed also within this subgroup a remarkable genotype heterogeneity even among patients with similar clinical presentation. However, an interesting finding of this study was the fact that while 72% of 122 GD3 patients included in the International Gaucher Registry carry the p.L444P/p.L444P genotype, only one out of 16 GD3 patients with PME presented this genotype, suggesting that the most frequent genotype found in GD3 patients would be underrepresented among GD3 patients with PME. In contrast, some rare mutants were encountered among GD3 patients with PME. In particular three point mutations seems to be associated with this phenotype, the V394L, N188S and G377S, suggesting that GD3 patients carrying one of these mutations in the absence of the N370S mutation should be carefully evaluated for PME (Park et al., 2003).

The correlation between the presence of N188S and the occurrence of PME in GD3 patients has been further supported by the work of Kowarz et al. showing a high frequency of the N188S mutation in a series of 17 GD3 patients with PME (Kowarz et al., 2005). In addition, the N188S/S107L genotype was also found in a GD3 patient with visual seizures and PME (Filocamo et al., 2004).

Mutation N188S was first described in Korean and Chinese Type I GD patients (Kim et al., 1996). Later, it was demonstrated by in vitro expression experiments that the GBA protein carrying the N188S mutation retained a high residual enzymatic activity (67% of control, Montfort et al., 2004). Furthermore, the residual GBA activity found in cultured fibroblasts obtained from a GD3 patient with PME who presented the N188S mutation was 24% of control (Park et al., 2003). The reasons for this apparent discordance between the residual activity and the clinical phenotype are not fully understood. However, the association between the presence of N188S mutation and PME in GD suggests that despite the high residual activity the mutation might alter the protein structure, binding, post-translational processing or might modify the role of other proteins involved in the ethiology of the PME.

3. Action myoclonus-renal failure syndrome (AMRF)

AMRF (MIM 254900) is a lethal inherited form of PME associated with renal failure. It was initially described in French- Canadians but it has been reported in patients with various ethnic origins (Andermann et al., 1986; Badhwar et al., 2004). It is caused by the deficiency of the lysosomal integral membrane protein type 2 (LIMP-2) (Berkovic et al., 2008, Balreira et al., 2008), an ubiquitously expressed transmembrane protein (Fujita et al. , 1992) mainly found in the lysosomes and late endosomes (Fukuda, 1991), that mediates the mannose 6-phosphate-independent targeting of GBA to the lysosomes (Reczek et al., 2007). The deficient activity of LIMP-2 leads to the mistarget of the GBA protein, which can not reach the lysosome. In fact, this condition is characterized by pathological levels of GBA activity in fibroblasts, normal or slightly reduced levels in leukocytes, but increased levels in plasma (Balreira et al., 2008; Dardis et al., 2009).

3.1 Clinical aspects

Clinically it presents at the age of 15-25 years with proteinuria evolving to renal failure and/or with neurological symptoms.

The renal pathology is characterized by focal glomerulosclerosis and sometimes with features of glomerular collapse, while the main neurological symptoms are tremor, action myoclonus, seizures and later ataxia without intellectual impairment.

In most ARMF patients reported until recently, the neurological and renal features developed simultaneously or the renal symptoms appeared first. However, mutations in the *SCARB2* gene (encoded LIMP-2 protein) have been demonstrated in a group of five AMRF patients who developed neurological symptoms before the appearance of the renal symptoms. When neurological symptoms develop first, the renal disease begun after 3 to 11 years and always by the age of 30 years (Dibbens et al., 2009, Dardis et al., 2009). These findings stressed the concept that a sorting defect of the GBA enzyme should be always considered in patients with PME of unknown etiology even in the absence of renal impairment (Dibbens et al., 2009, Dardis et al., 2009)

3.2 Molecular aspects

LIMP-2 is a 478 residue type III transmembrane protein (Fujita et al., 1991) comprised of about 400 aminoacid luminal domain, two transmembrane domais and a cytosolic domain of 20 residues. It presents a highly glycosylated loop within the lysosomal lumen (Eskelinen et al., 2003). It has been recently demonstrated that the binding region to the GBA protein is located between amonoacids 145 and 288 within the luminal domain of LIMP-2 , which probably mediates the binding in a carbohydrate independent manner (Blanz et al., 2010).
In humans LIMP-2 is encoded by the *SCARB2* gene (NM_005506) located on chromosome 4q13-21 (Reczek et al., 2007). To date, 12 mutations in the *SCARB2* gene have been reported in 11 patients affected by AMRF (Berkovic et al., 2008; Balreira at al., 2008; Dardis et al., 2009; Dibbens et al., 2009). Among these mutations, five are located in intronic regions and may affect the mRNA splicing process, three are non sense, three are small deletions or insertions that cause a shift in the reading frame and one is missense.
The impact of two nonsense mutations, W178X (c.533G.A) and Q288X (c.862C.T), one frameshift mutation, W146SfsX16 (c.435_436insAG), and the missense mutation H363N, on the LIMP-2 traffiking and binding properties was analyzed in vitro. Both nonsense mutations and the frameshift mutation led to the synthesis of truncated proteins that were retained in the endoplasmic reticulum. When the interaction between these LIMP-2 mutants and the GBA was analyzed, it was found that while the Q288X mutant retained its binding capacity, the mutants W146SfsX16 and W178X, lost their ability to bind the GBA almost entirely.
The H363N mutant protein was retained in the ER and its expression level was reduced with respect to wild-type. Unexpectedly, the H363N mutant seems to bind GBA even more efficiently than wild-type LIMP-2 (Blanz et al., 2010).
Although the number of patients affected by AMRF studied to date is quite limited it seems that there is no correlation between the genotype and the clinical presentation of the disease. Studies in large series of patients as well as longer periods of clinical follow up are needed to better understand the molecular bases and the phenotypic expression of this disease.

4. Neuronal ceroid lipofuscinoses

The neuronal ceroid lipofuscinosis (NCLs) are a group of severe progressive neurodegenerative diseases, which present an incidence in Scandinavian countries of 1:12000 live births while the worldwide incidence is 1:100000 (Santavuori, 1988). NCLs are caused by mutations in at least ten human genes, eight of which have been characterized (*CLN1, CLN2* , *CLN3* , *CLN5* , *CLN6* , *CLN7* , *CLN8* , *CLN10*) (Jalanko et al., 2009). Although they constitute a genetically heterogeneous group, they share some clinical and histopatological characteristics. All NCLs present a degeneration of nerve cells mainly in the cerebral and cerebelar cortex and the accumulation of autofluorescent ceroid lipopigments both in the neural and peripheral tissues.
NCLs are considered lysosomal diseases since the ceroid lipopigments accumulate within the lysosomes and many proteins that are deficient in the NCLs are localized within the lysosomes (Futerman et al., 2004; Kyttala et al., 2006). However, the accumulated material is not a disease specific substrate and the main storage material is the c subunit of the mitochondrial ATP synthase or the sphingolipid activator proteins A and D (saposine A and D) (Tyynela et al., 1993; Elleder et al., 1997).

4.1 Clinical aspects

Clinically, they are progressive neurological diseases characterized almost in all cases by a combination of retinopathy, dementia and epilepsy. They have been originally clinically classified according to the age at onset in four main forms: infantile (INCL), late infantile (LINCL), juvenile (JNCL) and adult (ANCL). However, they are currently classified on the bases of the genetic defect (Wisniewski et al., 2001; Haltia, 2003, Mole et al., 2005, Jalanko et al., 2009, Kohlschütter & Schulz, 2009) (Table 1).

The clinical spectrum of NCL1 includes all four forms. Patients with NCL2 can present the late infantile or juvenile phenotype. The late infantile presentation has been reported in NCL5, NCL6, NCL7, NCL 8; the juvenile presentation has been reported in NCL3 and NCL9 and the adult phenotype has been reported in CLN4 (Table 1).

The ultrastructural pattern of accumulated lipopigment is different in different types of NCL: NCL1 and NCL10 present a pattern referred as granular osmiophilic deposits (GROD), while NCL2 and NCL3 are characterized by the presence of curvilinear (CLP) and fingerprint (FPP) profiles, respectively. The other forms, NCL4, NCL 5, NCL 6, NCL 7, and NCL8, show a mixed combination of CLP, FPP and rectilinear profiles (RLP) (Table 1).

Despite the wide molecular heterogeneity, the clinical findings are quite monomorfic. In fact, neuromotor impairment (tremor, ataxia, myoclonus, dysarthria, speech loss), ocular involvement (pigmentary retinal degeneration, optic atrophy, blindness), myoclonic epilepsy, progressive mental deterioration and behavior modifications are common clinical signs shared by all forms of NCLs. The main clinical signs and symptoms are summarized in table 1.

NCL	**Clinical phenotype**	**Storage pattern**	**Clinical signs**
NCL1	ICLN LINCL/JNCL ANCL	GROD	muscular hypotonia, growth impairment, psychomotor deterioration, ataxia, myoclonic jerks, seizures, retinal blindness, microcephaly. ataxia, myoclonic jerks, seizures, vision deterioration, mental deterioration. ataxia, parkinsonism, verbal impairment, pigmentary retinopathy, tunnel vision, depression, hallucinations, mental deterioration
NCL2	LINCL/JNCL	CLP	spasticity, ataxia, myoclonus, seizures, optic atrophy, rapid mental deterioration, dementia; no vaculated lymphocytes
NCL 3 (Batten disease)	JNCL	FPP	motor deterioration, dysarthria, parkinsonism, myoclonus, seizures, pigmentary retinopathy, optic atrophy with rapid visual loss, early mental deterioration
NCL4	ANCL		motor deterioration, athetoid movements, myoclonic epilepsy (in type A), tonic-clonic seizures, hearing impairment, mental deterioration, dementia, psychosis, stupors. No visual impairment (generally).

NCL	Clinical phenotype	Storage pattern	Clinical signs
NCL5 (Finnish variant)	LINCL	CLP, FPP	loss of strength, tremor, language deterioration, ataxia, myoclonic epilepsy, visual failure, blindness, behavioral changes, mental retardation. Rapid disease progression
NCL6	LINCL	RLP, FPP	ataxia, myoclonic jerks, seizures, vision deterioration, mental deterioration
NCL 7	LINCL	RLP, FPP	axial rigidity, hesitation in movement initiatio, coarse postural tremor, myoclonus, speech impairment, loss of vision, aggressive behaviour, memory impairment, mental deterioration
NCL8	LINCL	CLP	motor impairment, myoclonus, seizures, speech impairment, loss of vision, behavioral changes, mental deterioration *Northern epilepsy variant*: progressive epilepsy with generalized tonic-clonic seizures, mental deterioration; No visual involvement
NCL9	JNCL		declining vision, ataxia, seizures, motor and language impairment, cognitive decline
NCL10	LINCL Congenital	GROD	ataxia, loss of motor functions at early school age progressive cognitive decline, loss of speech;, pigmentary retinopathy, retinal atrophy, rigidity, tremor,status epilepticus, apnea, microcephaly, precocious death

INCL: infantile, LINCL: late infantile, JNCL: juvenile, ANCL: adult, GROD: granular osmiophilic deposits; CLP: curvilinear profiles; FPP: fingerprint profiles; RLP: rectilinear profiles.

Table 1. NCLs classification, age at onset, storage pattern and clinical signs.

As other neurodegenerative disorders, which manifest during the first year of life, generalized hypotonia and psychomotor regression are the first clinical signs of classic INCL. They are generally accompanied by head growth impairment (leading to microcephaly), seizure and myoclonic jerks. Behavior and sleep disturbance are frequently reported. Disease progression leads to visual and language deterioration. Death usually occurs within the first decade of life (Williams et al., 2006).

The late-infantile forms present with a similar clinic phenotype, showing progressive neurological deterioration during pre-school age. The classical late-infantile form of NCL2, generally begins during the second year of life, with slow cognitive regression and language deterioration. Epilepsy appears later, becoming rapidly intractable and accompanied with cognitive loss, myoclonic jerks and retinopathy. Patient autonomy is completely lost within the age of 6-8 and death occurs within adolescence period (Zhong et al., 2000; Steinfeld et al., 2002; Kohan et al., 2009).

Two major distinct phenotypes have been described for classical juvenile phenotype of NCL3 (Batten disease), according to the patient's genotype: a. patients carrying the 1-kb deletion in homozygous, (firstly described in Finland and Northern Europe), and b. patients carrying a compound of 1-kb deletion with other mutations (Munroe et. al., 1997).

In homozygous patients, visual impairment represent the onset sign, appearing during the first school years, with a pigmentary retinopathy; frequently a first diagnosis of retinitis pigmentosa or cone dystrophy is made. Often the cognitive skills are normal until teenage period, with subsequent deterioration and development of generalized or partial epilepsy, responsive to therapy. Behavior becomes aggressive; mood disturbance and psychotic symptoms are present. With disease progression, motor skills regress as well as speech articulation and parkinsonism and myoclonus become prominent.

In compound heterozygous patients, visual impairment is also the first accused symptom, but cognitive and motor deterioration are less pronounced and slower. Some patient have been reported as completely free from motor and cognitive signs (Lauronen et al. 1999, Jarvela et al. 1999).

Adult phenotypes are described in NCL1 and in the very rare form of NCL4 (Kukfs disease) (Martin, 1991; Ruchoux & Goebel, 1996). In the NCL1 patients, neurological and mental degeneration, depression, retinal and optic atrophy have been described, while the ocular involvement is not present in NCL4.

Absence of visual impairment, has also been reported in NCL8. This form comprises a subgroup of patients (described as Northern Epilepsy Variant) who develop generalized tonic-clonic epilepsy during early school age, followed by progressive mental retardation. With ageing epilepsy severity decreases but cognitive deterioration is maintained. Survival may last to fifth-sixth decade (Herva et al., 2000) .

Finally, a rare congenital form of NCL has been described in NCL10 (Siintola et al., 2006). Clinical course is characterized by microcephaly and severe neurological involvement (rigidity, tremor, status epilepticus) in the first hours of life. Respiratory insufficiency and apnea crisis follow with precocious death (generally within the first weeks of life).

Electrophysiological exams (EEG, ERG,VEP, ABR, SSP) show a wide spectrum of abnormalities in the different phenotypes (Topçu et al., 2004; Weleber et al., 2004; Caraballo et al., 2005; Collins et al., 2006). While brain imaging studies show a variable degree of cerebral and cerebellum atrophy accompanied with abnormalities in the signal pattern of the periventricular white matter and other brain areas (thalami, basal ganglia and putamen) (D'Incerti , 2000; Santavuori et al., 2001; Vanhanen et al., 2004).

4.2 Molecular aspects

NCLs are caused by mutations in at least 10 different recessively inherited human genes. Eight of them have been identified. These genes encode soluble or transmembrane proteins localized to the endoplasmic reticulum (ER) or the endosomal/lysosomal organelles.

The genes involved in the NCLs, their chromosomal localization, the encoded proteins and the storage materials are summarized in table 2.

The human ***CLN1*** gene has been located to chromosome 1p32 and encodes a palmitoyl protein thioesterase (PPT1), an enzyme that removes palmitate residues from proteins (Vesa et al., 1995). The enzyme consists in a 306 aminoacid polypeptide including a N-terminal signal sequence which is cleaved cotraslationally. Overexpressed PPT1 is directed to late-endosomes/lysosomes via mannose-6-pèhosphate receptor (M6PR) mediated pathway in non neuron cells (Verkruyse & Hofmann, 1996; Hellsten et al., 1996). It has not been demonstrated that this pathway is utilize to target the PPT1 in neurons. However, PPT1 has been found as part of the human brain mannose 6-phosphoproteasome (Sleat et al., 2005).

Most NCL1 patients accumulate autofluorescent lysosomal deposits, consisting mainly in sphingolipids activation proteins A and D.
In neurons palmitoylation targets proteins for transport to nerve terminals and regulates trafficking at synapses (Huang et al., 2005). It is worth of note that PPT1 has been detected in non lysosomal compartments such as cells soma, varicosities and presynaptic terminals (Lehtovirta et al., 2001; Ahtiainen et al., 2003).

Gene	**Chromosome**	**Protein**	**Main storage material**
CNL1	1p32	palmitoyl protein thioesterase (PPT1), lysosomal enzyme	Saposins A and D
CNL2	11p12	ripeptidil peptidase 1 (TPP1), lysosomal enzyme	Subunit c of ATP synthase
CNL3	16p12	CNL3, lysosomal transmembrane protein	Subunit c of ATP synthase
CNL5	13q21-q32	CNL5, lysosomal soluble protein	Subunit c of ATP synthase
CNL6	15q23	CNL6, transmembrane ER protein	Subunit c of ATP synthase
CNL7	4q28.1-q28.2	CNL7, lysosomal transmembrane protein	Subunit c of ATP synthase
CNL8	8p23	CNL8, transmembrane ER protein	Subunit c of ATP synthase
CNL10	11p15.5	CTSD, cathepsin D, lysosomal enzyme	Saposins A and D

Table 2. NCL genes, localization, encoded proteins and storage materials (Jalanko & Braulke, 2009)

To date, 48 disease causing mutations distributed throughout the entire *CLN1* gene have been described (http://www.ucl.ac.uk/ncl) , most of them have been found in individual families. The only exception is represented by the missense mutation (c.364A>T, R122W), which has been found in most Finnish families. Most mutations cause the severe infantile form of NCL (MIM256730). However, mutations causing late infantile, juvenile and adult form have also been reported. No clear correlation between the phenotype and the genotype has been demonstrated (Das et al., 1998; Mitchison et al., 1998; van Diggelen et al., 2001; Williams et al., 2006).

The human ***CLN2*** gene has been located to chromosome 11p12 and encodes the CLN2 protein tripeptidil peptidase 1 (TPP1) (Sleat et al., 1997), a lysosomal hydrolase that removes tripeptides from the N-terminus of small polypeptides (Golabek et al., 2006) such as the subunit c of mitochondrial ATP synthase. TPP1 consists in a 563 aminoacids, which includes a 19 aminoacid signal peptide and a 176 aminoacid prosegment that is autocatalytically cleaved within the lysosomes (Golabek et al., 2003). It is transported to the lysosomes in a M6PR-dependent manner (Chang et al., 2008).

The storage bodies contain mainly the subunit c of mitochondrial ATP synthase and to a less extent saposin A and D.

To date, 72 disease-causing mutations have been reported (http://www.ucl.ac.uk/ncl) leading to the classic late infantile NCL or Jansky-Bielschowsky disease (MIM 204500). Among them, the splice site mutation c.509-1G>C and the nonsense mutation c.622C>T (R208X) are quite frequent (Mole et al., 2005) and they result in very similar phenotypes.

The human **CLN3** has been located to chromosome 16p12 and encodes an integral membrane glycoprotein of 438 aminoacids (International Batten Disease Consortium, 1995). It possesses six transmembrane domains and the glycosilation varies in different tissues (Ezaki et al., 2003; Storch et al., 2007). Overexpressed CLN3 protein is localized in the lysosomes in non neuronal cells while it is detected in the endosomal/lysosomal structures and in the synaptosome in neurons (Kyttala et al., 2004; Luiro et al., 2001). In addition, CLN3 protein has also been detected in the plasma membrane and in lipid rafts (Rakheja et al., 2004; Rusyn et al., 2008). Many different functions have been attributed to CLN3 protein, including lysosomal acidification (Holopainen et al., 2001), lysosomal import of basic aminoacids (Kim et al., 2003), autophagy (Cao et al., 2006), membrane fusion, vesicular transport, , cytoskeletal organization (Brooks et al., 2003; Luiro et al., 2006) and apoptosis (Persaud-Sawin & Boustany, 2005; Wang et al., 2011).

The storage deposits contain mainly subunit c of the mitochondrial ATP Synthase (Lake & Hall, 1993). NCL3 is the only NCL typified by vacuolated lymphocytes (Mole et al., 2005)

So far, 49 disease causing mutations have been described in the *CLN3* gene (http://www.ucl.ac.uk/ncl), causing the juvenile NCL or Batten disease (MIM 204200). Many patients present the ancestral 1 kb deletion mutation, which results in the deletion of 2 exons. This mutation is predicted to produce an inactive truncated protein. However, it has been recently proposed that this mutated protein may retain some degree of residual function (Kitzmuller at al, 2008).

The human ***CLN5*** gene has been located to chromosome 13q21-q32 and encodes a 407 aminoacid polypeptide. Sequence analysis shows the presence of four initiation methionines and the production of four different polypeptides with a molecular weight ranging from 39 to 47 kDa has been described (Vesa et al., 2002). The human CLN5 contains mannose-6-phosphate residues on high-mannose type oligosaccharides, suggesting that at least some variants would be soluble. (Sleat et al., 2006). Overexpressed protein is localized to lysosomes, however it has also been detected in axons in neuronal cells (Holmberg et al., 2004). It has been demonstrated that CLN5 interacts with both NCL2 and NCL3 (Vesa et al., 2002).

The main storage component in NCL5 patients is the subunit c of the mitochondrial ATP Synthase (Tyynela et al., 1997).

Mutations in the *CLN5* gene cause the Finnish variant form of late infantile NCL (MIM 256731). Twenty seven mutations have been reported to date (http://www.ucl.ac.uk/ncl). A frequent mutation consists in a 2bp deletion in exon 4 (c.1175delAT) and has been found in 94% of Finnish NCL5 alleles.

The human **CLN6** gene has been located to chromosome 15q23 and encodes a 311 amoniacid non glycosilated membrane protein. It is localized in the ER and in neuronal cells it is additionally found along neural extension in subdomains of a tubular ER network. It contains a N-terminal cytoplasmic domain, seven putative transmembrane domains and a C-terminal luminal domain (Heine et al., 2004; Mole et al., 2004).

The main storage component in NCL6 cells is the subunit c of the mitochondrial ATP Synthase (Elleder et al.., 2006).

Forty six disease mutations have been described to cause a late infantile variant of NCL (MIM601780) (http://www.ucl.ac.uk/ncl). The nonsense mutation c.214G>T (p.E72X) has been demonstrated to be highly frequent in patients from Costa Rica probably due to founder effect (Gao et al, 2002; Wheeler et al., 2002).

The human **CLN7** gene has been recently located to chromosome 4q28.1-q28.2 and encodes a transmembrane protein of 518 aminoacids. The CLN7 protein belongs to the major facilitator superfamily (MFS), which transport specific substrates. However, its specific substrate has not been identified yet (Kasho et al., 2006). Overexpressed CLN7 is located in lysosomes (Siintola et al., 2007).

Mutations in the CLN7 gene cause a variant late infantile NCL (MIM610951). Twenty-three disease-causing mutations have been described to date (http://www.ucl.ac.uk/ncl). Mutations in CLN7 gene have been initially described in Turkish patients (Siintola et al, 2007) and therefore it has been considered the Turkish variant late infantile NCL. However, it has been recently shown that CLN7 defects are geographically widespread (Aiello et al., 2009; Aldahmesh et al., 2009; Stogmann et al., 2009; Kousi et al., 2009). The missense mutation c.881C>A (p.T294K) was found in most patients of Romany origin previously studied by Elleder et al. (Elleder et al., 1997). Haplotype analysis of these patients was consistent with the existence of a common founder effect (Kousi et al., 2009).

The human **CLN8** gene has been located to chromosome 8p23 (Ranta et al., 1999). It encodes a non glycosylated membrane protein of 286 aminoacids. The CLN8 protein belongs to the TRAM-Lag1p-CLN8 (TLC) family. Members of this family are involved in the biosynthesis, metabolisms, transport and sensing of lipids (Winter & Ponting, 2002). However, the function of the CLN8 is not known.

The overexpressed protein has been localized in the ER but it seems to shuttle between ER and the ER-Golgi intermediate complex (ERGIC) (Lonka et al., 2000). The storage material in NCL8 patients consists mainly in the subunit c of the mitochondrial ATP Synthase.

Sixteen mutations in the *CLN8* gene have been reported to date (http://www.ucl.ac.uk/ncl). They have been identified in Finnish families with Northern Epilepsy (Ranta et al., 1999) and in patients of other ethnic origins affected with a more severe variant of NCL (Ranta et al., 2004; Cannelli et al., 2006; Vantaggiato et al., 2009; Kousi et al., 2009; Reinardt et al., 2010; Zelnik et al., 2007; Mole et al., 2005) . All but one Finnish patient present the missense mutation c.70C>G (p.R24G)in homozygous, suggesting that this mutation would be associated to a protracted and atypical NCL (Ranta et al., 1999).

The human **CLN10** gene has been located to chromosome 11p15.5 and encodes the major lysosomal aspartic protease cathepsine D (CTSD). The CLN10 protein consists in 412 aminoacids and it is synthesized as a preproenzyme, which becomes posttranslationally modified by glycosilation and proteolysis leading to intermediates and mature forms (Gieselmann et al., 1985). Depending on the cell type it is trafficking to the lysosomes as a M6PR dependent or independent manner (Dittmer et al., 1999). CTSD is involved in limited proteolysis in the lysosomes and several proteins function as CTSD substrates, including

prosaposin that can be cleaved to saposins A, B, C and D (Gopalakrishnan et al., 2004). Most patients accumulate autofluorescent lysosomal deposits with GRODs.
Only four disease-causing mutations have been described to date (http://www.ucl.ac.uk/ncl).

5. Sialidosis

Sialidosis (MIM#256550) is a LSD caused by the inherited deficiency of the lysosomal enzyme alpha-N-acetyl-neuraminidase-1 (NEU1), which cleaves the terminal sialic acid residues of several oliogosaccharides and polypeptides.
Therefore, the deficiency of NEU1 leads to the accumulation of sialic acid (N-acetylneuraminic acid) covalently linked to oligosaccharides and/or glycoproteins. This aspect distinguishes sialidoses from sialurias, in which the neuraminidase activity is normal or elevated with a storage and excretion of 'free' sialic acid, rather than 'bound' forms.

5.1 Clinical aspects

A systematic classification of Sialidosis has been provided by Lowden and O'Brien in 1979, who divided them in two main clinical variants: Type I, the milder form of the disease, which lacks the physical changes (normosomatic) and Type II, a more severe form with an earlier onset, which can be subdivided in 2 different phenotypes: congenital/neonatal and juvenile forms.
Patients affected with type I sialidosis, (normomorphic or 'cherry-red-spot, myoclonus syndrome'), generally manifest first clinical signs during school-age period or early adulthood. Progressive reduction of visual acuity, red-green and night blindness, bilateral cherry-red spots, punctate corneal opacity and nistagmus, are prominent symptoms. Ocular involvement is accompanied or followed by the appearance of motor impairment, with walking difficulties and myoclonus. Same cases may present seizures. In contrast with type II forms, these patients generally do not present dysmorphisms or bone dysplasia and they have a normal intelligence. Survival is usually long.
Type II congenital sialidosis may manifest in utero with foetal hydrops or foetal ascites while the neonatal form is characterised by diffused edema, hepatosplenomegaly, ascites and Hurler's like clinical signs: facial dysmorphisms, umbilical and inguinal hernias, short trunk with a prominent sternum, kyphosis, and dysostosis multiplex (Froissart et al., 2005). Severe dysmrphisms (coarse facies, pectus carinatum, short trunk, exaggerated toracic kyphosis, and wadding gait) as well as growth delay characterize also infantile phenotypes, cherry-red spot, corneal opacity, hearing loss, progressive neurodegeneration and cognitive deterioration with myoclonic seizures. Skeletal imaging shows dysostosis multiplex with vertebral abnormalities and generalized osteoporosis. Renal involvement, nephrosialidosis, may be present in some patients with proteinuria evolving to nephrotic syndrome (Okada et al., 1983).
Juvenile onset is charactrized by less pronounced dysmorphic signs with muscular hypotonia and hypotrophy, ataxia, and myoclonic seizures. Cherry-red spots and corneal opacities are constantly present, as well as hearing loss. Pyramidal syndrome with cerebellar anomalies and peripheral neuropaty have been described. Mental retardation is costant. Survival rarely exceed the second, third decade of life (Winter et al., 1980; Caciotti et al., 2009; Canafoglia et al., 2011).

5.2 Molecular aspects

The human *NEU1* gene (Gen Bank AF040958) has been located to chromosome 6p21.3 within the region of the major histocompatibility complex (Bonten et al., 1996; Pshezhetsky et al., 1997). It contains 6 exons and spans approximately 3.5 kb of genomic DNA (Milner et al., 1997).

The *NEU1* gene encodes a protein of 415 aminoacids including a signal sequence, a central hydrophobic core and a more polar c-terminal domain (Bonten et al., 1996). After the removal of the signal peptide and glycosilation the protein would have a molecular mass of 45 kD. In fact, western blot studies have demonstrated the presence of two major bands of 44 -45 kD which yielded a 40 kD protein after de-glycoslation (Bonten et al., 1996). NEU1 exists as a multienzyme complex with at least two other proteins, β-galactosidase and the protective protein/cathepsin A (PPCA) (d'Azzo et al., 2001). The association with PPCA is necessary for its enzymatic activity. The association with PPCA stabilizes the active conformation of NEU1 in lysosomes. Moreover, since NEU1 is poorly mannose 6-phosphorylated, it depends on PPCA for its correct compartmentalization and catalytic activation in lysosomes (van der Spoel et al., 1998; van der Spoel et al., 2000; Yamamoto et al., 1987).

About 45 different mutations in *NEU1* gene have been reported to date (http://www.hgmd.org/). Almost all of them have been found in single families and most of them are missense mutations. Bonten et al. have studied the impact of some missense mutations on NEU1 protein distribution and catalytic activity and they classified these mutant proteins in 3 groups: 1-catalytically inactive and not lysosomal; 2-catalytically inactive and lysosomal and 3-catalytically active and lysosomal. A good correlation between the residual activity of mutant proteins and the severity of the disease has been found. In fact, patients with the severe type II infantile form presented mutations from group 1 while those with a mild form of type I disease had at least one mutation from group 3. Mutations from group 2 were found mainly in patients with the juvenile form of type II sialidosis with an intermediate phenotype (Bonten et al., 2000).

6. Niemann pick type C (NPC) disease

Niemann Pick type C (NPC) disease (NPC1, MIM 257220; NPC2, MIM 607625) is an autosomal recessive neurodegenerative lysosomal storage disorder, caused by the abnormal function of NPC1 or NPC2 protein. Both proteins are involved in the intracellular trafficking of cholesterol and other lipids. The deficiency of either of them leads to the accumulation of the endocytosed unesterified cholesterol within the lysosomes (Patterson et al., 2001).

Endocyted low density lipoproteins are delivered to the late endosomes/lysosomes where they are hydrolized. In normal cells, free cholesterol is transported to the plasma membrane or to the endoplasmic reticulum through the action of NPC1 and NPC2 proteins. In NPC cells cholesterol accumulate within the lysosomes and the subsequent induction of all low-density lipoprotein cholesterol-mediated homeostatic responses, including cholesterol esterification, is compromised.

In addition NPC-deficient cells also accumulate gangliosides and other GSLs. These findings show that the defect in NPC cells encompasses a global transport error. In fact, while unesterified cholesterol is the main lipid accumulated in peripheral tissues, GM_3, GM_2 and glucosylceramide are the mayor lipids accumulated in brain of NPC patients (Zervas et al., 2001a).

Approximately 95% of NPC patients present mutations in *NPC1* gene (MIM 607623) (Carstea et al., 1993; Vanier et al., 1996) , while the other 5% of patients present mutations in *NPC2* gene (MIM 601015) (Naureckiene et al., 2000)
The incidence of NPC disease has been difficult to assess. Estimates of incidences ranging from 0,66 to 0,83 per 100000 were proposed for France, UK and Germany based on the diagnoses made over a period 1988-2002. This incidence is probably underestimated since the wide clinical spectrum of NPC disease was not recognized until the early 90's and no specific laboratory testing was available until the mid 80s. A probably more realistic incidence of 0,96/100000 was recently calculated considering the total amount of cases diagnosed in France from 2000-2009 (including prenatal cases from terminated pregnancies) vs the number of birth during the same period. However, this data is likely to be still underestimated due to the presence of atypical phenotypes that may not be recognized, in particular among adult patients (Patterson, 2001; Vanier and Millat, 2003).

6.1 Clinical aspects

Clinically, NPC disease presents a highly variable phenotype ranging from fetal to adult age. It is classically a neurovisceral condition, characterized by liver and/or spleen enlargement, and neurological or psychiatric manifestations. Systemic disease, when present, always precedes the neurological symptoms. However, it is absent in about 15% of patients and in about half of the adult onset patients (Vanier 2010).
It is important to point out that the course of the systemic signs is independent of that of the course of the neurological symptoms and that disease progression and lifespan are always correlated with the age at onset of the neurological symptoms.
Even if initial manifestations may be systemic, neurological, or psychiatric, the disease has been classified according to the age at onset of neurological symptoms. Although the neurological forms of the disease may be considered as a continuous of phenotypes, the disease has been classically classified in a severe infantile form (onset before 2 y of age), a late infantile form (onset between 3-5 y of age), a juvenile form (onset between 5 and 16 y) and an adult form (onset at age>16 y) (Patterson et al., 2001; Vanier & Millat, 2003).
A perinatal form of NPC has also been described. This form is characterized by the presence of prolonged neonatal cholestatic icterus, appearing within the first weeks of life and often associated with progressive hepatosplenomegay (Kelly et al., 1993; Vanier et al., 1998; Yerushalmi et al., 2002). In most cases, the icterus spontaneously resolves at 2-4 month of age while the hepatosplenomegaly remains for a variable period. In about 10% of patients the icterus worsens leading to liver failure and dead within the first 6 month of age (Vanier et al., 1998). Some patients, in particular those presenting mutations in *NPC2* gene, may present with hepatosplenomegay in association with a severe respiratory insufficiency, which in most cases is fatal. It is important to note that NPC patients do not present neurological symptoms during the neonatal period. However, an important observation to consider during the genetic counseling is the fact that in many cases patients who die during the perinatal period have siblings affected with the infantile or juvenile neurological form (Vanier & Susuki, 1998; Vanier and Millat, 2003).
Patients affected with early infantile form (3 month to < 2 years) almost invariable present with isolated hepatosplenomagaly during the first month of age followed by delay of development motor milestones, which presents at around 8-9 month of age, and central hypotonia. Subsequent clinical course includes loss of acquired motor skills, spasticity with

pyramidal tract involvment, hearing loss (Wraith et al., 2009). Seizures are uncommon in these patients and they usually die during the first 5 years of age (Vanier 2010).

In late infantile forms (2 to <6 years), hepatosplenomegaly is usually present. Language delay is frequent and these children often present gait problems, frequent falls and clumsiness. Cataplexy is quite frequent and vertical supranuclear gaze palsy (VSGP) is usually present but it may not be recognized at this early stage. Progressive ataxia is followed by dystonia, dysphagia, dysarthria and central hypotonia. Hearing loss has been described (Wraith et al., 2009; Vanier 2010). A significant proportion of patients develop seizures, partial, generalized or both. In general these patients respond to standard antiepileptic treatment but some cases may be refractory to therapy. Severe epilepsy has a bad prognosis and shortens the lifespan of patients. As disease progress patients develop pyramidal signs, spasticity and swallowing problems. In most cases patients die between 7 to 12 years of age (Vanier 2010).

The juvenile form (6 to 15 years is in many countries the most frequent form of the disease. Moderate splenomegaly or hepatosplenomegaly is frequently present and may have been detected at early time. However, in at least 10% of the cases organomegaly is not present. School failure, learning disability and behavioral problems are the most common signs. VSGP is almost invariabile present and may be the first sign. As the disease progress the children present frequent falls, clumsiness and develop progressive ataxia, dysarthria, dystonia, dysphagia. Cataplexy and myoclonus are other common symptoms. About half of the patients with this form develop seizures (partial and/or generalized). At late stage patients develop Pyramidal signs, spasticity and swallowing problems (Wraith et al., 2009; Vanier 2010).

Even if during the last years many patients affected with the adult form (>15 years) of the disease have been reported, this diagnosis has been probably underestimated. Organomegaly or isolated splenomegaly are rare in adult patients and VSGP is usually present. The most common clinical presentation is similar to that of a juvenile form but attenuated. However, it is worth of note that about one third of patients present with psychiatric signs that may appear several years before the onset neurological symptoms. During this period the neurological examination may be normal. Among the psychiatric signs, paranoid delusions and auditory or visual hallucinations are the most commonly described. Other psychiatric signs that may be present in these patients are depressive syndrome, behavioral problems with aggressiveness, social isolation, bipolar disorders, obsessive compulsive disorders. Epilepsy is not very common in this group of patients (15%) and the course is similar to that in the juvenile form (Vanier 2010).

6.2 Molecular aspects

As mentioned above, two disease-causing genes, *NPC1* (NM000271) and *NPC2* (NM006432) have been identified (Steinberg et al., 1994; Vanier et al., 1996 ; Cartsea et al., 1997). About 95% of human NPC disease is caused by mutations in the *NPC1* gene (Naureckiene et al., 2000). *NPC1* gene, located on chromosome 18q11-q12, encodes a large membrane glycoprotein of 1278 aminoacids containing 13 transmembrane domains and located predominantly in late endosomes (Davies & Ioannou, 2000). It presents a sterol sensing domain (SSD), which shows extensive homology with the sterol sensing domains (SSD) found in SREBP cleavage activating protein (SCAP) and 3-hydroxy-3-methyl-glutaryl coenzyme A (HMG-CoA) reductase, two cholesterol regulated proteins. The SSD domain appears to have important functional significance (Watari, et al., 1999). Two luminal functional important domains have been identified: a cysteine-rich loop with a ring-finger motif which harbours about 1/3 of the mutations described in patients and a highly conserved N-terminal domain with a leucine zipper motif which has been shown to possess a cholesterol-binding domain (Davies & Ioannou, 2000). In fact, it has recently been demonstrated that a water soluble fragment of NPC1 is able to bind cholesterol and oxysterols (Infante et al., 2008a; Infante et al., 2008b). The mature NPC1 protein has 14 potential glycosilation sites and shows a size of 170 and 190 kDa *NPC2* gene is mapped to chromosome 14q24.3 and encodes a small soluble protein present in the lumen of the lysosomes (Naureckiene et al., 2000, Vanier & Millat 2004).

It possess a hydrophobic pocket that has the property to bind cholesterol (Vanier & Millat, 2004).

Although it is well known that NPC1 and NPC2 participate together in mediating the egress of cholesterol from endo/lysosomes, the precise mechanism by which these proteins function is not fully understood. It has been demonstrated that a water soluble fragment of NPC1 binds cholesterol in an orientation opposite to NPC2. Based on these results, the following working model was proposed to explain the egress of cholesterol derived from receptor mediated endocytosis of LDL from lysosomes: after liberation from LDL, cholesterol is bound by NPC2 which carries it to the lysosomal membrane, where it transfers to the N-terminal domain of the membrane bound *NPC1* (Kwon et al., 2009).

The mutational spectrum of *NPC1* gene is very heterogeneous and to date more than 290 mutations have been reported (http://npc.fzk.de/; Runz et al., 2008). Among them, the mutant allele I1061T is quite frequent in Western Europe and US (Millat et al. 1999, Sun et al. 2001, Park et al. 2003) where it accounts from 20-25% of the alleles. However, it seems to be much less frequent in Italy and Spain (Fernandez- Valero et al., 2005; Fancello et al., 2009; Macias-Vidal et al., 2010), suggesting that there is a gradient of increasing frequency of the p.I1061T mutation from southeast to northwest Europe.

Two other relatively frequent mutations, p.P1007A and p.G992W, have been reported to be associated to the biochemical "variant phenotype" (see section 9), characterized by a milder cholesterol trafficking impairment. The p.G992W mutation is typical of patients from Nova-Scotia but it has been found in patients from other origins (Millat et al., 2001; Ribeiro et al., 2001; Fernandez- Valero et al., 2005; Fancello et al., 2009).

Phenotype-genotype correlation studies are quite difficult to perform due to the very limited number of patients carrying the same genotype. However, some general consideration can be made. It has been shown that the genotype correlates with the neurological form of the disease and not with the systemic manifestations. While a good correlation has been found between the nonsense or frameshift mutations and the more severe infantile form of the disease, the phenotype is more variable in patients carrying missense mutation. However, the presence of missense mutations in the sterol sensing domain of the protein correlates with the more severe form of the disease.

It has been proposed that in the homoallelic state mutation I1061T is associated with a severe impairmet of cholesterol trafficking and correlates with the juvenile neurologic form of the disease, while in the heteroallelic state, the final phenotype depends on the mutation present in the second allele but until recently it had never been found in the severe infantile neurologic form. However, a study performed in a Spanish cohort of 30 patients affected with NPC has demonstrated the presence of the p.I1061T mutation in homozygosis in a patient affected with the severe infantile form (Macias-Vidal, 2010).

So far, only 19 mutations have been reported in the *NPC2* gene. Among them the most frequent mutation is the p.E20X. A good correlation between the severity of the mutation and the clinical course of the disease has been found.
Most reported patients affected with mutations in the *NPC2* gene presented a very severe fatal form of the disease leading to dead within the first years of life. Only few patients presenting a slower disease progression and a longer survival have been described so far (Klunemann et al., 2002; Millat et al., 2001; Millat et al., 2005).

7. GM2 gangliosidosis

GM2 gangliosidoses are a group of recessive disorders characterized by accumulation of GM2 ganglioside in neuronal cells due to the deficient activity of human β-hexosaminidases (β-N-acetylhexosaminidase, EC3.2.1.52, Hex), ysosomal hydorlases that cleave the terminal N-acetylhexosamine residues from GM2 gangliosides bound to the GM2 activator protein. Two major isoenzymes exist: Hex A consisting of one α and one β subunit encoded by *HEXA* and *HEXB* genes, respectively, and Hex B consisting of two β subunits. In vivo, the GM2/GM2 activator complex is a substrate only for the Hex A isoenzyme. Mutations in either *HEXA* or *HEXB* genes or in the *GM2A* gene (that encodes for the GM2 activator protein) result in GM2 gangliosidosis.
In particular, mutations in the *HEXA* gene cause Tay Sachs disease (TSD; MIM 272800), characterized by deficiency of Hex A activity, while mutations in the *HEXB* gene lead to Sandhoff disease (SD; MIM 26880), characterized by combined deficiency of Hex A and Hex B activities. On the other hand, mutations in the *GM2A* gene cause GM2 activator deficiency, characterized by normal Hex A and Hex B activities but the inability to form a functional GM2/GM2 activator complex. Only few patients with a defect in the *GM2A* gene have been reported whereas most patients affected by GM2 gangliosidosis present mutations in *HEXA* or *HEXB* genes.
While SD disease is panethnic, the incidence of TSD is about one in 3600 Ashkenazi Jewish, corresponding to a carrier frequency of 1 in 30. Among Sephardic Jews and all non-Jews, the disease incidence has been observed to be about 100 times less common, corresponding to a tenfold lower carrier frequency (between 1/250 and 1/300).

7.1 Clinical aspects

The clinical phenotypes associated with each biochemical variant vary widely from the infantile onset of rapidly progressive neurodegenerative forms, leading to death before the fourth year of life, to the later onset forms, a progressive neurological condition compatible with survival into childhood or long survival (Gravel et al., 2001)
For TSD, three main phenotypes have been identified: classic infantile, juvenile and chronic or adult forms. Signs of the classic infantile TSD are generally evident within the first semester of life. In general noise hypersensitivity with startle response precedes psychomotor retardation, generalized hypotonia, growing of head circumference leading to macrocephalia, amurosis and myoclonic epilepsy. Cherry red spots may be present at funduscopic examination. The peripheral organs are spared from storage process. Disease progression leads to a very severe neurological degeneration until decerebration state. The juvenile form has a later onset, generally between the age of 2-6 years, presenting with behavior modifications and progressive cognitive impairment. Ataxia become evident and

the disease progresses to decerebrate rigidity. Unlike classic form, blindness is not obligatory. Death occurred between ages 5 and 15 years. Finally, in the adult phenotype the disease may be silent for a prolonged period, becoming evident during school-age. However, the diagnosis may be delayed until adulthood. Clinical presentation is variegated, some patients present with symptoms of atypical Friedreich ataxia, while in others a clinical picture suggestive of Kugelberg-Welander phenotype (progressive leg weakness and fasciculations) was described. A different pattern of motor impairment (including: ataxia, progressive gait disturbance, clumsiness, generalized weakness, mild spasticity, dystonia, dysarthria, tremor involuntary jerks) and cognitive deterioration (loss of memory and comprehension, dementia) has been detected. In some patients mental capacity and behaviour are normal (Neudorfer et al., 2005; Maegawa et al., 2006).

Imaging studies on TSD patients showed different findings in the three different forms, an involvement of basal ganglia and thalamus with cortical atrophy has been detected in classic infantile form, while both juvenile and adult phenotypes do not present basal ganglia abnormalities but show a cortical and cerebellar atrophy, the later characteristic of adult form (Grosso et al., 2003; Inglese et al., 2005; Aydin et al., 2005; Maegawa et al. 2006).

Neurophysiological studies showed a variable pattern of EEG abnormalities with an early progressive loss of the VEP in infantile form. Saccadic abnormalities and impairment of smooth pursuit have also been observed at the evaluation of eye movements in some patients (Rapin 1986; Rucker et al. 2004).

In SD clinical findings are indistinguishable from those of TSD. In infantile onset, startle reaction, psychomotor deterioration, early blindness, macrocephaly, cherry red spots are all present. The course of the disease is rapidly fatal, with death within the third year of life. In late-onset forms, cognitive and mental involvement (school difficulties, emotional lability, intermittent psychosis, confusional state) as well as neurological deterioration (muscle weakness, muscle atrophy, fasciculations, supranuclear gaze palsy, muscular atrophy, hyperreflexia, myoclonic jerks, seizures) have been described. Imaging and neurophysiological studies are similar to TSD (Yüksel et al., 1999; Alkan et al., 2003; Hendriksz et al., 2004; Jain et al., 2010)

7.2 Molecular aspets

The human ***HEXA*** gene (MIM# 606869) is located on chromosome 15q23-q24 and contains 14 exons. More than 100 mutations have been identified to cause TSD disease, including single base substitutions, small deletions, small duplications/insertions, partial gene deletions, splicing alterations and complex gene rearrangements (http://www.hexdb.mcgill.ca/hexadb; http://www.hgmd.org/; Stenson et al., 2003). Most of these alterations are "private" mutations and have been detected in single or very few families. Others are present in small isolated populations and only a few have been frequently found in diverse populations. In the Ashkenazi Jewish population three distinct *HEXA* mutations are responsible for 98% of all mutant alleles: the most common four-bases duplication c.1274_1277dupTATC and the splicing mutation c.1421+1G>C (IVS12+1G>C) account for 81% and 15% of alleles, respectively; the alteration in exon 7 c.805G>A (p.G269S), associated with the late onset form of the disease, has been found in approximately 2% of alleles (Kaback et al., 1993). Among the non-Jewish populations the mutation pattern is completely different. Only 30% of the alleles are due to the duplication c.1274_1277dupTATC, none present the IVS12+1G>C and about 5% carry the G269S mutation (Kaback et al., 1993). By contrast, the abnormal splicing mutation c.1073+1G>A (IVS9+1G>A), absent among the Jewish population, is found in about 15% of the non-Jewish carriers (Akerman et al., 1992). There are mutations in the *HEXA* gene causing the B1 Variant, associated with the late onset form of TSD. This biochemical phenotype is characterized by a Hex A isoenzyme catalytically inactive against the physiological substrate, GM2 ganglioside, but active towards commonly used synthetic substrate (4-methylumbelliferyl β-Nacetylglucosaminide) (Tutor, 2004). Concerning the *HEXA* mutations associated with the B1 Variant, the most common is the c.533G>A (p.R178H) that was first found predominantly in Portuguese patients (dos Santos et al., 1991; Gravel et al., 2001) and which has been subsequently detected in individuals with different European backgrounds (Montalvo et al., 2006).

Human ***HEXB*** gene has been located to chromosome 5q13 (MIM 26880) and contains 14 exons distributed over about 40 kb of DNA. To date, about 40 different mutations have been identified to cause SD, most of the have been identified in individual families (http://www.hexdb.mcgill.ca/hexadb; http://www.hgmd.org/). However, a common mutation found in patients with different ethnic backgrounds is a deletion at the 5' end of the gene that removes 16 kb of DNA including the HEXB promoter, exons 1–5, and part of intron , which account for about 27% of SD alleles (Neote et al., 1988; Bolhuis & Bikker, 1992) . This mutation seems to be quite unfrequent in Italian SD patients. Among this population the most frequent mutation is the c.850C>T (p.R284X) present in 27% of the affected alleles. The high frequency of this mutation is probably due to a founder effect (Zampieri et al., 2009).

Although the number of SD patients characterized to date is quite small to perform an analysis of phenotype/genotype correlation, it is of note that missense mutations p.P504S, p.R505Q and p.R533H, seem to be associated to the late onset form of the disease (Maegawa et al., 2006). In addition, the missense mutation p. D459A has been recently discovered in six patients with a rare juvenile SD variant (Wang et al., 2008).

8. Differential diagnosis

The diagnosis of the specific LSD present in patients affected with PME may be challenging. However, the correct diagnosis is crucial in order to implement the best available therapeutic options and to provide an accurate genetic counselling.

Although each LSD presents with specific sings and symptoms, some general features should prompt the physician to suspect the presence of a LSD in a patient with PME:

1- a familiar history suggestive of a genetic disease, 2- association with other signs of neurological impairment, 3- the presence of visceral involvement.

The visceral and neurologic signs most frequently associated to PME in LSD are shown in table 3. At physical examination, dysmorphism is a constant feature of sialidosis type II. Visceral storage represents a major sign of GD and sialidosis, while is generally less evident in NPC, where protracted jaundice is a highly suggestive sign that must be searched during patient anamnesis. Macrocephaly is a diagnostic sign in the infantile TSD, where abnormal growing of head circumference becomes evident with disease progression. With disease progression, ataxic motor impairment is generally detected in all of them, with dystonic movements evident in NPC, NCL and GM2 gangliosidosis, while dysarthria is detectable in AMRF, NPC and GM2 gangliosidosis. Parkinsonian syndrome may be present in adult patients with NCL. Involvement of ocular system is widely described in many LSD, both at functional and tissue storage levels. Supranuclar gaze palsy is patognomonic in NPC, but is also present in GD3 and AMFR, while blindness affects particularly infantile TSD and NCL (infantile NCL1 and late-infantile NCL Finnish variant, CLN5); green-red and nocturnal visual loss may be present in type 1 sialidosis. Signs of retinal storage are detectable in form of cherry-red spot (in Sialidosis and GM2), pigmentary degeneration (diagnostic sign in NCL) and optic atrophy (NCL and GM2 gangliosidosis). Degeneration of mental capacities with different grade of severity are constantly present in all these pathologies, while skeleton is severely involved by in sialidosis and usually mildly affected in GD3. Finaly, renal failure characterized the late phase of AMFR, but in form of nephritic syndrome may affect sialidosis type 2.

	GD3	AMRF	NPC	NCL	Sialidosi	GM2 gangliosidosis
dysmorphisms		-	-	-	+	-
visceral storage	+	-	+	-	+	-
protracted joundice	-	-	+	-	-	-
macrocephaly	-	-	-	-	-	+
ataxia	+	+	+	+	+	+
dystonia	-	-	+	+	-	+
dysarthria	-	+	+	-	-	+
parkinsonism	-	-	-	+	-	-
gaze palsy	+	+	+	-	-	-
blindness	-	-	-	+	+	+
cherry red spot	-	-	-	-	+	+
retinal degeneration	-	-	-	+	-	-
optic atrophy	-	-	-	+	-	+
mental deterioration	+	+	+	+	+	+
skeletal involvement	+	-	-	-	+	-
renal involvement	-	+	-	-	+	-

Table 3. visceral and neurologic signs most frequently associated to PME in LSD

8.1 Laboratory diagnosis

Routine laboratory tests result usually normal in patients with LSDs, with just few exceptions summarized in table 4.

On the other hand, in patients with PME in whom the presence of a LSD is suspected, some relative simple tests may be performed (Table 4). The assessment of chitotriosidase activity in serum, a marker of macrophage activation, is substantially elevated in patients affected with GD and may be slightly elevated in patients with NPC disease. In addition, a recent report described the presence of high levels of chitotriosidase activity in 2 patients affected

with sialidosis type II (Caciotti et al., 2009). However, about 30% of individual from various genetic origins carry a chitotriosidase gene with a 24 bp duplication that prevents the production of the enzyme. Therefore, about 6% of the population is homozygous for this mutant allele and completely lack chitotriosidase activity.
Patients affected with sialidosis excrete increased amount of several oligosaccharides and sialylglycopeptides derived from glycoproteins. Since the metabolic defect in these patients results in the inability to cleave sialic acid, the accumulated oligosaccharides are rich in sialic acid. Thus, a first screening test that may be performed when a sialidosis is suspected is the analysis of oligosaccharides in urine by thin layer chromatography (TLC). Staining of oligosaccharides resolved by TLC reveals a abnormal pattern in affected patients. However, abnormal patters of urine oligosaccharides are also found in patients affected with other disorders of glycoprotein degradation. In addition it is also possible to analyze the presence of sialic acid containing oligosaccharides by staining the TLC plates with resorcinol (Holmes & O'Brien, 1979).

LSD	**Non specific laboratory findings**
Gaucher	Anemia, thrombocytopenia, Minor elevation of liver enzymes Elevation of acid phosphatase, angiotensin converting enzyme (ACE) and ferritin Elevation serum chitotriosidase acivity
AMRF	Proteinuria
Niemann Pick type C	Reduced plasma levels of HDL-cholesterol Moderate elevation of serum chitotriosidase acivity
Sialidosis	Elevation of serum chitotriosidase. Abnormal pattern of urin oligosaccharides

Table 4. Non specific laboratory findings in patients affected with LSDs that may present with PME.

The presence of glycolipid-laden macrophages in various tissues is a hallmark of GD. In particular the presence of these "Gaucher cells" in bone marrow aspirates provide a strong support for this diagnosis. However, these cells have to be distinguished from those present in other disorders that exhibit pathological macrophages as a hallmark, such as the sea blue histiocyte syndrome or NPC disease. In addition, foam cells my also be present in bone marrow samples of patients affected with sialidosis. Although the examination of bone marrow aspiration may be useful for the diagnosis of GD, NPC disease and sialidosis, it should not be necessarily the initial diagnostic test considering the invasiveness of the procedure.

8.1.1 Specific test

A schematic approach to the laboratory diagnosis of the specific LSDs discussed in this chapter is represented in figure 1.
The suspect of **GD** can be confirmed by the assessment of GBA activity in peripheral blood leukocytes or cultured fibrobalsts. A residual activity below 15 % of the mean normal activity is diagnostic.
However, it is important to keep in mind that **AMRF is** caused by a mistargeting of GBA enzyme due to a defect in its receptor LIMP-2 and therefore patients affected by this disorder

also show low levels of GBA activity in fibroblasts but slightly reduced or normal in peripheral blood leukocytes. AMRF should always be considered in patients with reduced intracellular GBA activity in the absence of other markers of Gaucher disease, such as elevated serum chitotriosidase activity or the presence of "Gaucher" cells in bone marrow.

The determination of GBA activity in serum should be perform in order to provide a differential diagnosis since it is elevated only in patients affected with AMRF (Dardis et al., 2009).

In both cases the molecular analysis of *GBA* or *SCARB-2* gene should be carried out in order to confirm the diagnosis and to provide a genetic counseling.

The diagnostic approach of **NCL** depends on the type of defect that is suspected. As shown in figure 1, the diagnosis of **NCL 1, NCL2 and NCL10** can be achieved by the assessment of PPT1, TPP1 or Cathepsin D activity in leukocytes or cultured fibroblasts. If **NCL3** is suspected, the diagnosis can be confirmed by the presence of typical vacuoles in the cytoplasm of the patient lymphocytes, which are detectable on a regular blood smear (Kohlschütter & Schulz, 2009).

In the case of **NCL5, NCL6, NCL7 and NCL8** it is advisable to investigate the presence of storage material by electron microscopic examination of skin biopsy material or isolated lymphocytes as a first approach and then procede to the molecular genetic studies. The definitive diagnosis in all cases is reached by the molecular analysis of the corresponding genes (Kohlschütter & Schulz, 2009).

The definitive diagnosis of **sialidosis** is achieved by measuring the NEU1 activity is fresh samples of blood leukocytes or cultured fibroblasts. Special care should be taken to ensure that the tissue to be examined has not been frozen or exposed to prolonged sonication since the neuraminidase is quite unstable (Den Tandt & Brossemer, 1984). The residual enzymatic activity is extremely low or absent in patients affected with sialidosis independently of the severity of the clinical phenotype. On the contrary, a good correlation between the genotype and the phenotype has been found, therefore the molecular analysis of the *NEU1* may provide useful information about disease severity and progression, which is particularly relevant to provide a better genetic counseling.

It is important to keep in mind that also the Galactiosialidosis, a LSD associated with combined deficiency of NEU1 and β–galactosidase due to the defect of the proteictive protein /cathepsin A (PPCA), results in reduced levels of NEU1 activity. However, in this case the levels of NEU1 are not as low as in sialidosis and they are associated with low levels of β–galactosidase activity.

The diagnosis of NPC disease may be quite challenging. It is time consuming and should be performed by specialized centers with the required experience.

The biochemical diagnosis is based on the demonstration of the impaired intracellular cholesterol transport and homeostasis in fibroblasts in culture. The filipin test is considered the more specific and sensitive assay. Cells are cultured in the presence of LDL enriched medium and then fixed and stained with filipin, a molecule that has a high affinity for unesterified cholesterol (Blanchette-Mackie et al., 1988). In patients with NPC disease, fluorescence microscopic examination of stained cells shows in most of them, the presence of strong fluorescent perinuclear vesicles evidencing the intralysosomal accumulation of cholesterol. The majority of NPC patients present this "classical" biochemical pattern. However, about 20% of NPC patients present a milder level of unesterified cholesterol storage, presenting the so called "variant" biochemical phenotype.The diagnosis in these

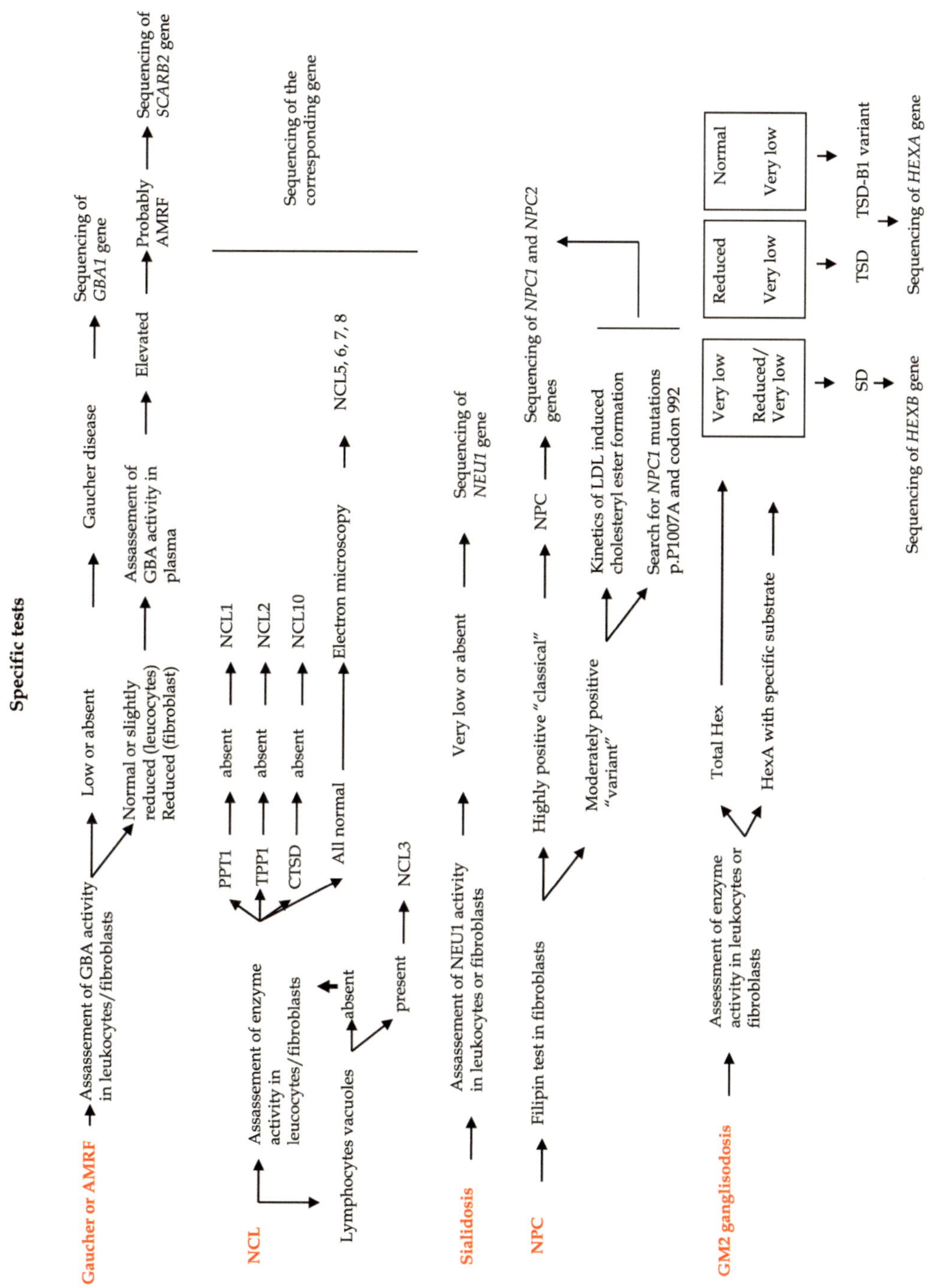

Fig. 1. Schematic representation of the laboratory diagnostic strategy in suspected cases of PME due to LSD

patients may be difficult. Measurement of the LDL-induced rate of cholesterol esterification may be used as a secondary test. However, while very low levels rates of esterification are detected in cell lines with a "classical" biochemical phenotype only a mild or non-significant impairment is detected in those with a "variant" phenotype. Therefore, in these cases mutational analysis of *NPC1* and *NPC2* are necessary in order to provide a definitive diagnosis. Since some mutations of *NPC1* gene have been associated to the variant biochemical phenotype (see 6.2), it is advisable to screen the presence of these mutations in patients presenting a variant phenotype.

Finally, the molecular analysis should be performed in all newly diagnosed patients since molecular genetic studies are the highly preferred strategy for prenatal diagnosis, and the only reliable one for identification of carriers in blood relatives (Vanier et al., 2010).

The suspect of **GM2 gangliosidosis** can be confirmed by the measurement of β-hexosaminidases activities in blood leukocytes or cultured fibroblasts. From the biochemical point of view, the differential diagnosis between SD and TSD, the most common causes of GM2 gangliosidosis, can be performed by the assessment of total Hex activity, the HEX activity after heat inactivation and the specific assay of the HexA isoenzyme in leukocytes or fibroblasts. The synthetic substrate usually used is the 4-methylumbelliferyl N- acetyl β-glucosaminide which can be digested by both HexA (α/β heterodimero) and HexB (β/β homodimero) isoenzymes and it is used to determine the total Hex activity. Since the HexA is thermolabile, it can be inactivated by heating the sample at 50°. The activity against the 4-methylumbelliferyl N- acetyl β-glucosaminide after heat inactivation is represented only by HexB. This value is used to determine the % of HexA and HexB activity The specific activity of Hex A isoenzyme can be measured using the synthetic substrate, 4-methylumbelliferyl N-acetyl β-glucosamine 6-sulfate (MUGS) (Bayleran, et al., 1984). Sandhoff disease is characterized by the impairment of both HexA and HexB activities and therefore total Hex activity is very low. A residual Hex A activity may be detected in these patients due the presence of HexS, consisting in two α subunits, which is not deficient in SD and is also active towards the synthetic substrate.

Tay Sachs disease is confirmed by the presence of reduced levels of total Hex and very low levels of HexA. It is important to keep in mind that the B1 variant of Tay Sachs is characterized by the presence of an Hex A isoenzyme catalytically inactive against the physiological substrate, GM2 ganglioside, but active towards commonly used synthetic substrate 4-methylumbelliferyl -N-acetyl β–glucosaminide (Tutor, 2004). Biochemical identification of these patients requires always the use of the specific substrate MUGS. (Bayleran et al., 1984).

In the case of normal Hex activities a deficiency of the GM2 activator protein should be suspected. In this case, the definitive diagnosis is achieved by the molecular analysis of the GM2A gene.

In patients with a biochemical diagnosis of SD and TSD it is advisable to perform the molecular analysis of *HEXA* or *HEXB* genes, respectively, in order to confirm the diagnosis and to provide genetic counseling. In addition in patients with a biochemical pattern compatible with a diagnosis of TSD disease it is important to exclude the presence of a pseudodeficiency due to specific mutations (p.R247W and p.R249W) in the *HEXA* gene. These protein variants are inactive towards the synthetic substrates but active towards the natural substrate, GM2 ganglioside (Triggs-Raine et al., 1992; Cao et al., 1993).

9. Therapeutic options

Twenty years ago the availability of enzyme replacement therapy (ERT) for GD opened a new era for the treatment of LSDs, giving to the patients a concrete hope for recovering (Brady, 2006; Connock et al. 2006). However, clinical history of GD demonstrated the limited effect of ERT on neurological phenotypes. The difficulty to cross the blood-brain barrier for macromolecule such glycoproteins prevent the neuronal access to the intravenous infused enzyme. Despite the good efficacy in correcting the visceral and hematological alterations of the disease also in neurological phenotypes, only a very limited number of patients seem to benefit from ERT, showing an improvement of EEG pattern and a stabilization of neurological conditions. Quite all of them carried the L444P mutation in homozygosis. On the contrary very few are GD3 patients presenting with myoclonic epilepsy that carry these mutation in homozygosis or heterozygosis with other rare mutations. Therefore, myoclonic epilepsy represents a unfavorable prognostic factor in GD3 (Altarescu et al., 2001). Despite the negative results obtained by Schiffmann et al. (2008), Capablo at al. (2007) showed an improvement of neurologic conditions and EEG pattern as well as a decrease of the epileptic crisis in patients who presented with myoclonic sezures and the L444P/E326K+N188S phenotype, after 12 month treatment with combined ERT and substrate reduction therapy (SRT). Recently, Accardo et al. (2010), demonstrated the recovery of saccades in two GD3 sisters in course of SRT. The availability of small molecules capable to cross the blood-brain barrier might widening therapeutic prospective in neuronopathic GD.

Glycosphingolipids reduction therapy may represent a strategy also for other glycosphingolipidosis, like NPC and GM2 gangliosidosis (Platt et al., 2005; Platt & Lachmann, 2009).

Different clinical experiences have been reported in literature concerning SRT in NPC patients. The results of clinical trials performed both in pediatric and adult patients showed a significant improvement of swallowing and saccades, as well as an overall stabilization of neurological conditions (Patterson et al. 2007; Galanaud et al. 2009). Substrate reduction therapy has also been used to reduce glicosphingolipids synthesis in GM2 gangliosidosis patients (Bembi et al., 2006;Shapiro et al., 2009), both in infantile and late-onset forms, without any evidence of measurable benefits.

Very recently a Clarke JT et al. (2011) have demonstrated an in vivo enhancement of Hex A activity in a group of late-onset GM2 patients (TSD and Sandhoff) treated with pyrimethamine for a period of 16 weeks. The study was aimed to analyze drug safety and no data on clinical results are available at present.

Apart from symptomatic and supportive therapy, no specific treatments are at present available for NCL and sialidosis, even if preclinical therapeutic programs are ongoing, based on enzyme and gene therapy, stem cell replacement and immunotherapy (Wang et al, 2005; Hobert & Dawson, 2006).

10. Conclusions

LSDs are the main cause of the inherited form of PME. However, they are poorly known as a cause of PME and the differential diagnosis might be challenging. An accurate diagnosis is crucial to provide the best therapeutic approach and an appropriate genetic counselling.

Therefore, in this chapter we have discussed the main clinical and molecular findings in patients with PME affected by LSDs.
It is important to highlight that even if each LDS present with specific sings, some general features should prompt the physician to suspect the presence of a LSD in a patient with PME, such as 1- a familiar history suggestive of a genetic disease, 2- association with other signs of neurological impairment, 3- the presence of visceral involvement.
In the suspect of a LSDs as a cause of PME, specific tests should be performed in specialized laboratories in order to provide an accurate biochemical diagnosis. In addition, the identification of the genes involved in most of these disorders offers the possibility to perform a molecular diagnosis. This type of analysis is quite laborious and time consuming since in most cases the complete sequencing of the affected gene is needed. However, molecular genetic studies are the only reliable tests for the identification of carriers in blood relatives and it is the highly preferred strategy for prenatal diagnosis.
Over the last years a lot of progresses in the understanding of the clinical features and the genetic bases of LSDs have been done. However, very little is known about their pathogenetic mechanisms. In fact, the elucidation of the molecular pathways leading to the neuronal degeneration and the development of therapeutic strategies for these diseases remain the main challenge for the future.

11. References

Accardo A., Pensiero S., Ciana G., Parentin F., Bembi B. (2010) Eye movement impairment recovery in a Gaucher patient treated with miglustat. *Neurology Research International*, Epub 2010 Sep 26, ISSN 2090-1852.

Ahtiainen L., Van Diggelen OP., Jalanko A. & Kopra O. (2003) Palmitoyl protein thioesterase 1 is targeted to the axons in neurons. *Journal of Comparative Neurology*, Vol. 455, No. 3 (Jan), pp. 368-77, ISSN 0021-9967.

Aiello C., Terracciano A., Simonati A., Discepoli G., Cannelli N., Claps D., Crow YJ., Bianchi M., Kitzmuller C., Longo D., Tavoni A., Franzoni E., Tessa A., Veneselli E, Boldrini R., Filocamo M., Williams RE., Bertini ES., Biancheri R., Carrozzo R., Mole SE. & Santorelli FM. (2009) Mutations in MFSD8/CLN7 are a frequent cause of variant-late infantile neuronal ceroid lipofuscinosis. *Human Mutation*, Vol. 30, No. 3 (Mar), pp. E530-40, ISSN 1059-7794.

Akerman BR., Zielenski J., Triggs-Raine BL., Prence EM., Natowicz MR., Lim-Steele JS., Kaback MM., Mules EH., Thomas GH., Clarke JT., et al. (1992) A mutation common in non-Jewish Tay-Sachs disease: frequency and RNA studies. *Human Mutation*, Vol. 1, No. 4, pp. 303-9, ISSN 1059-7794.

Aldahmesh MA., Al-Hassnan ZN., Aldosari M. & Alkuraya FS. (2009) Neuronal ceroid lipofuscinosis caused by MFSD8 mutations: a common theme emerging. *Neurogenetics*, Vol. 10, No. 4 (Oct), pp. 307-11, ISSN 0167-7063.

Alkan A., Kutlu R., Yakinci C., Sigirci A., Aslan M. & Sarac K. (2003) Infantile Sandhoff's disease: multivoxel magnetic resonance spectrosecopy findings. Child Neurology, Vol. 18, No. 6 (Jun), pp. 425-8, ISSN 0887-8994.

Altarescu G., Hill S., Wiggs E., Jeffries N., Kreps C., Parker CC., Brady RO., Barton NW. & Schiffmann R. (2001) The efficacy of enzyme replacement therapy in patients with chronic neuronopathic Gaucher's disease. *Journal of Pediatrics*, Vol. 138, No. 4 (Apr), pp. 539-47, ISSN 0022-3476.

Andermann E., Andermann F., Carpenter S., Wolfe LS., Nelson R., Patry G., & Boileau J. (1986) Action myoclonus-renal failure syndrome: a previously unrecognized neurological disorder unmasked by advances in nephrology. *Advances in Neurology*, Vol. 43, pp. 87-103, ISSN 0091-3952.

Applegarth DA., Toone JR, & Lowry RB. (2000) Incidence of inborn errors of metabolism in British Columbia, 1969-1996. *Pediatrics*, Vol. 105, No. 1 (Jan), pp. e10, ISSN 1098-4275.

Aydin K., Bakir B., Tatli B., Terzibasioglu E. & Ozmen M. (2005) Proton MR spectroscopy in three children with Tay-Sachs disease. *Pediatric Radiology*, Vol. 35, No. 11 (Nov), pp. 1081-5, ISSN 0301-0449.

Badhwar A., Berkovic SF., Dowling JP., Gonzales M., Narayanan S., Brodtmann A., Berzen L., Caviness J., Trenkwalder C., Winkelmann J., Rivest J., Lambert M., Hernandez-Cossio O., Carpenter S., Andermann F., & Andermann E. (2004) Action myoclonus-renal failure syndrome: characterization of a unique cerebro-renal disorder. *Brain*, Vol 127, No. 10 (Oct), pp. 2173-82, ISSN 0006-8950.

Balreira A., Gaspar P., Caiola D., Chaves J., Beirão I., Lima JL., Azevedo JE., & Miranda MC. (2008) A nonsense mutation in the LIMP-2 gene associated with progressive myoclonic epilepsy and nephrotic syndrome. *Human Molecular Genetics*, Vol. 17, No. 14 (Jul), pp.2238-43, ISSN 0964-6906.

Bayleran J., Hechtman P. & Saray W. (1984) Synthesis of 4-methylumbelliferyl-beta-D-N-acetylglucosamine-6-sulfate and its use in classification of GM2 gangliosidosis genotypes. *Clinica Chimica Acta*, Vol. 143, No. 2 (Nov), pp. 73-89, ISSN 0009-9120.

Bembi B., Marchetti F., Guerci V., Ciana G., Addobbati R., Grasso D., Barone R., Cariati R., Fernandez-Guillen L., Butters T. & Pittis MG. (2006) Substrate reduction therapy in the infantile form of Tay-Sachs disease. *Neurology*, Vol. 66, No. 2 (Jan), pp. 278-80, ISSN 0028-3878.

Berkovic SF, Dibbens LM, Oshlack A, Silver JD, Katerelos M, Vears DF, Lüllmann-Rauch R, Blanz J, Zhang KW, Stankovich J, Kalnins RM, Dowling JP, Andermann E, Andermann F, Faldini E, D'Hooge R, Vadlamudi L, Macdonell RA, Hodgson BL, Bayly MA, Savige J, Mulley JC, Smyth GK, Power DA, Saftig P, Bahlo M. (2008) Array-based gene discovery with three unrelated subjects shows SCARB2/LIMP-2 deficiency causes myoclonus epilepsy and glomerulosclerosis. *The American Journal of Human Genetics*, Vol.82, No. 3 (Mar), pp. 673-84, ISSN 0002-9297.

Beutler E. & Grabowski G.A. (2001) Gaucher disease. The Metabolic and Molecular Basis of Inherited Disease Vol. III, 8th ed. Scriver CR., Beaudet AL., Sly WS., Valle D., editors, 3635–68, NY, McGraw-Hill, New York.

Beutler E., & Gelbart T. (1993) Gaucher disease mutations in non-Jewish patients. *British Journal of Haematology*, Vol. 85, No. 2 (Oct), pp.401-5, , ISSN 0007-1048.

Beutler E., Nguyen NJ., Henneberger MW., Smolec JM., McPherson RA., West C., & Gelbart T. (1993) Gaucher disease: gene frequencies in the Ashkenazi Jewish population. The American Journal of Human Genetics, Vol. 52, No. 1 (Jan), pp. 85-8, ISSN 0002-9297.

Blanchette-Mackie EJ., Dwyer NK., Amende LM., Kruth HS., Butler JD., Sokol J., Comly ME., Vanier MT., August JT., Brady RO. & Penchev P. (1988) Type-C Niemann-Pick disease: low density lipoprotein uptake is associated with premature cholesterol accumulation in the Golgi complex and excessive cholesterol storage in lysosomes. *Proceedings of the National Academy of Science U S A*, Vol. 85, No. 21 (Nov), pp. 8022-6, ISSN 0073-6600.

Blanz J., Groth J., Zachos C., Wehling C., Saftig P., & Schwake M. (2010) Disease-causing mutations within the lysosomal integral membrane protein type 2 (LIMP-2) reveal the nature of binding to its ligand beta-glucocerebrosidase. *Human Molecular Genetics*, Vol. 19, No. 4 (Feb), pp. 563-72, ISSN 0964-6906.

Bolhuis PA. & Bikker H. (1992) Deletion of the 5'-region in one or two alleles of HEXB in 15 out of 30 patients with Sandhoff disease. *Human Genetics*, Vol. 90, No. 3 (Nov), pp. 328-9, ISSN 0340-6717.

Bonten E., van der Spoel A., Fornerod M., Grosveld G., & d'Azzo A. (1996) Characterization of human lysosomal neuraminidase defines the molecular basis of the metabolic storage disorder sialidosis. *Genes & Development*, Vol. 10, No. 24 (Dec), pp. 3156-69, ISSN 0890-9369.

Bonten EJ., Arts WF., Beck M., Covanis A., Donati MA., Parini R., Zammarchi E., & d'Azzo A. (2000) Novel mutations in lysosomal neuraminidase identify functional domains and determine clinical severity in sialidosis. *Human Molecular Genetics*, Vol. 9, No. 18 (Nov), pp. 2715-25, ISSN 0964-6906.

Brady RO. (2006) Enzyme replacement for lysosomal diseases. *Annual Review of Medicine*, Vol.57, pp. 283-96, ISSN 0066-4219.

Brooks AI., Chattopadhyay S., Mitchison HM., Nussbaum RL. & Pearce DA. (2003) Functional categorization of gene expression changes in the cerebellum of a Cln3-knockout mouse model for Batten disease. *Molecular Genetics and Metabolism*, Vol. 78, No. 1 (Jan), pp. 17-30, ISSN 1096- 7192.

Caciotti A., Di Rocco M., Filocamo M., Grossi S., Traverso F., d'Azzo A., Cavicchi C., Messeri A., Guerrini R., Zammarchi E., Donati MA. & Morrone A . (2009) Type II sialidosis: review of the clinical spectrum and identification of a new splicing defect with chitotriosidase assessment in two patients. *Journal of Neurology*, Vol. 256, No. 11 (Nov), pp. 1911-5, ISSN 0340-5354.

Cannelli N., Cassandrini D., Bertini E., Striano P., Fusco L., Gaggero R., Specchio N., Biancheri R., Vigevano F., Bruno C., Simonati A., Zara F. & Santorelli FM. (2006) Novel mutations in CLN8 in Italian variant late infantile neuronal ceroid lipofuscinosis: Another genetic hit in the Mediterranean. *Neurogenetics*, Vol. 7, No. 2 (May), pp. 111-7, ISSN 0167-7063.

Cao Y., Espinola JA., Fossale E., Massey AC., Cuervo AM., MacDonald ME & Cotman SL. (2006) Autophagy is disrupted in a knock-in mouse model of juvenile neuronal ceroid lipofuscinosis. *Journal of Biological Chemistry*, Vol. 281, No. 29 (Jul), pp. 20483-93, ISSN 0021-9258.

Cao Z., Natowicz MR., Kaback MM., Lim-Steele JS., Prence EM., Brown D., Chabot T. & Triggs-Raine BL. (1993) A second mutation associated with apparent beta-hexosaminidase A pseudodeficiency: identification and frequency estimation. *The American Journal of Human Genetics*, Vol. 53, No. 6 (Dec), pp. 1198-205, ISSN 0002-9297.

Capablo JL., Franco R., de Cabezón AS., Alfonso P., Pocovi M. & Giraldo P. (2007) Neurologic improvement in a type 3 Gaucher disease patient treated with imiglucerase/miglustat combination. *Epilepsia*, Vol. 48, No. 7 (Jul), pp. 1406-8, ISSN 0013-9580.

Caraballo R., Sologuestua A., Ruggieri VL., Monges S., Cersósimo R., Taratuto AL., Medina C. & Fejerman N. (2005) Clinical and electroencephalographic aspects of late infantile neuronal ceroid lipofuscinosis. *Revista de Neurologia*, Vol. 40, No. 3 (Feb) , pp. 135-40, ISSN 0210-0010.

Carstea ED., Polymeropoulos MH., Parker CC., Detera-Wadleigh SD., O'Neill RR., Patterson MC, Goldin E., Xiao H., Straub RE., Vanier MT., et al. (1993) Linkage of Niemann-Pick disease type C to human chromosome 18. *Proceedings of the National Academy of Science* U S A, Vol. 90, No. 5 (Mar), pp. 2002-4, ISSN 0073-6600.

Chang M., Cooper JD., Sleat DE., Cheng SH., Dodge JC., Passini MA., Lobel P & Davidson BL. (2008) Intraventricular enzyme replacement improves disease phenotypes in a mouse model of late infantile neuronal ceroid lipofuscinosis. *Molecular Therapy*, Vol. 16, No. 4 (Apr), pp. 649-56, ISSN 0969-7128.

Clarke JT., Mahuran DJ., Sathe S., Kolodny EH., Rigat BA., Raiman JA. & Tropak MB. (2011) An open-label Phase I/II clinical trial of pyrimethamine for the treatment of patients affected with chronic GM2 gangliosidosis (Tay-Sachs or Sandhoff variants). *Molecular Genetics and Metabolism*, Vol. 102, No. 1 (Jan), pp. 6-12, ISSN 1096-7192.

Collins J., Holder GE., Herbert H. & Adams GG. (2006) Batten disease: features to facilitate early diagnosis. *British Journal of Ophthalmology*, Vol. 90, No. 9 (Sep), pp.1119-24, ISSN 0007-1161.

Connock M., Burls A., Frew E., Fry-Smith A., Juarez-Garcia A., McCabe C., Wailoo A., Abrams K., Cooper N., Sutton A., O'Hagan A. & Moore D. (2006) The clinical effectiveness and cost-effectiveness of enzyme replacement therapy for Gaucher's disease: a systematic review. *Health Technology Assessement*, Vol 10, No. 24 (Jul), pp. :iii-iv, ix-136, ISSN 1366-5278.

Cox TM., & Schofield JP. (1997) Gaucher's disease: clinical features and natural history. *Bailliere's Clinical Haematology*, Vol. 10, No. 4 (Dec), pp. 657-89, ISSN 0950-3536.

Dardis A., Filocamo M., Grossi S., Ciana G., Franceschetti S, Dominissini S., Rubboli G., Di Rocco M., & Bembi B. (2009) Biochemical and molecular findings in a patient with myoclonic epilepsy due to a mistarget of the beta-glucosidase enzyme. *Molecular Genetics and Metabolism*, Vol. 97, No. 4 (Aug), pp. 309-11, ISSN 1096-7192.

Das AK., Becerra CH., Yi W., Lu JY., Siakotos AN., Wisniewski KE. & Hofmann SL. (1998) Molecular genetics of palmitoyl-protein thioesterase deficiency in the U.S. *Journal of Clinical Investigation*, Vol. 15, No.2 (Jul), pp. 361-70, ISSN 0021-9738.

Davies JP. & Ioannou YA. (2000) Topological analysis of Niemann-Pick C1 protein reveals that the membrane orientation of the putative sterol-sensing domain is identical to those of 3-hydroxy-3-methylglutaryl-CoA reductase and sterol regulatory element binding protein cleavage-activating protein. *Journal of Biological Chemistry*, Vol. 275, No. 32 (Aug), pp. 24367-74, ISSN 0021-9258.

d'Azzo A., Andria G., Strisciuglio P. & Galjaard H. (2001). Galactosialidosis. The Metabolic and Molecular Basis of Inherited Disease Vol. III, 8th ed. Scriver CR., Beaudet AL., Sly WS., Valle D., editors, 3811–26, NY, McGraw-Hill, New York.

Den Tandt WR. & Brossmer R. (1984) Determination of methylumbelliferyl-N-acetylneuraminic acid sialidase for clinical purposes. *Journal of Clinical Chemistry and Clinical Biochemistry,* Vol. 22, No. 2 (Feb), pp. 189-93, ISSN 0939-4974.

Dibbens LM., Michelucci R., Gambardella A., Andermann F., Rubboli G., Bayly MA., Joensuu T., Vears DF., Franceschetti S., Canafoglia L., Wallace R., Bassuk AG., Power DA., Tassinari CA., Andermann E., Lehesjoki AE., & Berkovic SF. (2009) SCARB2 mutations in progressive myoclonus epilepsy (PME) without renal failure. *Annals of Neurology,* Vol. 66, No. 4 (Oct), pp. 532-6, ISSN 0364-5134.

D'Incerti L. (2000) MRI in neuronal ceroid lipofuscinosis. *Neurological Science,* Vol. 21, (3 Suppl), pp. S71-3, ISSN 1590-1874.

Dionisi-Vici C., Rizzo C., Burlina AB., Caruso U., Sabetta G., Uziel G. & Abeni D. (2002) Inborn errors of metabolism in the Italian pediatric population: a national retrospective survey. *Journal of Pediatrics,* Vol. 140, No. 3 (Mar), pp. 321-7, ISSN 0022-3476.

Dittmer F., Ulbrich EJ., Hafner A.., Schmahl W., Meister T., Pohlmann R. & von Figura K. (1999) Alternative mechanisms for trafficking of lysosomal enzymes in mannose 6-phosphate receptor-deficient mice are cell type-specific. *Journal of Cell Science,* Vo. 112, Vol. 10 (May), pp. 1591-7, ISSN 0021-9533.

dos Santos MR., Tanaka A., sá Miranda MC., Ribeiro MG., Maia M. & Suzuki K. (1991) GM2-gangliosidosis B1 variant: analysis of beta-hexosaminidase alpha gene mutations in 11 patients from a defined region in Portugal. *The American Journal of Human Genetics,* Vol. 49, No. 4 (Oct), pp. 886-90, ISSN 0002-9297.

Elleder M., Franc J., Kraus J., Nevsímalová S., Sixtová K. & Zeman J. (1997) Neuronal ceroid lipofuscinosis in the Czech Republic: analysis of 57 cases. Report of the 'Prague NCL group'. *European Journal of Paediatric Neurology,* Vol. 1, No. 4, pp. 109-14, ISSN 1090-3798.

Erikson A. (1986) Gaucher disease-Norrbottnian type (III). Neuropaediatric and neurobiological aspects of clinical patterns and treatment. *Acta Paediatric Scandinavica Supplement,* Vol. 326, pp. 1-42, ISSN 0300-8843.

Eskelinen EL., Tanaka Y., & Saftig P. (2003) At the acidic edge: emerging functions for lysosomal membrane proteins. *Trends in Cell Biology,* Vol. 13, No. 3 (Mar), pp. 137-45, ISSN 0962-8924.

Ezaki J., Takeda-Ezaki M., Koike M., Ohsawa Y., Taka H., Mineki R., Murayama K., Uchiyama Y, Ueno T. & Kominami E.(2003) Characterization of Cln3p, the gene product responsible for juvenile neuronal ceroid lipofuscinosis, as a lysosomal integral membrane glycoprotein. *Journal of Neurochemistry,* Vol. 87, No 5 (Dec), pp. 1296-308, ISSN 0022-3042.

Fancello T., Dardis A., Rosano C., Tarugi P., Tappino B., Zampieri S., Pinotti E., Corsolini F., Fecarotta S., D'Amico A., Di Rocco M., Uziel G., Calandra S., Bembi B. & Filocamo M. (2009) Molecular analysis of NPC1 and NPC2 gene in 34 Niemann-Pick C Italian patients: identification and structural modeling of novel mutations. *Neurogenetics,* Vol. 10, No. 3 (Jul), pp. 229-39, ISSN 0167-7063.

Fernandez-Valero EM., Ballart A., Iturriaga C., Lluch M., Macias J., Vanier MT., Pineda M. & Coll MJ. (2005) Identification of 25 new mutations in 40 unrelated Spanish Niemann-Pick type C patients: genotype-phenotype correlations. *Clinical Genetics,* Vol. 68, No. 3 (Sep), pp. 245-54, ISSN 0009-9163.

Filocamo M., Mazzotti R., Stroppiano M., Grossi S., Dravet C., & Guerrini R. (2004) Early visual seizures and progressive myoclonus epilepsy in neuronopathic Gaucher disease due to a rare compound heterozygosity (N188S/S107L). *Epilepsia*, Vol. 45, No. 9 (Sep), pp.1154-7, ISSN 0013-9580.

Franceschetti S., Uziel G., Ciano C., Scaioli V., Guerrini R., Visani E. & Panzica F. (2011) Characterization of severe action myoclonus in sialidoses. *Epilepsy Research*, Vol. 94, No. 1-2 (Mar), pp. 86-93, ISSN 0920-1211.

Froissart R., Cheillan D., Bouvier R., Tourret S., Bonnet V., Piraud M. & Maire I. (2005) Clinical, morphological, and molecular aspects of sialic acid storage disease manifesting in utero. *Journal of Medical Genetics*, Vo. 42, No. 11 (Nov), pp. 829-36, ISSN 00222593.

Fujita H., Tanaka Y., Noguchi Y., Kono A., Himeno M., & Kato K. (1991) Isolation and sequencing of a cDNA clone encoding rat liver lysosomal cathepsin D and the structure of three forms of mature enzymes. *Biochemical and Biophysical Research Communications*, Vol. 179, No. 1 (Aug), pp.190-6, ISSN 0006-291X

Fukuda M. (1991) Lysosomal membrane glycoproteins. Structure, biosynthesis, and intracellular trafficking. *Journal of Biological Chemistry*, Vol. 266, No. 32 (Nov), pp.1327-30, ISSN 0021-9258.

Futerman AH. & van Meer G. (2004) The cell biology of lysosomal storage disorders. *Nature Reviews Molecular Cell Biology*, Vol. 5, No. 7 (Jul), pp. 554-65, ISSN 1471-0072.

Galanaud D., Tourbah A., Lehéricy S., Leveque N., Heron B., Billette de Villemeur T., Guffon N., Feillet F., Baumann N., Vanier MT. & Sedel F. (2009) 24 month-treatment with miglustat of three patients with Niemann-Pick disease type C: follow up using brain spectroscopy. *Molecular Genetics and Metabolism*, Vol. 96, No. 2 (Feb), pp. 55-8, ISSN 1096-7192.

Gao H., Boustany RM., Espinola JA., Cotman SL., Srinidhi L., Antonellis KA,. Gillis T., Qin X., Liu S., Donahue LR., Bronson RT., Faust JR., Stout D., Haines JL., Lerner TJ & MacDonald ME. (2002) Mutations in a novel CLN6-encoded transmembrane protein cause variant neuronal ceroid lipofuscinosis in man and mouse. *The American Journal of Human Genetics*, Vol. 70, No. 2 (Feb), pp. 324-35, ISSN 0002-9297.

Garvey MA., Toro C., Goldstein S., Altarescu G., Wiggs EA., Hallett M., & Schiffmann R. (2001) Somatosensory evoked potentials as a marker of disease burden in type 3 Gaucher disease. *Neurology*, Vol. 13, No. 56 (Feb), pp. 391-4, ISSN 0028-3878.

Gieselmann V., Hasilik A. & von Figura K. (1985) Processing of human cathepsin D in lysosomes in vitro. *Journal of Biological Chemistry*, Vol. 260, No. 5 (Mar), pp. 3215-20, ISSN 0021-9258.

Golabek AA & Kida E. (2006) Tripeptidyl-peptidase I in health and disease. *Biological Chemistry*, Vol. 387, No 8 (Aug), pp. 1091-9, ISSN 1431-6730.

Golabek AA., Kida E., Walus M., Wujek P., Mehta P & Wisniewski KE. (2003) Biosynthesis, glycosylation, and enzymatic processing in vivo of human tripeptidyl-peptidase I. *Journal of Biological Chemistry*, Vol. 278, No 9 (Feb). pp. 7135-45, ISSN 0021-9258.

Gopalakrishnan MM., Grosch HW., Locatelli-Hoops S., Werth N., Smolenová E., Nettersheim M., Sandhoff K. & Hasilik A. (2004) Purified recombinant human prosaposin forms oligomers that bind procathepsin D and affect its autoactivation. *Biochemical Journal*, Vol. 383, No. 3 (Nov), pp. 507-15, ISSN 0264-6021.

Grabowski GA., & Horowitz M. (1997) Gaucher's disease: molecular, genetic and enzymological aspects. *Baillieres in Clinical Haematology*, Vol. 10, No. 4 (Dec), pp.635-56, ISSN 0950-3536.

Gravel RA., Kaback MM., Proia RL., Sandhoff K., Suzuki K. & Suzuki K. (2001) The GM2 gangliosidoses. *The Metabolic and Molecular Bases of Inherited Diseases* Vol. III, 8th ed. Scriver CR., Beaudet AL., Sly WS., Valle D., editors, 3827-76, NY, McGraw-Hill, New York.

Grosso S., Farnetani MA., Berardi R., Margollicci M., Galluzzi P., Vivarelli R., Morgese G. & Ballestri P. (2003) GM2 gangliosidosis variant B1 neuroradiological findings. *Journal of Neurology*, Vol. 250, No. 1 (Jan), pp. 17-21, ISSN 0340-5354.

Haltia M. (2003) The neuronal ceroid-lipofuscinoses. *Journal of Neuropathology & Experimental Neurology*, Vol. 62, No. 1 (Jan), pp. 1-13, ISSN 0022-3069.

Heine C., Koch B., Storch S., Kohlschütter A., Palmer DN. & Braulke T. (2004) Defective endoplasmic reticulum-resident membrane protein CLN6 affects lysosomal degradation of endocytosed arylsulfatase A. *Journal of Biological Chemistry*, Vol. 279, No 21 (May), pp. 22347-52, ISSN 0021-9258.

Hellsten E., Vesa J., Olkkonen VM., Jalanko A. & Peltonen L. (1996) Human palmitoyl protein thioesterase: evidence for lysosomal targeting of the enzyme and disturbed cellular routing in infantile neuronal ceroid lipofuscinosis. *EMBO Journal*, Vol. 15, No. 19 (Oct), pp. 5240-5, ISSN 0261-4189.

Hendriksz CJ., Corry PC., Wraith JE., Besley GT., Cooper A. & Ferrie CD. (2004) Juvenile Sandhoff disease--nine new cases and a review of the literature. *Journal of Inherited Metabolic Disease*, Vol. 27, No. 2, pp. 241-9, ISSN 0141-8955.

Herva R., Tyynelä J., Hirvasniemi A., Syrjäkallio-Ylitalo M. & Haltia M. (2000) Northern epilepsy: a novel form of neuronal ceroid-lipofuscinosis. *Brain Pathology*, Vol. 10, No. 2 (Apr), pp. :215-22, ISSN 1015-6305.

Hobert JA. & Dawson G. (2006) Neuronal ceroid lipofuscinoses therapeutic strategies: past, present and future. *Biochimica et Biophysica Acta*, Vol. 1762, No. 10 (Oct), pp. 945-53, ISSN 0304-4165.

Holmberg V., Jalanko A., Isosomppi J., Fabritius AL., Peltonen L. & Kopra O. (2004) The mouse ortholog of the neuronal ceroid lipofuscinosis CLN5 gene encodes a soluble lysosomal glycoprotein expressed in the developing brain. *Neurobiology of Disease*, Vol. 16, No. 1 (Jun), pp. 29-40, ISSN 0969-9961.

Holmes EW. & O'Brien JS. (1979) Separation of glycoprotein-derived oligosaccharides by thin-layer chromatography. *Analytical Biochemistry*, Vol. 93, No. 1 (Feb), pp. 167-70, ISSN 0003-2697.

Holopainen JM., Saarikoski J., Kinnunen PK & Järvelä I. (2001) Elevated lysosomal pH in neuronal ceroid lipofuscinoses (NCLs). *European Journal of Biochemistry*, Vol. 268, No. 22 (Nov), pp. 5851-6, ISSN: 0014-2956.

Horowitz, M., Wilder S., Horowitz Z., Reiner O., Gelbart T., & Beutler E. (1989) The human glucocerebrosidase gene and pseudogene: structure and evolution. *Genomics*, Vol 4, No. 1 (Jan), pp. 87-96, ISSN 0888-7543.

Huang K. & El-Husseini A. (2005) Modulation of neuronal protein trafficking and function by palmitoylation. *Current Opinion in Neurobiology*, Vol. 15, No. 5 (Oct), pp. 527-35, ISSN 0959-4388.

Infante RE., Abi-Mosleh L., Radhakrishnan A., Dale JD., Brown MS. & Goldstein JL. (2008a) Purified NPC1 protein. I. Binding of cholesterol and oxysterols to a 1278-amino acid membrane protein. *Journal of Biological Chemistry,* Vol. 283, No. 2 (Jan), pp. 1052-63, ISSN 0021-9258.

Infante RE., Radhakrishnan A., Abi-Mosleh L., Kinch LN., Wang ML., Grishin NV., Goldstein JL. & Brown MS.(2008b) Purified NPC1 protein: II. Localization of sterol binding to a 240-amino acid soluble luminal loop. *Journal of Biological Chemistry,* Vol. 283, No. 2 (Jan), pp. 1064-75, ISSN 0021-9258.

Inglese M., Nusbaum AO., Pastores GM., Gianutsos J., Kolodny EH. & Gonen O. (2005) MR imaging and proton spectroscopy of neuronal injury in late-onset GM2 gangliosidosis. *American Journal of Neuroradiology,* Vol. 26, No. 8 (Sep), pp. 2037-42, ISSN 0195-6108.

International Batten Disease Consortium. (1995) Isolation of a novel gene underlying Batten disease, CLN3. The International Batten Disease Consortium. *Cell,* Vol. 82, No. 6 (Sep), pp. 949-57, ISSN 0092-8674.

Jain A., Kohli A. & Sachan D. (2010) Infantile Sandhoff's disease with peripheral neuropathy. *Pediatric Neurology,* Vol. 42, No. 6 (Jun), pp. 459-61, ISSN 1098-3600.

Jalanko A. & Braulke T. (2009) Neuronal ceroid lipofuscinoses. *Biochimica et Biophysica Acta,* Vol. 1793, No. 4 (Apr), pp. 697-709, ISSN 0304-4165.

Järvelä I., Autti T., Lamminranta S., Aberg L., Raininko R. & Santavuori P. (1999) Clinical and magnetic resonance imaging findings in Batten disease: analysis of the major mutation (1.02-kb deletion). *Annals of Neurology,* Vol. 42, No. 5 (Nov), pp. 799-802, ISSN 0364-5134.

Kaback M., Lim-Steele J., Dabholkar D., Brown D., Levy N. & Zeiger K. (1993) Tay-Sachs disease--carrier screening, prenatal diagnosis, and the molecular era. An international perspective, 1970 to 1993. The International TSD Data Collection Network. *JAMA,* Vol. 270, No. 19 (Nov), pp. 2307-15, ISSN 00987484.

Kasho VN., Smirnova IN. & Kaback HR. (2006) Sequence alignment and homology threading reveals prokaryotic and eukaryotic proteins similar to lactose permease. *Journal of Molecular Biology,* Vol. 358, No. 4 (May), pp. 1060-70, ISSN 0022-2836.

Kelly DA., Portmann B., Mowat AP., Sherlock S. & Lake BD. (1993) Niemann-Pick disease type C: diagnosis and outcome in children, with particular reference to liver disease. *Journal of Pediatrics,* Vol. 123, No. 2 (Aug), pp. 242-7, ISSN 0022-3476.

Kim JW., Liou BB., Lai MY., Ponce E., & Grabowski GA. (1996) Gaucher disease: identification of three new mutations in the Korean and Chinese (Taiwanese) populations. *Human Mutation,* Vol. 7, No. 3, pp.214–218, ISSN 1059-7794.

Kim Y., Ramirez-Montealegre D. & Pearce DA. (2003) A role in vacuolar arginine transport for yeast Btn1p and for human CLN3, the protein defective in Batten disease. *Proceedings of the National Academy of Science U S A,* Vol. 100, No. 26 (Dec), pp. 15458-62, ISSN 0073-6600.

Kitzmüller C., Haines RL., Codlin S., Cutler DF. & Mole SE. (2008) A function retained by the common mutant CLN3 protein is responsible for the late onset of juvenile neuronal ceroid lipofuscinosis. *Human Molecular Genetics,* Vol. 17, No.2 (Jan), pp. 303-12, ISSN 0964-6906.

Klünemann HH., Elleder M., Kaminski WE., Snow K., Peyser JM., O'Brien JF., Munoz D., Schmitz G., Klein HE. & Pendlebury WW. (2002) Frontal lobe atrophy due to a mutation in the cholesterol binding protein HE1/NPC2. *Annals of Neurology*, Vol. 52, No. 6, pp. 743-9, ISSN 0364-5134.

Kohan R., Cismondi IA., Kremer RD., Muller VJ., Guelbert N., Anzolini VT., Fietz MJ., Ramírez AM. & Halac IN. (2009) An integrated strategy for the diagnosis of neuronal ceroid lipofuscinosis types 1 (CLN1) and 2 (CLN2) in eleven Latin American patients. *Clinical Genetics*, Vol. 76, No. 4 (Oct), pp. 372-82, ISSN 0009-9163.

Kohlschütter A & Schulz A. (2009) Towards understanding the neuronal ceroid lipofuscinoses. *Brain & Development*, Vol. 31, No. 7 (Aug), pp. 499-502, ISSN 0387-7604.

Kousi M., Siintola E., Dvorakova L., Vlaskova H., Turnbull J., Topcu M., Yuksel D., Gokben S., Minassian BA., Elleder M., Mole SE. & Lehesjoki AE. (2009) Mutations in CLN7/MFSD8 are a common cause of variant late-infantile neuronal ceroid lipofuscinosis. *Brain*, Vol. 132, No. 3 (Mar), pp. 810-9, ISSN 0006-8950.

Kowarz L., Goker-Alpan O., Banerjee-Basu S., LaMarca ME., Kinlaw L., Schiffmann R., Baxevanis AD., & Sidransky E. (2005) Gaucher mutation N188S is associated with myoclonic epilepsy. *Human Mutation*, Vol. 26, No. 3 (Sep), pp. 271-3, ISSN 1059-7794.

Kraoua I., Sedel F., Caillaud C., Froissart R., Stirnemann J., Chaurand G., Flodrops H., Tari S., Gourfinkel-An I., Mathieu S., Belmatoug N., Billette de Villemeur T., & Mignot C. (2010) French experience of type 3 Gaucher disease: Phenotypic diversity and neurological outcome of 10 patients. *Brain & Development*, Vol. 33, No. 3 (Feb), pp. 131-9, ISSN 0387-7604.

Kwon HJ., Abi-Mosleh L., Wang ML., Deisenhofer J., Goldstein JL., Brown MS. & Infante RE. (2009) Structure of N-terminal domain of NPC1 reveals distinct subdomains for binding and transfer of cholesterol. *Cell*, Vol. 137, No. 7 (Jun), pp. 1213-24, ISSN 0092-8674.

Kyttälä A., Ihrke G., Vesa J., Schell MJ. & Luzio JP. (2004) Two motifs target Batten disease protein CLN3 to lysosomes in transfected nonneuronal and neuronal cells. *Molecular Biology of the Cell*, Vol. 15, No. 3 (Mar), pp. 1313-23, ISSN 1059-1524.

Kyttälä A., Lahtinen U., Braulke T. & Hofmann SL. (2006) Functional biology of the neuronal ceroid lipofuscinoses (NCL) proteins. *Biochimica et Biophysica Acta*, Vol. 1726, No. 10 (Oct), pp. 920-33, ISSN 0304-4165.

Lake BD & Hall NA. (1993) Immunolocalization studies of subunit c in late-infantile and juvenile Batten disease. *Journal of Inherited Metabolic Disease*, Vol. 16, No. 2, pp. 263-6, ISSN 0141-8955.

Lauronen L., Munroe PB., Järvelä I., Autti T., Mitchison HM., O'Rawe AM., Gardiner RM., Mole SE., Puranen J., Häkkinen AM., Kirveskari E. & Santavuori P. (1999) Delayed classic and protracted phenotypes of compound heterozygous juvenile neuronal ceroid lipofuscinosis. *Neurology*, Vol. 52, No. 2 (Jan), pp. 360-5, ISSN 0028-3878.

Lehtovirta M., Kyttälä A., Eskelinen EL., Hess M., Heinonen O. & Jalanko A. (2001) Palmitoyl protein thioesterase (PPT) localizes into synaptosomes and synaptic vesicles in neurons: implications for infantile neuronal ceroid lipofuscinosis (INCL). *Human Molecular Genetics*, Vol. 10, No. 1 (Jan), pp. 69-75, ISSN 0964-6906.

Leonova T., & Grabowski GA. (2000) Fate and sorting of acid beta-glucosidase in transgenic mammalian cells. *Molecular Genetics and Metabolism*, Vol. 70, No. 4 (Aug), pp: 281-94, ISSN 1096-7192.

Lonka L., Kyttälä A., Ranta S., Jalanko A. & Lehesjoki AE. (2000) The neuronal ceroid lipofuscinosis CLN8 membrane protein is a resident of the endoplasmic reticulum. *Human Molecular Genetics*, Vol. 9, No. 11 (Jul), pp. 1691-7, ISSN 0964-6906.

Lowden JA. & O'Brien JS. (1979) Sialidosis: a review of human neuraminidase deficiency. *American Journal of Human Genetics*, Vol. 31, No. 1 (Jan), pp. 1-18, ISSN 0002-9297.

Luiro K, Kopra O, Lehtovirta M, Jalanko A. (2001) CLN3 protein is targeted to neuronal synapses but excluded from synaptic vesicles: new clues to Batten disease. *Human Molecular Genetics*, Vol. 10, No. 19 (Sep), pp. 2123-31, ISSN 0964-6906.

Luiro K., Kopra O., Blom T., Gentile M., Mitchison HM., Hovatta I., Törnquist K. & Jalanko A. (2006) Batten disease (JNCL) is linked to disturbances in mitochondrial, cytoskeletal, and synaptic compartments. *Journal of Neuroscience Research*, Vol. 84, No. 5 (Oct), pp. 1124-38, ISSN 0360-4012.

Macías-Vidal J., Rodríguez-Pascau L., Sánchez-Ollé G., Lluch M., Vilageliu L., Grinberg D., Coll MJ.; the Spanish NPC Working Group. (2010) Molecular analysis of 30 Niemann-Pick type C patients from Spain. *Clinical Genetics,* Jul 6. [Epub ahead of print], ISSN 0009-9163.

Maegawa GH., Stockley T., Tropak M., Banwell B., Blaser S., Kok F., Giugliani R., Mahuran D. & Clarke JT. (2006) The natural history of juvenile or subacute GM2 gangliosidosis: 21 new cases and literature review of 134 previously reported. *Pediatrics*, Vol. 118, No. 5 (Nov), pp. 1550-62, ISSN 0031-4005.

Marseille Consensus Group. (1990) Classification of progressive myoclonus epilepsies and related disorders. *Annals of Neurology*, Vol. 28, No. 1 (Jul), pp. 113-6, ISSN 0364-5134.

Martin JJ. (1991) Adult type of neuronal ceroid lipofuscinosis. *Developmental Neuroscience*, Vol. 13, No. 4-5, pp.331-8, ISSN 0378-5866.

Meikle PJ., Hopwood JJ., Clague AE., & Carey WF. (1999) Prevalence of lysosomal storage disorders. *Journal of American Medical Association*, Vol. 281, No. 3 (Jan), pp. 249-54, ISSN 0098-7484.

Millat G., Marçais C., Rafi MA., Yamamoto T., Morris JA., Pentchev PG., Ohno K., Wenger DA. & Vanier MT. (1999) Niemann-Pick C1 disease: the I1061T substitution is a frequent mutant allele in patients of Western European descent and correlates with a classic juvenile phenotype. *The American Journal of Human Genetics*, Vol. 65, No. 5 (Nov), pp. 1321-9, ISSN 0002-9297.

Millat G., Baïlo N., Molinero S., Rodriguez C., Chikh K. & Vanier MT. (2005) Niemann-Pick C disease: use of denaturing high performance liquid chromatography for the detection of NPC1 and NPC2 genetic variations and impact on management of patients and families. *Molecular Genetics and Metabolism*, Vol. 86, No. 1-2 (Sep-Oct), pp. 220-32, ISSN 1096-7192.

Millat G., Chikh K., Naureckiene S., Sleat DE., Fensom AH., Higaki K., Elleder M., Lobel P. & Vanier MT. (2001) Niemann-Pick disease type C: spectrum of HE1 mutations and genotype/phenotype correlations in the NPC2 group. *The American Journal of Human Genetics*, Vol. 69, No. 5 (Nov), pp. 1013-21, ISSN 0002-9297.

Milner CM., Smith SV., Carrillo MB., Taylor GL., Hollinshead M., & Campbell RD. (1997) Identification of a sialidase encoded in the human major histocompatibility complex. *Journal of Biological Chemistry*, Vol. 272, No. 7 (Feb), pp. 4549-58, ISSN 0021-9258.

Mistry P. & Germain DP. Therapeutic goals in Gaucher disease. (2006) *Revue de médecine interne*. Vol. 27, Suppl 1 (Mar), pp. S30-8, ISSN 0248-8663.

Mitchison HM., Hofmann SL., Becerra CH., Munroe PB., Lake BD., Crow YJ., Stephenson JB., Williams RE., Hofman IL., Taschner PE., Martin JJ., Philippart M., Andermann E., Andermann F., Mole SE., Gardiner RM. & O'Rawe AM. (1998) Mutations in the palmitoyl-protein thioesterase gene (PPT; CLN1) causing juvenile neuronal ceroid lipofuscinosis with granular osmiophilic deposits. *Human Molecular Genetics*, Vol. 7, No 2 (Feb), pp. 291-7, ISSN 0964-6906.

Mole SE., Michaux G., Codlin S., Wheeler RB., Sharp JD. & Cutler DF. (2004) CLN6, which is associated with a lysosomal storage disease, is an endoplasmic reticulum protein. *Experimental Cell Research*, Vol. 298, No. 2 (Aug), pp. 399-406, ISSN 0014-4827.

Mole SE.., Williams RE & Goebel HH. (2005) Correlations between genotype, ultrastructural morphology and clinical phenotype in the neuronal ceroid lipofuscinoses. *Neurogenetics*, Vol. 6, No. 3 (Sep), pp. 107-26, ISSN 0167-7063.

Montalvo AL., Filocamo M., Vlahovicek K., Dardis A., Lualdi S., Corsolini F., Bembi B. & Pittis MG. (2005) Molecular analysis of the HEXA gene in Italian patients with infantile and late onset Tay-Sachs disease: detection of fourteen novel alleles. *Human Mutation*, Vol. 26, No. 3 (Sep), pp. 282-90, ISSN 1059-7794.

Montfort M., Chabás A., Vilageliu L., & Grinberg D. (2004) Functional analysis of 13 GBA mutant alleles identified in Gaucher disease patients: Pathogenic changes and "modifier" polymorphisms. *Human Mutation*, Vol. 23, No. 6 (Jun). pp. 567-75, ISSN 1059-7794.

Munroe PB., Mitchison HM., O'Rawe AM., Anderson JW., Boustany RM., Lerner TJ., Taschner PE., de Vos N., Breuning MH., Gardiner RM., Mole SE. (1997) Spectrum of mutations in the Batten disease gene, CLN3. *American Journal of Human Genetics*, Vol. 61, No. 2 (Aug), pp. 310-6, ISSN 0002-9297.

Naureckiene S., Sleat DE., Lackland H., Fensom A., Vanier MT., Wattiaux R., Jadot M., & Lobel P. (2000) Identification of HE1 as the second gene of Niemann-Pick C disease. *Science*, Vol. 290, No. 5500 (Dec), pp. 2298-301, ISSN 0036-8075.

Neote K., Bapat B., Dumbrille-Ross A., Troxel C., Schuster SM., Mahuran DJ. & Gravel RA. (1988) Characterization of the human HEXB gene encoding lysosomal beta-hexosaminidase. *Genomics*, Vol. 3, No. 4 (Nov), pp. 279-86, ISSN 0888-7543.

Neudorfer O., Pastores GM., Zeng BJ., Gianutsos J., Zaroff CM. & Kolodny EH. (2005) Late-onset Tay-Sachs disease: phenotypic characterization and genotypic correlations in 21 affected patients. *Genetics in Medicine*, Vol. 7, No. 2 (Feb), 119-23, ISSN 1098-3600.

Okada S., Sugino H., Kato T., Yutaka T., Koike M., Dezawa T., Yamano T. & Yabuuchi H. (1983) A severe infantile sialidosis (beta-galactosidase-alpha-neuraminidase deficiency) mimicking GM1-gangliosidosis type 1. *European Journal of Pediatrics*, Vol. 140, No. 4 (Sep), pp. 295-8, ISSN 0340-6199.

Park JK., Orvisky E., Tayebi N., Kaneski C., Lamarca ME., Stubblefield BK., Martin BM., Schiffmann R., & Sidransky E. (2003) Myoclonic epilepsy in Gaucher disease: genotype-phenotype insights from a rare patient subgroup. *Pediatric Research*, Vol. 53; No. 3 (Mar), pp. 387-95, ISSN 0971-9032.

Park WD., O'Brien JF., Lundquist PA., Kraft DL., Vockley CW., Karnes PS., Patterson MC. & Snow K. (2003) Identification of 58 novel mutations in Niemann-Pick disease type

C: correlation with biochemical phenotype and importance of PTC1-like domains in NPC1. *Human Mutation*, Vol. 22, No. 4 (Oct), pp. 313-25, ISSN 1059-7794.

Pasmanik-Chor M., Elroy-Stein O., Aerts H., Agmon V., Gatt S., & Horowitz M. (1996) Overexpression of human glucocerebrosidase containing different-sized leaders. *Biochemical Journal*, Vol.1, No. 317 (Jul), pp.81-8, ISSN 0264-6021.

Patterson MC, Vanier MT, Suzuki K, Morris JA, Carstea E, Neufeld EB., Blanchette-Mackie JE. & Pentchev P. (2001). Niemann- Pick Disease type C: a lipid trafficking disorder. *The metabolic and molecular bases of inherited disease* Vol. III, 8th ed. Scriver CR., Beaudet AL., Sly WS., Valle D., editors, 3611–34. 3635–68, NY, McGraw-Hill, New York.

Patterson MC., Vecchio D., Prady H., Abel L. & Wraith JE. (2007) Miglustat for treatment of Niemann-Pick C disease: a randomised controlled study. *Lancet Neurology*, Vol. 6, No. 9 (Sep), pp. 765-72, ISSN 1474-4422.

Persaud-Sawin DA. & Boustany RM. (2005) Cell death pathways in juvenile Batten disease. *Apoptosis*, Vol. 10, No. 5 (Oct), pp. 973-85, ISSN 1360-8185.

Pinto R., Caseiro C., Lemos M., Lopes L., Fontes A., Ribeiro H., Pinto E., Silva E., Rocha S., Marcão A., Ribeiro I., Lacerda L., Ribeiro G., Amaral O. & Sá Miranda MC. (2004) Prevalence of lysosomal storage diseases in Portugal. *European Journal of Human Genetics*, Vol. 12, No. 2 (Feb), pp. 87-92, ISSN 1018-4813.

Platt FM. & Lachmann RH. (2009) Treating lysosomal storage disorders: current practice and future prospects. *Biochimica et Biophysica Acta*, Vol. 1793, No. 4 (Apr), pp. 737-45, ISSN 0304-4165.

Platt FM., Jeyakumar M., Andersson U., Dwek RA. & Butters TD. (2005) New developments in treating glycosphingolipid storage diseases. *Advances in Experimental Medicine and Biology*, Vol. 564, pp. 117-26, ISSN 0065-2598.

Poorthuis BJ., Wevers RA., Kleijer WJ., Groener JE., de Jong JG., van Weely S., Niezen-Koning KE. & van Diggelen OP. (1999). The frequency of lysosomal storage diseases in The Netherlands. *Human Genetics*, Vol. 105, No. 1-2, (Jul-Aug), pp. 151-6, ISSN 0340-6717.

Poupetová H., Ledvinová J., Berná L., Dvoráková L., Kozich V. & Elleder M. (2010) The birth prevalence of lysosomal storage disorders in the Czech Republic: comparison with data in different populations. *Disease*, Vol. 33, No. 4 (Aug), pp. 387-96, ISSN 0141-8955.

Pshezhetsky AV., Richard C., Michaud L., Igdoura S., Wang S., Elsliger MA., Qu J., Leclerc D., Gravel R., Dallaire L., & Potier M. (1997) Cloning, expression and chromosomal mapping of human lysosomal sialidase and characterization of mutations in sialidosis. *Nature Genetics*, Vol.15, No. 3 (Mar), pp. 316-20, ISSN 1061-4036.

Rakheja D., Narayan SB., Pastor JV. & Bennett MJ. (2004) CLN3P, the Batten disease protein, localizes to membrane lipid rafts (detergent-resistant membranes). *Biochemical and Biophysical Research Communication*, Vol. 317, No. 4 (May), pp. 988-91, ISSN 0006-291X.

Ranta S., Topcu M., Tegelberg S., Tan H., Ustübütün A., Saatci I., Dufke A., Enders H., Pohl K., Alembik Y., Mitchell WA., Mole SE. & Lehesjoki AE. (2004) Variant late infantile neuronal ceroid lipofuscinosis in a subset of Turkish patients is allelic to Northern epilepsy. *Human Mutation*, Vol. 23, No. 4 (Apr), pp. 300-5, ISSN 1059-7794.

Ranta S., Zhang Y., Ross B., Lonka L., Takkunen E., Messer A., Sharp J., Wheeler R., Kusumi K., Mole S., Liu W., Soares MB., Bonaldo MF., Hirvasniemi A., de la Chapelle A.,

Gilliam TC. & Lehesjoki AE. (1999) The neuronal ceroid lipofuscinoses in human EPMR and mnd mutant mice are associated with mutations in CLN8. *Nature Genetics*, Vol. 23, No. 2 (Oct), pp. 233-6, ISSN 1061-4036.

Rapin I. (1986) Myoclonus in neuronal storage and Lafora diseases. *Advances in Neurology*. Vol. 43, pp. 65-85, ISSN 0091-3952.

Reczek D., Schwake M., Schröder J., Hughes H., Blanz J., Jin X., Brondyk W., Van Patten S., Edmunds T., & Saftig P. (2007) LIMP-2 is a receptor for lysosomal mannose-6-phosphate-independent targeting of beta-glucocerebrosidase. *Cell*, Vol. 131, No. 4 (Nov), pp. 770-83, ISSN 0092-8674.

Reinhardt K ., Grapp M., Schlachter K., Brück W., Gärtner J. & Steinfeld R. (2010) Novel CLN8 mutations confirm the clinical and ethnic diversity of late infantile neuronal ceroid lipofuscinosis. *Clinical Genetics*, Vol. 77, No. 1 (Jan), pp. 79-85, ISSN 0009-9163.

Ribeiro I., Marcão A., Amaral O., Sá Miranda MC., Vanier MT. & Millat G. (2001) Niemann-Pick type C disease: NPC1 mutations associated with severe and mild cellular cholesterol trafficking alterations. *Human Genetics*, Vol. 109, No. 1 (Jul), pp. 24-32, ISSN 0002-9297.

Ruchoux MM. & Goebel HH. (1996) Diagnostic (clinical and morphological) criteria for adult neuronal ceroid-lipofuscinosis (Kufs' disease). *Neuropathology and Applied Neurobiology*, Vol 23, No. 3 (Jun), pp. 262-3, ISSN 0305-1846.

Rucker JC., Shapiro BE., Han YH., Kumar AN., Garbutt S., Keller EL. & Leigh RJ. 2004 Neuro-ophthalmology of late-onset Tay-Sachs disease (LOTS). *Neurology*, Vol. 63, No. 10 (Nov), pp. 1918-26, ISSN 0028-3878.

Runz H., Dolle D., Schlitter AM. & Zschocke J. (2008) NPC-db, a Niemann-Pick type C disease gene variation database. *Human Mutation*, Vol. 29, No. 3 (Mar), pp. 345-50, ISSN 1059-7794.

Rusyn E., Mousallem T., Persaud-Sawin DA., Miller S. & Boustany RM. (2008) CLN3p impacts galactosylceramide transport, raft morphology, and lipid content. *Pediatric Research*, Vol. 63, No. 6 (Jun), pp. 625-31, ISSN-0971-9032.

Santavuori P. (1988) Neuronal ceroid-lipofuscinoses in childhood. *Brain & Development*, Vol. 10, No. 2, pp. 80-3, ISSN 0387-7604.

Schiffmann R., Fitzgibbon EJ., Harris C., DeVile C., Davies EH., Abel L., van Schaik IN., Benko W., Timmons M., Ries M. & Vellodi A. (2008) Randomized, controlled trial of miglustat in Gaucher's disease type 3. *Annals of Neurology*. Nov, Vol. 64, No.5, pp: 514-22, ISSN 0364-5134.

Seeman PJ., Finckh U., Höppner J., Lakner V., Liebisch I., Grau G., & Rolfs A. (1996) Two new missense mutations in a non-Jewish Caucasian family with type 3 Gaucher disease. *Neurology*. Vol. 46, No. 4 (April), pp. 1102-7, ISSN 0028-3878.

Shapiro BE., Pastores GM., Gianutsos J., Luzy C. & Kolodny EH. (2009) Miglustat in late-onset Tay-Sachs disease: a 12-month, randomized, controlled clinical study with 24 months of extended treatment. *Genetics in Medicine*, Vol. 11, No. 6 (Jun), pp. 425-33, ISSN 1098-3600.

Siintola E., Partanen S., Strömme P., Haapanen A., Haltia M., Maehlen J., Lehesjoki AE. & Tyynelä J. (2006) Cathepsin D deficiency underlies congenital human neuronal ceroid-lipofuscinosis. *Brain*, Vol. 129, No. 6 (Jun), pp. 1438-45, ISSN 0006-8950.

Siintola E., Topcu M., Aula N., Lohi H., Minassian BA., Paterson AD., Liu XQ., Wilson C., Lahtinen U., Anttonen AK. & Lehesjoki AE. (2007) The novel neuronal ceroid lipofuscinosis gene MFSD8 encodes a putative lysosomal transporter. *The American Journal of Human Genetics*, Vol. 81, No. 1 (Jul), pp. 136-46, ISSN 0002-9297.

Sleat DE., Donnelly RJ., Lackland H., Liu CG., Sohar I., Pullarkat RK. & Lobel P. (1997). Association of mutations in a lysosomal protein with classical late-infantile neuronal ceroid lipofuscinosis. *Science*, Vol. 277, No 5333, (Sep), pp. 1802-5, ISSN 0036-8075.

Sleat DE., Lackland H., Wang Y., Sohar I., Xiao G., Li H. & Lobel P. (2005) The human brain mannose 6-phosphate glycoproteome: a complex mixture composed of multiple isoforms of many soluble lysosomal proteins. *Proteomics*, Vol.5, No. 6 (Apr), pp. 1520-32, ISSN 1615-9861.

Sleat DE., Zheng H., Qian M. & Lobel P. (2006) Identification of sites of mannose 6-phosphorylation on lysosomal proteins. *Molecular & Cellular Proteomics*, Vol. 5, No. 4 (Apr), pp. 686-701, ISSN 1535-9476.

Sorge J., West C., Westwood B., & Beutler E. (1985) Molecular cloning and nucleotide sequence of human glucocerebrosidase cDNA. *Proceedings of the National Academy of Science USA*, Vol. 82, No. 21 (Nov.), pp. 7289-93, ISSN 0073-6600.

Sorge JA., West C., Kuhl W., Treger L., Beutler E. (1987) The human glucocerebrosidase gene has two functional ATG initiator codons. *The American Journal of Human Genetics*, Vol. 41, No. 6 (Dec), pp.1016-24, ISSN 0002-9297.

Staretz-Chacham O., Lang TC., LaMarca ME., Krasnewich D. & Sidransky E. (2009) Lysosomal storage disorders in the newborn. *Pediatrics*, Vol. 123, No. 4 (Apr), pp. 1191-207, ISSN 0031-4005.

Steinberg SJ., Ward CP. & Fensom AH. (1994) Complementation studies in Niemann-Pick disease type C indicate the existence of a second group. *Journal of Medical Genetics*, Vol. 31, No. 4 (Apr), pp. 317-20, ISSN 0022-2593.

Steinfeld R., Heim P., von Gregory H., Meyer K., Ullrich K., Goebel HH. & Kohlschütter A. (2002) Late infantile neuronal ceroid lipofuscinosis: quantitative description of the clinical course in patients with CLN2 mutations. *American Journal of Medical Genetics*, Vol 112, No. 4 (Nov), pp. 347-54, ISSN 1552-4841.

Stenson PD., Ball EV., Mort M., Phillips AD., Shiel JA., Thomas NS., Abeysinghe S., Krawczak M., & Cooper DN. (2003) Human Gene Mutation Database (HGMD): 2003 update. *Human Mutation, Vol.* 21 No. 6, pp. 577-81, ISSN 1059-7794.

Stogmann E., El Tawil S., Wagenstaller J., Gaber A., Edris S., Abdelhady A., Assem-Hilger E., Leutmezer F., Bonelli S., Baumgartner C., Zimprich F., Strom TM & Zimprich A. (2009) A novel mutation in the MFSD8 gene in late infantile neuronal ceroid lipofuscinosis. *Neurogenetics*, Vol. 10, No. 1 (Feb), pp. 73-7, ISSN 0167-7063.

Storch S., Pohl S., Quitsch A., Falley K. & Braulke T. (2007) C-terminal prenylation of the CLN3 membrane glycoprotein is required for efficient endosomal sorting to lysosomes. *Traffic,* Vol. 8, No. 4 (Apr), pp. 431-44, ISSN 1398-9219.

Sun X., Marks DL., Park WD., Wheatley CL., Puri V., O'Brien JF., Kraft DL., Lundquist PA., Patterson MC., Pagano RE. & Snow K. (2001) Niemann-Pick C variant detection by altered sphingolipid trafficking and correlation with mutations within a specific domain of NPC1. *The American Journal of Human Genetics,* Vol. 68, No. 6 (Jun), pp. 1361-72, ISSN 0002-9297.

Topçu M., Tan H., Yalnizoğlu D., Usubütün A., Saatçi I., Aynaci M., Anlar B., Topaloğlu H., Turanli G., Köse G. & Aysun S. (2004) Evaluation of 36 patients from Turkey with neuronal ceroid lipofuscinosis: clinical, neurophysiological, neuroradiological and histopathologic studies. *Turkish Journal of Pediatrics,* Vol. 46, No. 1 (Jan-Mar), pp. 1-10, ISSN 0041-4301.

Triggs-Raine BL., Mules EH., Kaback MM., Lim-Steele JS., Dowling CE., Akerman BR., Natowicz MR., Grebner EE., Navon R., Welch JP., et al. (1992) A pseudodeficiency allele common in non-Jewish Tay-Sachs carriers: implications for carrier screening. *The American Journal of Human Genetics,* Vol. 51, No. 4 (Oct), pp. 793-801, ISSN 0002-9297.

Tutor JC. (2004) Biochemical characterization of the GM2 gangliosidosis B1 variant. *Brazilian Journal of Medical and Biological Research,* Vol. 37, No. 6 (Jun), pp. 777-83.

Tylki-Szymańska A., Vellodi A., El-Beshlawy A., Cole JA., & Kolodny E. (2010) Neuronopathic Gaucher disease: demographic and clinical features of 131 patients enrolled in the International Collaborative Gaucher Group Neurological Outcomes Subregistry. *Journal of Inherited Metabolic Diseases,* Vol. 33, No. 4 (Aug), pp. 339-46, ISSN 0141-8955.

Tyynelä J., Palmer DN., Baumann M. & Haltia M. (1993) Storage of saposins A and D in infantile neuronal ceroid-lipofuscinosis. *FEBS Letters,* Vol. 330, No. 1 (Sep), pp. 8-12, ISSN 0014-5793.

Tyynelä J., Suopanki J., Santavuori P., Baumann M. & Haltia M. (1997) Variant late infantile neuronal ceroid-lipofuscinosis: pathology and biochemistry. *Journal of Neuropathology & Experimental Neurology,* Vol. 56, No. 4 (Apr), pp. 369-75, ISSN 0022-3069.

Van der Spoel A., Bonten E., & d'Azzo A. (1998) Transport of human lysosomal neuraminidase to mature lysosomes requires protective protein/cathepsin A. *EMBO Journal,* Vol. 17, No. 6 (Mar), pp. 1588-97, ISSN 0261-4189.

van der Spoel A., Bonten E., & d'Azzo A. (2000) Processing of lysosomal beta-galactosidase. The C-terminal precursor fragment is an essential domain of the mature enzyme. *Journal of Biological Chemistry* , Vol. 275, No. 14 (Apr), pp. 10035-40, ISSN 0021-9258.

van Diggelen OP., Thobois S., Tilikete C., Zabot MT., Keulemans JL., van Bunderen PA., Taschner PE., Losekoot M. & Voznyi YV. (2001) Adult neuronal ceroid lipofuscinosis with palmitoyl-protein thioesterase deficiency: first adult-onset patients of a childhood disease. *Annals of Neurology,* Vol. 15, No.2 (Aug), pp. 269-72, ISSN 0364-5134.

Vanhanen SL., Puranen J., Autti T., Raininko R., Liewendahl K., Nikkinen P., Santavuori P., Suominen P., Vuori K. & Häkkinen AM. (2004) Neuroradiological findings (MRS, MRI, SPECT) in infantile neuronal ceroid-lipofuscinosis (infantile CLN1) at different stages of the disease. *Neuropediatrics,* Vol. 35, No. 1 (Feb), pp. 27-35, ISSN 0174-304X.

Vanier MT& Millat G. (2003) Niemann-Pick disease type C. *Clinical Genetics,* Vol. 64, No. 4

Vanier MT. & Millat G. (2004) Structure and function of the NPC2 protein. *Biochimica et Biophysica Acta,* Vol. 1685, No. 1-3 (Oct), pp. 14-21, ISSN 0304-4165.

Vanier MT. & Suzuki K.(1998) Recent advances in elucidating Niemann-Pick C disease. *Brain Pathology,* Vol 8, No. 1 (Jan), pp. 63-74, ISSN 1015-6305.

Vanier MT. (2010) Niemann-Pick disease type C. *Orphanet Journal of Rare Diseases,* Vol. 5, 16 (Jun), ISSN 1750-1172.

Vanier MT., & Suzuki K. (1998) Recent advances in elucidating Niemann-Pick C disease. *Brain Pathology*, Vol. 8, No. 1 (Jan), pp. 163-74, ISSN 1015-6305.

Vanier MT., Duthel S., Rodriguez-Lafrasse C., Pentchev P., & Carstea ED. (1996) Genetic heterogeneity in Niemann-Pick C disease: a study using somatic cell hybridization and linkage analysis. *The American Journal of Human Genetics,* Vol. 58, No. 1 (Jan), pp. 118-25, ISSN 0002-9297.

Vantaggiato C., Redaelli F., Falcone S., Perrotta C., Tonelli A., Bondioni S., Morbin M., Riva D., Saletti V., Bonaglia MC., Giorda R., Bresolin N., Clementi E. & Bassi MT. (2009) A novel CLN8 mutation in late-infantile-onset neuronal ceroid lipofuscinosis (LINCL) reveals aspects of CLN8 neurobiological function. *Human Mutation*, Vol. 30, No. 7 (Jul), pp. 1104-16, ISSN 1059-7794.

Verkruyse LA. & Hofmann SL. (1996) Lysosomal targeting of palmitoyl-protein thioesterase. *Journal of Biological Chemistry*, Vol. 271, No. 26 (Jun), pp. 15831-6, ISSN 0021-9258.

Vesa J., Chin MH., Oelgeschläger K., Isosomppi J., DellAngelica EC., Jalanko A.& Peltonen L. (2002) Neuronal ceroid lipofuscinoses are connected at molecular level: interaction of CLN5 protein with CLN2 and CLN3. *Molecular Biology of the Cell*, Vol. 13, No.7 (Jul), pp. 2410-20, ISSN 1059-1524.

Vesa J., Hellsten E., Verkruyse LA., Camp LA., Rapola J., Santavuori P., Hofmann SL. & Peltonen L. (1995) Mutations in the palmitoyl protein thioesterase gene causing infantile neuronal ceroid lipofuscinosis. *Nature*, Vol. 376, No. 6541 (Aug), pp. 584-7, ISSN 0028-0836.

Wang D., Bonten EJ., Yogalingam G., Mann L. & d'Azzo A. (2005) Short-term, high dose enzyme replacement therapy in sialidosis mice. *Molecular Genetics and Metabolism*, Vol. 85, No. 3 (Jul), pp. 181-9, ISSN 1096-7192.

Wang SZ., Cachón-González MB., Stein PE., Lachmann RH., Corry PC., Wraith JE. & Cox TM. (2008) A novel HEXB mutation and its structural effects in juvenile Sandhoff disease. *Molecular Genetics and Metabolism*, Vol. 95, No. 4 (Dec), pp. 236-8, ISSN 1096-7192.

Watari H., Blanchette-Mackie EJ., Dwyer NK., Watari M., Neufeld EB., Patel S., Pentchev PG. & Strauss JF 3rd. (1999) Mutations in the leucine zipper motif and sterol-sensing domain inactivate the Niemann-Pick C1 glycoprotein. *Journal of Biological Chemistry*, Vol. 274, No 31 (Jul), pp. 21861-6, ISSN 0021-9258.

Weleber RG., Gupta N., Trzupek KM., Wepner MS., Kurz DE. & Milam AH. (2004) Electroretinographic and clinicopathologic correlations of retinal dysfunction in infantile neuronal ceroid lipofuscinosis (infantile Batten disease). *Molecular Genetics and Metabolism*, Vol. 83, No. 1-2 (Sep-Oct), pp. 128-37, ISSN 1096-7192.

Wheeler RB., Sharp JD., Schultz RA., Joslin JM., Williams RE. & Mole SE. (2002) The gene mutated in variant late-infantile neuronal ceroid lipofuscinosis (CLN6) and in nclf mutant mice encodes a novel predicted transmembrane protein. *The American Journal of Human Genetics*, Vol. 70, No. 2 (Feb), pp. 537-42, ISSN 0002-9297.

Williams RE., Aberg L., Autti T., Goebel HH., Kohlschütter A. & Lönnqvist T. (2006) Diagnosis of the neuronal ceroid lipofuscinoses: an update. *Biochimica et Biophysica Acta*, Vol. 1762, No. 10 (Oct), pp. 865-72, ISSN 0304-4165.

Winter E. & Ponting CP. (2002). TRAM, LAG1 and CLN8: members of a novel family of lipid-sensing domains? *Trends Biochemical Science*, Vol. 27, No. 8, (Aug), pp. 381-3, ISSN 0968-0004.

Winter RM., Swallow DM., Baraitser M. & Purkiss P. (1980) Sialidosis type 2 (acid neuraminidase deficiency): clinical and biochemical features of a further case. *Clinical Genetics,* Vol. 18, No. 3 (Sep), pp. :203-10, ISSN 0009-9163.

Wisniewski KE., Kida E., Golabek AA., Kaczmarski W., Connell F. & Zhong N. (2001) Neuronal ceroid lipofuscinoses: classification and diagnosis. *Advances in Genetics,* Vol. 45, pp. 1-34, ISSN 0065-2660.

Wraith JE., Baumgartner MR., Bembi B., Covanis A., Levade T., Mengel E., Pineda M., Sedel F., Topçu M., Vanier MT., Widner H., Wijburg FA. & Patterson MC. (2009) Recommendations on the diagnosis and management of Niemann-Pick disease type C. *Molecular Genetics and Metabolism,* Vol. 98, No. 1 (Sep-Oct), pp. 152-65, ISSN 1096-7192.

Yamamoto Y., & Nishimura K. (1987) Copurification and separation of beta-galactosidase and sialidase from porcine testis. *International Journal of Biochemistry,* Vol. 19, No. 5, pp. 435-42, ISSN 0020-711X.

Yerushalmi B., Sokol RJ., Narkewicz MR., Smith D., Ashmead JW. & Wenger DA. (2002) Niemann-pick disease type C in neonatal cholestasis at a North American Center. *Journal of Pediatric Gastroenterology and Nutrition,* Vol. 35, No. 1 (Jul), pp. 44-50, ISSN 1536-4801.

Yüksel A., Yalçinkaya C., Işlak C., Gündüz E. & Seven M. (1999) Neuroimaging findings of four patients with Sandhoff disease. *Pediatric Neurology,* Vol. 21, No. 2 (Aug), pp. 562-5, ISSN 0887-8994.

Zelnik N., Mahajna M., Iancu TC., Sharony R. & Zeigler M. (2007) A novel mutation of the CLN8 gene: is there a Mediterranean phenotype? *Pediatric Neurology,* Vol. 36, No. 3 (Jun), pp. 411-3, ISSN 0887-8994.

Zervas M., Dobrenis K., & Walkley SU. (2001) Neurons in Niemann-Pick disease type C accumulate gangliosides as well as unesterified cholesterol and undergo dendritic and axonal alterations. *Journal of Neuropathology & Experimental Neurology,* Vol. 60, No. 1 (Jan), pp 49-64, ISSN 0022-3069.

Zhong N., Moroziewicz DN., Ju W., Jurkiewicz A., Johnston L., Wisniewski KE. & Brown WT. (2000) Heterogeneity of late-infantile neuronal ceroid lipofuscinosis. *Genetics in Medicine,* Vol. 2, No. 6 (Nov-Dec), pp. 312-8, ISSN 1098-3600.

Zimran A., Gelbart T., Garver P., Thurston D., Saven A., & Beutler E. (1992) Gaucher disease. Clinical, laboratory, radiologic, and genetic features of 53 patients. *Medicine (Baltimore),* Vol. 71, No. 6 (Nov.), pp. 337-53, ISSN 0025-7974.

14

Social Cognition in Epilepsy

Jane McCagh
Liverpool Hope University
England

1. Introduction

There is a paucity of research which has investigated social cognition in epilepsy, this is surprising given the abundance of evidence that exists in relation to the difficulties that people with epilepsy (PWE) have in relation to social functioning (McCagh et al., 2009).

The study of social cognition in epilepsy will lead to a greater understanding of the social cognitive deficits of the epileptic condition. This may in turn lead to more effective psychological interventions to enable the smoother functioning of people with epilepsy in society.

The aim of this chapter is to provide a detailed critical review of research which has investigated socio-cognitive functioning in people with epilepsy to date. Throughout the chapter, the impact of epilepsy related variables in relation to socio-cognitive processing will be considered.

The final part of the chapter will explore why people with epilepsy may have social cognitive deficits and will go on to summarise limitations in past research. The author will conclude by providing the rationale and aims of their current research in this area and suggestions for future work.

Abbreviations

AED	Antiepileptic drug
BF	Bifrontal
EEG	Electroencephalogram
EI	Emotional intelligence
FHI	Frontal Head Injury
FL	Frontal lobe
FLE	Frontal lobe epilepsy
FSIQ	Full Scale Intelligence Quotient
HADS	Hospital Anxiety and Depression Scale
HC	Healthy Controls
IGE	Idiopathic generalised epilepsy
IQ	Intelligence Quotient
LT	Left temporal lobe
LTLE	Left temporal lobe epilepsy
LF	Left frontal lobe
LFT	Left fronto-temporal
LH	Left hemisphere
MME	Mini Mental State Examination

MTLE	Medial temporal lobe epilepsy
MRI	Magnetic resonance imaging
NC	Normal control group
QoL	Quality of Life
OFC	Orbito-frontal cortex
QoL	Quality of life
PFC	Prefrontal cortex
PWE	People with epilepsy
RF	Right frontal lobe
RFT	Right fronto-temporal
RH	Right hemisphere
RT	Right temporal lobe
RTLE	Right temporal lobe epilepsy
TASITS	The Awareness of Social Inference Task
ToM	Theory of mind
TL	Temporal lobe
TLE	Temporal lobe epilepsy
WAIS	Wechsler Adult Intelligence Scale
WTAR	Wechsler Test of Adult Reading
VM PFC	Ventromedial prefrontal cortex

2. Social cognition

Essentially social cognition is concerned with how people process social information and how they use this information in social situations. Social cognitive processing involves the perception and interpretation of social information and the ability to provide an appropriate response to it.

2.1 Theory of mind (ToM)

The ability to comprehend social information and to participate effectively in social interactions is reliant on 'the adequate functioning of a mental mechanism termed theory of mind (ToM)' (Mazza et al., 2007, p.257). This term was first established by Premack and Woodruff (1978). It is the socio-cognitive ability which normal functioning individuals have to effectively infer the thoughts, beliefs and intentions of other people. It allows them to appreciate that people's thoughts behaviour may be based upon beliefs and knowledge that are different from their own. This skill facilitates successful social communication and the cohesive functioning of individuals in society. ToM skills enable people to interpret their own mental states as well as the mental states of others, consequently one can understand and make predictions about behaviour. ToM is used to understand what another person intends or means in social situations where these may not be immediately clear. For example, when someone makes an ironic statement, drops a hint or tells a joke.

ToM is seen to consist of both 'cold cognition' the ability to make inferences about others' cognitive states such as knowledge, desires and beliefs and 'hot cognition' the ability to make inferences about the affective states (emotions and preferences) of other people (Brothers & Ring, 1992; Stone, 2000).

2.2 Assessment of theory of mind

Researchers have used a variety of assessment techniques to tap into ToM functioning. The most common measures and those which are most relevant to the studies which will be discussed in this chapter will be outlined.

The most established and validated measure of ToM has utilised the concept of false belief. Dennett (1978) argued that the best evidence for an understanding of other people's minds is the ability to attribute a "false belief" to another person. Detection of false belief requires that you can appreciate that another person has misconceived an event as a result of incorrect reasoning. Many subsequent empirical tests of ToM are based on this criterion and assessment of false belief is regarded as the 'litmus test' of ToM functioning. This method is widely used and validated because it establishes whether an individual can attribute beliefs to others that may differ from their own. As Astington (2001) highlights, false belief is 'an unequivocal marker of mentalistic understanding' (p.685).

Typically false belief has been assessed at first order and second order levels of intentionality. Appreciation of first order false belief usually develops by the age of four and by the age of seven, children should be able to pass second order false belief tasks (Perner & Wimmer, 1985; Wellman et al., 2001; Wimmer & Perner, 1983). Often such tests are developed within the context of ToM stories, which are often accompanied by story boards to aid the participant in following the story. First order stories involve a character having a false belief about the state of the world. The tasks require the individual to understand that another person may not have access to information about the world which they themselves have and as a consequence that the other person's viewpoint is mistaken. Typically first order stories involve a protagonist leaving an object in one location and then leaving a room upon which the object is moved to a new location. Demonstration of intact first order false belief would involve the participant appreciating that the protagonist will look for the object in the old location on re entering the room. To master first order false belief the participant must appreciate that reality and another person's perception of reality can be different.

Second order stories are more complex and involve one character having a false belief about the belief of another character in a story. The age of developing false belief skills has been shown to be the same across cultures and continents (Avis & Harris, 1991; Wellman et al., 2001; Wellman & Lagattuta, 2000). Generally adults score at ceiling on both first and second order false belief tasks (Stone et al., 1998a) so designing tests which tap in to ToM in adults can be challenging.

Deception has also been used as another way of testing mentalising ability. As Baron-Cohen (2000) proposes, deception is important in understanding another's mind as it involves trying to make a person believe something that is untrue. It involves being aware that beliefs can be manipulated and people will base these beliefs on knowledge derived from what they have heard or observed.

More advanced tests of ToM involve being able to appreciate non-literal language or figurative speech. An appreciation of the pragmatics of language is needed to understand such things as sarcasm, irony, humour, metaphor and hinting and consequently paradigms using these concepts have been applied to assess ToM performance. By reference to contextual information, the listener must go beyond the literal meaning of the words that are used and comprehend the intentions of the speaker and the meaning they are trying to convey.

A number of paradigms have been used in studies to assess these higher order ToM abilities. These include: appreciation of irony (Shamay-Tsoory et al., 2003; Shamay-Tsoory et al., 2005a), sarcasm (Shamay-Tsoory et al., 2002; Shamay-Tsoory et al.,2005 a; Shamay-

Tsoory et al., 2005 b), hinting (Corcoran et al., 1995; Corcoran & Frith, 2003), faux pas (Farrant et al.,2005; Schacher, et al., 2006; Shaw et al.,2007; Stone et al., 1998a; Shamay-Tsoory et al., 2005 a) humour (Winner et al.,) and metaphor (Van Lancker & Kemper, 1987) to name a few.

Another unconventional ToM task that has proved popular was developed by Baron-Cohen et al. (1997). The Reading the Mind in the Eyes task (RME) involves the participant identifying complex mental states (emotions) by looking at photographs of the eye region only. Participants are provided with four words depicting emotions and are required to select the word corresponding to the emotion expressed by the eyes.

2.3 Testing considerations

In order to make sure that measures reflect ToM functioning and not other cognitive skills, a number of control measures need to be considered when assessing ToM. Most studies incorporate a measure of general cognitive ability (such as an IQ test) to make sure that apparent deficits in ToM are not a simple consequence of general cognitive dysfunction. To minimise the load on working memory, tasks utilize devices such as pictorial story boards (in ToM stories) or participants are allowed to refer to the relevant text/stimuli throughout testing. As well as questions which assess ToM ability, tasks usually incorporate 'reality' or comprehension questions to ensure that the relevant prose has been understood and to guard against the possibility that poor performance on the task simply reflects memory or comprehension difficulties. In order to achieve this, tasks will typically include some questions requiring general inferential ability (such as making inferences about physical states). These complement the key questions which assess the participant's ability to make inferences about the mental states of others. All these precautions are designed to ensure that the impairments that are observed reflect ToM difficulties as distinct from problems in other cognitive domains.

3. Epilepsy and social cognition

Some of the psychological problems associated with epilepsy have their origins in the ability of people with epilepsy (PWE) to engage in meaningful and appropriate social interactions. PWE often report difficulties in social functioning (McCagh et al., 2009), yet research investigating the socio-cognitive skills of this group has been sparse. Impairments in social competence in children, adolescents and adults with epilepsy are also evident (Austin et al.,1994; Caplan et al. 2005; Herman et al., 1981; Jalava et al., 1997). Schilbach et al. (2007) argue that social competence has a considerable effect on quality of life yet the study of social cognition in epilepsy has been largely neglected. A number of studies have shown that quality of life (QoL) scores increase after surgery but often these measures do not adequately assess improvements in social functioning (Kirsch, 2006).

Epilepsy may affect social cognition in many ways that are hard to quantify. Kirsch (2006) suggests that frequent seizures may interfere with the development of interpersonal skills in children or adolescents, such that they may not always be able to participate in situations where they can develop such skills due to ictal and post ictal disruption to functioning. Medication may impact on their ability to respond effectively in interpersonal conversation to subtle social cues. The child's social networks may be reduced due to stigmatisation, lack of self esteem or because parents are more protective over the child and consequently this reduces their exposure to social environments where they may learn the intricate social skills that are necessary to achieve social competence. Children with epilepsy have been shown to under perform on measures of social competence in comparison to children without epilepsy as indicated by their parents in a number of studies (Dorenbaum et al., 1985; McCusker et al., 2002; Williams et al., 1996).

Exactly why PWE have social difficulties is not entirely clear but is likely to be a consequence of a number of complex interrelated psychosocial factors that impact on the person with epilepsy. These include the impact of stigma, unemployment or underemployment, anxiety and depression, cognitive dysfunction, poor self esteem, social isolation and difficulties in interpersonal relationships (McCagh et al., 2009).

'Despite many years of speculation, it remains unclear to what extent psychosocial difficulties are related to the fact that patients are living with a chronic and stigmatising condition and to what extent they are related to neuropathology' (Walpole et al., 2008, p.1470).

Whether social maladjustments in PWE can be attributed to social cognitive deficits remains uncertain (Schacher et al., 2006).

3.1 Research studies

To date there have been seven studies, some of which have also looked at recognition of emotion as well as ToM in PWE, though it is not the purpose of the chapter to review research which has assessed emotion recognition in epilepsy per se. One study has investigated emotional intelligence in people with active epilepsy (who have not undergone surgery) and because of its relevance to the area it will be included in the review. The latter part of the chapter will provide a critical review of the methodology used in research to date. Throughout the chapter, the impact of epilepsy related variables in relation to socio-cognitive processing will be highlighted.

3.1.1 Temporal lobe epilepsy

3.1.1.1 Emotional intelligence and emotion recognition

Walpole et al. (2008) investigated emotional intelligence (EI) and emotion recognition in temporal lobe epilepsy (TLE). Sixteen patients with TLE were compared with 14 healthy controls (HC). People with TLE were only included in the study if they did not have any history of psychiatric illness (excluding anxiety and depression), head injury, hypoxia, personality disorder, neurological condition or autistic spectrum disorder. People with TLE who had undergone surgery for epilepsy were excluded from the study.

Participants were assessed on a range of background measures including the Wechsler Test of Adult Reading (WTAR; Wechsler, 2001), cognitive intelligence as assessed by the Full Scale IQ (FSIQ) score on the Wechsler Abbreviated Scale of Intelligence (WASI; Wechsler, 1999) the Hospital Anxiety and Depression Scale (HADS; Zigmond & Snaith, 1983) and Quality of Life in Epilepsy 31 (QOLIFE-31; Cramer et al., 1998). Participants were also assessed on emotional intelligence (EI) using the Emotional Quotient Inventory (EQ-I; Bar On, 1997) and identification of emotional expression using Ekman and Friesen (1976) 60 photographs of facial expressions.

This study found that the TLE group were significantly impaired on total EI score but not cognitive intelligence (FSIQ). The TLE group made significantly more errors when identifying emotional expression than the control group. Significant negative correlations were found between EI (total score) and anxiety and depression as measured by the HADS. Higher QoL scores were associated with higher EI in the TLE group, though this relationship was not significant. No significant differences in EI were established between people with LTLE (N=7) and RTLE (N=9) and EI was not significantly associated with duration of illness or number of seizures. The author concludes that the psychosocial problems in TLE may well be associated with low EI which may be a consequence of epilepsy-related disruption to the functions of the medial temporal lobe.

Walpole et al. (2008) conducted their study under the premise that impairments in a study on EI were present in people with lesions to the ventro medial prefrontal cortex (VM PFC) and to the amygdala or insular cortices, brain areas that have also been implicated in social cognition (Bar On et al., 2003). Walpole et al. (2008) argue that EI is closely related to social cognition in that it involves being able to discriminate between and monitor 'one's own feelings and those of others 'and being able to use 'this information to guide responding' (p. 1470).

Evaluation: This study would have benefited by recruiting a frontal lobe epilepsy (FLE) group to establish if EI was impaired in this sample in line with evidence in the literature which implicates the importance of the frontal lobes in social cognition (Rowe et al., 2001; Shamay-Tsoory et al., 2005a; Stone et al., 1998; Stuss et al., 2001). Walpole et al. (2008) do acknowledge the need to study EI in other types of epilepsy to determine if EI impairment is specific to TLE. This study can be criticised for not stating whether people had refractory TLE, where participants were recruited from, what AEDs they were on and how many they were taking.

Differences in RTLE and LTLE were not established in this study, though this may or may not have been impeded by the small sample size of each of the groups. It should be noted that a recent study by Gawryluk and McGlone (2007) which investigated PWE who had TL resections did not find any evidence of laterality of EI, although it needs to be emphasised that these participants did not have active epilepsy.

Quality of life (QoL) was assessed in the study and was not significantly related to EI although Walpole et al. (2008) acknowledge that the role of seizure related variables and the impact of epilepsy need to be studied in more depth in relation to EI. If a larger sample was recruited, relationships between these variables may have been more evident.

3.1.1.2 Theory of mind and emotion recognition

Shaw et al. (2007) assessed 19 PWE on ToM tasks and emotion recognition before and after anterior temporal lobectomy (excision of the amygdala occurred in all cases as did removal of anterior parts of the hippocampus) for refractory epilepsy. Those with TLE (10 RTLE and 9 LTLE) had amygdala damage as a consequence of gliosis, neuronal loss or focal lesions. Seizures had stopped or there was a marked reduction in seizures post surgery. Testing took place 1-3 months prior to surgery and 4-6 months post-surgery. Patients who underwent surgery were on the same AEDs post surgery. Nineteen healthy controls with no history of neurological or psychiatric disorders were also assessed on the same measures twice, six months apart.

Participants were assessed on a range of background measures including IQ and the Benton Facial Recognition task (Benton et al., 1983). This task entailed matching images of faces of identical people. These images were taken at different angles or levels of illumination. The Hayling and Brixton tests assessed executive functioning (Burgess & Shallice, 1996a, 1996b). The Hayling test assesses the ability to inhibit predominant responses and speed of task initiation and the Brixton test assesses set shifting and rule detection.

The two main experimental measures were recognition of facial expressions and emotions and appreciation of ToM. The Ekman and Friesen (1976) pictures of facial emotion were used and participants had to rate the intensity of one of six basic emotions (sad, happy, surprise, anger, fear, disgust) in two male and female faces who displayed all six emotions. A faux pas test by Stone et al. (1998a) and Happé's Strange Stories (Happé, 1994) assessed ToM. Happé's Strange Stories depict characters that do not literally mean what they say, participants are required to illustrate that they understand what the character really means and their true motivations. The faux pas test required participants to identify that a faux pas had taken place, why the comment was inappropriate and the affect that the faux pas may have had on the character in the story (how it would have made them feel). A control question was incorporated to assess comprehension.

Verbal and performance IQ was significantly lower in the RTLE (N = 10) and LTLE (N = 9) operative groups in relation to controls. Duration of epilepsy did not differ between these groups. Scores on the Benton Facial Recognition Test and measures of executive functioning did not differ between groups or significantly change as a consequence of surgery in either group.

Shaw et al. (2007) found that there were no significant differences in scores pre or post surgery in Happé's Strange Stories or for detection of faux pas or in either RTLE or LTLE, nor was there a significant change in scores from pre to post surgery in relation to these two groups. When RTLE and LTLE groups were combined there was no significant difference in change scores on either of the ToM measures. Change scores in executive function and ToM tasks were not correlated with each other so changes in executive function were unrelated to changes in ToM performance. Prior to surgery patients with LTLE were impaired in recognising facial expressions depicting fear but improved after surgery which the authors suggest may be accounted for by removing a hyper-excitable amygdala. Another explanation they consider is that epileptogenic tissue in the LTLE may inhibit the emotion recognition network prior to surgery which would account for improvements post surgery, such improvements have occurred in executive processes after anterior temporal lobectomy (Hermann & Sedenberg, 1995; Martin et al., 2000).

Evaluation: Whilst differences in ToM performance pre and post surgery were not evident, the small sample size in the study will have reduced statistical power to detect changes in ToM performance. The ToM tests used in this study may not be sensitive enough to detect a change in performance pre and post operatively or differences between right and left TLE in such a small sample. These tests have also not demonstrated functional activation in the amygdala in past research. Past research has shown that bilateral damage is typically found with ToM impairment in adults (Stone et al., 2003), yet participants only had unilateral damage in this study. Memory and learning effects of the tasks may have improved performance after surgery, as the same tests were administered pre and post surgery. Such effects are not controlled for and are hard to quantify, this could be overcome if different tasks were matched in terms of the amount of socio-cognitive processing involved.

Schilbach et al. (2007) also investigated ToM and emotion recognition in TLE. Their study recruited 10 right handed females with LTLE from an epilepsy monitoring unit and an outpatient clinic. Two participants had MTS (mesial temporal sclerosis); there were no detectable structural abnormalities in the other eight. All had a history of complex partial seizures. Ten right handed healthy volunteers with no neurological or psychiatric history were also recruited. All participants included in the study had an MMSE (Mini Mental State

Examination) score within the normal range and were assessed for depression by the Beck Depression Inventory (BDI). Two of the epilepsy participants had scores of 16 or above so all further analysis took account of this.

Participants were presented with video scenarios involving virtual reality characters depicting facial expressions. The expressions were either socially relevant and the character was intending to initiate interpersonal relations with either the participant or another virtual character. Alternatively the facial expressions were arbitrary and socially irrelevant. Self involvement in the scenarios was also manipulated such that the characters either looked at the participant or looked away. Participants were required to answer two questions after presentation of each video scenario (there were 100 trials), which evaluated their perception of self involvement and required them to rate how much social interaction was present in each scenario using a four point Likert scale.

The TLE sample group all illustrated the same trend in how they rated social intent despite the different type and number of AEDs that were being taken across the sample. They rated a scenario as more socially relevant if they were more involved in the interaction, this trend was also apparent even if the facial expression was arbitrary. The authors suggest that over reacting to self involvement in social interactions may be a way that people with TLE compensate for their socio cognitive difficulties in interpreting facial expressions and the mental states (intention) of others.

Evaluation: The study can be criticised as the sample was biased towards females, the sample was small and that only people with LTLE were tested. Another weakness is that the study did not evaluate the impact of epilepsy related variables (age at onset, seizure type or seizure frequency) on social cognition.

Schacher et al. (2006) investigated ToM in TLE. They assessed the ability to detect faux paux in 27 people with MTLE (medial temporal lobe epilepsy) of which 16 were investigated prior to surgical resection, and 11 after anterior temporal lobectomy or selective amygdalohippocamectomy (12-18 months after surgery). They also recruited 27 people who had extra mesiotemporal epilepsy (extra MTLE) but not FLE (frontal lobe epilepsy) and 12 healthy controls (HC) with no history of psychiatric or neurological disorder. PWE were recruited from an in patient epilepsy centre in Switzerland and had refractory epilepsy. MTLE and unilateral seizure onset was determined by EEG and MRI. Testing on PWE and healthy controls took place in hospital, all PWE including post surgical MTLE were being treated with AEDs.

Participants were administered with a shortened version of the faux pas test by Stone et al. (2003). Participants read the story themselves whilst having a copy of the story in front of them to reduce the working memory demands of the task. Participants were asked four questions, three questions assessed inferences about affective and cognitive mental states and one question was a control question to assess that the story had been comprehended correctly. All participants in the study had intact language comprehension as assessed by the Chapman-Cook test (Chapman, 1923) and correct answers on the faux pas comprehension question and IQ were also measured. Participants were required to understand the faux pas correctly and infer the mental state and emotions of another person.

The MTLE (pre and post op) were significantly impaired on faux pas in relation to the extra MTLE group or healthy controls, task performance between these two groups was comparable. No differences between the pre op MTLE and post op MTLE were established. In the MTLE group as a whole (R= 14 and L=13) people with right sided onset performed significantly worse than those with a left sided onset. There was an interaction between gender and side of onset such that male patients with LMTLE performed better than females with LMTLE and males with RMTLE. Beyond the above noted epilepsy-related differences, faux pas performance was not associated with IQ, age, age at seizure onset or duration of epilepsy. IQ may have mediated faux pas performance in healthy controls as they showed a trend for higher faux pas scores when IQ was a covariate in the analysis, this mediating effect was not apparent when comparing performance in the MTLE and extra MTLE group on faux pas. Schacher et al. (2006) argue that this refutes the idea that a general cognitive deficit impairs ToM performance and supports Frith and Frith (2003) proposal that ToM skills are independent from other cognitive domains. Impairments in faux pas can not be attributed to language or comprehension as these factors were controlled in the study. The authors suggest that the effect of AEDs is unlikely to account for the observed deficits as the extra MTLE who performed in a similar manner to healthy controls had refractory epilepsy and were receiving AED therapy.

The authors conclude that MTLE plays a role in higher-order aspects of social cognition. They emphasise the role of the amygdala in emotional and socio-cognitive functioning and highlight that this is often impaired in MTLE. MTLE may impact on socio-cognitive skills by disrupting the integration of temporolimbic and frontal systems which have been implicated in social cognitive functioning.

Evaluation: This study would have benefited by recruiting a FLE group to establish if appreciation of faux pas was impaired in this sample in line with evidence in the literature which implicates the importance of the frontal lobes in social cognition (Rowe et al., 2001; Shamay-Tsoory et al., 2005a; Stone et al., 1998; Stuss et al., 2001). This would also help establish if people with MTLE has a specific deficit in appreciating faux pas.

4. The right hemisphere

4.1 ToM and emotion recognition in the right hemisphere

Fournier et al. (2008) investigated social cognition in two patients, one who underwent a right hemispherectomy (S.M.) and one who underwent a left hemispherectomy (J.H.) to treat intractable epilepsy. Both participants underwent surgery in adolescence and were assessed 30 years after surgery on emotion recognition, formation of social inferences and advanced socio- cognitive judgements. Their performance was compared to normative data collected on the measures.

J.H. (LH) no longer experienced seizures after surgery and was no longer on AED therapy, post surgical recovery was excellent. S.M. (RH) still experienced complex partial seizures after surgery, though these were considerably reduced, and he was still taking AEDs. Both participants experienced hemianopsia and hemiplegia on the contralateral side to surgery.

The two participants were assessed on a variety of background measures to examine IQ, executive functioning, language, construction skills and visual perception. FSIQ scores were comparable and differences in performance on typically RH tasks (attention and visuospatial processing) and LH tasks (verbal working memory, speeded verbal processing) were as expected. The MMSE Examination was also administered and performance was in the normal range for both participants.

The Awareness of Social Inference Task (TASITS) which assesses ToM judgements, emotion recognition and how people make social inferences in daily life was used to assess social cognition (McDonald et al., 2003). This test uses video recordings in which actors engage in scenes of everyday life. The first part of the test (Emotion Evaluation test) requires participants to recognise common emotional expressions in 28 short video vignettes. Happy, sad, disgust, anger, fear, surprise or neutral expressions are demonstrated on four separate occasions that are randomly administered. Participants have to choose one of the seven emotions and match them to each of the vignettes.

The second and third part of the TASITS involves identifying whether conversations between individuals are sincere; such that conversations can be understood in terms of their literal meaning or that they are counterfactual, where there are discrepancies in the literal content of the conversation and its context. The counterfactual vignettes involve the participant having to infer the underlying meaning of the conversational exchange. In the second part of the test (Social Inference - Minimal) the participant must detect sincere or sarcastic exchanges in 15 vignettes. To detect sarcasm involves appreciating prosody, body language and facial expressions and participants are asked four questions after each vignette. These questions assess participant's ability to detect what the protagonist was thinking, doing, saying and feeling. Two of the questions probe what the protagonist was intending and feeling, these assess both first and second order levels of ToM.

In the third part of the test (Social - Inference Minimal) 16 short vignettes are administered with similar content to part two of the test, the only difference is that participants are provided with extra information regarding the conversational exchange before and after the video. Participants are expected to comprehend the true nature of the exchange whilst integrating the additional information provided to them so that they can determine the protagonist's intention. The probe questions asked after the video assess appreciation of deception (lies) and sarcasm. Both participants were also administered the Reading the Mind in the Eyes test (Baron-Cohen et al. 2001).

The participant who underwent RH (S.M.) surgery was impaired in recognising negative emotional expressions and surprise, in appreciation of sarcasm, lies, detecting others intentions and their emotions. The participant who underwent (J.H.) LH surgery was competent in interpersonal situations and was mildly impaired when recognising emotional disgust or anger but performed well on parts two and three of the TASITS.

Fournier et al. (2008) argue that their findings emphasise the importance of the RH in reasoning and social cognition:

'taken together, the results suggest a strong role of the right hemisphere in social cognition and processing of information related to the understanding of basic emotional expressions, attributions of the beliefs and intensions of others, as well as the meaning of specific types of conversational inferences' (p. 468).

Evaluation: This study was unique in that it is the first of its kind to establish the long term effects of right and left hemispherectomy on social cognition with reference to ToM. An additional strength of the study is that it utilised an ecologically valid measure of ToM and emotion recognition by using the TASITS. The main criticism is that ToM was not evaluated prior to surgery so the observed impairments cannot be conclusively related to the surgery itself. S.M. who underwent RH surgery was still experiencing seizures and being treated by AEDs at the time of testing which may have accounted for some of the impairments observed.

As MMSE performance was normal and examines general neurocognitive functions the authors argue that the observed socio-cognitive impairments were not specific to any modality (visual, motor or auditory). Attention deficits and general cognitive impairment could account for the impairment in appreciating sarcasm and the intentions of the protagonist observed in S.M. (RH). Fourier et al. (2008) argue that this is unlikely as both the sincere and sarcastic vignettes did not differ greatly in terms of attentional demands. Also J.H. (LH) demonstrated deficits on verbal working memory but showed no difficulty in correctly identifying the true nature of social exchange in the vignettes, her performance on the comprehension questions were comparable to that of healthy controls.

As this research adopted a case study approach this study did not evaluate the impact of epilepsy related variables (AED therapy, duration of epilepsy, seizure type or seizure frequency) on social cognition. Consequently the findings cannot be generalised to the wider epilepsy population.

5. Frontal lobe epilepsy

5.1 ToM and emotion recognition

Farrant et al. (2005) investigated facial emotion recognition and ToM in 14 people with FLE (8 LFLE, 5 RFLE and 1 Bilateral) and 14 healthy controls. The FLE group were recruited from a specialist epilepsy unit and were being assessed for surgery. Groups did not differ significantly on age, gender ratio, years of education, premorbid IQ or long term memory. Executive functioning was assessed using the Trail Making Task (Reitan & Wolfson, 1993) to assess sequencing (part A) and mental flexibility (part B). The FLE group were significantly slower on the sequencing aspect of this task. The Hayling and Brixton tests (Burgess & Shallice, 1996a, 1996b) were administered and the FLE were significantly slower on the section 1 of the Hayling Test though there were no group differences on response inhibition, the FLE did make more mistakes on the task. The FLE were significantly impaired in relation to controls on a verbal fluency task.

ToM was measured using Happé's Strange Stories (Happé et al., 2001; Happé et al., 1999). The ToM stories all involved human interaction where double bluff, mistakes, white lies or persuasion were evident (with two examples or each of these), participants were asked a question which required them to make an inference about the mental states of people in the story. Faux pas was assessed using a version of the task by Stone et al. (1998a). Participants were assessed on their ability to make inferences about affective and cognitive mental states and their comprehension of the stories (as a control measure).

Humour was assessed via a cartoon task which required the participant to infer the mental state of a character in six cartoons (ToM) or to acknowledge a physical anomaly or a violation of a social norm (non ToM) in six cartoons. The memory load of the ToM stories, faux pas and humour tasks was reduced as participants had a copy of the story/cartoon in front of them whilst being asked questions. The Reading the Mind in the Eyes Task by Baron-Cohen et al. (2001) was administered where participants had to match correct emotions to the photographs displayed. Recognition of facial emotion was assessed using Ekman and Friesen (1976) pictures of facial emotion depicting the following emotions; sad, happy, surprise, anger, fear, disgust. Twelve pictures were displayed, one male and female picture for each emotion and participants were required to match the correct verbal labels to the emotions displayed.

FLE did not show deficits on the story task or appreciation of faux pas though they did illustrate a trend towards impairment. FLE were impaired in both the mental state and physical state cartoons, on emotion recognition and perception of eye gaze expression. ToM was intact but appreciation of humour and emotional expression was not. Mild impairments were observed except in the appreciation of emotion expression where impairment was substantial. These impairments were in relation to recognising sadness, anger and fear. Verbal second order ToM was intact in the FLE group (as examined in the story task). Age of onset was not correlated with any of the socio-cognitive measures. Executive functions were not correlated with socio-cognitive tasks in the FLE group but verbal fluency was correlated with the eyes task and the non ToM cartoons in the control group.

Evaluation: It is unlikely that the observed deficits in social cognition can be attributed to memory or IQ or deficits in executive functioning in the FLE group. As has been supported in studies of cognitive dysfunction in FLE the sample in this study exhibited specific as opposed to general deficits in social cognition. This may be because some tests are more sensitive to detecting impairment than others, though it should be noted that a large sample may have detected more impairments across the tasks. Specific areas in the FL may support different aspects of social cognition, consequently deficits in performance may reflect those areas of damage in the brain in the FLE group. This is the main criticism of the study as it did not report any analysis based on whether people had RFLE or LFLE, due to the small sample size of the groups. The exact site of seizure foci could only be established in 9 of the 14 FLE group (6 with medial and 3 with dorsolateral abnormalities), there were no patients with orbitofrontal involvement. Consequently whether different regions of damage within the FL are associated with specific impairments in the social cognition could not be fully explored. The study did not recruit people with MTLE to compare performance on tests of social cognition in relation to FLE.

This study can also be criticised as it does not provide the reader with any background information about seizure frequency, seizure type, duration of epilepsy or AED treatment in the FLE group, all of which could impact on functioning. Analysis has not been considered in light of these epilepsy related variables.

5.2 ToM and pragmatic language

Corcoran et al. (cited in Corcoran, 2000) conducted a small scale study (unpublished) in the Chalfont Centre for Epilepsy in 1999. They compared the performance of epilepsy patients on their appreciation of veiled intention in a Hinting Task (Corcoran et al., 1995), a ToM measure. Five patients with right frontal or right fronto-temporal foci, 3 with left frontal and left fronto-temporal foci, 3 with bilateral frontal foci and 23 normal controls were tested. Despite the small sample size differences were found between the groups on performance of the Hinting Task. The right fronto-temporal group appeared to perform worse than normal controls on the Hinting Task independent of group differences in IQ.

Evaluation: This study had a very small sample size and consequently hinting ability was not evaluated in relation to any epilepsy related variables.

6. Methodological difficulties of past research

In critically evaluating their study Farrant et al. (2005) suggest that a larger sample is needed to enable seizure foci in FLE and social cognition to be fully explored. People with FLE need to be compared with other focal epilepsies particularly MTLE to establish if there are specific socio cognitive deficits observed in FLE. Executive impairments have been illustrated in both FLE and TLE, so it is important to determine the nature of socio-cognitive dysfunction in epilepsy. Farrant et al. (2005) also highlight that a larger sample would enable comparison of performance between right and left FLE.

Most of the studies are cross sectional in that they either investigate social cognition post surgery or pre surgery. Consequently these studies cannot differentiate between social cognitive deficits as a consequence of surgery or the pre-existing epilepsy syndrome (Kirsch, 2006).

One main criticism with all the studies cited in this review is that no single study has compared people with TLE and FLE, so none of the studies can conclusively determine whether socio-cognitive deficits are characteristic of TLE and/or FLE. Studies that have attempted to investigate the impact of side of seizure onset can all be criticised for having small sample sizes and consequently findings cannot be generalised or the power to detect an effect is greatly reduced. None of the studies reviewed recruited a group of patients with idiopathic generalised epilepsy (IGE) who could act as a clinical control group to help to establish the impact of focal epilepsy on these skills. The added advantage of using an IGE group is that they have active epilepsy, take AEDs and will also be affected by epilepsy related variables such as seizure frequency, seizure type, age of onset and duration. None of the studies that have investigated social cognition in FLE recruited a frontal head injured group without epilepsy in order to determine the impact of FLE on socio-cognitive functioning. The studies reviewed have also not evaluated socio-cognitive performance in relation to social functioning in PWE.

There is a general lack of research investigating social cognition in epilepsy as highlighted in the literature (Schacher et al., 2006; Kirsch, 2006). Research that has been conducted has not utilised designs that can adequately explore socio-cognitive functioning in focal epilepsy. The impact that socio-cognitive skills have in relation to everyday social functioning in PWE needs to be investigated (Walpole et al., 2008; Schacher et al., 2006; Farrant et al., 2005). Such research could provide valuable insight into the socio-cognitive deficits associated with epilepsy and may ultimately improve social functioning in PWE.

7. Current research

In light of the methodological problems highlighted in previous studies, the author and colleagues (McCagh et al., unpublished) designed a study to explore socio-cognitive functioning in people with seizure foci in the RF, LF, RT, LT lobes. To overcome previous sample size difficulties the minimum number of people within each group was 11. As well as a healthy control group, this study recruited an IGE and FHI (frontal head injured) group to establish the impact that focal epilepsy and in particular FLE have on these skills, as Farrant et al. (2005) argue, social cognition has not been fully explored in FLE. Information was also collected on relevant epilepsy related variables (age at onset, AEDs, seizure frequency and duration of epilepsy) in relation to the sample. The study also aimed to establish the impact that socio-cognitive functioning may have on the every day life of PWE by assessing social cognitive performance in relation to perceived impact of epilepsy using the Impact of Epilepsy Scale (Jacoby et al., 1993).

Appreciation of false belief and deception in ToM stories and understanding veiled intentions in the Hinting Task were assessed across all clinical groups. All epilepsy groups were administered the Impact of Epilepsy Scale to compare task performance in relation to the perceived impact of epilepsy, this could then help to establish how socio-cognitive skills are related to social functioning in real life.

To date this is the largest lesion study to investigate ToM and the largest study within the field of epilepsy to investigate social cognition. The findings of this research are currently being written up for publication. A major outcome from the study is that the RF epilepsy group consistently under performed on ToM tasks. They illustrated deficits across two different ToM paradigms, appreciation of first and second order false belief and deception and appreciation of non-literal language in the Hinting Task in relation to the other experimental groups. These findings indicate that impaired ToM may be a particular feature of right frontal lobe pathology. The extent of the RF mentalising deficit is evident in their performance on one of the most basic assessment measures of ToM, first order ToM (Stone, 2000).

This deficit in first order ToM cannot be attributed to the impact of immediate story recall or level of education, nor is it a consequence of group differences in IQ, number of AEDs, age of onset or duration of epilepsy. The RF group also appear to have difficulty in making inferences based on non-literal language. They were significantly worse on this task than all of the other experimental groups, though further analyses revealed that this deficit was mediated by immediate story recall. The LT were impaired on second order ToM tasks and appreciation of hints though both of these deficits were mediated by immediate story recall. NC performed significantly better on the Hinting Task than all of the patient groups.

The results did not show a significant difference between the epilepsy groups on the Impact of Epilepsy score. Only a subgroup of participants were included in this analysis as this questionnaire was administered part way through recruitment. Therefore this sub sample may not have been representative of the entire target population, though there is no specific evidence to suggest this was the case. The RF group did rate the impact of epilepsy higher than any of the other groups but given the small cell sizes, there may not have been sufficient power to detect significant differences between the groups and so it is necessary to exercise caution in interpreting these findings. PWE do not appear to have insight into their social functioning difficulties, which may well reflect underlying pathology. Interestingly there was a significant negative correlation between impact of epilepsy score and level of education suggesting that the more educated the individual was the more likely they were to realise the social restraints of their condition.

The exact site of lesion within the frontal and temporal lobes is not analysed in relation to task performance. Whilst seizure foci and lateralisation are clearly established, there was no more detailed information available for the PWE included in this study to further localise the exact anatomical site of the seizure focus. Thus the information obtained for this study was not detailed enough to make generalisations about how important specific anatomical locations were within the frontal and temporal lobes in the processing of the tasks used.

8. Directions for future research

Small sample sizes have reduced the statistical power of findings in many of the studies discussed in the literature review (Farrant et al., 2005; Schilbach et al., 2007; Shaw et al., 2007; Walpole et al., 2008), clearly there is a need for studies with larger sample sizes that will enable comparisons across anatomical lesion sites in the frontal and temporal lobes. None of the epilepsy studies that were reviewed recruited a suitable control group or assessed both right and left frontal and temporal groups. The authors current research, recruited an IGE group, who were also taking AEDs to reduce the possibility that the impact of medication might confound the results. Future study designs need to consider these issues. Lesion studies have to date mostly focused on assessing ToM in either patients with frontal or temporal lobe damage but as this study (McCagh et al., unpublished) and brain imaging studies have shown (Brunet et al., 2000; Fletcher et al.,1995; Gallagher et al., 2000;

Goel et al., 1995; Saxe & Kanwisher, 2003; Vogeley et al., 2001), both lobes would appear to be implicated in the processing of ToM. Therefore future research should incorporate patients with unilateral lesions to both the frontal and temporal lobes.

Often it has been too difficult to compare the findings of studies which employ different ToM paradigms. Harrington et al. (2005) reviewed 30 studies testing ToM in schizophrenia and concluded that ToM deficits are apparent but that comparison of results was difficult due to the fact that a variety of ToM measures were used to test the same construct e.g. irony and picture board stories, deception, false belief, hinting etc. As Baron-Cohen et al. (1995) suggest, ToM may be underpinned by a network of many neural structures which could represent different aspects of ToM abilities and differing task demands. Consequently this may account for the disparity in research findings. Therefore future research should endeavour to administer ToM test batteries that assess ToM using techniques that are validated and incorporate measures of general inferential ability, executive function and memory. This will help to establish if ToM abilities are domain general or domain specific skills. Immediate story recall mediated some of the ToM deficits observed in the authors research and so should be accounted for when assessing ToM in future studies. To enable more fruitful comparison between research findings, future research needs to use similar ToM tasks across different populations or to carefully monitor variations in task demand with corresponding active brain regions.

Studies should further explore the effects of brain damage at different stages of development to ToM (Happé et al., 1999). This would differentiate the importance of specific structures in the development of ToM and in online ToM abilities in adulthood. Whilst some studies have attempted to do this (Shaw et al., 2004) there is lack of research in this area.

Inconsistent findings across studies using adult samples may in part be due to the difficulty in finding appropriate measures to assess ToM in adult populations. Tests need to be hard enough to 'generate errors yet simple enough that errors are not merely due to more general processing demands' (Apperley et al., 2004, p.1774.). Future work could endeavour to develop more sophisticated measures. Studies should utilise more ecological valid measures of testing which reflect the complex subtle social cues that are apparent in human social interaction (Lough et al., 2006). To date most research which has investigated socio-cognitive functioning specifically in relation to ToM has used vignettes depicting social interactions or photographs illustrating different emotional expressions. Traditional measures are easy to administer but may not necessarily tap into the complex perceptual processes that occur when we interpret social interactions. Future work should use ecologically valid measures of dynamic social interaction as it occurs in everyday life. It has been asserted that the TASITS is a much more ecologically valid measure of emotion recognition and social inference than traditional measures. This test might be incorporated into future research as it may be particularly sensitive in detecting impairments in social functioning. It has been used in one epilepsy study to date (Schilbach et al., 2007) and has been shown to be a valid measure of social cognition in people with head injury in past research (McDonald et al., 2003).

One of the main problems in investigating social cognition in epilepsy is that it is difficult to differentiate between the impact of development, the epileptic foci, AED therapy and surgery on the social abilities of PWE (Kirsch 2006). A number of studies have shown that quality of life scores increase after surgery but often these measures do not adequately assess improvements in social functioning (Kirsch, 2006). As Schilbach et al. (2007) argue, social competence has a considerable effect on quality of life yet the study of social cognition in epilepsy has been largely neglected. Future research needs to continue to explore the impact that socio-cognitive dysfunction has on social functioning and quality of life in FLE and TLE. This could be achieved by administering a wide range of measures that utilise different paradigms in social cognition. Future work should include objective ratings of social functioning to see if real life behaviour is related to socio cognitive task performance. Quality of life measures that fully explore the impact of epilepsy on social functioning that are not self report measures but objective measures completed by significant others need to be employed. This may help resolve the difficulty of insight that appears to be apparent in FLE.

Future research which assesses social cognition before and after surgery is needed (Fournier et al., 2008). Surgery may help reduce seizures activity and reduce the amount of AEDs taken which in turn may improve social cognitive performance. Shaw et al. (2007) found improvements in social cognition (facial expression recognition) in people with left TLE after surgery. There is need for longitudinal research which establishes the impact of surgery on social cognition to establish whether epilepsy surgery is beneficial in improving such skills.

Further research should focus on trying to rehabilitate PWE after surgery where they may find themselves in new social situations that they have not previously experienced and may have difficulty adjusting (Bladin, 1992; Wilson, Bladin & Saling, 2004). PWE may have new found independence which can impact on interpersonal relationships, causing friction and resentment. This may be particularly problematic if parental over protectiveness was a feature before surgery.

9. Conclusion

ToM deficits may also provide some explanation for the complex psychosocial difficulties apparent in PWE. Such difficulties include the experience of stigma, unemployment or underemployment, anxiety and depression, poor self esteem, social isolation and difficulties in interpersonal relationships (Austin & de Boer, 1997; Collings, 1990; De Souza & Salgado, 2006; Fisher et al., 2000; Grabowska-Grzyb et al., 2006; Jacoby et al., 1996; McCagh et al., 2009; McCagh, 2010; Mensah et al., 2007; Morrell, 2002; Suurmeijer et al., 2001.).

Current quality of life measures rely on patients to self report improvements in functioning after surgery which may be problematic as this will rest on how well the patient has insight into their social difficulties. This could pose a particular problem for patients with RH lesions where sense of self may be impaired. (Kirsch, 2006) Discrepancies between self report and objective measures of social functioning reports by significant others and or carers of social functioning in PWE on quality of life measures have been evident Hays et al. (1995). This evidence and the findings of the authors study imply that self report measures are not reliable so clinicians need to consider alternative ways of measuring social functioning in PWE.

Presurgical neuropsychological evaluation plays a major role in determining potential outcomes and treatment intervention after surgery. Recent research have demonstrated that PWE have difficulties with socio cognitive functioning (Corcoran et al., 2000; Farrant et al., 2005; Fournier et al., 2008; Schacher et al., 2006; Schillbach et al., 2007; Walpole et al., 2008). It is becoming clear that neuropsychological assessment during clinical audit needs to consider assessing socio cognitive functioning in PWE and that such an assessment should be part of the pre and post surgical evaluation of potential surgical candidates. It is recommended that an instrument such as the TASITS which is more ecologically valid and likely to be more sensitive to socio cognitive impairment in real life, should be incorporated with more traditional measures to accurately establish the impairments of social perception in PWE. Such assessments should be complemented by an effective measure of the actual social difficulties that PWE experience in everyday life. A number of authors criticise current measures of social functioning used on PWE, currently these measures do not fully explore the impact that surgery has on interpersonal relationships or social competence (Kirsch, 2006; Schilbach et al., 2007). Therefore development of more appropriate measures is needed.

The authors' current research lateralises socio-cognitive dysfunction to the right frontal lobe and left temporal lobe, further study in this area may be able to support the lateralisation of these skills. If this is the case then socio-cognitive assessment may provide clinicians with a useful and inexpensive tool for lateralising the site of seizure foci in patients, particularly where anterior foci are suspected. This may be particularly valuable as there are few neuropsychological tests which can lateralise damage in the prefrontal cortex. The effects of lateralisation or localisation have not been found in studies which assess cognitive functioning in FLE (Helmstaedter et al., 1996; Upton & Thompson, 1996). Tests of social cognition may provide the clinician with an objective measure of deficits in social competence particularly as patients with FLE may lack insight into their impairments. Patients who are at risk of reduced social competence can be identified and may possibly benefit from treatment intervention. Future investigations should assess the efficacy of such interventions in epilepsy.

Social cognition is an important but neglected area of study in the field of epilepsy. The study of ToM in epilepsy will lead to a greater understanding of the social cognitive deficits of the epileptic condition. This may in turn lead to more effective psychological interventions to enable the smoother functioning of people with epilepsy in society.

10. References

Apperly, I. A., Samson, D., Chiavarino, C., & Humphreys, G. W. (2004). Frontal and temporo-parietal lobe contributions to theory of mind: Neuropsychological evidence from a false-belief task with reduced language and executive demands. *Journal of Cognitive Neuroscience, 16,* 1773-1784.

Astington, J.W. (2001). The future of theory-of-mind research: understanding motivational states, the role of language, and real-world consequences. *Child Development, 72* (3), 685-7.

Austin, K., Smith, M.S., Risinger, M.W., & McNelis, A.M. (1994). Childhood epilepsy and asthma: comparison of quality of life. *Epilepsia, 35* (3), 608-615.

Austin, K. and deBoer, H. (1997). Disruptions in social functioning and services facilitating adjustment for the child and adult. In: Engel Jr. J., Pedley, T.A. (Eds.). *Epilepsy: A Comprehensive Textbook* (pp. 2191–2201). Philadelphia: Lippincott-Raven.

Avis, J.and Harris, P. (1991). Belief-desire reasoning among Baka children: evidence for a universal conception of mind. *Child Development, 62,* 460-467.

Bar-On, R. (1997). *The emotional quotient inventory (EQ-I): a test of emotional intelligence.* Multi-Health Systems, Toronto, Canada.

Bar-On, R., Tranel, D., Denburg, N., & Bechara, A. (2003). Exploring the neurological substrate of emotional and social intelligence. *Brain, 126,* 1790–800.

Baron-Cohen, S., Leslie, A. Frith, U. (1995). Does the autistic child have a theory of mind? *Cognition, 21,* 37-46.

Baron-Cohen, S., O'Riorden, M, Stone, V. E., Jones, R., Plaisted, K. (1997). Recognition of mental state terms: clinical findings in children with autism and a functional neuroimaging study of normal adults. *British Journal of Psychiatry, 165, 640-649.*

Benton, A.L., Sivan, A.B., Hamsher, K., Varney, N.R., & Spreen, O. (1983). *Benton facial recognition test.* New York: Oxford University Press.

Bladin, P.F. (1992). Psychosocial difficulties and outcome after temporal lobectomy. *Epilepsia, 33*:898–907.

Brothers, L. and Ring, B. (1992). A neuroethological framework for the representation of minds. *Journal of Cognitive Neuroscience, 4, 107*-118.

Brunet, E., Sarfati, Y., Hardy-Bayle, M., & Decety, J. (2000). A PET investigation of the attribution of intentions with a nonverbal task. *Neuroimage*, 11, 157-166.

Burgess, P. W. and Shallice, T. (1996a). Bizarre responses, rule detection and frontal lobe lesions. *Cortex, 32* (2), 241–259.

Burgess, P.W. and Shallice,T. (1996b). Response suppression, initiation and strategy use following frontal lobe lesions. *Neuropsychologia, 34* (4), 263–272.

Caplan, R., Sagun, J., Siddarth, P., Gurbani, S., Koh, S., et al. (2005). Social competence in paediatric epilepsy: insights into underlying mechanisms. *Epilepsy & Behavior, 6,* 218–28.

Chapman, J. (1923). *Chapman-Cook speed of reading test.* University Press, Ames Iowa State.

Collings, J. A. (1990). Psychosocial well-being and epilepsy: an empirical study. *Epilepsia 31,* 418-426.

Corcoran, R., Mercer, G. & Frith, C.D. (1995). Schizophrenia, s symptomatology and social inference: investigating theory of mind in people with schizophrenia. *Schizophrenia Research, 17,* 5-13.

Corcoran, R. (2000). Theory of mind in other clinical conditions: is a selective theory of mind deficit exclusive to autism? In Baron-Cohen, S., Tager-Flusberg, H.,& Cohen D.J. (Eds.). *Understanding other minds: Perspectives from developmental cognitive neuroscience* (2nd ed.) (pp. 391-421). Oxford: Oxford University Press.

Corcoran, R. and Frith, C. D. (2003). Autobiographical memory and theory of mind: evidence of a relationship in schizophrenia. *Psychological Medicine, 33,* 897-905.

Cramer, J.A., Perrine, K., Devinsky, O., Bryant-Comstock, I., Meador, K., Hermann, B.P. (1998). Development and cross-cultural translation of a 31-item quality of life questionnaire (QOLIFE-31). *Epilepsia, 39,* 81-88.

De Souza, .E.A.P. and Salgado, P.C.B. (2006). A psychosocial view of anxiety and depression in epilepsy. *Epilepsy & Behavior, 8,* 232-8.

Dennett, D. (1978). Beliefs about beliefs. *Behavioral and Brain Sciences,* 4, 568-570.

Dorenbaum, D., Cappelli, M., Keene, D., McGrath, P, (1985). Use of a child behavior checklist in the psychosocial assessment of children with epilepsy. *Clinical Paediatrics, 24,* 634-637.

Ekman, P. and Friesen, W. V. (1976). *Pictures of facial affect.* Palo Alto, CA: Consulting Psychologists Press.

Fournier, N.M., Claverley, K.L., Wagner, J.P., Poock, J.L., & Crossley, M (2008). Impaired social cognition 30 years after hemispherectomy for intractable epilepsy: the importance of the right hemisphere in complex social functioning. *Epilepsy & Behavior, 12,* 460-471.

Frith, U. and Frith, C.D. (2003). Development and neurophysiology of mentalizing. *Philosophical Transactions of the Royal Society of London. Series B, Biological Sciences,* 358, 459–473.

Gawryluk, A. and McGlone, J. (2007). Does the concept of emotional intelligence contribute to our understanding of temporal lobe resections? *Epilepsy & Behavior 11,* 421–426.

Goel,V., Grafman,J,. Sadato,N., & Hallett, M.(1995). Modeling other minds. N*euroreport, An International Journal for the Rapid Communication of Research in Neuroscience, 6,*(13). , 1741-1746.

Grabowska-Grzyb, A., Jędrzejczak, J., Nagańska , E., & Fiszer, U. (2006). Risk factors for depression in patients with epilepsy. *Epilepsy & Behavior, 8,* 411-417.

Happé, F. (1994). An advanced test of theory o mind: Understanding of story characters' thoughts and feelings by able autistic, mentally handicapped, and normal children and adults. *Journal of Autism and Developmental Disorders, 24* (2), 129-154.

Happé , F., Brownell, H., & Winner, E. (1999). Acquired 'theory of mind' impairments following stroke. *Cognition, 70* (3), 211–240.

Happé, F., Malhi, G. S.,& Checkley, S. (2001). Acquired mind-blindness following frontal lobe surgery? A single case study of impaired theory of mind in a patient treated with stereotactic anterior capsulotomy. *Neuropsychologia, 39,* 83–90.

Harrington, L., Siegert, R., & McClure, J. (2005). Theory of mind in schizophrenia: A critical review. *Cognitive Neuropsychiatry, 10,* (4), 249-286.

Helmstaedter, C., Gleissner, U., Zentner, J., & Elger, C.E. (1998). Neuropsychological consequences of epilepsy surgery in frontal lobe epilepsy. *Neuropsychologia, 36,* 681-9.

Herman, B.P., Black, R.B., & Chhabria, S. (1981). Behavioral problems and social competence in children with epilepsy. *Epilepsia, 22,* 703-710.

Hermann, B. P. and Seidenberg, M. (1995). Executive system dysfunction in temporal lobe epilepsy: effects of nociferous cortex versus hippocampal pathology. *Journal of Clinical & Experimental Neuropsychology, 17* (6), 809–819.

Jacoby, A., Baker, G.A., Smith, D., Dewey, M & Chadwick, D.W. (1993). Measuring the impact of epilepsy: the development of a novel scale. *Epilepsy Research, 16,* 83-88.

Jacoby, A., Baker, G.A., Steen, N., Potts, P., & Chadwick, D.W. (1996). The clinical course of epilepsy and its psychosocial correlates: findings from a U.K. community study. *Epilepsia, 37,*148–61.

Jalava, M., Sillpanää, M., Camfield., C. & Camfield, P. (1997). Social adjustment and competence 35 years after onset of childhood epilepsy: a prospective study. *Epilepsia, 38,* (6), 708-715.

Kirsch, H.E. (2006). Social cognition and epilepsy surgery. *Epilepsy and Behavior, 8,* 71–80.

Martin, R.C., Sawrie, S.M., Edwards, R., Roth, D. L., Faught, E., et al. (2000). Investigation of executive function change following anterior temporal lobectomy: Selective normalization of verbal fluency. *Neuropsychology, 14* (4), 501–508.

McCagh, J., Fisk, J.E., & Baker, G.A. (2009). Epilepsy, psychosocial and cognitive functioning. *Epilepsy Research 86* (1), 1-14.

McCagh, J. (2010). Epilepsy, Myths, Stereotypes & Stigma. In: Simon, E.L.(Ed.)Psychology of Stereotypes (pp265-278): New York: Nova Science Publishers.

McCusker, C., Kennedy, P., Anderson, J., Hicks, E., & Harahan, D. (2002). Adjustment in children with intractable epilepsy: importance of seizure duration and family factors. *Developmental Medicine & Child Neurology, 44,* 687-687.

McDonald, S. (1996). Exploring the process of inference generation in sarcasm: a review of normal and clinical studies. *Brain & Language, 68,* 486-506.

Mensah, S.A., Beavis, J.M., Thapar, A.K., & Kerr, M.P. (2007). A community study of the presence of anxiety order in people with epilepsy. *Epilepsy & Behavior, 7,* 438–46.

Morrell, M.J. (2002). Stigma and epilepsy. *Epilepsy & Behavior, 3,* S21–5.

Perner, J. and Wimmer, H. (1985). John thinks that Mary thinks that…., attribution of second-order false beliefs by 5 to 10 year old children. *Journal of Experimental Child Psychology, 5,* 125-137.

Premack, D. and Woodruff, G. (1978). Does the chimpanzee have a 'theory of mind?'*Behavioural and Brain Sciences. 1,* 515-526.

Rowe, A. D., Bullock, P. R., Polkey, C. E., & Morris, R. G. (2001). 'Theory of mind' impairments and their relationship to executive functioning following frontal lobe excisions. *Brain,* 124, 600-616.

Saxe, R., and Kanwisher, N. (2003). People thinking about thinking people.The role of the temporoparietal junction in ''theory of mind''. *Neuroimage, 19,* 1835-1842.

Schacher, M., Winkler, R., Grunwald, T., Kraemer, G., Kurthem, M., & Reed, V. (2006). Mesial temporal lobe epilepsy impairs advanced social cognition. *Epilepsia, 47,* 2141–6.

Schilbach, L., Koubeissi, M.Z., David, N., Vogeley, K.,& Ritzl, E.K. (2007). Being with virtual others: Studying social cognition in temporal lobe epilepsy. *Epilepsy & Behavior,* 316-323.

Shamay-Tsoory, S. G., Tomer, R., Yaniv, S., & Aharon- Peretz, J. (2002). Empathy deficits in Aspergers syndrome: A cognitive profile. *Neurocase, 8,* 245-252.

Shamay-Tsoory, S. G., Tomer, R., Berger, B. D., & Aharon-Peretz, J. (2003). Characterization of empathy deficity following prefrontal brain damage: The role of the right ventromedial prefrontal cortex. *Journal of Cognitive Neuroscience, 15*(3), 324–337.

Shamay-Tsoory S.G., Tomer, R., Berger, B.D., Goldsher, D., & Aharon- Peretz, J. (2005a). Impaired "affective theory of mind" is associated with right ventromedial prefrontal damage. *Cognitive & Behavioral Neurology,* 18, (1), 55-67

Shamay-Tsoory S.G., Tomer, R., & Aharon-Peretz, J. (2005b). The neuroanatomical basis of understanding sarcasm and its relationship to social cognition. *Neuropsychology. 19* (3), 288-300.

Shaw, P., Lawrence, E., Radbourne, C., Bramham, J., Polkey, C.E., & David, A.S. (2004). The impact of early and late damage to the human amygdala on 'theory of mind' reasoning. *Brain, 127*(7):1535-48.

Shaw, P., Lawrence, E., Bramham, J., Brierley, B., Radbourne, C., & David, A.S. (2007). A prospective study of the effects of anterior temporal lobectomy on emotion recognition and theory of mind. *Neuropsychologia, 45,* 2783-90.

Stone, V. E., Baron-Cohen, S., & Knight, R. T. (1998a). Frontal lobe contributions to theory of mind. *Journal of Cognitive Neuroscience, 10* (5), 640–656.

Stone, V.E. (2000). The role of the frontal lobes and the amygdala in theory of mind. In Baron-Cohen, S., Tager-Flusberg, H., & Cohen D.J. (Eds.). *Understanding other minds: Perspectives from developmental cognitive neuroscience* (2nd ed.) (pp. 253-273). Oxford: Oxford University Press.

Stone, V.E., Baron-Cohen, S., Calder, A., Keane, J., & Young, A. (2003). Acquired theory of mind impairments in individuals with bilateral amygdala lesions. *Neuropsychologia, 41,* 209–220.

Stuss, D. T., Gallup, G. G., & Alexander, M. P. (2001). The frontal lobes are necessary for theory of mind. *Brain,* 124, 279-286.

Suurmeijer, T.P., Reuvekamp, M.F., & Aldenkamp, B.P. (2001). Social functioning, psychological functioning and quality of life in epilepsy. *Epilepsia, 42,* 1160–8.

Upton, D. and P. J. Thompson. (1996).Epilepsy in the frontal lobes: neuropsychological characteristics. *Journal of Epilepsy, 9,* 215-222

Van Lancker, D.R. and Kemper, D. (1987) Comprehension of familiar phrases by left- but not by right-hemisphere damaged patients *Brain & Language,* 32 (2), 265-77.

Vogeley, K., Bussfeld, P., Newen, A., Herrmann, S., Happ´e, F., et al. (2001). Mind reading: Neural mechanisms of theory of mind and self-perspective. *Neuroimage, 14,* 170-181.

Walpole, P., Isaac, C.L., & Reynders, H.J. (2008). A comparison of emotional and cognitive intelligences in people with and without temporal lobe epilepsy. *Epilepsia, 49* (8), 1470-1474.

Wechsler, D. (1999). *Wechsler Abbreviated Scale of Intelligence.* San Antonio: The Psychological Corporation.

Wechsler, D. (2001). *Wechsler Test of Adult Reading - UK Adaptation (WTAR – UK).* San Antonio: The Psychological Corporation.

Wellman, H.M. and Lagattuta, K.H. (2000). Theory of mind and executive ffunction, is there a developmental relationship? In Baron-Cohen,S., Tager-Flusberg, H., &Cohen D.J. (Eds.). *Understanding other minds: Perspectives from developmental cognitive neuroscience* (2nd ed.) (pp. 21-49). Oxford: Oxford University Press.

Wellman, H.M., Cross, D., & Watson, J. (2001). Meta-analysis of theory-of-mind development: The truth about false belief. *Child Development, 72,* 655-684.

Williams, J., Sharp, G., Bates, S., Griebel, & M. Lange, B., et al. (1996). Academic achievement and the behavioral ratings in children with absence and complex partial epilepsy. *Education & Treatment of Children,* 19, 143–52.

Wilson, S.J., Bladin, P.F., & Saling, M.M. (2004). Paradoxical results in the cure of chronic illness: the "burden of normality" as exemplified following seizure surgery. *Epilepsy & Behavior, 5,*13–21.

Wimmer, H. and Perner, J. (1983). Beliefs about beliefs, representation and constraining function of wrong beliefs in young children's understanding of deception. *Cognition, 13,* 103-128.

Winner, E., Brownell, H., Happé, F., Blum, A., & Pincus, D. (1998). Distinguishing lies from jokes: Theory of mind deficits and discourse interpretation in right hemisphere brain-damaged patients. *Brain & Language, 62,* 89-106.

Zigmond, A. and Snaith, R. (1983). The hospital anxiety and depression scale. *Acta Psychiatrica Scandinavia, 67,* 361–70.

15

Epilepsy in Mitochondrial Disorders

Silvana Franceschetti[1], Graziella Uziel[2],
Eleonora Lamantea[3], Gianfranco Carrara[3],
Carlo Antozzi[4], Massimo Zeviani[3] and Laura Canafoglia[1]
[1]From the Department of Neurophysiopathology and Epilepsy Centre,
[2]Child Neurology,
[3]Biochemistry and Medical Genetics,
[4]Myopathology, IRCCS Foundation Neurological Institute Carlo Besta, Milan,
Italy

1. Introduction

Mitochondrial encephalopathies (MEs) are characterized by an extreme clinical heterogeneity since they can involve different systems and manifest at distinct ages with variable course. Many affected individuals display a cluster of clinical features that fall into discrete syndromes - among syndromic pictures, epilepsy is relevant in myoclonic epilepsy with ragged-red fibers (MERRF), mitochondrial encephalomyopathy with lactic acidosis and stroke-like episodes (MELAS), neurogenic weakness with ataxia and retinitis pigmentosa (NARP), Alpers' encephalopathy and Leigh syndrome (LS). However, many patients do not fit neatly into one particular syndrome, due to "overlapping" presentations (sharing symptoms of different syndromes) or atypical clusters of symptoms.
Epilepsy is a frequent symptom also in non-syndromic patients, sometimes dominating the clinical presentation.

2. Genetics

Mitochondrial disorders derive from mutations of mitochondrial (mtDNA) or nuclear DNA (nDNA), which lead to the impairment of the mitochondrial respiratory chain activity or mitochondrial ATP synthesis. Mitochondrial disorders typically involve tissues or organs with high energy demand including peripheral nervous system (PNS), central nervous system (CNS), eyes, ears, heart, endocrine system, kidney, guts, and liver. Fever, infection and stress may aggravate the neurological symptoms.
Generally, the genotype-phenotype correlation in mitochondrial disorders is poor, since the clinical phenotype is not only dependent on the type and pathogenicity of the DNA mutation, but it may also derive from other genetic and environmental factors.
A possible mechanism of inheritance is maternal transmission of the mutations located in the mtDNA. It is noteworthy that variable amounts of the mutated mtDNA (mutation load) usually coexist with wild-type molecules in the different tissues, resulting in a "heteroplasmic state". Moreover, the phenotypic expression of mtDNA mutations may be dependent on a threshold effect, which can be dissimilar in different tissues, in relation to

specific energy demand. Nuclear "modifier" genes, environmental factors, mtDNA haplotypes (polymorphisms) or clusters of mtDNA variants could also influence the expression of mtDNA.

The mtDNA contains 37 genes: 13 encoding for subunits of the respiratory chain complexes I (ND1-6, ND4L), III (cytochrome b), IV (COX I-III) and V (ATPase6, ATPase8) (oxidative phosphorylation system, OXPHOS); 22 encoding for transfer RNAs (tRNAs); 2 for ribosomial RNAs (rRNAs). The mitochondrial genetic code differs from the universal genetic code since mtDNA is not protected by any repair mechanism, thus resulting prone to mutations; indeed mutation rates of mtDNA are 10 times higher than those of nDNA.

MtDNA mutations are classified as either large-scale rearrangements (partial deletions or duplications) or point mutations. Rearrangements are frequently sporadic, while point mutations are commonly inherited.

The nuclear genome encodes more than 95% of all proteins located in the mitochondria. An increasing number of clinical conditions have been associated with nDNA mutations, which may involve different genes. These genes have been divided into four groups, according to their function. First group includes genes encoding for structural components of the respiratory chain; second group genes encoding for assembly factors of the respiratory chain complexes; third group genes responsible for factors of mtDNA stability; fourth group genes involved in biogenesis of mitochondria (Finsterer, 2006). Mutations of the nDNA are inherited by autosomal mechanism.

Nuclear-mitochondrial interactions play a fundamental role in cellular homeostasis. The optimal interaction between nuclear and mitochondrial encoded factors is essential for transcription and translation of mtDNA and also for the correct assembly and function of the OXPHOS system.

In both maternal and autosomal inherited MEs, single or multiple defects of the respiratory chain can be detected in the blood cells or muscular specimens. However, biochemical analysis can also identify defective activity of the respiratory chain complexes (in particular complex I and IV) in case of mitochondrial DNA depletion (see for example the mtDNA depletion syndrome 4A, due to mutation in the nuclear gene encoding for mitochondrial polymerase gamma) or multiple deletions.

3. Maternally inherited syndromes with epilepsy, associated with mtDNA mutations

Among MEs characterized by maternal inheritance, generalized seizures and myoclonus are the main symptoms of *MERRF* (myoclonus epilepsy with ragged-red fibers) syndrome (MIM ID #545000). This syndrome, initially described by Fukuhara et al (1980), is characterized by myoclonus, seizures, progressive cerebellar syndrome, and ragged-red fibers in muscle biopsy. It can be due to mutations in more than one mitochondrial gene, e.g. MTTK, MTTL1, MTTH, MTTS1, MTTS2, MTTF and MTND5. However, a specific mtDNA mutation of the tRNA(Lys) gene (MTTK), implying an A-to-G transition at nucleotide 8344, accounts for 80 to 90% of MERRF cases (Shoffner and Wallace, 1992). Biochemically, this mutation produces multiple deficiencies in the enzyme complexes of the respiratory chain (typically complexes I and IV), consistent with a defect in translation of all mtDNA-encoded genes.

A typical MERRF picture was observed in a patient bearing a mutation of the MTTF gene which codes tRNA(Phe) (Mancuso et al, 2004).

Myoclonus epilepsy may manifest at variable age and can associate with other symptoms including general weakness, muscle wasting, deafness, dementia, short stature, optic atrophy, peripheral neuropathy, cardiomyopathy, myoglobinuria and renal tubular dysfunction (Wu et al, 2010).

As an example of the heterogeneity affecting also well defined ME with epilepsy, we report here some features of a MERRF family, bearing the common MTTK mutation, including four affected siblings with similar symptoms, but clinically different severity. The proband, previously described by Roger et al. (1982), had typical and severe progressive myoclonus epilepsy associated with optic atrophy. His brother showed occasional seizures and photoparoxysmal EEG response. His sister had late-onset action myoclonus and photoparoxysmal EEG response (figure 1).

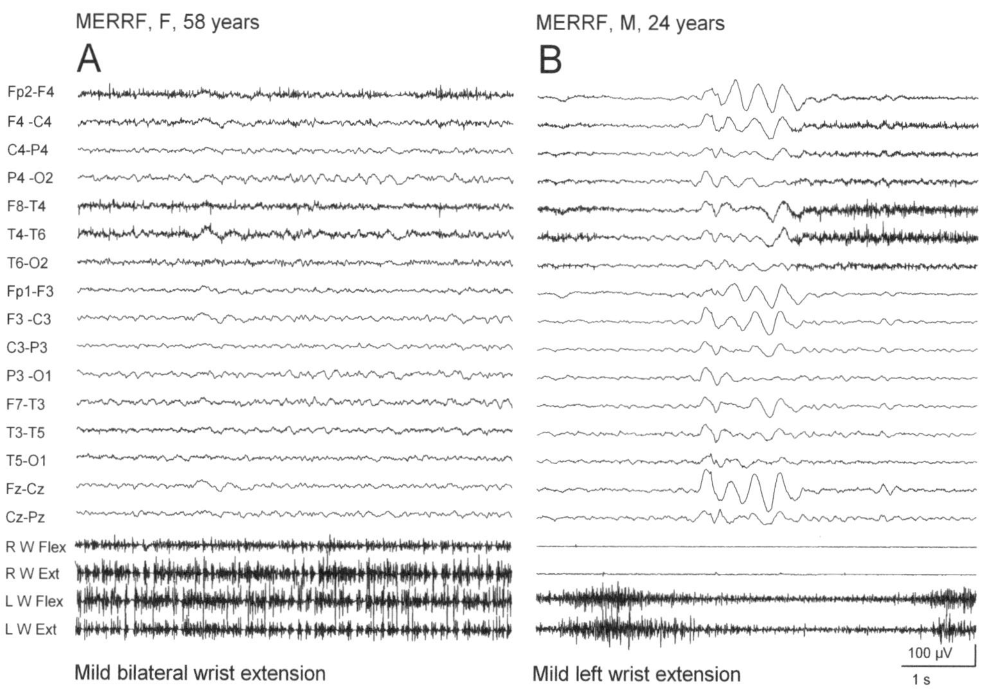

A: EEG recording of a 58 years-old female patient with MERRF syndrome showing slow background activity and diffuse slow waves; EMG recording includes positive and negative myoclonic jerks. B: EEG recording of the 24 years-old son of the previous patient showing a sequence of diffuse slow waves; in this case, EMG shows regular muscular contraction.

Fig. 1. Heterogeneous EEG-EMG features in the same family with MERRF syndrome

His nephew showed decreased visual acuity, associated with photosensitive (but not action-induced) myoclonus (figure 2).

MELAS (MIM ID #540000) syndrome is characterized by mitochondrial myopathy, encephalopathy, lactic acidosis, and stroke-like episodes. The disorder is characterized by symptoms and signs of central nervous system involvement, including seizures, migraine, hemiparesis, hemianopsia, cortical blindness, and episodic vomiting. Other common symptoms are: hearing loss, reduced statural growth, diabetes (Ciafaloni et al, 1992).

MELAS syndrome can be caused by mutation in several genes of the mtDNA coding for tRNA or polypeptides, including MTTL1, MTTQ, MTTH, MTTK, MTTS1, MTND1, MTND5, MTND6, and MTTS2. The 3243A-G transition in the MTTL1 gene can be found in about 80% of the patients (Goto et al, 1992).

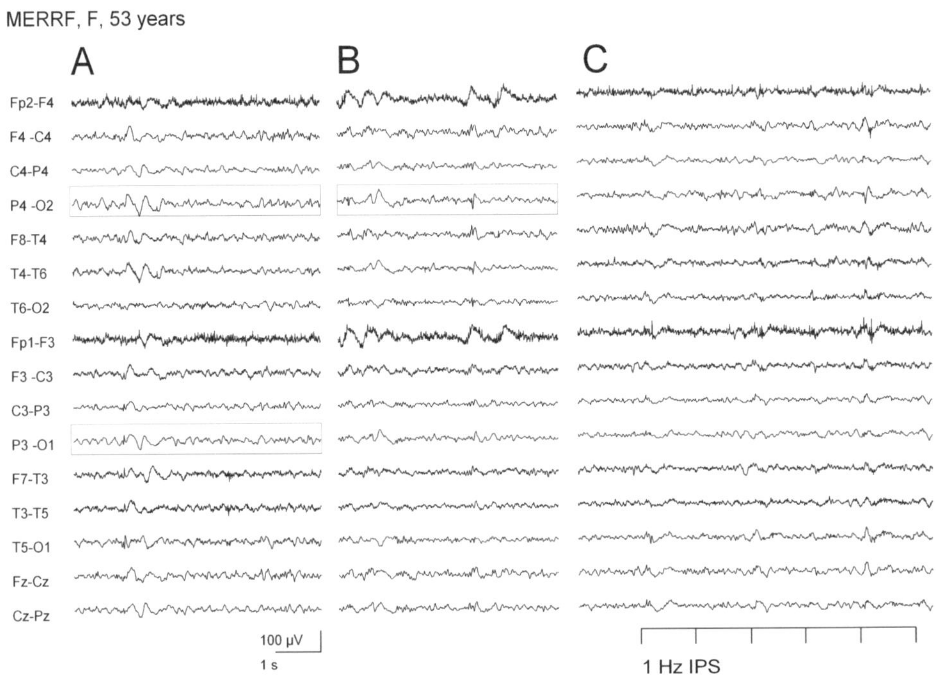

A and B: EEG recording of a female patient with MERRF syndrome showing diffuse spike and slow waves prevalent on posterior derivations (boxes) with occasional spontaneous occurrence. C: Intermittent photic stimulation (IPS) induces an increase of the epileptic discharges.

Fig. 2. Spontaneous and photically-induced epileptiform abnormalities in MERRF syndrome

In MELAS syndrome, epilepsy is a frequent symptom; seizures are often of motor type and can be grouped in clusters (until the extreme picture of *epilepsia partialis continua*) even without the evidence of concomitant new acute brain insult (Canafoglia et al, 2004). However, a relationship between clusters of seizures and stroke-like episodes is common: focal neuronal hyperexcitability or epileptic activity may cause an increase of ATP demand which can be followed by depletion of ATP and consecutive vasogenic edema (Iizuka et al, 2002 ; 2003). Finally, the vasogenic edema turns into laminar necrosis indicated by T1 hyperintensity at cerebral MRI. Another explanation suggests that stroke like episodes are due to metabolic derangement, spreading beyond an ischemic focus. Figure 3 shows the dramatic change of EEG activity after repeated seizures, indicated by the appearance of subcontinuous focal slow waves, in a patient with MELAS syndrome.
A syndrome characterized by features of both MERRF and MELAS (*overlap MERRF-MELAS*) has been described by Zeviani et al. (1993) in association with a point mutation at nucleotide 8356 (T-to-C transition) in the MTTK gene. The phenotype was characterized by myoclonic epilepsy, neural deafness, ataxia, stroke-like episodes in the majority of the affected siblings

or rarely by the association of seizures with other symptoms. In other families with an overlap MERFF-MELAS, Nakamura et al. (1995) identified a heteroplasmic mutation in the MTTS1 gene, while Melone et al. (2004) reported a heteroplasmic mutation in the MTTH gene.

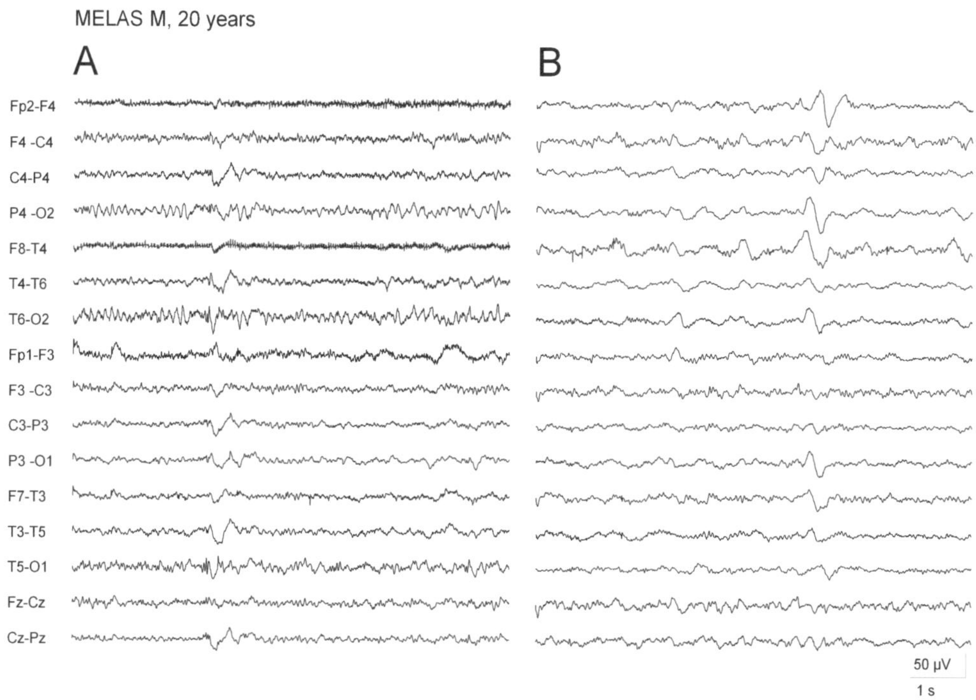

A: EEG recording of a patient with MELAS syndrome showing asymmetric background activity and occasional diffuse spike and waves with posterior prevalence.
B: After repeated seizures, the EEG recording of the same patient shows diffuse attenuation of the background activity and the appearance of subcontinuous slow waves on posterior derivations.

Fig. 3. EEG changes in a patient with MELAS syndrome after repeated seizure occurrence

Neurogenic muscle weakness, ataxia, and retinitis pigmentosa (NARP) syndrome typically presents with proximal motor neuropathy, sensory disturbances, cerebellar ataxia, and retinitis pigmentosa. More rare features include developmental delay, mental retardation, dementia, epilepsy, or cardiomyopathy.

In some patients, NARP may clinically overlap with Leigh syndrome (NARP/MILS overlap) due to point mutations in the mitochondrial ATPase6 gene, presumably resulting in impaired ATP synthesis. In this syndrome usually associated with T8993G mutation, have been described infantile spasms with hypsarrithmia (Desguerre at al, 2003)

4. Autosomal inherited syndromes with epilepsy, associated with nDNA mutations

Other mitochondrial syndromes causing epilepsy are associated with multiple mtDNA deletions or tissue-specific depletions. These conditions are due to nuclear gene defects involved in controlling the nuclear-mitochondrial intergenomic signaling (Spinazzola and Zeviani, 2005).

These conditions include the following syndromes:

Developmental delay or dementia, lactic acidosis, cyclic vomiting, seizures, failure to thrive, hearing loss, myopathy, liver failure, renal tubular acidosis, pancreatitis, manifesting at 1-3 months, characterize childhood myo-cerebro-hepatopathy spectrum (MCHS).

Myoclonic epilepsy, myopathy, sensory ataxia (MEMSA) is characterized by epilepsy, myopathy, ataxia without ophthalmoplegia (previously defined as spinocerebellar ataxia with epilepsy: SCAE).

Ataxia neuropathy spectrum (ANS) is characterized by ataxia and neuropathy, seizures (reported in two-thirds of the patients), ophthalmoplegia (one-half), clinical myopathy (rare). This disorder was previously defined as recessive ataxia syndrome: MIRAS and sensory ataxia neuropathy dysarthria and ophthalmoplegia: SANDO.

Autosomal Recessive progressive external ophthalmoplegia (arPEO) and Autosomal Dominant progressive external ophthalmoplegia (adPEO) are characterized by myopathy, variable sensorineural hearing loss, axonal neuropathy, ataxia, depression, parkinsonism, hypogonadism, and cataracts (previously defined as CPEO plus). Seizures are uncommon; however, few patients may have signs reminding those observed in MELAS syndrome, including stroke-like episodes and seizures (Deschauer et al, 2007). These syndromes are typically associated with mutations in the nuclear-encoded DNA polymerase-gamma gene (gene map locus: 15q25).

The syndrome variably defined as Alpers' disease, Alpers' syndrome, Alpers-Huttenlocher's disease, progressive neuronal degeneration of childhood, progressive sclerosing poliodystrophy or progressive infantile poliodystrophy is characterized by neuronal degeneration of the cerebral cortex and elsewhere, caused by recessive mutations in nDNA, coding for the mitochondrial DNA polymerase-gamma. In this syndrome, the onset is usually before age four years and up to age 25-35; often there is pre-existing developmental delays of variable severity. The syndrome is characterized by seizures, episodic psychomotor regression, liver dysfunction or failure, which may follow exposure to certain antiepileptic medication. The electro-clinical pattern is typically characterized by periodic EEG and epilepsia partialis continua.

5. Leigh syndrome

Leigh syndrome also defined as "subacute necrotizing encephalomyelopathy" is characterized by focal, bilateral, and symmetric necrotic lesions associated with demyelination, vascular proliferation, and gliosis in the brain stem, diencephalon, basal ganglia, cerebellum, and (occasionally) cerebral white matter.

The syndrome has early onset with hypotonia, failure to thrive, psychomotor regression, and brain stem and basal ganglia dysfunction with ataxia, ocular movement abnormalities, dystonia, and swallowing and respiratory disturbances. It can be inherited as autosomal recessive trait or as autosomal dominant or X-linked mechanism, while other patients show maternal inheritance (MILS). It can be associated with functional or molecular defects in several enzyme systems (pyruvate dehydrogenase complex: PDHC), respiratory chain complexes I-IV (cytochrome c oxidase: COX), and mitochondria-encoded ATPase 6 subunit of complex V.

Molecular exams could identify heterogeneous mutations in various mitochondrial and nuclear genes coding for complex I, complex III and complex IV and complex V gene. Mutations have been found also in genes encoding mitochondrial tRNA proteins (MTTV, MTTK, MTTW, and MTTL1) and in components of the pyruvate dehydrogenase complex (e.g. PDHA1: X-linked Leigh syndrome). The French-Canadian (or Saguenay-Lac Saint Jean) type of Leigh syndrome with COX deficiency (LSFC) is caused by mutation in the LRPPRC gene. Deficiency of coenzyme Q10 can present as Leigh syndrome.
In the Leigh syndrome, both generalized and focal seizures have been described, according to genetic and biochemical heterogeneity.

6. Non-syndromic pictures

Seizures can manifest in many patients with infantile MEs, who were diagnosed on the bases of their biochemical defects but still not classified genetically. Epilepsy may manifest as catastrophic neonatal forms, neonatal myoclonic encephalopathies, infantile spasms, refractory status epilepticus, epilepsia partialis continua, myoclonic epilepsy (El Sabbagh et al , 2010), Landau Kleffner, Lennox-Gastaut syndromes, unclassified generalized epilepsy or partial epilepsy (Canafoglia et al, 2001; Lee et al, 2008). Thus, epilepsy may be either focal or generalized and its severity varies in different case series, though the appearance of drug-resistant seizures possibly marks a severe turn in the disease with high risk of neurological deterioration and fatal outcome (El Sabbagh et al , 2010).
Among various biochemical defects, it's worth noting complex I deficiency. Complex I deficiency, due to mutations in mtDNA genes coding for ND subunits, has been described in patients with heterogeneous syndromic (MELAS, Leigh) and non-syndromic MEs, frequently associated with severe epilepsy (Antozzi et al, 1995; Malfatti et al, 2007).
Mitochondrial dysfunctions may be implicated also in sporadic forms of partial epilepsy such is temporal lobe epilepsy, since severe impairment of the respiratory chain activity has been detected *in vitro* on hippocampus samples from patients with drug resistant epilepsy. This observation was also supported by various evidences obtained *in vivo* using neuroimaging techniques (Zsurka and Kunz, 2010).

7. Pyruvate dehydrogenase (PDH) Deficiency (MIM ID #312170)

Pyruvate dehydrogenase complex (PDHC) is a mitochondrial matrix enzyme complex that catalyzes the oxidative decarboxylation of pyruvate to acetyl CoA, nicotinamide adenine dinucleotide (the reduced form, NADH), and CO2. This reaction constitutes the bridge between anaerobic and aerobic cerebral energy metabolism. The great majority of PDH complex deficiencies results from mutations in the X-linked pyruvate dehydrogenase (E1) alpha subunit gene (PDHA1). Gene map locus: *Xp22.2-p22.1*.
The clinical severity can vary from early neonatal presentation with severe lactic acidosis to a progressive disease with mental retardation and neurological complications. Some females are only mildly affected or asymptomatic in relation to the pattern of X-inactivation.
Epilepsy has been reported with a high frequency in children with PDH deficiency (Canafoglia et al, 2001; Kang et al, 2007). Epilepsy is frequently severe and may have variable characteristics including some forms of epileptic encephalopathy.

8. Guidelines for the recognition of patients with mitochondrial DNA disease

Guidelines for recognition of patients with mitochondrial DNA disease should include the detection of the classic syndromes; however, in non-syndromic cases, may be useful the recognition of characteristic clinical features (for example, myoclonus) or specific combinations of symptoms (for example, strokes and migraine and seizures and ataxia). Typically, in the mitochondrial encephalopathies, the observed symptoms may be referred to the involvement of many organ systems, for example, diabetes and deafness.

Besides the clinical observation, characteristic MRI findings may orientate the diagnostic work-up.

Laboratory exams should include the determination of the lactic acidaemia, which is frequently elevated in children in case of mitochondrial encephalopathy. Finally, the muscle biopsy may reveal ragged-red fibres or cytochrome c oxidase-deficient fibres. (Falk, 2010)

Among other symptoms, epileptic presentation may include isolated seizure or isolated status, intermittent seizures or status, severe epilepsies, focal or multifocal epilepsies, generalized seizures and myoclonus (mainly progressive myoclonus epilepsies).

Though not always associated with MEs, myoclonus, epilepsia partialis continua, status epilepticus and intractable epilepsy should be considered common symptoms of these disorders.

9. References

Antozzi C, Franceschetti S, Filippini G, Barbiroli B, Savoiardo M, Fiacchino F, Rimoldi M, Lodi R, Zaniol P, Zeviani M. Epilepsia partialis continua associated with NADH-coenzyme Q reductase deficiency. J Neurol Sci. 1995;129:152-61.

Canafoglia L, Franceschetti S, Antozzi C, Carrara F, Farina L, Granata T, Lamantea E, Savoiardo M, Uziel G, Villani F, Zeviani M, Avanzini G. Epileptic phenotypes associated with mitochondrial disorders. Neurology. 2001;56:1340-6.

Ciafaloni E, Ricci E, Shanske S, Moraes CT, Silvestri G, Hirano M, Simonetti S, Angelini C, Donati MA, Garcia C, Martinuzzi A, Mosewich R, Servidei S, Zammarchi E, Bonilla E, DeVivo DC, Rowland LP, Schon EA, DiMauro S. MELAS: clinical features, biochemistry, and molecular genetics. Ann Neurol 1992;31: 391-398.

Deschauer M, Tennant S, Rokicka A, He L, Kraya T, Turnbull DM, Zierz S, Taylor RW. MELAS associated with mutations in the POLG1 gene. Neurology 2007;68: 1741-1742.

Desguerre I, Pinton F, Nabbout R, Moutard ML, N'Guyen S, Marsac C, Ponsot G, Dulac O. Infantile spasms with basal ganglia MRI hypersignal may reveal mitochondrial disorder due to T8993G MT DNA mutation. Neuropediatrics. 2003;34:265-9.

Falk MJ. Neurodevelopmental manifestations of mitochondrial disease. J Dev Behav Pediatr. 2010;31:610-21. Review.

Finsterer J. Central nervous system imaging in mitochondrial disorders. Can J Neurol Sci 2009;36:143-53. Review.

Fukuhara N, Tokiguchi S, Shirakawa K, Tsubaki T. Myoclonus epilepsy associated with ragged-red fibres (mitochondrial abnormalities): disease entity or a syndrome?

Light-and electron-microscopic studies of two cases and review of literature. J Neurol Sci 1980;47:117-33

Goto Y, Horai S, Matsuoka T, Koga Y, Nihei K, Kobayashi M, Nonaka I. Mitochondrial myopathy, encephalopathy, lactic acidosis, and stroke-like episodes (MELAS): a correlative study of the clinical features and mitochondrial DNA mutation. Neurology 1992;42: 545-550.

Iizuka T, Sakai F, Suzuki N, Hata T, Tsukahara S, Fukuda M, Takiyama Y. Neuronal hyperexcitability in stroke-like episodes of MELAS syndrome.Neurology 2002;59:816–24.

Iizuka T, Sakai F, Kan S, Suzuki N. Slowly progressive spread of the stroke-like lesions in MELAS. Neurology 2003;61:1238–44.

Kang HC, Kwon JW, Lee YM, Kim HD, Lee HJ, Hahn SH. Nonspecific mitochondrial disease with epilepsy in children: diagnostic approaches and epileptic phenotypes. Childs Nerv Syst. 2007;23:1301-7.

Lee YM, Kang HC, Lee JS, Kim SH, Kim EY, Lee SK, Slama A, Kim HD. Mitochondrial respiratory chain defects: underlying etiology in various epileptic conditions. Epilepsia. 2008;49(4):685-90.

Malfatti E, Bugiani M, Invernizzi F, de Souza CF, Farina L, Carrara F, Lamantea E, Antozzi C, Confalonieri P, Sanseverino MT, Giugliani R, Uziel G, Zeviani M. Novel mutations of ND genes in complex I deficiency associated with mitochondrial encephalopathy. Brain. 2007;130:1894-904.

Mancuso M, Filosto M, Mootha VK, Rocchi A, Pistolesi S, Murri L, DiMauro S, Siciliano GA. novel mitochondrial tRNA-phe mutation causes MERRF syndrome. Neurology 2004;62:2119-2121.

Melone MAB, Tessa A, Petrini S, Lus G, Sampaolo S, di Fede G, Santorelli FM, Cotrufo R. Revelation of a new mitochondrial DNA mutation (G12147A) in a MELAS/MERFF phenotype. Arch Neurol 2004;61: 269-272.

Nakamura M, Nakano S, Gato Y-i, Ozawa M, Nagahama Y, Fukuyama H, Akiguchi I, Kaji R, Kimura, J. A novel point mutation in the mitochondrial tRNA (ser(UCN)) gene detected in a family with MERRF/MELAS overlap syndrome. Biochem Biophys Res Commun 1995;214: 86-93.

Roger J, Pellissier JF, Dravet C, Bureau-Paillas M, Arnoux M, Larrieu JL. Spinocerebellar degeneration, optic atrophy, epilepsy, myoclonus and mitochondrial myopathy: a case report. Rev Neurol (Paris) 1982;138:187-200.

Shoffner JM, Wallace DC. Mitochondrial genetics: principles and practice. Am J Hum Genet 1992;51:1179-1186.

Spinazzola A, Zeviani M. Disorders of nuclear-mitochondrial intergenomic signaling. Gene. 2005 Jul 18;354:162-8. Review.

Tiranti V, Hoertnagel K, Carrozzo R, Galimberti C, Munaro M, Granatiero M, Zelante L, Gasparini P, Marzella R, Rocchi M, Bayona-Bafaluy MP, Enriquez JA, Uziel G, Bertini E, Dionisi-Vici C, Franco B, Meitinger T, Zeviani M. Mutations of SURF-1 in Leigh disease associated with cytochrome c oxidase deficiency. Am J Hum Genet. 1998;63:1609-21.

Wu S-B Ma YS, Wu YT, Chen YC, Wei YH. Mitochondrial DNA mutation-elicited oxidative stress, oxidative damage, and altered gene expression in cultured cells of patients with MERRF syndrome. Mol Neurobiol. 2010;41(2-3):256-66. Review.

Zsurka G, Kunz WS. Mitochondrial dysfunction in neurological disorders with epileptic phenotypes. J Bioenerg Biomembr 2010;42(6):443-8. Review.

16

Social and Psychological Issues in Patients with Epilepsy

Tai Sharon
University of Malaya
Malaysia

1. Introduction

1.1 Background and purpose

Patients with epilepsy commonly have associated psychological, psychiatric and social issues. The objective is to look into the psychosocial problems that are encountered by the patients with epilepsy.

1.2 Methods

The literature on psychosocial issues of patients with epilepsy will be reviewed. The differences of the issues between the two genders are also explored. We also would like to look into the literature regarding the differences in the social and psychological issues in the western countries as compared to the Asian countries.

1.3 Results

A high number of patients with epilepsy have depressive illness and psychosis. They also have higher rate of suicidal attempts or ideation. They also have negative social skills and impaired coping mechanisms. Unemployment and higher anxiety states are more frequent for women with epilepsy as compared to men with epilepsy. Female patients have more difficulty finding life partners and have higher rate of divorce compared with males. Women with epilepsy rarely use constructive coping methods, and thus have poor psychosocial status and adjustment within the family and society.

1.4 Conclusions

Patients with epilepsy have higher risk of psychiatric problems with behavioural changes. Female patients tend to have more mood disorders and social problems in comparison to male patients.

2. Epileptic patients with social and psychological issues

Epilepsy is a common illness in the world. Epilepsy affects 50 million people worldwide. (1) Epilepsy is a chronic illness. The disease results 1% of days lost to ill health globally. (2) Epilepsy is characterised as recurrent, intermittent seizures unprovoked by any acute medical condition or transient brain disorder. (2) Epilepsy is the fourth most common neurologic disease. (3) One in 26 people develops epilepsy during the lifetime. (3)

Epilepsy is one of the most common serious neurological diseases in childhood. (4) Epilepsy is ranked second in a range of health conditions.(5) The incidence of epilepsy is slightly higher in male patients with epilepsy.(6)

Patients with epilepsy commonly have multiple psychological, psychiatric and social problems due to their illness. (7, 8, 9) and also due to medication. There is significant psychological and social impact of epilepsy.(1)

Epilepsy is associated with increased mortality, including increased risk of sudden unexpected death. (2) Epilepsy can also result in morbidity which may be physical occurring directly from seizures. (2) The patients can also have cognitive delay, speech difficulties, language difficulties or learning disabilities. (2) Epilepsy can also result in aggressive behaviour or psychosocial issues.(2)

Patients frequently have poor knowledge of epilepsy. (10) Thus, they are more prone to having low self-esteem.

Epileptic patients feel stigmatised by the society and they develop social maladjustment as well. (11) They have multiple social problems such as social withdrawal, ostracism and low self-esteem. (7, 12) These issues may be due to attitude and perception of the society. (7) People with epilepsy are wrongly perceived as having mental health and also being antisocial. (1)

Twenty-five percent of adults having epilepsy describe social stigma as a result of their epilepsy (1) The patients fear rejection from their peers and from other people. (1) Many a times, they feel lonely (1) and feel being outcast from society.

Stigma is associated with poor psychosocial health outcomes in people with epilepsy. (13) Epilepsy stigma can be categorised into internalized, interpersonal, and institutional. (14) The stigma is based on misunderstandings and wrong conception that are present for many years. (1) Despite modernisation of society, there are still wrong concepts and ideas about patients with epilepsy, resulting in difficult social environment for the patients. (14)

Some people may have wrong beliefs and stereotypes with negative expectations of patients with epilepsy. (5) There is an association between stigma and poor quality of life. (14)

However, there are some improvements in public attitudes towards epilepsy as compared to before. (14, 15) A study in France showed that there is improvement of public attitudes towards epilepsy. (16)

The majority of people in the public in France who participated in the survey felt that people with epilepsy should have the opportunity to get married and that children with epilepsy should be allowed to go to school with others. (16) However, there are still gaps of wrong beliefs and knowledge among the men, elderly and people from the lower educational group.(16)

In a Middle Eastern country Jordan, a study was done where 16,044 people from different areas in the country were interviewed with questionnaire. (17) Eighty-eight percent of the people interviewed had knowledge about epilepsy. (17) About 85% of the people surveyed, believed that epilepsy is a neurological disease. (17)

Around 80% of the participants in Jordan thought that there is loss of consciousness with epilepsy. (17) The younger participants and those with higher education had more knowledge on causes and symptoms of epilepsy with statistically significance. (17)

The Jordanian participants also believed that people with epilepsy are able to have children and to have high educational level, such as degrees. (17) However, about 10% of respondents had negative attitudes, and believed that patients with epilepsy have mental disorder. (17)

A large proportion of Jordanian participants (88.5%) objected to the marriage of epileptic patients with epilepsy to the participants' children. (17) One third of the respondents believed that epilepsy is more serious compared to diabetes mellitus and hypertension. (17) The knowledge and attitudes of Jordanians towards epilepsy is almost similar to the results from Asia. However the results are more negative than results from the West.(17)

There was a study done in New Zealand. (15) A survey of community knowledge and attitudes toward epilepsy was carried out. (15) Telephone interviews were conducted on 400 people aged more than 17 years old from a provincial town.(15) Attitudes toward people with epilepsy were favorable.(15) Ninety-five percent of the participants had knowledge about epilepsy.(15)

The respondents who were less knowledgeable were the younger people, the people with less education and lower socioeconomic status with those of Maori or non-European ethnicity.(15) Only 5% of the respondents objected to their children marrying an epileptic patient. (15) Less positive attitudes were found among the older people. (15) People in New Zealand have good knowledge of epilepsy.(15) The attitudes of New Zealanders to epilepsy are positive.(15)

There was another study done in Hungary with recruitment of 1000 respondents from the general public who interviewed with questionnaire in 1994 and in 2000. (18) The participants had prejudice towards employment of patients with epilepsy.(18) However, in recent years, there was a significant decrease in stigmatisation towards regarding marriage of people with epilepsy.(18) There could be culture-specific characteristics of understanding epilepsy.(18)

The patients, relatives and the general public may have misunderstanding or wrong conception about the disease and therefore, have unnecessary fear about the disease and consequences of disease and therapy. (7) One study reported that social skills are inversely proportionate to depression and negative social skills are inversely associated with anxiety. (19)

Financial issue is a major problem for the patients. (20) Most epileptic live with their parents, foster homes or institutions as reported by a Dutch study. (21) The longer the duration of epilepsy is, the worse the psychological issues are. (22) They have impaired quality of life, such as loneliness. (23)

Epileptic patients have poor education and achievement later on in life. (21) Patients who have epilepsy at school age have worse learning achievement. (21)

Learning disorders are disorders that interfere with academic performance or with daily activities that require reading, writing or mathematical skills in subjects with a normal intelligence quotient. (4)

Learning disorders are more common in children with epilepsy than in the general population. (4) Therefore, the risk of cognitive impairment in children with epilepsy is high. (4) Learning disorders are affected by the type of epileptic syndrome, the age of onset and the antiepileptic treatment.(4)

Even some children who have relatively benign form of epilepsy such as, benign childhood epilepsy with centrotemporal spikes (BECTS), they have delayed reading, counting or spelling ability by about one academic year. (24)

Some children with BECTS have poorer drawing and visuo-spatial skills and visuo-spatial memory compared to children of normal population.(24) However, their verbal functions and memory remain intact.(24)

Adolescent patients with epilepsy have more depression, anhedonia, social anxiety and obsessive symptoms than patients in general population of same age group. (25) They have low self- esteem. (10) Generally, higher seizure frequency is associated with low self-esteem. (25)

Patients with tonic-clonic seizures have higher levels of depression. (25) Poor knowledge of epilepsy is significantly associated with higher level of depression, lower self-esteem and higher level of social anxiety. (25)

They have problems with finding their self- identity. (13) They also are more prone to being stigmatized by the society. (13) There are significant negative attitudes in the adolescent public globally worldwide, resulting in loneliness and social avoidance in school.(1)

Vocational issue is common in epileptic patients, as they have high unemployment rates and frequently work in underpaid jobs. (7) One of the reasons for employment problems of patients with epilepsy is the attitude of employers. (26)

The problem is worse in the female patients as they have a higher rate of unemployment. (27) Epileptic patients have difficulty in finding life partners or have children. (21) There is a tendency for them to be single. (7) They also have difficulties in achieving independence in their life. (7)

A study was done in South Korea regarding employment of people with epilepsy. (28) People with epilepsy have higher rate of unemployment (five times higher) at around 30% compared to general population.(28) The people with epilepsy who are unemployed have significantly lower quality of life than the employed ones.(28)

The employability of people with epilepsy was influenced by the frequency and severity of seizures, age at onset, interseizure psychosocial disabilities including self-esteem, personality, and problem-solving style and social discrimination.(28) There was stigmatization and misconception in employment of people with epilepsy. (28)

Nearly one quarter of the participants thought that they were treated unfairly at work or when trying to look for jobs. (28) More than half of those who disclosed their disease to employers said that they were refused jobs due to their illness.(28) About 75% of the patients mentioned that they did not reveal their disease when applying for job.(28)

There was a study done in United Kingdom looking at the attitudes of employers to people with epilepsy. (26) There were 204 respondents. (26) Nearly one quarter of the participants had experience of employing patients with epilepsy. (26) Sixteen percent considered that there were no jobs in their company suitable for people with epilepsy. (26) About 20% of the respondents thought that by employing people with epilepsy, it would be "a major issue." (26)

Employers believed that patients with epilepsy, even when in remission, should inform the condition of their illness to the employer. (26) Seizure severity and frequency are important when employers consider epileptic patients for employment, as half of the employers are worried of work-related accidents. (26) They are willing to give flexible working hours to epileptic patients. (26) Company size and type of company influence employability of people with epilepsy.(26)

Epilepsy is associated with reduced quality of life. (29) Patients with epilepsy generally have impaired coping skills or mechanisms especially female patients. (30) Patients who have seizures that are well controlled have better coping skills and better quality of life. (21) However, socioeconomic status can be an additional protective factor. (29)

Important predictors of good outcome are good quality of life at the beginning and few side effects of therapy. (29) Significant predictors of poor outcome were poor health perception and presence of depression. (29)

Patients on antiepileptic medications, also have worse social functioning. (21) Emotional problems are prevalent in the patients in the West and in Asia. (7, 11) Education plays an important role in assisting the patients cope with their illness. (30) In an interesting study in Holland, patients with epilepsy cope well with their epilepsy despite having worse psychosocial consequences than general population. (21)

A high number of patients with epilepsy have depressive illness (31) and psychosis. They also have problems with interpersonal relationship. (7) They also have higher rate of suicidal attempts or ideation. (32, 33)

Suicide in people with epilepsy is about four times more common than healthy people. (32) The major risk factors for suicidal ideation in epilepsy are depression and psychiatric symptoms. (33) Male patients with temporal lobe epilepsy have higher risk for suicidal behaviour. (34)

Patients with epilepsy are more anxious. (35) Different types of epilepsy can present with different types of psychiatric disorders. (19) Patients who suffer from juvenile myoclonic epilepsy tend to have anxiety and mood disorders. (19) Patients with mesial temporal sclerosis more commonly have psychotic disorders. (19)

Male patients with epilepsy have less sexual desire and lower erectile function compared to normal population.(36) They have higher sex hormone binding globulin levels and lower dehydroepiandrosterone level.(36)

There are gender-specific issues with regards to patients with epilepsy. Worsening anxiety is more frequent for women with epilepsy. (27) Female patients tend to have more mood disorders and social problems in comparison to male patients. (27)

Women with epilepsy have more comorbidities. (27) Female patients with epilepsy have more difficulty finding life partners compared with male patients. (27) They have more problems with marriage and therefore have increased risk of divorce. (27)

Female patients with epilepsy have increased risk of seizure at certain phases of menstrual cycle. (6) There is an increase in seizures during the second half of the menstrual cycle. (37) During menopause, about 40% of women report worsening of their seizure disorder, 27% improve, and a third had no change. (38) Hormone replacement therapy in postmenopausal women can also worsen the seizures. (6)

In a study in India, female patients with epilepsy in India between 15-40 years old had little quality of life. (30) Female patients have more difficulty finding life partners and have higher rate of divorce compared with males. Women with epilepsy rarely use constructive coping methods and they use less problem solving techniques. (30) As a result there is poor psychosocial status and adjustment within the family and society.

Epilepsy and the anticonvulsant therapy have effect on female reproductive function such as menstruation and fertility. (39) Both the disease and medication can cause menstrual disorder and infertility. (39) There is also an increase in polycystic ovaries and hyperandrogenism associated with sodium valproate therapy.(40)

In another recent study in India, 38.4% of 375 women with epilepsy had infertility. (41) The most common causes of infertility were treatment with numerous antiepileptic drugs, older age, and lower education. (41)

This association between low education and was in contrast to the observations from population studies where higher education status is associated with lower fertility. (41) A study in Great Britain showed that women with treated epilepsy from 25 to 39 years of age had 33% reduction in fertility. (42)

Antiepileptic medication which are liver-enzyme inducers, reduce the serum concentration of bioactive sex steroids. (43) Anticonvulsant treatment such as sodium valproate, which is liver enzyme inhibitor, increases the serum concentration of androgens. (43)

There can also be potential drug interaction between antiepileptic drugs and oral contraceptive pills. (44) This drug interaction can cause worsening of frequency of seizure or unplanned pregnancies. (44) There are potential drug interactions between the combined oral contraceptive pills and liver microsomal-inducing anti-epileptic medication such as, phenytoin, barbiturates, carbamazepine, topiramate (at dose>200 mg daily), oxcarbazepine and lamotrigine.(37) Antiepileptic medication which are liver-enzyme inducers, reduce the serum concentration of bioactive sex steroids. (43)

Nonenzyme-inducing AEDs (sodium valproate, benzodiazepines, ethosuximide and levetiracetam) do not show drug interaction with the combined oral contraceptive pill. (38) Anticonvulsant treatment such as sodium valproate, which is liver enzyme inhibitor, increases the serum concentration of androgens. (43)

There are no contraindications to the use of non-hormonal methods of contraception in women with epilepsy.(38)

There is also a decrease in childbirth rates in patients with epilepsy. (41) The childbirth rate in female patients with epilepsy is 25% lower compared to women in the general population. (39) Female patients with epilepsy have reduced sexual interest. (45) In some female patients with epilepsy, the desire and arousal phases may be inhibited.(38)

As for treatment during pregnancy, the teratogenic risks of anticonvulsant drugs such as spina bifida and the seizure control of the pregnant mothers need to be balanced. (6) Pre-conception counselling should be given to women with epilepsy who are thinking about getting pregnant. (37) Female patients with epilepsy should be informed about certain issues, including methods and consequences of prenatal screening, labour, breast feeding and care of a child. (37)

Preconceptional folic acid (at least 0.4 mg) is given to prevent major congenital malformations in the babies of women with epilepsy who are taking anticonvulsant medications. (46) During pregnancy, the lowest effective dose of the most appropriate anticonvulsant drug should be given. (37) There is more teratogenesis with sodium valproate is than carbamazepine.(37) The combination of sodium valproate and lamotrigine is especially teratogenic. (37)

Pregnancy probably causes increased amount in the clearance and decreased concentration of lamotrigine, phenytoin, and to a lesser extent carbamazepine. (46) Pregnancy possibly decreases the concentration of levetiracetam and the active oxcarbazepine metabolite, the monohydroxy derivative. (46)

The majority of infants are delivered healthy with no increased risk of obstetric complications in female patients with epilepsy. (37) Monitoring of lamotrigine, carbamazepine, and phenytoin levels during pregnancy should be considered.(46) Monitoring of levetiracetam and oxcarbazepine (as monohydroxy derivative) levels may be considered.(46)

Breastfeeding is not contraindicated in babies of female patients with epilepsy. (37) The antiepileptic medication concentration in breast milk follows the plasma concentration curve. (37) The total amount of drug transferred to babies via breast milk is much smaller than the amount transferred via the placenta during pregnancy. (37) However, repeated administration of lamotrigine via breast milk may lead to accumulation in the baby. (37)

Primidone and levetiracetam probably transfer into breast milk in amounts that may be clinically important. (46) Sodium valproate, phenobarbital, phenytoin, and carbamazepine probably are not transferred into breast milk in clinically important amounts. (46)

The risk of the child being harmed depends on the type of seizure and its severity and frequency.(38) The risk is small if the mothers and caregivers are trained in safety precautions.(38)

Female patients with epilepsy may have problems with bone health. (37) Women with epilepsy are at increased risk of fractures, osteoporosis and osteomalacia.(37)

In a study in Zimbabwe, it is uncertain whether epileptic patients living in the rural areas have more disability compared to the urban location. (47) In another African country, Nigeria, epilepsy is considered as a stigmatizing disease. (48) The Nigerian patients who have epilepsy face social discrimination in the areas of employment, marriage, housing and education similar to patients from other parts of the world. (48)

Patents with epilepsy need proper and adequate management. Management of psychosocial problems of epileptic patients includes adequate counseling therapy. (11) Social support is beneficial for patients with epilepsy as they have problems with social integration. (49)

Formation of social support groups will benefit the patients. (11) Social support groups can provide assistance in terms of important emotional and social support. (23) These groups can provide resources for the patient in helping them communicate with the society. (23)

This is a good type of professional support given to patients. (33) This support can be given as an addition to conventional therapy. (23) This will help improve patients' quality of life. (33)

Family counseling will also be helpful. (7) Social network and access to information about epilepsy should be given to patients. (25) Educational campaigns are necessary to improve public perception about epilepsy.(17)

Psychosocial interventions are important for the patients. (50) Psychosocial interventions are useful to increase self-mastery and promote positive adjustment to a diagnosis, which therefore will improve the patients' quality of life.(29)

A study which was done on adolescent patients with epilepsy showed that educational intervention can lead to improvement in knowledge of illness and attitude to the disease with statistical significance. (10) The patients enjoyed the sessions and found them invaluable. (10)

To be able to assist people with epilepsy, doctors should be aware of social resources and social welfare systems that are available for the patients. (49) Medical doctors should also perform thorough screening of epilepsy patients for depression and other psychiatric problems. (33) If they have any psychiatric issues, they need to be given treatment early and managed appropriately.

Proper treatment should be given to these patients to reduce suicidal behaviour. (33) In summary, rehabilitation in epilepsy is important in prevention and treatment of psychosocial disorders. (7)

Epilepsy self-management interventions which address issues such as, health care needs, medical adherence, depression, anxiety, employment, and sleep problems have been investigated. (51) Programmes such as, self-management programmes involving face-to-face individual or group meetings led by an epilepsy professional can be organized.(51)

Sessions that focus on education sessions such as, managing disability and leading a healthy lifestyle can be done. (51) Emotional coping strategies and emotional self-management can also be organized. (51)

3. Conclusion

In conclusion, patients with epilepsy irrespective of location in the world generally have numerous psychosocial problems related to disease and treatment. Women with epilepsy have more mood disturbance and social problems compared to male patients.

4. References

[1] Bandstra NF, Camfield CS, Camfield PR. Stigma of epilepsy. *Can J Neurological Science.* 2008 Sep;35(4):436-40.

[2] Maree L Hackett, Nicholas S Glozier, Alexandra L Martiniuk, Stephen Jan, Craig S Anderson. Sydney epilepsy incidence study to measure illness consequences: the SESIMIC observational epilepsy study protocol. *BMC Neurol.* 2011; 11: 3.

[3] D.C. Hesdorffer, G. Logroscino, E.K.T. Benn, N. Katri, G. Cascino, W.A. Hauser. Estimating risk for developing epilepsy: A population-based study in Rochester, Minnesota. *Neurology.* 2011;76:23–27.

[4] Pavlou E, Gkampeta A. Learning disorders in children with epilepsy. *Chils Nerv Syst.* 2011 Mar;27(3):373-9.

[5] Jacoby A, Gorry J, Gamble C, Baker GA. Public knowledge, private grief: a study of public attitudes to epilepsy in the United Kingdom and implications for stigma. *Epilepsia.* 2004 Nov;45(11):1405-15.

[6] Pennell PB, Thompson P. Gender-specific psychosocial impact of living with epilepsy. *Epilepsy Behav.* 2009 Jun; 15 Suppl 1:S20-5.

[7] Alvarado L, Ivanovic-Zuvic F, Candia X, et al. Psychosocial evaluation of adults with epilepsy in Chile. *Epilepsia.* 1992;33: 651–6.

[8] Kogeorgos J, Fonagy P, Scott DF. Psychiatric symptom patterns of chronic epileptics attending a neurological clinic: a controlled investigation. *Br J Psychiatry.* 1982;140: 236–43.

[9] Hermann B, Jacoby A. The psychosocial impact of epilepsy in adults. *Epilepsy Behaviour.* 2009 Jun; 15 Suppl 1:S11-6.

[10] Frizzell CK, Connolly AM, Beavis E, Lawson JA, Bye AM. Personalised epilepsy education intervention for adolescents and impact on knowledge acquisition and psychosocial function. *J Paediatric Child Hea*lth. 2011 Jan 18.

[11] Vanessa W. Y. Lau, Tatia M. C. Lee, Philip K. K. Ng, Virginia C. N. Wong. Psychosocial Adjustment of People with Epilepsy in Hong Kong. *Epilepsia.* 2001 Sep;42(9):1169–1175.

[12] Collings, J. The impact of epilepsy on self-perceptions. *J Epilepsy* 1990;8: 164–71.

[13] MacLeod JS, Austin JK. Stigma in the lives of adolescents with epilepsy: a review of the literature. *Epilepsy Behav.* 2003 Apr;4(2):112-7.

[14] Jacoby A, Austin JK. Social stigma for adults and children with epilepsy. *Epilepsia.* 2007;48 Suppl 9:6-9.

[15] Hills MD, MacKenzie HC. New Zealand community attitudes toward people with epilepsy. *Epilepsia.* 2002 Dec;43(12):1583-9.

[16] Rafael F, Dubreuil CM, Burbaud F, Tran DS, Clement JP, Preux PM, Nubukpo P. Knowledge of epilepsy in the general population based on two French cities: implications for stigma. *Epilepsia.* 2010 Jan;17(1):82-6.

[17] Daoud A, Al-Safi S, Otoom S, Wahba L, Alkofahi A. Public knowledge and attitudes towards epilepsy in Jordan. *Seizure*. 2007 Sep;16(6):521-6.

[18] Mirnics Z, Czikora G, Závecz T, Halász P. Changes in public attitudes toward epilepsy in Hungary: results of surveys conducted in 1994 and 2000. *Epilepsia*. 2001 Jan;42(1):86-93.

[19] Ma TM, Hou WK, Hung A, Lee TM. Personality traits and social behaviors predict the psychological adjustment of Chinese people with epilepsy. *Seizure*. 2010 Oct; 19(8):493-500.

[20] Dodrill CB, Beier R, Kasparick M, Tacke I, Tacke U, Tan S-Y. Psychosocial problems in adults with epilepsy: Comparison of findings from four countries. *Epilepsia*. 1984;25: 176–83.

[21] Sachin S, Padma MV, Bhatia R, Prasad K, et al. Psychosocial impact of epilepsy in women of childbearing age in India. *Epileptic Disorder*. 2008 Dec;10(4):282-9.

[22] Shackleton DP, Kasteleijn-Nolst Trenite DGA, de Craen AJM, Vandenbroucke JP, Westerndorp RGJ. Living with epilepsy:Long term prognosis and psychosocial outcomes. *Neurology*. 2003;61:64-70.

[23] Chaplin J, Yepez R, Lasso S, et al. National general practice study of epilepsy: the social and psychosocial effects of a recent diagnosis of epilepsy. *Br Med J*. 1992;304: 1416–8.

[24] Theo P. B. M. Suurmeijer, Marieke F. Reuvekamp, Bert P. Aldenkamp. Social Functioning, Psychological Functioning, and Quality of Life in Epilepsy. *Epilepsia*. 2001;42(9):1160-1168.

[25] Pinton F, Ducot B, Motte J, Arbuès AS, Barondiot C, Barthez MA, Chaix Y, Cheminal R, Livet MO, Penniello MJ, Peudenier S, de Saint-Martin A, Billard C. Cognitive functions in children with benign childhood epilepsy with centrotemporal spikes (BECTS). *Epileptic Disord*. 2006 Mar;8(1):11-23.

[26] Baker GA, Spector S, McGrath Y, Soteriou H. Impact of epilepsy in adolescence: a UK controlled study. *Epilepsy Behav*. 2005 Jun;6(4):556-62.

[27] Jacoby A, Gorry J, Baker GA. Employers' attitudes to employment of people with epilepsy: still the same old story? *Epilepsia*. 2005 Dec;46(12):1978-87.

[28] Gopinath M, Sarma PS, Thomas SV. Gender-specific psychosocial outcome for women with epilepsy. *Epilepsy Behav*. 2011 Jan;20(1):44-7.

[29] Lee SA. What we confront with employment of people with epilepsy in Korea. *Epilepsia*. 2005;46 Suppl 1:57-8.

[30] Taylor J, Jacoby A, Baker GA, Marson AG, Ring A, Whitehead M. Factors predictive of resilience and vulnerability in new-onset epilepsy. *Epilepsia*. 2011 Mar;52(3):610-8.

[31] Robertson MM, Trimble MR, Townsend HRA. Phenomenology of depression in epilepsy. *Epilepsia*. 1987;28: 364–72.

[32] Matthews WS & Barabas G. Suicide and epilepsy: a review of the literature. *Psychosomatics*. 1981;22: 515–24.

[33] Lim HW, Song HS, Hwang YH. Predictors of suicidal ideation in people with epilepsy living in Korea. *J Clin Neurol*. 2010 Jun;6(2):81-8.

[34] Kalinin VV, Polyanskiy DA. Gender and suicidality prediction in epilepsy. *Epilepsy Behav*. 2005;7:657–663.

[35] Collings J. Psychosocial well-being and epilepsy: an empirical study. *Epilepsia*. 1990;31: 418–26.

[36] James A. Talbot, Russell Sheldrick, Helen Caswell, Susan Duncan. Sexual function in men with epilepsy:How important is testosterone? *Neurology*. 2008;70:1346–1352.
[37] Crawford PM. Managing epilepsy in women of childbearing age. *Drug Saf.* 2009;32(4):293-307.
[38] Crawford P. Best practice guidelines for the management of women with epilepsy. *Epilepsia*. 2005; 46 Suppl 9:117-24.
[39] Gerhard Luef. Female issues in epilepsy: A critical review. *Epilepsy and Behavior*. 2009;15:78-82.
[40] Isojarvi JI, Laatkainen TJ, Pakarinen AJ, et al. Polycystic ovaries and hyperandrogenism in women taking valproate for epilepsy. *N Engl J Med*. 1993; 329:1383-8.
[41] Sapna Cheravalloor Sukumaran, P. Sankara Sarma, Sanjeev V. Thomas. Polytherapy increases the risk of infertility in women with epilepsy. *Neurology*. 2010;75:1351–1355.
[42] Wallace H, Shorvon S, Tallis R. Age-specific incidence and prevalence rates of treated epilepsy in an unselected population of 2,052,922 and age-specific fertility rates of women with epilepsy. *Lancet*. 1998; 352:1970 –1973.
[43] Isojarvi J. Disorders of reproduction in patients with epilepsy: antiepileptic drug related mechanisms. *Seizure*. 2008; 17:111-9.
[44] Sabers A. Pharmacokinetic interaction s between contraceptives and antiepileptic drugs. *Seizure*. 2008; 17:141-50.
[45] Bergen D, Daugherty S, Eckenfels E. Reduction of sexual activities in females taking antiepileptic drugs. *Psychopathology*. 1992; 25:1-4,
[46] Harden CL, Pennell PB, Koppel BS, Hovinga CA, Gidal B, Meador KJ, Hopp J, Ting TY, et al. Practice parameter update: management issues for women with epilepsy--focus on pregnancy (an evidence-based review): vitamin K, folic acid, blood levels, and breastfeeding: report of the Quality Standards Subcommittee and Therapeutics and Technology Assessment Subcommittee of the American Academy of Neurology and American Epilepsy Society. *Neurology*. 2009 Jul 14;73(2):142-9.
[47] Gerhard Luef. Female issues in epilepsy: A critical review. *Epilepsy and Behavior*. 2009;15:78-82.
[48] Akinsulore A, Adewuya A. Psychosocial aspects of epilepsy in Nigeria: a review. *Afr J Psychiatry (Johannesburg)*. 2010 Nov; 13(5):351-6.
[49] Kubota H. Social support for people with epilepsy. *Brain Nerve*. 2011 Apr; 63(4):401-409.
[50] Schachter SC. Quality of life for patients with epilepsy is determined by more than seizure control: the role of psychosocial factors. *Expert Rev Neurother*. 2006 Jan;6(1):111-8.
[51] Fraser RT, Johnson EK, Miller JW, Temkin N, Barber J, Caylor L, Ciechanowski P, Chaytor N. Managing epilepsy well: self-management needs assessment. *Epilepsy Behav*. 2011 Feb;20(2):291-8.

17

Epilepsy Secondary to Parasitic Zoonoses of the Brain

Humberto Foyaca-Sibat
*Walter Sisulu University, Nelson Mandela Academic Hospital,
Division of Neurology Mthatha,
South Africa*

1. Introduction

In spite of natural disaster like the one we are seeing today in Japan (March 20, 2011) where thousand of peoples died due to earthquake and tsunami and some food are contaminated by radioactivity , and other disasters caused by human beings by different modalities of war like the one we are seeing today at the North of Africa plus different modalities of terrorism, destruction of their environment and so forth; world population continues to grow and there has been ever increasing need to develop and maintain food products with a high protein content (particularly livestock and fish) under intensive farming situations, which is inevitably leading to a greater spread of animal diseases and their transmission to humans (McCarthy & Moore 2000; Keiser & Utzinger 2005).

Improved diagnosis and/or recognition of neglected human infections can account for some diseases apparently emerging or re-emerging in recent times (e.g. Human fascioliasis). Climate change has also been suggested as a cause for disease spread and is a concern for the future (McCarthy & Moore 2000); thousand of wild or domestic animals are becoming sick and birds that usually migrate from one continent to another one they don't do it today. It will bring serious consequences to humans being by the increment of the number of infectious disease is transmitted from animals to humans (known by zoonotic diseases). Zoonotic infectious agents are among the most prevalent on earth and are thought to be responsible for more than 60 per cent of all human infections and 75 per cent of emerging human infectious diseases (Cunningham 2005). The success and widespread epidemiology of these infections can be attributed to a range of human factors including social and dietary changes as well as an increased mobility of the human population (McCarthy & Moore 2000; Vorou *et al.* 2007).

Some zoonotic diseases are grouped as neglected tropical diseases (NTD) which are uncommonly recognized or diagnosed in developed countries; are less well understood than more common infections due to a of lack of research interest and/or insufficient funding; and, lastly, remain mysterious or unknown to health care providers because of minimal or no instruction regarding the diseases during medical students training. However, certain food-borne trematode infections in particular remain "neglected" NTD, according to the World Health Organization. These include clonorchiasis (Chinese liver fluke disease), fascioliasis (sheep liver fluke disease), opisthorchiasis (fish liver fluke disease), and paragonimiasis (lung fluke disease). These diseases most often significantly

affect large numbers of poverty-stricken individuals, generally in resource-limited regions, and receive very little interest from funding or government agencies. As these diseases have complex life cycles and are rarely encountered in the developed world, they receive little attention in the education of physicians, which furthers their enigmatic status.(Tolan, 2011)
For human, domestic animal and wildlife health, key effects of directional climate change include the risk of the altered occurrence of infectious diseases. Many parasite zoonoses have high potential for vulnerability to the new climate, in part because their free-living life-cycle stages and ectothermic hosts are directly exposed to climatic conditions. For these zoonoses, climate change can shift boundaries for ecosystem components and processes integral to parasite transmission and persistence, and these shifts can impact host health. The vulnerable boundaries include those for spatial distributions, host-parasite assemblages, demographic rates, life-cycle phenologies, associations within ecosystems, virulence, and patterns of infection and disease (Polley & Thomson, 2009)
Zoonotic infections of humans are caused by a wide variety of agents including viruses (e.g. avian influenza and rabies), bacteria (e.g. brucellosis and salmonellosis), parasites (e.g. leishmaniasis, schistosomiasis, neurocysticercosis and toxocariasis) and others 'unconventional' agents such as prions (e.g. Bovine spongiform encephalopathy and its variant: Creutzfeldt–Jakob disease). As we previously reported (Foyaca-Sibat et al., 2010), the infectious agent may be transmitted in a variety of ways, as can be seen in Table 1

Direct contact with animal flesh (Tularemia)
Drinking of cows or goats milk ((TB and Brucellosis)
Inhalation of dust particles contaminated by animal excreta or products (Q Fever & Anthrax)
Eating of insufficiently cooked infected flesh (Anthrax, Trichinosis, Taeniosis-*T solium)*
A bite by insect vectors (Plague, Scrub Typhus and Equine Encephalomyelitis) or a bite from a diseased animal (Rabies)
Others ways

Table 1. Some zoonotic infections and its way of transmission

A seizure complication of zoonotic infections can consist of a single seizure or can go on to become chronic epilepsy. Seizures can arise as an acute, sub-acute, or long- term consequence of an infectious states. Seizures are temporary abnormal electro-physiologic phenomena of the brain, resulting in abnormal synchronization of electrical neuronal activity. They can manifest as an alteration in mental state, tonic, clonic or tonic-clonic movements, and various other psychic symptoms (such as déja vu, jamais vu, etc.).
A seizure can last from a few seconds to more than 20 minutes like: status epilepticus, a continuous seizure that will not stop without intervention and patients does not regain their normal level of consciousness between the attacks.
Sometimes, a seizure can also be as subtle as marching numbness of a part of the body, a brief loss of memory, sparkling of flashes, sensing an unpleasant odour, a strange epigastric sensation, a sensation of fear, levitation, laryngeal constriction, peribucal paresthesiae and dysphagia (last four seen in insular seizures).Therefore seizures are typically classified as motor, sensory, autonomic, emotional or cognitive. The type of epileptic complication and

when it arises from an infection depend on the nature of the infectious illness, its duration, and the type and extent of damage to the brain but in general antisezures and antiepileptic treatment follow the same pattern describe for epilepsy secondary to neurocysticercosis(NC). We recommend to readers to consult our book about " Treatment approach to epilepsy"

Human infections caused by parasitic helminths are of particular importance given the relatively recent acknowledgement of a number of species as important human pathogens (McCarthy & Moore 2000; Mas-Coma et al. 2005; Garcia et al. 2007). The main aim of this chapter is to review all information related to parasitic zoonoses of the brain causing epilepsy based on our personal experience and the medical literature and the way forward of toxocariasis (Robinson, 2009).

1.1 Zoonotic diseases

Around the world the three major components of climate change already evident and escalating in magnitude and significance are; 1) warming; 2) altered patterns of precipitation; and 3) an increased incidence of extreme climatic events. For the structure and function of ecosystems, the impacts of climate change vary with place and with time, and among the key outcomes are shifting boundaries for many components and processes within the systems. Among these components are pathogens and infectious diseases, including those caused by helminth, arthropod and protozoan parasites in people, domestic animals, and wildlife (Polley, 2010)

1.1.1 Rabies

From viral zoonotic infections, rabies keeps the leadership in mortality rate. The word "rabies" is derived from a Latin word which means "madness" or "rage" - the very characteristic of people with this disease. A person with this illness usually dies of fatal encephalitis. This disease is caused by the bullet shaped rhabdovirus which is commonly called the rabies virus. The virus is transmitted to a human being when he or she is bitten by an infected animal, usually with dogs. There are reports which claim that even the saliva of those infected animals could cause rabies. Rabies virus from saliva could enter skin scratches and the eyelids. In fact, aerosols of bat secretions in caves have caused rabies to some researchers. Workers who have macerated infected tissues in the laboratory for analysis have acquired the virus and developed the disease; probably aerosols from the macerated tissue entered the workers' mouth, nose, or eye linings. (Sace, 2009) Rabies presents about 30 days after contact with a rabid animal. A nonspecific prodrome of fever, headache, sore throat, and abdominal pain progresses to an agitated, hallucinatory delirium followed by coma and death. Seizures occur in about 10% of cases (Goldstein & Harden, 2002) and rabies vaccine therapy has been excluded as antiseizures treatment many years ago (Inkeman et al., 1938)

1.1.2 Avian influenza

Avian influenza viruses do not typically replicate efficiently in humans, indicating direct transmission of avian influenza virus to humans is unlikely. However, since 1997, several cases of human infections with different subtypes (H5N1, H7N7, and H9N2) of avian influenza viruses have been identified and raised the pandemic potential of avian influenza virus in humans. A better understanding of the biological and genetic basis of host restriction of influenza viruses is a critical factor in determining whether the introduction of a novel influenza virus into the human population will result in a pandemic. (Lee & Saif, 2009) Epilepsy is not a known complication in this group and its presence suggests reviewing the clinical diagnosis.

1.1.3 Slow virus infections

Slow virus infections are also known as prion diseases. Prions are proteinaceous infectious particles (PrPs). The brain pathology of prion diseases consists of a vacuolar (spongiform) degeneration of the neuropil, cortical neurons, and subcortical gray matter with neuronal loss and gliosis. Early diagnosis is difficult, in part because prions do not have nucleic acids, making conventional nucleic acid–based viral detection systems ineffective. PrPs also elude detection by not producing a humoral immune response (Johnson & Gibbs, 1998) As part of this group is: bovine spongiform encephalopathy (BSE) which is thought to have originated in Great Britain where it was first observed (April 1985) and was officially diagnosed. Control measures have since reduced incidence of the disease, and currently fewer than 100 new cases are reported per week. It occurs in cattle between two and eight years old and is always fatal.
A transmissible spongiform encephalopathy of adult cattle, transmitted by feed containing protein in the form of meat and bone meal derived from infected animals. Affected adults may have seizures as part of the serious neurological illness. Renkawek et al (1992), hypothesized that a defect of Na^+/K^+ -ATPase of the astrocytes could be the most common pathogenetic factor for the congenital convulsive status and for the spongy state.
Cellular prion protein (PrP^c) plays an essential role in maintaining neurotransmitter homeostasis in the central nervous system. This discovery has been made possible by the observation that both a deficiency and an excess of the protein have a considerable effect on this homeostasis. Surprisingly, in both cases, the central nervous excitability threshold is altered to such an extent that an epileptic seizure may result. Thanks to this discovery, we now have more tools at our disposal that can help us to deepen our basic understanding of epilepsy. (IBEC, 2009)
As under normal conditions the protein is found in adequate concentrations, it was expected that greater amounts of PrP^c would provide greater protection against seizures. Surprisingly, however, the study showed that this is not the case. With an excessive amount of the protein, the level of excitability of the central nervous system is increased even more than in the absence of PrP^c, due to the fact that both the excitatory and inhibitory mechanisms are altered. Such alterations further increase the possibility of suffering severe epileptic seizures. The protein, when present at adequate concentrations, is essential for maintaining neurotransmitter homeostasis or equilibrium in the central nervous system. The researchers of IBEC who participated in the study are currently involved in developing a description of the possible differences in the expression and modification of the cellular prion protein in epileptic patients. (IBEC, 2009)

1.1.4 Neurobrucellosis

Brucellosis is a major ubiquitous zoonosis transmitted from livestock to humans. It is a public health problem in developing countries. The estimated mean incidence of neurobrucellosis is 4% with clinical manifestations that are variable and often multi-focal in the same patient. (Guenifi et al., 2010)
Neurobrucellosis is a rare form of systemic brucellosis, a disease acquired through ingestion of unpasteurized dairy products, it can affect any part of the nervous system and can mimic any neurological disease which may manifest as stroke, encephalitis, meningitis, or

psychiatric disorders and should suspected in individuals with pyrexia of unknown origin so that early detection and treatment could prevent long-term sequelae such as focal neurologic deficits, hydrocephalus, transient ischemic attack, intracerebral vasculopathy granulomas, seizures, paralysis of sixth and seventh cranial nerves and psychiatric illness and seizures responding well to first AED, doxycycline, rifampin, and ceftriaxone (Obiako et al., 2010; Asuman et al., 2010; Türel et al., 2010).

Early detection and treatment is the only predictor of a favourable outcome of neurobrucellosis, but there is no standardized treatment protocol. Neurobrucellosis may be difficult to diagnose especially in patients with atypical syndromes. Therefore, it should be suspected in patients who experience inexplicable neurological and psychiatric problems and the CSF must be adequately analysed. It should be kept in mind and to be included in differential diagnosis for any patient presenting central or peripheral neurological manifestations especially in the endemic zones. (Guenifi et al., 2010 Tekin-Koruk et al., 2010)

1.1.5 Neurosalmonellosis

Salmonella serotypes *typhi, typhimurium,* and *enteritidis* occurred most frequently. The precipitating factors of these infections included meningitis, trauma, and intracranial hematoma. Focal intracranial infections are unusual manifestations of salmonellosis. In one hundred years only 43 such infections have been reported in the world literature. Brain abscess occurred more often in adults; in contrast, subdural empyema presented more often in children and fever, signs and symptoms of increased intracranial pressure, change in mental status, seizures, and focal neurologic deficits were the commonest clinical features.(Rodriguez et al,. 1986)

2. Zoonotic parasites

Zoonotic parasites are separated into four categories, such as direct-zoonotic, meta-zoonotic, cyclo-zoonotic , and sapro-zoonotic parasites. Direct-zoonotic parasites, such as, *C. parvum, T. gondii,* and *P. carinii* have been prevalent in endemic areas and places where the prevalence of HIV/AIDS is increasing. Meta-zoonotic parasites can infect humans from invertebrate intermediate hosts, such as, *Babesia bovis, Babesia divergens, Plasmodium schwetzi, Clonorchis sinensis, Fasciola hepatica, Paragonimus westermani, Diphyllobothrium latum, Dipylidium caninum, Dirofilaria immitis, Brugia malayi, Onchocerca gibsoni,*and *Polymorphus boschadis* and some of them like *C. sinensis, H. nocens,M. yokogawai, P. westermanii,* and sparganum (*Spirometra* spp.), remain prevalent among people who consume raw freshwater fish or crabs in endemic areas. Cyclo-zoonotic parasites have vertebrate intermediate hosts, such as, *Taenia multiceps, Echinococcus granulosus, Taenia saginata, Taenia solium,* sparganum (*Spirometra* spp.), *Porrocaecum crassum, Contracaecum osculatum, Capillaria hepatica,* and *Gnathostoma spinigerum.* Cyclo-zoonotic parasites, such as, *T. saginata, T. solium,* and *T. asiatica,* are still prevalent in peoples who consumed raw cattle or pig meat and there is a tendency to increase and spread all over the world due to globalization. Sapro-zoonotic parasites mean that parasites can infect humans from soil or water, such as, *Ancylostoma caninum, Ascaris suum, Capillaria hepatica, Strongyloides stercoralis, Trichuris vulpis,* and *Hypoderma bovis.*

Many of carnivorous parasites are zoonotic parasites because dogs and cats have lived with humans for a long period of time. On the other hand, anthroponotic parasites mean that the parasites can be transmitted from humans to animals. Some examples of these are *E. histolytica, C. sinensis, D. latum,* and *Trichuris trichiura.* (Youn H, 2009). On the other hand, along with social, epidemiological and environmental changes, together with improvements in our ability to diagnose helminth infections, several neglected parasite species are now fast-becoming recognized as important zoonotic diseases of humans, e.g. anasakiasis, several fish-borne trematodiasis and fasciolosis.Direct zoonotic parasites infect humans directly from animals, such as:

2.1.1 Neuroamebiasis

There is about 65,000 species of protozoan parasites worldwide. Unicellular organisms, almost all protozoa, live by holozoic nutrition. Protozoa are divided into 5 phyla, Sarcomastigophora, Apicomplexa, Microspora, Myxozoa, and Ciliophora. Sarcomastigophora have flagella or pseudopodia for locomotive organs, reproduce by binary fission, and include *Trichomonas* spp., *Giardia* spp., and amoeba (including *Endolimax nana, Entamoeba coli, E. histolytica,* and *Iodamoeba bu_tschlii*). Amebae can invade the central nervous system, causing rare but fatal infections and seizures can complicate any of the amoeba-caused clinical syndromes.

Although, epidemiologic data are inadequate to comment on the seizure incidence and prevalence is well-known that intracranial infection by *Entamoeba histolytica* can cause brain abscess (Shah et al., 1994) with an associated focal neurological signs, and other signs due to raised intracranial pressure such as: abducens palsy which can be identified ipsilateral or contralateral of the infective mass. Some micro abscess located near to the cerebral cortex can cause partial, partial with secondary generalization or generalized motor seizures but no only *E histolytica* cause neurological manifestation as can be seen in the Table 2.

Zoonotic protozoa	Neurological complications	Clinical features
Entamoeba histolytica	Amebic brain abscess (resembles brain abscess, tumours, chronic meningitis, or a combination of these)	Meningeal sings Focal signs Seizures
Naegleria fowleri	Primary amebic meningoenchephalitis (acute meningoenchephalitis)	Meningeal signs Seizures Stupor/coma
Acanthamoeba or Hartmannella	Granulomatous amebic encephalitis (resembles brain abscess, tumour, chronic meningitis, or a combination of these)	Meningeal signs Seizures Focal deficits Stupor/coma
Plasmodium falciparum. (*P. malariae* and *P. vivax* are infrequent causes of CNS malaria.)????	Cerebral malaria*	Epileptic seizures Coma

*There are concerns that endemic infections and infestations, such as malaria and neurocysticercosis, could be responsible for the increased incidence of epilepsy in the developing world. (Sander & Perucca, 2003)

Table 2. Some protozoans than can infect cerebral hemispheres

2.1.2 Cryptosporidiasis

Cryptosporidial infection can thus be transmitted from fecally contaminated food and water, from animal-person contact, and via person-person contact. The probability of transmission from just a small amount of contamination is fairly high, (DuPont, *et al.*, 1995). Infection is by ingestion of infective oocysts (*Cryptosporidium*) from the environment or from contaminated food or water.

Climate change has the potential to alter survival rates for the cysts and oocysts (which are infective when voided by the hosts) and, because both parasites are found in surface water, shifts in local and regional hydrology may alter parasite distributions and the risks of human and animal exposure. In human settlements altered patterns of precipitation and extreme climatic events may disrupt the integrity of the infrastructure, particularly water supplies and sewage disposal, increasing the risk of human infection. Risk for epilepsy is not certain in most of the cases. In addition, these elements of the climate change may result in increased run-off and contamination of water with animal feces, and increased risk of zoonotic transmission. (Polley, 2010).

2.1.3 Neurotoxoplasmosis

The most important zoonotic protozoa recently are *T. gondii, C. parvum,* and *Pneumocystis carinii* (Hong, 1991; Chai et al., 1996; Choi et al., 1997). The first one affects the nervous system more than others. Before AIDS, reactivation of neurotoxoplasmosis occurred most often in patients with hematologic malignancies. Because many of these patients receive immunosuppressive therapy, the relative contribution of immune dysfunction from malignancy versus immune suppression from drugs is difficult to define. (Dukes, 1997). neurotoxoplasmosis can also occur in patients receiving immunosuppressive chemotherapy after organ transplantation or for collagen vascular disorders. *Toxoplasma gondii* is a causal agent. *T.gondii* is an intracellular protozoan parasite. Most human infections with *T. gondii* are asymptomatic, but it can potentially cause four syndromes as can be seen in Table 3:

Meningoenchephalitis during primary infection of an immunocompetent host
Epilepsy, intracerebral mass lesions or encephalitis in immunocompromised hosts
Retinochoroiditis associated with primary infection or reactivation of an earlier infection
Congenital toxoplasmosis, encephalitis, and retinochoroiditis as a result of transplacental fetal infection. (McCabe et al., 1987)

Table 3. Clinical presentation of neurotoxoplasmosis

The only definitive host for T. gondii is domestic cats. Transmission of T. gondii to humans occurs commonly, usually by eating undercooked meat or by inadvertent ingestion of oocysts from cat feces. Systemic parasitemia occurs after the invasion of the gut lining by toxoplasma and it is certainly associated with seizures and it is one of the most common opportunistic infections in advanced stage of HIV infections, so cases of neurotoxoplasmosis have increased dramatically since 1981. Neurotoxoplasmosis is responsible for over one-third of neurologic symptoms in AIDS patients. (Dukes, 1997). (In contrast, both primary CNS and metastatic lymphoma account for approximately 5% each.) More than 95% of toxoplasmic encephalitis in patients with AIDS is due to reactivation of chronic latent infection. For most HIV-infected patients, toxoplasmic encephalitis develop after the CD4 count falls below 100. (Dukes, 1997). In the United States, 10–40% of AIDS patients are latently infected, and 30–50% of these will develop toxoplasmic encephalitis. (Dukes, 1997)

Clinical manifestations are variable, ranging from an insidious process to an acute confusional state. Reported seizure rates range from 18% to 29% and may include partial, complex partial, and generalized seizures (Porte & Sande, 1992; Ragnaud et al., 1993). Detection of antibodies to Toxoplasma in sera from patients suffering from recurrent unprovoked seizures were performed using "in-house" indirect hemagglutination assay and by commercially available anti-Toxoplasma immunoglobulin G and immunoglobulin M enzyme-linked immunosorbent assays. Serum antibody to toxoplasmosis were detected in 12.3% and 15.3% by indirect hemagglutination assay and enzyme-linked immunosorbent assays and respectively. Controls showed seropositivity of 5.7% for antibodies to Toxoplasma using the same methods. Seropositivity was higher in children compared to adults. Individuals with rural background (living in relatively unhygienic conditions) were more commonly affected compared to people living in urban areas. (Mirdha, 2003)

The presence of positive antibody titters to *Toxoplasma* and *Toxocara* in an adult epileptic population has been examined in relation to other observations of aetiological importance. With *Toxoplasma,* and more particularly with *Toxocara,* a higher incidence of positive antibody titters were recorded than in non-epileptic populations. Comparison with previous studies in childhood epilepsy indicate that the incidence of positive titres increased with age throughout adult life. Reported seizure rates range from 18% to 29% and may include partial, complex partial, and generalized seizures. (http://professionals.epilepsy.com/page/infectious_toxoplas.html)

Despite attention to the age of onset of epilepsy, presumed etiological factors, and electroencephalographic and clinical observations, no causal relationship between parasitic infection and the etiology of epilepsy was established (Critchley et al., 1982). However, Stommel et al. (2001) found a statistically significant correlation between chronic *T. gondii* infection and cryptogenic epilepsy in a group of patients with cryptogenic epilepsy and they proposed that the dormant *T. gondii* cysts containing bradyzoites are responsible for some cases of cryptogenic epilepsy, although other explanations for this finding exist: (a) The cryptogenic subpopulation could be more susceptible to the parasitic infection for reasons unrelated to epilepsy; or (b) The cryptogenic epilepsy patients could be more susceptible to *T. gondii* infection and have intrinsic immunologic differences that predispose them to epilepsy, implying an immune basis to the epilepsy. Because there are certainly multiple etiologies for cryptogenic epilepsy, any statistical analysis may only partially reflect an etiology. In any case, antiparasitic and antiepileptic treatment is mandatory. For more detailed information about antiepileptic and antiseizures medicine please consult our book: "Treatment approach of epilepsy" ISBN 978-953-307-678-2

Therapy for toxoplasmic encephalitis is the combination of pyrimethamine and sulfadiazine. Clindamycin can be used as an alternative to sulfadiazine. Serial neuroimaging provides the best follow-up to assess treatment progress. Maintenance anticonvulsant therapy is usually required. Newborns of women contracting toxoplasmosis during pregnancy should be treated with clindamycin to reduce the likelihood of developing late neurologic sequelae, including seizures.(Georgiev, 1994)

2.1.4 Neurohymenolepiasis

Hymenolepis nana is also known as the Dwarf Tapeworm and it is the cestode that most commonly infects humans, especially school-aged children when they ingest infective eggs from accidental ingestion of insects (immature fleas, flour beetles, meal worms, cockroaches) that carry the parasite in their body cavities, most commonly by direct fecal-oral exposure. Infective eggs are ingested by insects and hatch in their guts. After hatching, they invade into the body cavity and become cysticercoid larvae, which are infectious for humans. After the insects are consumed and digested, the larvae are released in the small intestine and mature within 25 days into 50-cm adults. When the adult tapeworm begins to pass eggs, insect hosts can become infected again.

Most infections produce no symptoms (Craip, 2007). Hymenolepis nana infestations are prevalent in highly populated areas where hygiene and sanitary conditions are poor. The symptom frequency seems to correlate with increasing worm burden and in order of decreasing frequency includes restlessness, irritability, diarrhea, abdominal pain, restless sleep, anal pruritus, and nasal pruritus. Rare symptoms include anorexia, increased appetite, vomiting, nausea, bloody diarrhea, hives, extremity pain, headache, dizziness, behavioural disturbances, and seizures. (Tolan, 2011; Chero et al., 2007).

2.1.5 Neurobaylisascariasis

Baylisascariasis is a rare parasitic infection caused by intestinal nematodes *Baylisascaris* procyonis, the raccoon roundworm (family Ascarididae) in the genus Baylisascaris. The three most pathogenic species are *Baylisascaris procyonis*, a parasite of raccoons (*Procyon lotor*), *B. melis*, which occurs in European badgers (*Meles meles*), and *B. columnaris*, which is found in skunks and was, at one time, thought to be the same species as *B. procyonis*. While fewer than 30 cases have been reported in the literature; the disease is likely under recognized. Raccoons have a high prevalence of infection and each worm is estimated to lay up to 179,000 eggs per day, and raccoons carry an average of 43-52 worms. Human infection occurs upon ingestion of viable eggs The larvae of these three species can cause extensive damage in their intermediate/paratenic hosts: they migrate extensively, continue to grow considerably within these hosts, and sometimes invade the brain (most often fatal) or the eye including permanent blindness when the worms migrate into the retina.

Neural larva migrans occurs when the parasites migrate through the brain. The initial signs may be mild, with subtle behavioral changes, lethargy, somnolence or irritability, weakness, speech defects and/or mild changes in vision, but they can rapidly become severe. A variety of symptoms including ataxia, seizures, paresis or paralysis, developmental regression, tremors, torticollis, nystagmus and coma have been reported. Epileptic seizures are quite common and partial, secondarily generalized or generalized from the beginning can be seen. The antiepileptic medication of choice is oral carbamazepine from 200mg three times a day.

The diagnosis of baylisascariasis is difficult in live patients; there is no available, non-invasive definitive test. Unless a brain biopsy is done and a larva is found, antemortem diagnosis usually depends on serology, with supporting evidence from other tests. In neural larva migrans, antibodies to *Baylisascaris* can be found in serum and cerebrospinal fluid (CSF); a rising titer is usually seen. An enzyme linked immunosorbent assay (ELISA), indirect immunofluorescence and immunoblotting (Western blotting) have been developed to detect anti-*Baylisascaris* antibodies.(Institute for International Cooperation in Animal Biologics, 2009). We have not experience in diagnosis based on CT/MRI images. Although

the potential for long-term sequelae is unknown, short-term recovery has been reported in anecdotic cases. (Pai et al., 2007).
List of parasitic zoonoses infecting the brain is increasing gradually by emergent and re-emergent infection as can be seen in Table 4

AGENT	DEFINITE HOST(S)	INTERMEDIATE HOST(S)	NEUROLOGICAL PROBLEMS
Taenia solium	Human	Pig	Epilepsy and other symptoms and signs due to neurocysticercosis
Toxocara canis (cati?)	Dogs, cats	NA	Epilepsy and manifestation due to neurotoxocariasis
Taenia (multiceps) serialis	Dogs, foxes and jackals	Sheep, goats	Epilepsy and other clinical manifestations of neurocoenurosis
Schistosoma japonicum	Mammals	Snails	Neuroschistosomiasis and seizures.
Gnathostoma spinigerum	Dogs, mammals	Crustacean copepod, freshwater fish, frogs	Epilepsy, and other manifestations of neurognathostomiasis.
Echinococcus granulosus	Dogs, other canidae	Domestic ungulates	Neuroechinoccosis included seizures
Cryptosporidium spp.	Cattle, dogs, cats, humans	NA	
Paragonimus spp.	Mammals, including humans	Snails (1^{ary}), crabs & crayfish (2^{ndary})	Epilepsy and other signs of neuroparagonimiasis.
Spirometra spp (Sparganum)*	Dogs and cats	Fish, reptiles, amphibians,	Epilepsy and other clinical manifestations of neurosparganosis
Baylisascaris procyonis	Raccoons, dogs	Small mammals and birds	Epilepsy, meningoenchephalitis, cranial nerve disorders
Paragonimus		Snail and crayfish	Epilepsy, blindness due to neuroparagonimiasis
Angiostrongylus cantonensis	Rats, Dogs	African giant land snails	Epilepsy and eosinophillic meningoencephalitis

*Spargana can live up to 20 years in the human host

Table 4. Some parasitic zoonoses reported as affecting the brain

Cerebral malaria is caused by the protozoan parasite Plasmodium, transmitted to humans via the Anopheles mosquito. The disease is endemic to large parts of Africa, South America, and Southeast Asia. Cerebral malaria is an encephalopathy occurring in approximately 2% of outpatients and 10% of inpatients infected with Plasmodium. The World Health Organization definition of cerebral malaria requires some feature that can be seen in Table 5.

Unarousable coma
Evidence of acute infection with P. falciparum
No other identifiable cause of coma

Table 5. Some clinical features of cerebral malaria

Clinical manifestations of cerebral malaria are diverse. Fever is nearly universal, as is comorbidity with clinical features of P. falciparum systemic infection. Clinicians working in tropical and subtropical regions regard any new CNS-attributable sign developing within the context of P. falciparum parasitemia as evidence of possible cerebral malaria. The cardinal feature is a disturbed level of consciousness, usually ranging from lethargy to stupor to coma, although an agitated delirium can also occur. To conform to the strict diagnosis of cerebral malaria, the patient must remain comatose for more than 6 hours after the seizure to distinguish the coma from postictal consciousness suppression. Generalized tonic-clonic seizures occur in more than 40% of adult patients. Partial seizures are uncommon. Seizures are associated with prolonged coma and increased risk of neurologic sequelae and death (Labar & Harden, 1997). Apart from brain edema other possible seizure causes are included in Table 6.

Cerebral hypoxia
Fever
Hypoglycemia
Lactic acidosis
Drugs (including antimalarials)

Table 6. Other possible causes of epileptic seizures due to malaria

Antimalarial medicine include: chloroquine and mefloquine. Other metabolic disturbances secondary to malarial systemic effects should be considered as a cause of seizures(Labar & Harden, 1997). Neurologic sequelae of cerebral malaria, including epilepsy, affect approximately 10% of survivors; for unclear reasons, children tend to be more frequently affected than adults (Marsden, 1975). Cerebral malaria is a medical emergency and treatment is tripartite:

Specific antimalarial therapy (quinine, quinidine, etc.)
Management of coexistent seizures
Treatment of associated superinfections.

Generalized seizures can be followed by rapid neurologic deterioration, so prompt treatment is required. Subclinical or nonconvulsive seizures should be suspected in patients with persistent coma.

2.2 Some major zoonotic trematodes (flukes)

There are 3 kinds of trematodes, such as monogenean, aspidogastrean, and digenean trematodes, with digenean being the only zoonotic trematodes. The characteristics of digenean trematodes are dorsoventrally flattened, unsegmented, and leaf-like worms and have 1 or 2 suckers (oral and ventral suckers), rarely armed with hooks or clamps. All digenean trematodes have 1or 2 intermediate hosts and first intermediate hosts are molluscs. Almost all zoonotic trematodes have the 2nd intermediate hosts, such as cyprinoid freshwater fish or crustacean (Young, 2009)

2.2.1 Neuroparagonimiasis

Paragonimiasis is a parasitic disease caused by *Paragonimus* trematodes, commonly known as lung flukes. Humans become infected by eating raw or undercooked crayfish (also known as crawfish and crawdads) or freshwater crabs that harbor the parasites. Paragonimiasis most frequently involves the lungs, but can affect other organs, including the brain and skin. In North America, *Paragonimus kellicotti* causes infections among dogs, cats, and wild carnivores, but rarely infects humans. After humans eat raw or undercooked crayfish that harbor *P. kellicotti,* the parasite penetrates through the intestinal wall into the peritoneal cavity, then through the diaphragm into the pleural space and lungs, and can migrate to other organs, including the brain (Chronic headache, epilepsy, etc.) and skin. Eggs laid in the lungs are excreted in the sputum, or swallowed and passed with stool. *Paragonimus* species are endemic in Africa, the Americas, and Asia, but the distribution of *P. kellicotti* is still being determined (Procop, 2009) Migration of the parasite to the brain can cause severe complications, including permanent blindness.

Liver and intestinal infections caused by fish-borne zoonotic trematodes (FZTs) are increasingly being recognized as serious public health problems and are especially widespread in Southeast Asia, including Vietnam, Lao People's Democratic Republic, Thailand, Cambodia, People's Republic of China, and North and South Korea . Liver flukes are associated with high incidence of bile duct cancer (WHO, 1995, 2002), and cause serious pathologic changes in the heart, brain, and spinal cord (Chai, 2005). The epidemiology of FZTs is complex because humans and reservoir hosts, such as dogs, cats, pigs, and fish-eating birds, harbor egg-shedding adult stages. (Thien et al., 2007;Chi et al., 2008; Phan et al., 2010)

2.2.2 Neuroschistosomiasis

Schistosomiasis is an important parasitic disease, occurring in more than 200 million people worldwide. Neuroschistosomiasis causes focal and generalized seizures; headache; and myeloradiculopathy with lower limb and back pain, bladder dysfunction, paresthesia, and weakness. Dizziness, nausea, and increased intracranial pressure can also occur in cerebellar schistosomiasis.(Wan et al., 2009). Visual scintillation from occipital mass has been described. (Fowler et al., 1999)

Schistosomiasis is endemic throughout much of the tropics. Three different schistosomal species (*S haematobium, S japonicum, and S mansoni*) can cause infection that involves the brain and spinal cord. Brain involvement is found in about 4% of all patients infected by *S mansoni*. The life cycle starts with cercariae, which penetrate the human skin and transform into schistosomulae. From there they migrate to the lungs and the liver. The organisms then mature into mating pairs of male and female worms, which settle in the mesenteric veins the adult worm laid eggs that are excreted with stool or urine. Different mechanisms of invasion of the brain have been discussed: the eggs may reach the brain through the valveless venous plexus of Batson, which joins the deep iliac veins and inferior vena cava with veins of the spinal cord and brain, or eggs may migrate to the brain via pulmonary arteriovenous shunts, or portalpulmonary arteriovenous shunts. Finally, the worms themselves may enter the cerebral veins and place their eggs directly at the ectopic site, which could be the cerebrum, cerebellum, leptomeninges, brainstem, or choroid plexus (Wan et al., 2009)

Neuroschistosomiasis usually follows the egg migration into the brain or spinal cord vasculature, leading to microinfarction or granuloma formation. Neurologic manifestations are rare, occurring in only 1- 2% of cases, but they can include a wide range of focal and nonfocal CNS symptoms, including seizures. . Neurologic disease during Katayama fever responds to steroids with or without antischistosomal therapy. Cerebral schistosomiasis may require surgical resection of the granuloma like masses. Praziquantel is the primary antischistosomal agent. Antiepileptic drugs are used as needed (Schachter, 2004).

2.2.3 Neurofascioliasis

Fascioliasis is a well-known parasite of herbivorous animals; it has a worldwide distribution on the animal reservoir host. A large variety of animals such as sheep, goat, cattle, buffalo, horses and rabbits show infection an rate that varies from 70% to 90% in some areas. Infection of the human host was very sporadic until the last two decades. However, it has now become an important trematode-borne infection of emerging concern until today. The estimated number of people infected is being estimated 2.4 million in 61 countries. An estimated number of populations at risk are considered more than 180 million throughout the world. Until today, largest number of infected people have been reported from Bolivia, China, Ecuador. Egypt, France Iran, Peru and Portugal. In Nepal's context, sporadic cases had been reported from human hospital since last decade,-while screening of human population has yet not been done. Same way in Iraq, Lebanon, Morocco, and Tunisia. (Karki, 2011).

Ectopic spinal localization of *Fasciola* may occur during the transmigration path of the parasite through the peritoneum or from the liver through the portal venous system and affect spinal cord causing paraplegia (Devendra et al., 2006). Park & Sohn (2010) reported the first case presenting cerebral lesions secondary to hepatic fascioliasis. Therefore seizures disorders does not represent a problem for this parasitism. CNS involvement can be associated with the hepatic stage of fascioliasis.

2.3 Some major zoonotic cestodes (tapeworms)

There are 2 kinds of cetodes, such as *Eucestoda* and *Cotyloda*. Cestodes are hermaphroditic and endoparasitic worms with an elongated flat body without a body cavity or alimentary canal. Their bodies are comprised of 3 parts, such as, scolex, neck, and strobila. *Eucestoda* have 1 intermediate host, but *Cotyloda* have 2 or more intermediate hosts. In Cheju (South Korea) many years ago, the pigsty was located below the toilet, so that pigs were raised to eat the stool and infected with the eggs of *Taenia* spp. Humans were habituated to eat raw pork products, especially the liver, so they became infected with the metacestodes of *Taenia* spp., *T. solium* and *Taenia asiatica*.

Min (1990) reported a review paper on cestode infections such as: the Pseudophyllidea, i.e., *D. latum*, *Diphyllobothrium yonagoense*, sparganum of *Spirometra erinacei*, and the

Cyclophyllidea, i.e., *H. diminuta, H. nana, Mesocestoides lineatus,T. saginata, T. solium,* and *E. granulosus.* He reported that the plerocercoid larva of *Spirometra* spp.(sparganum) infects humans through 16 kinds of animal hosts, such as, snakes, frogs, and so on.
Sparganosis first reported in swine in 1911 in Indochina. It is a disease found in snakes, reptiles, and mammals, including swine and man. It is caused by migration of the second larval stage (spargana) of the cestode *Spirometra.* (Mueller, 1974). Human sparganosis occurs worldwide. The majority of cases has been reported from China, Korea, Japan, and Southeast Asia. Approximately 70 cases of human sparganosis have been reported from the United States, most from the Southeast region of the country. Transmission to humans has occurred through intact mucous membranes, by the ingestion /handling of frogs and snakes, poultry, and pork, and by ingestion of contaminated water. Disease in man can produce subcutaneous, cerebral, ocular, visceral, and metastatic forms depending upon the migration of the parasite. (Pullar &McLenan 1949; Gordon, 1954; Gray et a., 1999).

2.3.1 Neuroechinoccosis

Echinococcosis is caused by tapeworms of the genus Echinococcus, common parasites of dogs and cats, who are the definitive hosts; humans can be intermediate hosts. The disease is endemic in countries around the Mediterranean: Greece, Turkey, and Lebanon have the highest prevalences. The small adult worms live in the definitive host's gut and discharge eggs into feces. If inadvertently ingested by a human, the eggs hatch in the human's gut, enabling the organism to penetrate the human's gut wall and spread hematogenously. Once located in a final tissue site, the organism forms a slowly enlarging cyst, a hydatid.When in the CNS, cysts usually locate in brain parenchyma. Clinical manifestations are secondary to this mass lesion, raised intracranial pressure, or both. Although praziquantel has activity against these organisms, the primary treatment of CNS hydatids is surgical. Antiepileptic management is a crucial adjunctive treatment. (Schachter, 2004)

2.3.2 Neurocoenurosis

Another parasitic zoonosis which shows similar symptoms to NC is coenuriasis, due to invasion of the brain by the larval stage knowing by *Coenuruses cerebralis* (CC) of the tapeworm *Multiceps multiceps.* Watson and Lurie (1956) from Edendale Hospital in PieterMarisberg, South Africa reported five cases from 1951 to 1956 and described their anatomic-pathological finding on post-mortem examinations. One year later also in South Africa, Plumber et al (1957) reported some cases and reviewed the medical literature. At the time that they reviewed the available English-language medical literature a total 14 case from South Africa were found. From his anatomopathological report we could not find gross different from racemose NCC and other descriptions about CC. At the veterinary side, two rare clinical manifestations of coenuriasis in sheep we reported in two lambs of 6–7 weeks old. In humans, symptoms include headaches, seizures, vomiting, paraplegia, hemiplegia, dysphasias, and epilepsy.

2.4 Some major zoonotic nematodes (roundworms)

Nematodes are characterized as free-living or parasitic, unsegmented, cylindrical, and elongated round worms with a body cavity and alimentary canal. Almost all nematodes are sex-separated and their life cycles are direct or indirect. The major intestinal nematodes are *Ascaris lumbricoides* (roundworm), *Enterobius vermicularis* (pinworm), hookworms, *Trichuris trichiura* (whipworm), *Trichostrongylus orientalis,* and *Strongyloides stercoralis.* As imported zoonotic nematode infections, loiasis cases due to the Loa loa. As indigenous infections, there have been several human *Thelazia callipaeda* infections. *Dirofilaria immitis* infections are very popular among dogs but very scanty medical information about this parasite in human beings is found.

2.4.1 Neuroangiostrongyliasis

Angiostrongyliasis is caused by the rat lungworm. *Angiostrongylus cantonensis* is endemic through Southeast Asia and the Pacific Islands. The infection in humans, an accidental host, is associated with eosinophilic meningitis. The dog tapeworm, Echinococcus granulosus, can infect humans with up to 2% of clinical cases presenting with brain cysts. The infection has a cosmopolitan distribution. Humans get infected with dog feces and CNS infection is usually associated with signs of increased intracranial pressure (Hughes & Biggs, 2002, 2002a) and epileptic seizures. There is no established antiparasitic treatment. Comorbid seizures are managed under the similar protocol for other parasitic zoonoses infecting the brain (Schachter, 2004).

2.4.2 Neurognathostomiasis

Gnathostomiasis is a parasitic infection caused by the third-stage larvae of the helminths *Gnathostoma spp.,* which are seen mostly in tropical and subtropical regions. The genus *Gnathostoma* belongs to the order *Spirurida,* one of the largest groups of nematodes. The genus has 12 species These groups are characterized biologically by requiring one or more intermediate hosts in their life cycles It is a food-borne zoonosis endemic in areas where people are accidental hosts in which the parasite fails to reach sexual maturity after eating raw freshwater fish or shellfish, especially Thailand and other parts of Southeast Asia, Japan, and increasingly Latin America, particularly Mexico. (Daengsvang, 1981; Nawa, 1991)

Visceral disease is more serious than the cutaneous manifestations and, in the case of central nervous system disease, may be fatal. (Herman & Chiodina, 2009). The main features of CNS involvement can cause radiculomyelitis, radiculomyeloencephalitis, eosinophilic meningitis, and subarachnoid hemorrhage. The hallmark symptoms are an acute onset of excruciating radicular pain and/or headache (subarachnoid hemorrhage or eosinophilic meningitis), with subsequent paralysis of the extremities and/or cranial nerve palsies. The typical clinical picture can be explained by the migratory pathway of the parasite, which gains entry to the spinal cord along nerve roots (cranial, cervical, thoracic, or lumbar), causing intense radicular pain (or headache in the case of cranial nerve or cervical root involvement) which usually lasts from 1 to 5 days. Cranial nerve palsies tend to occur after the onset of paralysis, and if multiple they signify a poor prognosis. Cerebral involvement is usually indicated by a depressed consciousness level or coma, but interestingly, mental confusion does not tend to occur (Herman & Chiodini, 2009).

The main differential diagnosis of neurognathostomiasis is with *Angiostrongylus cantonensis,* another highly prevalent parasite in Southeast Asia. This may produce a similar eosinophilic menigoencephalitis, but the acute nerve root pain, signs of spinal cord compression, and hemorrhagic or xanthochromic spinal fluid seen in gnathostomiasis are absent with *Angiostrongylus* infection (Herman & Chiodini, 2009). The *Gnathostoma* larva is more invasive than that of *Angiostrongylus* and therefore produces more frequent focal neurological signs.

In contrast, the *Angiostrongylus* larva, which is considerably smaller (120 μm wide and 12 mm long) and usually multiple, more commonly causes a menigoencephalitis, and although neurotropic, it is rarely fatal (Herman & Chiodini, 2009).

The triad of eosinophilia, migratory lesions, and obvious exposure risk are highly suggestive of the diagnosis of gnathostomiasis. Eosinophilia of the cerebrospinal fluid (CSF) is also highly supportive of neurognathostomiasis, with reported levels of 5 to 94% and a total CSF white cell count of up to $500/mm^3$ (range, 20 to $1420/mm^3$), but may also be found with several other parasites, e.g., *Angiostrongylus cantonensis, Toxocara canis, Strongyloides stercoralis, Ascaris lumbricoides, Paragonimus westermani, Fasciola hepatica,* and *Trichinella spiralis* and with schistosomiasis, cystercercosis, and other infections such as coccidiodomycosis and aspergillus infection Because no single area of the nervous system is inaccessible to the highly invasive gnathostome lava and multiplicity and/or rapid progression of lesions beyond the degree of cerebral edema explained by further migration of the parasite. Therefore epileptic seizures and epilepsy can be expected and treated accordingly. Multiple cranial nerve palsies are signs of poor prognosis. (Boongird et al., 1977)

2.4.3 Neurotrichinellosis

Trichinellosis also called trichinosis, trichinellosis or trichiniasis (Trich from Greek *thrix* meaning hair) is an infection due to nematodes of the genus *Trichinella,* most commonly *T spiralis.* Infection is initiated by ingestion of viable larvae in raw or undercooked meat. Digestive action liberates the larvae. The liberated larvae develop into adults in the duodenum and jejunum, where they mate and bear offspring. The adult worms are expelled in the stool. Eosinophilia develops in response to the presence of the worm. Patients who develop neurologic and cardiac dysfunctions have marked eosinophilia associated with arteriolar microthrombi, often simply from the numbers of larvae, leading to areas of cerebral and myocardial infarction.

Neurological involvement may occur in 0.2%-52% of cases with trichinellosis spirallis, generally in the most severely affected patients. However, another author refers that involvement of the central nervous system occurs in 10-20% and mortality rates may then approach 50% (Clausen, 1996). Apart from *Trichinella spiralis* other parasitic infections that may cause abnormal mental status and eosinophilia include toxocariasis (Despommier, 2003), angiostrongyloidiasis, and baylisascariasis (Gavin et al., 2005). Clinical signs and symptoms are meningitis, encephalitis, cranial nerve deficits, paresis, aphasia, convulsions and coma (Fourestie et al., 1993; Gay et al., 1982) Small hypodense areas in the white matter and in the cortex have been reported long time ago (Ellrodt et al., 1987). Absence of pets at home or contact with raccoons, the lack of eosinophils in the CSF, and the lack of ocular larva migrans on examination argue against trichinellosis. (Madariaga, 2007) Treatment of choice is thiabendazole and steroids. Epileptic seizures and epilepsy are managed following same protocol used routinely. For more details please consult the book : "Treatment approach for epilepsy" ISBN 978-953-307-678-2.

May dogs cause epilepsy?

Of course no, I always remember my parents when they said: "El perro es el mejor amigo del hombre" (The dog is the best man's friend) and they were right, I had a very good one because I also had a very good veterinarian friend. Without any doubt dogs are the most common pet animals worldwide and they perform a range of cultural, social, and economic functions at home and in our society. Dogs were domesticated from wolves as recently as 15000 years ago (Morey, 2006), or perhaps as early as 100000 years ago based on recent genetic fossil and DNA evidence (Savolainen *et al.*, 2002, Lindbald-Toh, 2005). Evidence suggests that dogs were first domesticated in East Asia, possibly China, and the first people to enter North America took dogs with them (Savolainen *et al.*, 2002).

Dogs are kept as pets and companions, for hunting, as guards, draught animals, for food, or for commercial purposes (Swai E et al., 2010). Some studies also suggest that keeping pets be associated with a higher level of self-esteem in children (Paul and Serpell, 1996; Knobel *et al.*, 2008). It is fairly common for a dog to become infected with an internal or external parasite at some point in their lifetime. Parasites can infect your pet any time of year and there is a long list of them. (See figure 1)

External parasites, such as fleas and ticks may be less prevalent outside during certain times of the year however they often survive in the house during the winter months, creating an uninterrupted life cycle. Other internal parasites such as worms may affect your pet all year long. Nevertheless, dogs have been living with humans since early civilization, studies of dog's parasitic zoonoses affecting the human brain in sub- Saharan Africa are scanty and very limited information is available in the medical literature. Dogs can carry over a dozen forms of zoonotic diseases mainly to their owners if they do not practice appropriate hygiene and disease-control measures. And to some peoples are at a higher risk of contracting zoonotic diseases such as: peoples with malignancies, young children, immunocompromised patients, and over expose persons. Some zoonotic diseases are fairly common in dogs, while others are exceedingly rare.

Apart from the tapeworm, other parasites can spread from dogs to humans (See figure 1). Hookworm and roundworm are both zoonotic infections that can be spread through the improper handling of contaminated dog feces. Several species of these parasites can thrive in the colons of both humans and dogs. Hookworm and roundworm can both be spread through the accidental ingestion of dog feces that is contaminated with parasite eggs or larvae. This can occur through improper handling of waste, and people may become infected by walking barefoot on soil that has been contaminated with infected dog feces. Nowadays, veterinary practices have the important responsibility of educating pet owners about the potential risk of zoonotic parasites and the different measures that can be taken for their control and prevention (CDC, 2004).

Another parasitic zoonosis associated with dogs and epilepsy is toxocariasis. The definitive hosts of *T. canis* and *T. cati* are dogs and cats, respectively. Infection in dogs is usually acquired in the uterus or through nursing. In the United States, it has been reported that up to 80% of puppies less than 6 weeks old are infected with *T. canis*. Hence, puppies are the most important sources of contamination of the environment. Cats of any age can contaminate the environment with *T. cati*. However, human infection with *T. cati* has been less often reported (Little, 2003).. Humans acquire the infection through ingestion of the eggs of the parasite that have been present in the environment for at least two weeks but that may have survived for several years. This make young children at a particularly high risk of infection due to their normal geophagy behavior. In the developing world, the environment is likely to be heavily contaminated with eggs that are infectious to humans.

The fact that most communities are largely agricultural, that most pet animals freely roam everywhere and that there is a lack of sanitation could lead to a high risk of infection in persons of all ages. Dogs without veterinarian care are not our best friend. The choice is yours advise is mine.

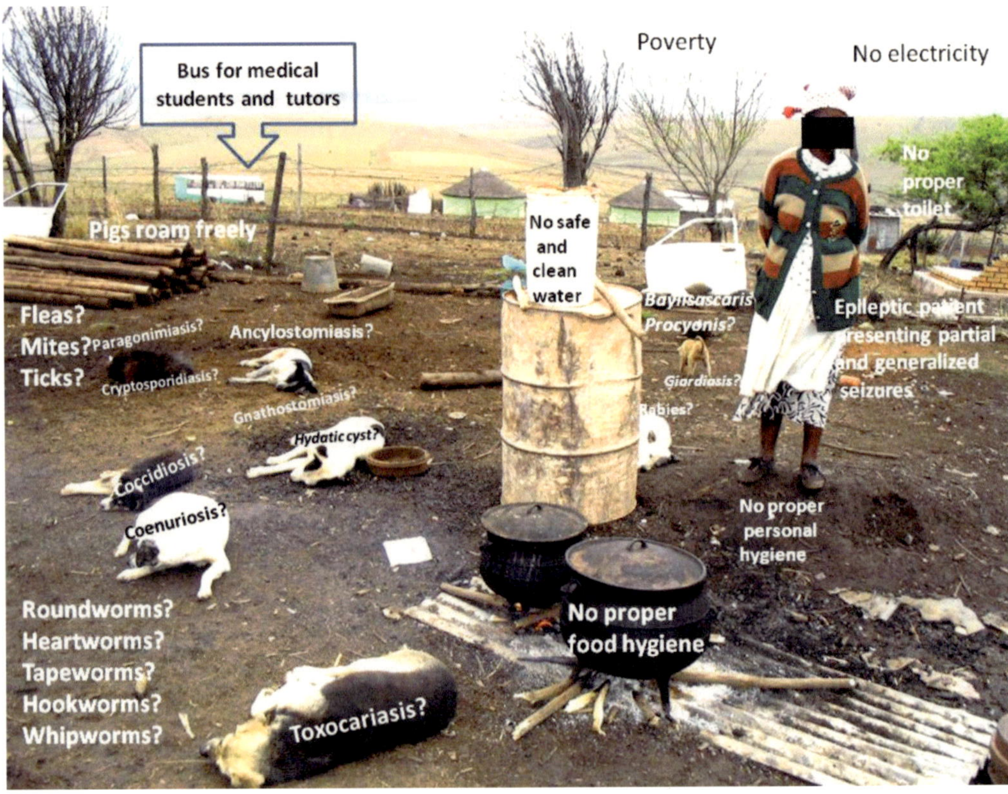

Fig. 1. Rural community at the former Transkei in South Africa.

2.5 Neuroborreliosis

Within days to weeks, *Borrelia burgdorferi* the causative agent of Lyme disease, spreads hematogenously and it probably enters the CNS at this time. One to two months postinfection, B. burgdorferi localizes and becomes sequestered in certain tissues. The nervous system is involved in up to 20% of untreated North American patients. Meningitis (typically lymphocytic) is the most common neuropathology abnormality in early disseminated of Lyme disease.

Neurologic deficits, including seizure, can be the initial clinical manifestation. Neurologic abnormalities that have been reported to be associated with early CNS Lyme disease include: acute aseptic meningitis, acute purulent meningitis chronic lymphocytic meningitis, recurrent meningitis, acute meningoenchephalitis, acute focal encephalitis, encephalomyelitis, leukoencephalitis, acute cerebellar ataxia, acute parkinsonian syndrome, acute transverse myelitis, subacute myelitis, cognitive deficits affective disturbance, and epileptic seizures. Lyme disease should be suspected in any patient with chronic lymphocytic meningitis or mild menigoencephalitis with associated cranial neuritis or radiculitis. Lab tests include serologic assays like immunofluorescent assay and enzyme-linked immunoassay tests for anti-B. burgdorferi antibodies. Specific anti-B. burgdorferi antibody also appears in CSF, where it can be detected even when serum antibody tests are negative. (To establish whether these antibodies are synthesized intrathecally, serum and CSF antibody levels should be measured simultaneously. Treatment for epilepsy did not differ from other parasitic zoonoses although epilepsy seems to be a minor problem in this condition even in HIV-positive patients (van Burgel et al., 2010; Henningsson et al., 2010).

2.6 Neuroccocidiosis

Coccidiosis is an intestinal disease that affects several different animal species including canines and humans. Coccidia is one of the most prevalent protozoal infections in North American animals, second only to giardia. Eimeria and Isospora are the two genera that are often referred to as "coccidia." These two genera contain a large number of species that infect a variety of animals throughout the world. The diseases caused by these microscopic protozoal parasites are referred to collectively as coccidiosis, and they vary tremendously in virulence. Some species cause diseases that result in mild symptoms that might go unnoticed (i.e., Mild diarrhea) and eventually disappear, while other species cause highly virulent infections that are rapidly fatal. The causative agent is a protozoan that has the ability to multiply rapidly. The major damage is due to the rapid multiplication of the parasite in the intestinal wall, and the subsequent rupture of the cells of the intestinal lining. Several stages of multiplication occur before the final stage, the oocyst, is passed in the feces. Oocysts are extremely resistant to environmental stress and are difficult to completely remove from the environment. Oocysts are frequent contaminants of feed and water and when the sporulated oocysts are ingested by other animals they start the life cycle over in the new host. Neurococcidiosis is characterized by epileptic seizures among other signs but it has been reported in calves and cows (Oliveira et al., 2009)

2.7 African trypanosomiasis

African trypanosomiasis, or sleeping sickness, is caused by Trypanosoma brucei. The tsetse fly is the arthropod vector. CNS involvement is the principal clinical consequence. An inflammatory nodule, a chancre, appears within several days at the site of parasite inoculations by the biting tsetse fly. Parasite replication and local tissue invasion are followed by lymphatic and bloodstream entry, causing a diffuse lymphadenopathy and parasitemia with high fever.

Recurrent cycles of hemo-lymphatic parasitemia follow, with corresponding bouts of fever alternating with periods of well-being. (African trypanosomiasis and malaria are two of the few causes of true intermittent fever. Trypanosomes eventually enter the CNS to cause meningoencephalitis, with a full range of neuropsychiatric signs and symptoms, including sleep-wake cycle abnormalities (e.g., Daytime drowsiness and nocturnal insomnia), from which the disease derived its name. Frequent episodes of awakening during sleep, blurring of sleep stages, and irregular bursts of rapid EEG activity during stage 4 sleep occur.

Generalized convulsions become common as the disease progresses to later stages. If untreated, mortality approaches 100%. Of the three drugs usually used for treatment (suramin, pentamidine, and melarsoprol), only melarsoprol penetrates the blood-brain barrier to be effective in CNS disease. Its use is complicated by an up to 18% incidence of severe, reactive arsenic encephalopathy, which can result in permanent neurologic damage or death. Consequently, melarsoprol should be used only in patients with CNS involvement. In a study of melarsoprol effects on patients with T. gambiense in the meningoencephalitic stage, EEG tracings before treatment showed marked abnormalities in the form of periodic delta outbursts. (Hamon & Camara, 1991)

2.8 American trypanosomiasis

American trypanosomiasis, also known as Chagas' disease, is an acute or chronic infection caused by *Trypanosoma cruzi* and occurs only in the western hemisphere. Chagas disease is the third most common parasitic infection worldwide after malaria and schistosomiasis. (WHO 2005). Seizures sometimes occur at stroke onset, and epilepsy is quite a frequent complication after chagasic stroke. Chronic vascular epilepsy, characterized by secondary generalised seizures, have been reported in around 20% of patients surviving chagasic stroke, whereas around 10% of stroke patients without the Chagas disease have seizures (Carod-Artal et al., 2005). The effect of uncontrolled seizures on cognition and disability in Chagas disease is unknown. No prospective epidemiological studies have addressed the risk of acute seizures and their recurrence in acute chagasic stroke (Carod-Artal & Gascon, 2010)

3. Other helminth parasitic infections to be considered

The capacity of climatic conditions to modulate the extent and intensity of parasitism is well known since long ago. Concerning helminths, among the numerous environmental modifications giving rise to changes in infections, climate variables appear as those showing a greater influence, so that climate change may be expected to have an important impact on the diseases they cause. However, the confirmation of the impact of climate change on helminthiases has been reached very recently. Only shortly before, helminthiases were still noted as infectious diseases scarcely affected by climate change, when compared to diseases caused by microorganisms in general: viruses, bacteria, and protozoans (Mas-Coma et al., 2009). In this group we have: neurocysticercosis as a leading cause of epilepsy in developing coutries and some developed places. (Foyaca-Sibat, 2011), and also sparganosis and toxocariasis among others.

3.1 Neurosparganosis

Sparganosis is a rare parasitic infection caused by the larval cestode of *Spirometra* that results from ingesting the plerocercoid harbored in frogs, snakes, and chickens. Reported worldwide, sparganosis is most prevalent in Southeast and Eastern Asia. The diagnosis is suggested by a wandering lesion, especially in endemic areas; the tunnel sign on a post contrast MRI is characteristic. The preferred treatment is the surgical removal of live worm.(Shirakawa et al., 2010) In the endemic area of sparganosis, where other neurological parasitic infestations (*e.g.* cysticercosis and gnathostomiasis) are also common, the clinical usefulness of MR imaging is very limited in providing a definitive diagnosis of cerebral sparganosis. A history of risky behaviour (*e.g.* drinking impure water, eating frog or snake meat, or using frog or snake meat as a poultice) might be a clue and offers supporting evidence for a presumptive diagnosis in cases of abnormal brain MR imaging results (Song et al., 2007; Chiu et al., 2010; Wiwanitkit, 2010). 4 cases had a history of eating raw frogs or snakes. 5 showed eosinophilia in peripheral blood, all with positive anti-Sparganum mansoni antibody in serum and cerebrospinal fluid. Cerebral MRI showed placeholder in all patients. Diagnosis was confirmed by pathological examination of operations and species identification. All patients were cured by operation removal and praziquantel treatment. (Chen & Shi, 2010).

3.2 Neurofilariasis

Filariasis and onchocerciasis are parasitic helminth diseases that constitute a serious public health issue in tropical regions. The filarial nematodes that cause these diseases are transmitted by blood-feeding insects and produce chronic and long-term infection through suppression of host immunity. Disease pathogenesis is linked to host inflammation invoked by the death of the parasite, causing hydrocoele, lymphoedema, and elephantiasis in lymphatic filariasis, and skin disease and blindness in onchocerciasis. (Taylor et al., 2011) As far we know, epilepsy secondary to filariasis has not been reported.

This capability, coupled with an integrated, multidisciplinary and ecological approach, makes possible the identification of parasitic infections and diseases likely to be particularly susceptible to climate change and, with adjustments for regional variations, the exploration of some of the possible consequences of accelerating climate change of the occurrence ofthese diseases and for animal and human health. This is a very urgent need, and without such an attempt to anticipate the possible, society is likely to be a more or less impotent spectator to the certainty of continual ecological calamities. (Polley, 2010).

3.3 Neurocysticercosis

Neurocisticercosis (NC) is a parasitic infection of central nervous system (CNS) caused by the larval stage (Cysticercus cellulosae) of the pig tapeworm Taenia solium. This is the most common helminth to produce CNS infection in human being. The occurrence of acquired epilepsy or the syndrome of raised intracranial pressure in a person living in or visiting a region where taeniasis is endemic or even in one living in close contact with people who have taeniasis should suggest a diagnosis of cysticercosis; the NC may remain asymptomatic for months to years and sometimes its diagnosis is made incidentally when neuroimaging is performed. Symptoms and signs are related both to the parasite which can show a different biological behavior from one place to another, and to the inflammatory-inmunological response of the host. NC is the most common cause of acquired epilepsy worldwide and most of the patients taking phenytoin or carbamazepine for a proper control of their seizures, respond very well NC is also an important cause of ischemic stroke secondary to infectious vasculitis (Foyaca-Sibat & Ibañez-Valdés, 2003). The most common cause of epilepsy due to NC is calcified lesion with or without evidence of perilesional edema. The prognosis of this situation is worse when there is an associated intraventricular cyst (Figure 2) that usually does not respond well to praziquantel and albendazole should be prescribe (Foyaca-Sibat & Ibañez-Valdés, 2003). More information about NC can be found in this book.

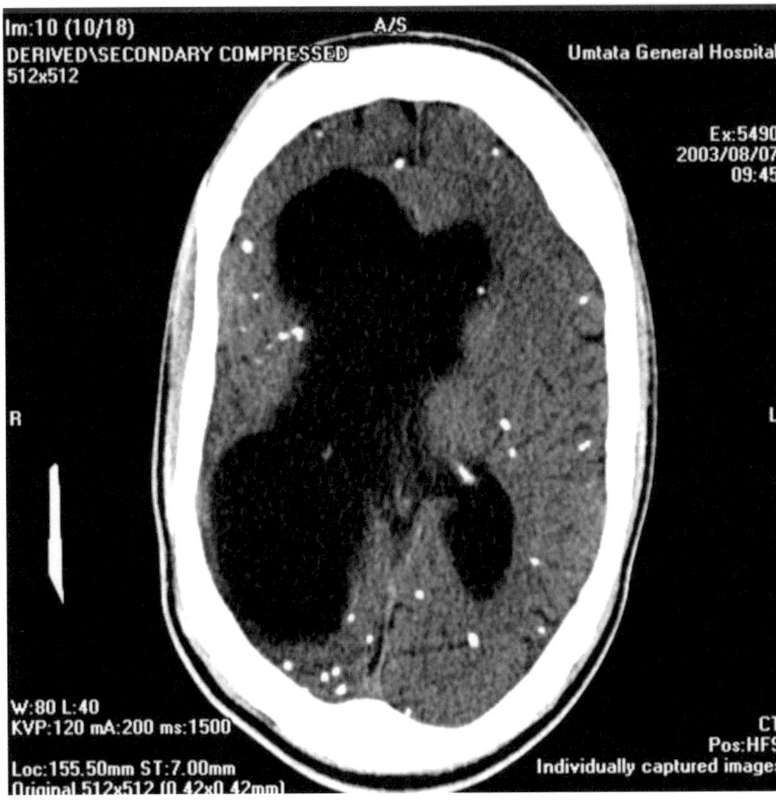

Fig. 2. Shows multiple intraparenchymal calcified NC with and without perilesional edema and hydrocephalus secondary to intraventricular NC.

4. Neurotoxocariasis and effect modification of HIV

4.1 Introduction

Human toxocariasis is usually contracted by exposure to contaminated soil. This disease is rarely transmitted by raw meat or giblets of paratenic animals, such as chickens, lambs, or cows. Hoffmeister et al, (2007) reported a case of isolated cerebral toxocariasis presumably caused by the consumption of the raw duck liver. Their patient, a 55-year-old woman had sudden-onset hemiparesis of the right leg, eosinophilia of 30%, and markedly elevated total serum IgE levels. Magnetic resonance imaging demonstrated multiple cerebral hyperintense lesions on T2-weighed images.

Tests for antibodies to Toxocara in serum and cerebrospinal fluid yielded highly positive results and repeated courses of albendazole and corticosteroids led to significant clinical improvement. Previously, Kim et al., (2003) reported a case of cerebral infarction which was caused by toxocariasis in adults, who had headache, abdominal pain and a right side weakness. He had only a history of ingestion of raw liver of deer. Although the seriousness of infection of *Toxocara canis* depends on the site of parasite migration, the aberrant larvae occasionally invade the CNS. Neurological problems, such as epilepsy, neuropsychological deficits, and ataxia have been observed clinically in humans and in the case of ocular larval migrans, vision loss and permanent blindness may result (Akao *et al.*, 2003; Nithiuthai *et al.*, 2004).

Three recent case-control studies conducted in rural Bolivia, Burundi and Italy (Nicoletti et al., 2002, 2007, 2008) reported a significant association between seropositivity to *T. canis* and epilepsy. The adjusted odds ratios (OR) in these three studies were 2.70 (95%CI=1.41-5.19), 2.13 (95%CI: 1.18-3.83) and 3.90 (95%CI: 1.91-7.98), in Bolivia, Burundi and Italy, respectively. Of particular interest, in 2 of the 3 studies, the OR of epilepsy associated with seropositivity to *Toxocara* spp. was higher among persons with partial seizures (OR=4.70, 95%CI=1.47-15.1 and OR=4.69, 95%CI: 2.24-9.80, respectively). The opposite was true in Burundi where the association was stronger among persons with generalized seizures (OR=2.52; 95%:1.01-6.26). Toxocariasis has also been associated with epilepsy in a study of children in Italy (Alpino et al., 1990). In this study, prevalence of antibody to *T. canis* was compared in 91 children with epilepsy younger than 18 years and 214 controls. The OR for seropositivity was estimated to 2.0 (95% CI=1.0-4.0). The association was present primarily in children less than 5 years of age. Whether exposure precedes the onset of seizures or is a result of behaviors such as geophagy in children with epilepsy is uncertain. However, there was no association between pica and seropositivity in the study by Alpino et al. (1990) and Nicoletti et al. (2002), the association between seropositivity and epilepsy was stronger for adults than for children and for those with partial seizures than for those with generalized seizures. These findings argue against exposure being a consequence of seizures rather than an antecedent. Pica had a protective effect in the most recent study of Nicoletti et al. conducted in Sicily (2008).

Recall bias is unlikely since an overestimation of the association rather than an underestimation was observed. Persons with early onset seizures (<15 years old) showed a stronger association between toxocariasis and epilepsy, which tends to support the hypothesis that young children are at higher risk of infection. The prevalence of infection with *Toxocara* spp. was 50.8% among the control group in Burundi, suggesting that the exposure to this zoonotic parasite in SSA is very high (Nicoletti et al., 2002).

We were unable to find a well-designed studies from countries where parasitic zoonoses are endemic that assessed the association between HIV infection, NC and cerebral toxocariasis. While it is possible that HIV infection may modify the association between known risk factors and parasitic zoonotic infections of the brain, to our knowledge, this has never been addressed (personal communication by Carabin H, 2010). More information about parasitic zoonoses of the brain and epilepsy can be found in our book entitled Epilepsy. Clinical manifestations. ISBN 978-953-307-1341-2

In 2004 and 2005, we conducted a pilot study at the St-Elisabeth hospital in Lusikisiki (ECP) which included 296 consecutive patients consulting the medical clinic for suspected new-onset seizures or existing epilepsy cases. Each week, four (4) randomly selected, consenting patients with confirmed seizure disorder were transported to Mthatha for CT scan of the brain. The prevalence of seropositivity to antigens of *T. solium* was 8% (95%CI: 4.5%-13%). A total of 92 patients with recurrent seizures and who also completed a questionnaire were referred to Mthatha for a CT-scan. Of these, 34 (37.0%, 95%CI: 27.1%-47.7%) had a definite diagnosis of neurocysticercosis (NCC), 14 of whom had active lesions visible on CT, 39 (42%) had no CT abnormality, and 19 (21%) had other, undefined non-NCC calcifications. Our results showed that serology alone cannot be used to diagnose NCC in this population (Foyaca-Sibat et al., 2009)

HIV status was available from 50 patients with confirmed seizures or epilepsy. Among the 47 patients with antibody ELISA results available, the antibody seroprevalence of *T. solium* was 30.0% among HIV positive patients and 48.1% among HIV negative patients. Interestingly, among the 33 patients with antigen ELISA results, the antigen seroprevalence of *T. solium* was 16.7% among the HIV positive patients but only 9.5% among the HIV negative patients. These preliminary results suggest that HIV patients may be less able to mount a detectable antibody response to cysticercosis and might be more likely to be infected with active cysts. A total of 22 of these patients (13 HIV negative and 9 HIV positive) were referred for a CT-scan. Of these, 5 HIV negative and 7 HIV positive patients had CT evidence of NC with 2 HIV negative and 5 HIV positive patients harboring active cysts. These very preliminary and imprecise results do suggest that there may be an association between NC and HIV infection. (Foyaca-Sibat et al., 2009)

4.1.1 The specific research aims of the current pilot study are

1. Conduct a pilot study to compare the cross-sectional seroprevalence of toxocariasis and cysticercosis in six groups: patients in the advanced stage of HIV, those who are HIV positive but not in the advanced stages, and HIV negative patients, each group being further subdivided into those with and without selected neurological disorders. Our research hypothesis was: the prevalence of parasitic zoonoses is higher among people with advanced HIV but CNS manifestations are more common among people in the early stages for HIV as compared to HIV negative people living in the Eastern Cape Province (ECP) of South Africa.
2. Conduct a pilot study to estimate the interaction between HIV and cysticercosis or toxocariasis in the occurrence of neurological complications in adolescents and adults with HIV infection. To estimate the interaction between HIV and cysticercosis and toxocariasis on the prevalence of neurological disorders and generate new, testable hypotheses about the biological mechanisms for such interactions.

The long-term goal of this project is to develop a multidisciplinary-based interventions to more effectively control preventable parasitic zoonotic infections that are associated with epileptic disorders and that may disproportionately affect people living with HIV/AIDS.

We did a pilot cross-sectional study comparing six groups of patients defined by HIV infection status (advanced HIV, HIV positive not in the advanced stages, and HIV negative) and the presence of clinical manifestations of selected CNS disorders (yes/no).

Advanced-stage HIV patients (groups 1 and 2) are individuals who have met the WHO definition of stage 3 HIV/AIDS in the past 12 months (WHO, 2005). Patients who have ever been diagnosed with stage 4 HIV/AIDS are excluded. Only stage 3 patients not yet on HAART at the time of the study were included. (See figure 3)

Newly (< 12 months) diagnosed HIV patients not in the advanced stage (Groups 3 and 4) are defined as persons living with HIV/AIDS (PLWH/A) under care who have CD4 counts >350 cells/mm^3 and who are not HIV stages 3 or 4 as defined by the WHO (WHO 2005) when the study starts or at the time of diagnosis of a neurological disorder. We needed to invite some of these patients to participate in the study during their first visit to the HIV clinic in order to recruit a sufficient number of these early stage patients.

Groups 1-4 were sampled from the Mthatha Hospital Complex's HIV/AIDS clinic which is likely to represent the largest source of PLWH/A under care in the ECP, Nelson Mandela Academic Hospital (NMAH) is included. Patients in Groups 1 and 3 have been diagnosed with epilepsy at any time following their diagnosis of advanced HIV (group 1) or HIV positivity (group 3) respectively. We used this inclusion criteria due to the possibility that co-infection with the study helminths may accelerate the progression of HIV infection to advanced stages.

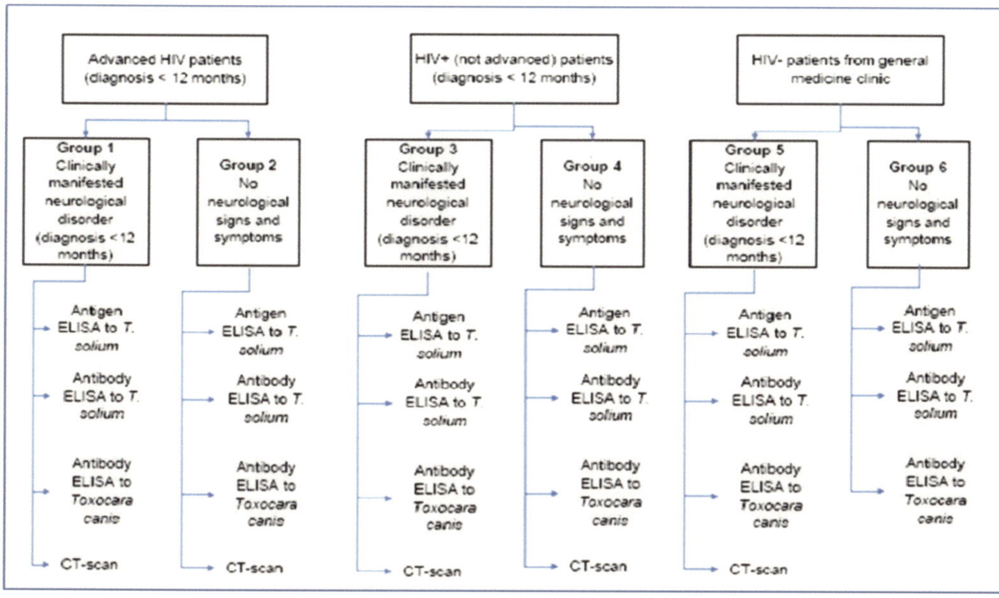

Fig. 3. Shows graphical composition of each group (Made by Prof. H Carabin from University of Oklahoma, USA)

Group 5 was sampled from the neurology/epilepsy/neurocysticercosis clinic at the NMAH. We took a random sample of clinic patients newly diagnosed with epilepsy within the previous 12 months and who tested negative for HIV at that time or anytime following the initial visit. Group 6 consisted of HIV negative patients referred to the general medicine clinic of the NMAH and who have no history of any neurological disorders. Group 6 had a negative HIV diagnostic test resulted in the past month. For Groups 5 and 6, if the patients had never been tested for HIV, we offered the test. Only those HIV seronegative was included in these groups. If tested participants do not wish to be informed about their HIV status (very common situation), we respected their choice. If they test positive and want to be informed, we do so and then refer them to the HIV/AIDS clinic for their care.
The sampling strategy depended on the expected number of patients available on each group, but we were aiming at sampling 50 patients in each group.

4.2 Statistical method

Data is analyzed to estimate the cross-sectional associations between HIV and infections with *T. solium* and *Toxocara spp.* and their potential interactions in clinically apparent neurological complications. The 6 groups, which are fixed by design, will be modeled as an interaction term between HIV status and the presence or absence of neurological disorders. Either the serological results or the presence of parasitic brain lesions on CT-scan (i.e., NC or neurological toxocariasis) are the "outcomes" in the statistical analyses since they are the random variables in this design. This approach allows us to test if there is indeed such interaction and if not, to assess the independent cross-sectional association between serological results (dependent variable) and HIV status and neurological disorders (independent variables).

We used three Bayesian multivariate logistic regressions with the presence/absence of antigen to cysticercosis, antibodies to cysticercosis and antibodies to *Toxocara* as outcomes. To estimate the association between the presence of NC and neurological toxocariasis (dependent variable) and HIV status among those with or without neurological disorders (independent variables), we used the same approach except that only groups 1-5 are represented. In all instances, we also run models adjusting for potential confounding variables such as age, gender, family history of epilepsy, area of residence, etc.

We want to emphasize that these analyses are also meant to direct our thinking in generating new hypotheses on the interaction between HIV and brain infection with parasitic zoonoses on neurological disorders in the developing world. We did not identify any causal relationships with data from a pilot cross-sectional study.Because of space limitation, power calculations cannot be presented here

4.3 Study design and methods

All patients meeting the inclusion criteria based on HIV stage and epilepsy have the opportunity to be included in this study. Thus, women and minorities meeting the eligibility criteria had the possibility of being included. For the CT-scan of the brain, pregnant women were excluded due to the risk to the fetus, but invited to come back to the exam after delivery.

4.3.1 Selection criteria

Fifty patients diagnosed with epilepsy in the past 12 months and receiving care at the neurology/epilepsy/neurocysticercosis clinic of the NMAH and who tested negative to HIV at that time or any time following the initial visit were invited to participate. Fifty HIV negative patients without neurological disorders, sampled from patients regularly attending a dermatology/general medicine clinic at the WSU hospital complex, were invited to participate by their physician who was informed of their eligibility by a member of the research team. Subjects included in the study were selected at random, and there are no selection criteria based on sex/gender or racial/ethnic groups.

The study is conducted in the former Transkei in South Africa where all population living in rural areas are black. Knowledge gained from this pilot study will assist in developing more definitive, prospective studies of the interaction between infections with parasitic zoonoses and HIV infection on the occurrence and clinical presentation of epilepsyat ECP of South Africa where HIV and cysticercosis are known as endemic.

A blood 10mL sample is collected on all participating subjects for the detection of antibodies to the larval stages of *T. solium* and of *Toxocara* spp and for the detection of the antigens to the larval stages of *T. solium*. Sera will be identified by their research identification numbers and stored in the NMAH laboratory. For HIV negative participants who have not been tested for HIV in the past 12 months, part of the sera will be used to test for HIV.

Each participant is assigned a research identification number. Data retained on participants will only be identified by their research ID. Information linking participants to their research ID will is stored in secured files in the research office. All of the biological specimens and the interview assessments listed above will be collected specifically for the purposes of the proposed research project.

Informed consent is obtained for all participants. All consent forms included a section in which the objectives of the study are clearly stated. This is followed by a description of what participation in the study involves for the subject. Because we know that a certain proportion of the population is illiterate, the explanation was read to the potential participants. Subjects that know how to sign asked to do it on a form that clearly explains, in simple words of either English or isi-Xhosa (local language in Mthatha), the objectives of the study. The culturally acceptable age at which individuals can be asked for either their assent or consent to participate is discussed with our local colleagues. The consent will clearly state that individuals may terminate participation at any time.

Persons who consent to participate in the study were identified by name and with an alphanumeric code. Only one coding sheet linking the names to the codes is created and it has a password protected. Every effort was made to keep the subject's personal data confidential. Until the end of the study, all data were entered into a password-protected database. All consent forms and the coding sheet were maintained in a locked file cabinet. Any data sent for data analysis was anonymous and with alphanumeric codes for the subjects names.

All investigators and collaborators completed the CITI training-course on the Protection of Human Research. All are sworn to the Hippocratic Oath and committed to respecting the norms of good clinical practice, as well as the requirements of the Helsinki Declaration.

The research protocol was evaluated and approved by Mthatha Umtata General Hospital, University of Transkei, and Walter Sisulu University IRB and the respective Ethical Committees (UGH:0001/99, UNITRA:0018/05, and WSU:0068/009).

Subjects who may require sedation for the CT-scan of the brain were excluded from this part of the study. Patients who do not know their HIV status or are HIV negative (groups 5 and 6) are offered an HIV test if they have not been tested in the past month. A diagnosis of HIV can be very upsetting and may lead to psychological distress. In order to assist newly diagnosed HIV positive participants, they were referred for counseling and treatment to the HIV clinic of the Mthatha Hospital Complex.

The benefits of the information gained from the study outweigh the minimal risk involved. All subjects either have already received or we offer a neurological examination and a CT-scan to determine the cause of their epilepsy, other neurological symptoms or the presence of silent CNS lesions. Individuals who have either never been tested or have not been recently tested for HIV it was given the opportunity to be tested.

4.4 Preliminary results

A brief summary about our preliminary findings can be seen in Table 6

Total = 48 participants enrolled with neurological disorders
46% Female, Median Age=29 Mean Age=33
98% Rural or semi-rural residence
Approx 60% HIV Positive
Of those with CT completed,
High proportion calcified lesions on CT
8 excluded due to CD4 counts>200

Table 6. Some preliminary results

4.5 Discussion, challenges to date, and conclusions

Our preliminary results were presented and discussed as: "Effect modification of HIV-associated central nervous system diseases by parasitic zoonoses in the Eastern Cape Province, South Africa" at 138th APHA Meeting.in Denver, Colorado. United States of America on November 9, 2010. (Abstract #222895).

Longer-term benefits of this study included a better understanding of the interaction between HIV and parasitic zoonoses on the development of seizure disorders. If the effects of parasitic zoonoses are more severe in HIV infected patients, future studies could be conducted to assess whether the risk factors for infection are the same in HIV positive and HIV negative patients, and control interventions to reduce the burden of these preventable causes of brain infection could be tested. Given that a very large proportion of HIV patients develops some neurological disorder in the course of their infection, being able to reduce the prevalence of some causes of these disorders would benefit patients themselves and the society as a whole by a reduction of medical costs and potential increase in productivity of these patients, especially in a region in which both HIV infection and parasitic zoonoses are highly prevalent.

Poor research capacity often means that there is a misunderstanding of the goals of the research and its ability to be combined with clinical and teaching services. A national political action strikes on campuses across South Africa escalated to violence, forcing the closure of WSU campus among others on four separate occasions. Though the majority of learners expressed their discontent peacefully, a small minority responded with violence. Campus activities were paralyzed on four occasions during the first phase of our study. The majority of the population speaks Isi-Xhosa (95% in ECP). Translations of study materials from English proved difficulties as few references exist containing vocabulary for scientific purposes.

There is a lack of knowledge regarding the interactions of HIV and helminthic infections, how their effects on immunological response affect risk of co-infection, and the role of altered immune responses that result from these infections.

Our pilot study is well underway and will lead to the development of new hypotheses on the interaction between HIV and parasitic infections of the brain.

5. Acknowledgment

We like to express our gratitude to those veterinarian doctors working in this field particularly: Professors Rosina "Tammi" Krecek, Albert Lee Willingham III, Linda Cowan, Samson Mukaratiwua and other members of our Cysticercosis Working Group for Eastern and Southern Africa (CWGESA) for their dedications and commitment.

Special thanks to Professor Helen Carabin from Department of Biostatistics and Epidemiology College of Public Health University of Oklahoma Health Sciences Center for her invaluable enthusiasm, persistence, and leadership in our research team.

We want to thanks to all radiologists and radiographers from Nelson Mandela Academic Hospital and Inkhosi Albert Luthuli Central Hospital in South Africa for their contribution to this study.

Many thanks are due to The Cuban Ministry of Health, The Institute of Tropical Medicine "Pedro Kouri", authorities of Faculty of Health Sciences, Directorate: Research Development from the Walter Sisulu University and some of mine colleagues from Nelson Mandela Academic Hospital for their unconditional support.

Special mention is made of Mrs Noluntu Funani. Research Coordinator at the Office of President. South Africa Medical Research Council, who gave me a valuable help.
We also acknowledge financial support from, Directorate of Research Development from Walter Sisulu University in South Africa, University of Oklahoma, and South African Medical Research Council.The founder had no role in study design, data collection and analysis, decision to publish, or preparation of this chapter.
I sincerely thank to INTECH open access publisher for supporting this chapter and to my beautiful friends Ms Dragana Manestar and Natalia Reinic for their kind attention and nice support.
My sweet wife Lourdes de Fátima was so patient with my late nights, and I want to thank her for her faithful support in writing this book. Words cannot express my gratitude to Lourdes for her advices, encouragement, and assistance in polishing this chapter.
Finally, I wish to declare my eternal, deepest love and gratitude to Lorna María Foyaca García, Thabo Humberto Jorge Foyaca Ibañez and Fátima Susana Adolfina Foyaca Ibañez, because without their love and unconditional support this chapter would not have been written.

6. References

Akao, N., M . Tomoda, E. Hayashi, R. Suzuki, M. Shimizu-Suganuma, K. Schichionohe and K. Cerebellar ataxia due to *Toxocara* infection in Mongolian gerbils, *Meriones unguiculatus*. Vet. Parasit., 113: 229-237, 2003.

Asuman I, Nurgul C, Ilknur E, Derya E, Seniha S, Seyfi O, Pasa G. Neurobrucellosis with transient ischemic attack, vasculopathic changes, intracerebral granulomas and basal ganglia infarction: a case report. Journal of Medical Case Reports 2010;4(1):340.

Bartolini A. Epilepsy and toxocariasis: a case-control study in Italy. Epilepsia 2008;49:594-599.

Bayliascariasis. Institute for International Cooperation in Animal Biologics. Iwoa State University College of Veterinary Medicine. Full article available at the URL: www.cfsph.iastate.edu/IICAB/.

Boongird, P., P. Phuapradit, N. Siridej, T. Chirachariyavej, S. Chuahirun, and A. Vejjajiva. 1977. Neurological manifestations of gnathostomiasis J. Neurol. Sci. 1977;31:279-291.

Carod-Artal FJ, Vargas AP, Horan TA, Nunes LG. Chagasic cardiomyopathy is independently associated with ischemic stroke in Chagas disease. *Stroke* 2005; 36: 965–70.

Carod-Artal FJ, Gascon J. Chagas disease and stroke. Lancet Neurol 2010; 9: 533–542

Chero JC, Saito M, Bustos JA, Blanco EM, Gonzalvez G, Garcia HH. Hymenolepis nana infection: symptoms and response to nitazoxanide in field conditions. *Trans R Soc Trop Med Hyg*. Feb 2007;101(2):203-205.

Centers for Disease Control and Prevention [homepage on the Internet] c-2005 Guidelines for veterinarians: prevention of zoonotic transmission of ascarids and hookworms of dogs and cats. National Center for Infectious Diseases, Division of Parasitic Diseases [updated 2011 March 22]. Available at the URL: http://www.cdc.gov/ncidod/dpd/parasites/ascaris/prevention.htm#pet_owners Last accessed 03/20/2011.

Clausen MR, Meyer CN, Krantz , Moseril C, Gommeg G, Kayser L, et al. *Trichinella* infection and clinical disease. *QJ Med* 1996; 89:631-636

Chai JY, Lee SH, Guk SM, Lee SH. An epidemiological survey of *Cryptosporidium parvum* infection in randomly selected inhabitants of Seoul and Chollanam-do. Korean J Parasitol 1996; 34:113-119.

Chai JY, Murrell KD, Lymbery AJ. Fish-borne parasitic zoonoses: status and issues. Int J Parasitol. 2005;35:1233–1254.

Chen XH, Shi GF. Clinical analysis of 6 cases with cerebral sparganosis mansoni. Zhongguo Ji Sheng Chong Xue Yu Ji Sheng Chong Bing Za Zhi. 2010 Oct 30;28(5):397-398

Chiu CH, Chiou TL, Hsu YH, Yen PS. MR spectroscopy and MR perfusion character of cerebral sparganosis: a case report. Br J Radiol 2010;83:e31–4

Choi WY, Nam HW, Kwak NH, Huh W, Kim YR, Kang MW, Cho SY, Dubey JP. Foodborne outbreaks of human toxoplasmosis. J Infect Dis 1997; 175: 1280-1282.

Craig P, Ito A. Intestinal cestodes. *Curr Opin Infect Dis.* Oct 2007;20(5):524-32Critchley EMR, Vakil SD, Hutchinson DN, Taylor P. *Toxoplasma, Toxocara,* and Epilepsy Epilepsy 982;23(3):315-321.

Daengsvang, S. Gnathostomiasis in Southeast Asia. Southeast Asian J. Trop. Med. Public Health.1981;12:319-332.

Devendra V, Shalini K, Vimala V, Priti V, Nuzhat H. Ectopic Fascioliasis in the Dorsal Spine: Case Report. Neurosurgery 2006;59(3):706-707.

Dukes CS, Luft BJ, Durack DT. Toxoplasmosis. In WM Scheld, RJ Whitley, DT Durack (eds), Infections of the Central Nervous System. Philadelphia: Lippincott–Raven, 1997;785–806

Fujita, 2003. Cerebellar ataxia due to *Toxocara* infection in Mongolian gerbils, Meriones unguiculatus. Vet. Parasitol., 113: 229-237. Despommier D, 2003. Toxocariasis: clinical aspects, epidemiology,medical ecology, and molecular aspects. *Clin Microbiol Rev 16:* 265–272.

Ellrodt A, Halfon P, Le Bras P, Halimi P, Bouree P, Desi M, Caquet R. Multifocal central nervous system lesions in three patients with trichinosis. *Arch Neurol* 1987; 44:432-4.

Foyaca-Sibat H, Ibañez-Valdés LdeF "Intraventricular neurocysticercosis in HIV patients" The Internet Journal of Neurology 2003;2(1):23-31 http://www.ispub.com/journal/the_internet_journal_of_neurology/volume_2_number_1_37/article/intraventricular_neurocysticercosis_in_hiv_positive_patients.html

Foyaca-Sibat H, Ibañez-Valdés LdeF."Pseudoseizures and Epilepsy in neurocysticercosis" Electron J Biomed 2003;2(2):20-29 Full free article available at the URL: http://www.uninet.edu/reb/2003/n2/2foyaca.html

Foyaca Sibat H, Ibañez-Valdés LdeF. Vascular dementia due to a Binswanger Disease in patients with active neurocysticercosis. Rev Electron Biomed / Electron J Biomed 2003;1(1):32-42. Full article available at the URL: http://biomed.uninet.edu/2003/n1/foyaca.html

Foyaca-Sibat H, Cowan LD, Carabin H, Serrano-Ocaña G, , Krecek RC, Willingham A. "Accuracy of the serological exam for the diagnosis of neurocysticercosis in outpatients with epilepsy, Eastern Cape Province, South Africa" PLOS Negleted Trop.Dis.Dec.2009;3(3):1-7

Foyaca-Sibat H, Ibañez-Valdés LdeF & J. Moré-Rodríguez : Parasitic Zoonoses Of The Brain: Another Challenger?. *The Internet Journal of Neurology.* 2010 Volume 12 Number 2 http://www.ispub.com/journal/the_internet_journal_of_neurology/volume_12_number_2_4/article/parasitic-zoonoses-of-the-brain-another-challenger.html

Fourestie V, Douceron H, Brugieres P, Ancelle T, Lejonc JL, Gherardi RK. Neurotrichinosis. A cerebrovascular disease associated with myocardial injury and hypereosinophilia. *Brain*. Jun 1993;116 (Pt 3):603-616.

Fowler R, Lee C, Keystone JS.The role of corticosteroids in the treatment of cerebral schistosomiasis caused by *Schistosoma mansoni*: Case report and discussion. *Am J Trop Med Hyg*.1999;6(1):47-50

Gavin PJ, Kazacos KR, Shulman ST, 2005. Baylisascariasis. ClinMicrobiol Rev. 2005;18:703–718

Garcia H. H., Moro P. L., Schantz P. M. Zoonotic helminth infections of humans: echinococcosis, cysticercosis and fascioliasis. Curr. Opin. Infect. Dis. 2007;20, 489–494.

Gay T, Pankey GA, Beckman EN, Washington P, Bell KA. Fatal CNS trichinosis. *JAMA* 1982; 247:1024-1025.

Georgiev V. Management of toxoplasmosis. Drugs 1994;48:79–88.

Chi TTK, Dalsgaard A, Turnbull JF, Tuan PA, Murrell KD. Prevalence of zoonotic trematodes in fish from a Vietnamese fish-farming community. J Parasitol. 2008;94:423–428

Gordon HM, Forsyth BA. Sparganosis in feral pigs in New South Wales. *Aust Vet J* 1954;30:135- 138.

Goldstein MA and Harden CL. Infectious states. In: Ettinger AB and Devinsky O, eds. Managing epilepsy and co-existing disorders. Boston: Butterworth-Heinemann; 2002;83-133.

Gray ML, Rogers F, Little S, et al. Sparganosis in feral hogs (*Sus scrofa*) from Florida. *J Am Vet Med Assoc* 1999;215(2):204-208.

Guenifi W, Rais M, Gasmi A, Ouyahia A, Boukhrissa H, Mechakra S, Houari M, Nouasria B, Lacheheb A Neurobrucellosis: description of 5 cases in Setif Hospital, Algeria. Med Trop (Mars). 2010;70(3):309-10.

Cunningham A. A. A walk on the wild side—emerging wildlife diseases. Br. Med. J. 2005;331: 1214–1215.

Hamon JF, Camara P. Electroencephalographic study of meningoencephalitis from Trypanosoma gambiense before and after treatment with melarsoprol. Neurophysiol Clin 1991;21:173–181.

Henningsson AJ, Malmvall BE, Ernerudh J, Matussek A, Forsberg P. Neuroborreliosis—an epidemiological, clinical and healthcare cost study from an endemic area of the south-east of Sweden Clinical Microbiology and Infection. 2010;16(8):1245–1251.

Herman JS, Chiodini PL. Gnathostomiasis, Another Emerging Imported Disease. Clinical Microbiology Reviews,2009;22(3):484-492.

Hoffmeister B; Glaeser S; Flick H; Pornschlegel S; Suttorp N; Bergmann F. Cerebral toxocariasis after consumption of raw duck liver.The Amer J Trop Med Hyg.2007;76(3):600-602.

Hong ST. Serologic response to Pneumocystis carinii of Seoul National University Hospital patients. Korean J Parasitol 1991; 29: 355-361.

Hughes AJ, Biggs BA. First report of human angiostrongyliasis acquired in Sydney. N Engl J Med 2002; 346: 668-675.Hughes A, Biggs B. Parasitic worms of the central nervous system: an Australian perspective. Intern Med J 2002; 32:541–553-539.

IBEC- Institute for Bioengineering of Catalonia. "Discovery of a new function of prion protein improves understanding of epilepsy. "ScienceDaily 31 December 2009. Full article is available at the URL: http://www.sciencedaily.com/releases/2009/11/091127175422.htm (Last review on 20 March, 2011)

Inkelman I, Arieff AJ, Schiller M. Rabies vaccine in the treatment of epilepsy. Am J Psychiatry.1938; 94:1363-1368.

Karki K. Human Fascioliasis an Emerging Zoonoses. The full article is available online at the URL: http://www.scribd.com/doc/3608468/Human-Fascioliasis-3 (Last review on March 18, 2011)

Keiser J., Utzinger J. Emerging foodborne trematodiasis. Emerg. Infect. *Dis. 2005;11, 1507–1514*Johnson RT, Gibbs CJ. Medical progress: Creutzfeldt-Jakob disease and related transmissible spongiform encephalopathies. N Engl J Med 1998;339:1994–2004

Kim YB, Ko YC, Jeon SH, Park HM, Shin WC, Lee YB, Ha KS, Shin DJ, Lim YH, Ryu JS, Chung MS. Toxocariasis: An Unusual Cause of Cerebral Infarction.*J Korean Neurol Assoc*. 2003 Dec;21(6):651-654

Lee CH, Saif YM. Avian influenza virus. Comparative Immunology, Microbiology and Infectious Diseases. 2009;32(4):301-310

Lindbald-Toh, K.Genome sequence, comparative analysis and halotype structure of the domestic dogs. Nature. 2005;38(7069): 803-819.

Little SE. Parasitic zoonoses: parasites transmitted from cats and dogs to children. Contemporary Pediatrics 2003;5:1-21

Labar DR, Harden C. Infection and Inflammatory Diseases. In J Engel Jr, TA Pedley (eds), Epilepsy: a Comprehensive Textbook. Philadelphia: Lippincott–Raven, 1997;2587–2596.

Madariaga MG, Cachay ER, Zarlenga DS. Case Report: A Probable Case of Human Neurotrichinellosis in the United States. Am. J. Trop. Med. Hyg.*2007*;77(2):347–349

Marsden PD, Bruce-Chwatt LJ. Cerebral malaria. Contemp Neurol Ser 1975;12:29–44.

Mas-Coma S., Bargues M. D.,Valero M. A. Fascioliasis and other plant-borne trematode zoonoses. Int. J. Parasitol.2005 35, 1255–1278.

Mas-Coma S, Valero MA, Bargues MD. Climate change effects on trematodiases, with emphasis on zoonotic fascioliasis and schistosomiasis. Veterinary Parasitology. 2009;163(4):264-280.

McCarthy J., Moore T. A.Emerging helminth zoonoses. Int. J. Parasitol.2000;30,1351–1360.

McCabe RE, Brooks RG, Dorfman RF, et al. Clinical spectrum in 107 cases of toxoplasmic lymphadenopathy. Rev Infect Dis 1987;9:754–774

Min DY. Cestode infections in Korea. Korean J Parasitol 1990; 28:123-144

Mirdha BR. Status of Toxoplasma gondii infection in the etiology of epilepsy. J Pediatr Neurol 2003; 1(2): 95-98

Morey, D., 2006. Burying key evidence: The social bond between dogs and people. J. Archaeol. Sci. 2006;33:158-175.

Mueller JF. The biology of Spirometra. *J Parasitol* 1974;60:3-14.Neghina R, Neghina AM, Marincu L,Iacobiciu L. Reviews on Trichinellosis (II): Neurological Involvement. Foodborne Pathogens and Disease 2010;10: 1089

Nawa Y. Historical review and current status of gnathostomiasis in Asia. Southeast Asian J. Trop. Med. Public Health 1991; 22(Suppl.):217-219.

Nicoletti A, Bartoloini A, Reggio A, et al. Epilepsy, cycticercosis, and toxocariasis. A population-based case-control study in rural Bolivia. Neurology 2002;58:1256-1261.

Nicoletti A, Bartolini A, Sofia V, Mantella A, Nsengiyumva G, Frescaline G, Preux P-M. Epielepsy and toxocariasis : a case-control study in Burundi. Epilepsia 2007;48:894-899.

Nicoletti A, Sofia V, Mantella A, Vitale G, Contrafatto D, Sorbello V, Biondi R, Preux P-M, Garcia HH, Zappia M, Nikolic S, Vujosevic M, Sasic M, et al. [Neurologic manifestations in trichinosis]. *Srp Arh Celok Lek*. May-Jun 1998;126(5-6):209-13. [Medline].

Nithiuthai, S., M.T. Anantaphrati, J. Waikagul and A. Gajadhar, 2004. Waterborne zoonotic helminthiases. Vet. Parasitol., 126: 167-193.

Obiako OR, Ogoina D, Danbauchi SS, Kwaifa SI, Chom ND, Nwokorie E. Neurobrucellosis--a case report and review of the literature. Niger J Clin Pract. 2010 Sep;13(3):347-50.

Oliveira, P. C. L.; Sampaio, R. L.; Lacerda, M. S.; Alvarenga, R. R.; Espinoza, M. F. Neurological coccidiosis in an adult Gir cow - case report. Ciência Animal Brasileira. 2009;10(1):322-329. Full article is available at the URL: http://www.revistas.ufg.br/index.php/vet/article/view/1145/4601 (Last review on March 20, 2011)

Pai PJ, Blackburn BG, Kazacos KR, Warrier RP, Bégué RE. Full recovery from Baylisascaris procyonis eosinophilic meningitis. Emerg Infect Dis. 2007 Jun;13(6):928-30.

Park SW, Sohn S. Cerebral Ischemia Caused by Hepatic Fascioliasis. Korean J Stroke 2010;12:33-35.

Paul, E. and J. Serpell, 1996. Obtaining a new pet dog: Effects on middle childhood children and their families. Appl. Anim. Behav. Sci. 1996;47:17-29.

Phan VT, Ersbøll KA, Nguyen VK, Madsen H, Dalsgaard A. Farm-level risk factors for fish-borne zoonotic trematode infection in integrated small-scale fish farms in northern Vietnam. PLoS Negl Trop Dis. 2010;4:742-746.

Plummer J, Kleaner H, Jobs K. Parasitic zoonoses in human brain. SA Med J 1957;10:78-87

Polley L, Thompson RCA. Parasite zoonoses and climate change: molecular tools for tracking shifting boundaries. Trends in Parasitology 2009; 25(6):285-291.

Polley L, Hoberg E, Kutz S. Climate change, parasites and shifting boundaries. *Acta Veterinaria Scandinavica* 2010; 52(1):0147-0152. The electronic version of this article can be found online at: http://www.actavetscand.com/content/52/S1/S1

Porter S, Sande M. Toxoplasmosis of the central nervous system in AIDS. N Engl J Med 1992;327:1643–1648

Procop GW. North American paragonimiasis (caused by *Paragonimus kellicotti*) in the context of global paragonimiasis. Clin Microbiol Rev 2009;22:415--446.

Pullar EM, McLenan GC. Sparganosis in a Victorian pig. *Aust Vet J* 1949;25:302-304.

Ragnaud J, Morlat P, Dupon M, et al. Cerebral toxoplasmosis in AIDS. Presse Med 1993;22:903–908.

Renkawek K, Renier WO, de Pont JHHM, Vogels OJM, Gabreëls FJM. Neonatal Status Convulsivus, Spongiform Encephalopathy, and Low Activity of Na^+/K^+ -ATPase in the Brain. Epilepsia 1992;33(1):58-64

Robinson MW, Dalton JP.Zoonotic helminth infections with particular emphasis on fasciolosis and other trematodiases. Phil. Trans. R. Soc. B 2009;364(1530): 2763-2776.

Rocha A, de Meneses AC, da Silva AM, et al. Pathology of patients with Chagas' disease and AIDS. Am J Trop Med Hyg 1994;50:261–268.

Rodriguez RE, Valero V, Watanakunakorn CH.Salmonella Focal Intracranial Infections: Review of the World Literature (1884–1984) and Report of an Unusual Case. Clin Infect Dis. (1986) 8 (1): 31-41.

Sace J.Rabies in Humans: Symptoms, Diagnosis, and Treatment.Edited & published by Leigh A. Zaykoski on Apr 10, 2009.

Schachter S C. Helminthic parasitic infections. Epilepsy.com Editorial Board. Available at the URL: http://professionals.epilepsy.com/wi/print_section.php?section=infectious_helminthic#helminthic_schistosom

Sander JW, Perucca E. Epilepsy and comorbidity: infections and antimicrobials usage in relation to epilepsy management.Acta neurological scandinavica 2003:108(180):16-22.

Savolainen, P., Y. Zang, J. Luo, J. Lundeberg and T. Leitner. Genetic evidence for an East Asian origin of domestic dogs. Science.2002; 298(5598):1610-1613.

Shah AA, Shaikh H, Karim M. Amoebic brain abscess: a rare but serious complication of Entamoeba histolytica infection. J. Neurol. Neurosurg. Psychiatr.1994; 57 (2): 240–241.

Shirakawa K, Yamasaki H, Ito A, Miyajima H, Hamamatsu D., Tokyo (H.Y.), and Asahikawa A.I., Cerebral sparganosis. The wandering lesion. Neurology 2010;74(2):

Song T, Wang WS, Zhou BR, et al. CT and MR characteristics of cerebral sparganosis. Am J Neuroradiol 2007;28:1700–1705

Stommel EW, Seguin R, Thadan VM, Schwartzman JD, Gilbert K, Ryan KA, Tosteson TD, Kasper LH. Cryptogenic Epilepsy: An Infectious Etiology? Epilepsia 2001;42(3):436-438.

Swai ES, Kaaya EJ, Mshanga DA, Mbise EW. A Survey on Gastro-Intestinal Parasites of Non-Descript Dogs in and around Arusha Municipality, Tanzania. Int. J. Anim. Veter. Adv. 2010;2(3): 63-67.

Thien PC, Dalsgaard AD, Thanh BN, Olsen A, Murrell KD. Prevalence of fishborne zoonotic parasites in important cultured fish species in the Mekong Delta, Vietnam. Parasitol Res. 2007;101:1277–84.

Tolan RW. Hymenolepiasis.eMedicine Speciallties.Jan 20, 2011. Full article available at the URL:http://emedicine.medscape.com/article/998498-overview

Taylor MJ, Hoerauf A, Bockarie MD The Lancet Seminar: Lymphatic filariasis and onchocerciasis The Lancet 2011;376(9747):1175-1185

Tolan RW Fascioliasis Due to *Fasciola hepatica* and *Fasciola gigantica* Infection: An Update on This 'Neglected' Neglected Tropical Disease. Laboratory Medicine. 2011;42(2):107-116

Tekin-Koruk S, Duygu F, Gursoy B, Karaagac L, Bayraktar M. A rare case of seronegative neurobrucellosis. Ann Saudi Med. 2010; 30(5): 412–414.

Türel Ö, Şanlı K, Hatipoğlu N, Aydoğmuş Ç,Hatipoğlu H, Şiraneci R. Acute meningoencephalitis due to Brucella: case report and review of neurobrucellosis in children. The Turkish Journal of Pediatrics 2010; 52: 426-429.

van Burgel ND, Oosterloo M, Kroon FP, van Dam VP. Severe course of Lyme neuroborreliosis in an HIV-1 positive patient; case report and review of the literature. *BMC Neurology* 2010;10:110-117.

Vorou R. M., Papavassiliou V. G., Tsiodras S. Emerging zoonoses and vector-borne infections affecting humans in Europe. Epidemiol. Infect. 2007;135:1231–1247.

Youn H. Review of Zoonotic Parasites in Medical and Veterinary Fields in the Republic of Korea. Korean J Parasitol 2009;47:133-141.

Wan H, Lei D, Mao Q. Cerebellar schistosomiasis: a case report with clinical analysis. *Korean J Parasitol*. Mar 2009;47(1):53-56.

Watson KC, Laurie W. Cerebral Coenuriasis in the Bantu. SA Med J. 1956;9:23-30

Wiwanitkit V. Cerebral sparganosis. British Journal of Radiology 2010;83:807

World Health Organization. Control of food borne trematode infections. WHO technical report series no. 849. Geneva: The Organization; 1995. p. 1–157

World Health Organization. Report: Joint WHO/FAO workshop on foodborne trematode infections in Asia: 2002 Nov 26–28 Ha Noi, Vietnam. Manila (Philippines): The Organization; 2004

WHO. Chagas disease. Seventeenth programme report UNDP/TDR. Geneva, Switzerland: World Health Organization, 2005. Full available at the URL:
http://www.who.int/tdrold/publications/publications/pdf/swg_chagas.pdf (Last acc